DONALDSONS' ESSENTIAL PUBLIC HEALTH

FOURTH EDITION

DONALDSONS' ESSENTIAL PUBLIC HEALTH

FOURTH EDITION

Liam J. Donaldson

Paul D. Rutter

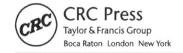

CRC Press
Taylor & Francis Group
Boca Raton London New York

CRC Press is an imprint of the
Taylor & Francis Group, an **informa** business

CRC Press
Taylor & Francis Group
6000 Broken Sound Parkway NW, Suite 300
Boca Raton, FL 33487-2742

© 2018 by Liam J. Donaldson
CRC Press is an imprint of Taylor & Francis Group, an Informa business

No claim to original U.S. Government works

Printed on acid-free paper

International Standard Book Number-13: 978-1-909-36895-8 (Paperback); 978-1-138-72201-9 (Hardback)

Library of Congress Cataloging-in-Publication Data

Names: Donaldson, Liam J., author. | Rutter, Paul D., author.
Title: Donaldsons' essential public health / Liam J. Donaldson and Paul D. Rutter.
Other titles: Essential public health
Description: Fourth edition. | Boca Raton : CRC Press, [2017] | Includes
bibliographical references and index.
Identifiers: LCCN 2016050366| ISBN 9781909368958 (pbk. : alk. paper) | ISBN 9781138722019 (hardback : alk. paper)
Subjects: | MESH: Public Health Practice | Preventive Health Services | Great Britain
Classification: LCC RA485 | NLM WA 100 | DDC 362.10941--dc23
LC record available at https://lccn.loc.gov/2016050366

Visit the Taylor & Francis Web site at
http://www.taylorandfrancis.com

and the CRC Press Web site at
http://www.crcpress.com

Contents

Preface

Since its first appearance in the early 1980s, as *Essential Community Medicine*, this book has remained in continuous print through several name changes and new editions. During these 33 years, the content has reflected the many shifts in the way that public health is understood, perceived and practised. Generally, the subject has become much broader based, more multidisciplinary and less dominated by the medical model, and has gained a greater emphasis on practical measures and action.

The text aims to bring together, in one volume, the principles and applications of epidemiology, the main health problems experienced by populations and by the main groups within them, the strategies for intervention to promote health and prevent disease, the main themes underlying health policy formulation and a description of the provision of health services.

This new edition is the biggest change to the book in 20 years. We have introduced an entirely new schedule of chapters, reflecting modern thinking on the scope of public health. Much of the content within them is entirely new too. We embraced the view that today's paradigm of public health is global, not purely national. As a result, each chapter is set in a global health context, while the core elements still cover the position for the United Kingdom. The opening chapter, 'Health in a Changing World', addresses the key ideas lying behind the concept of health, describes the burden of disease and addresses the main themes in global health, including the impact of globalization, population growth and migration, poverty, development, global health architecture and regulatory mechanisms.

Chapter 2, on epidemiology, sets out the ways in which health and disease can be described in populations using the concepts, rules and tools of the science of epidemiology. The sources, strengths and limitations of routinely available data are described, with many illustrative examples. The growing availability of large repositories of information that have not been collected for health purposes, yet are relevant to describing health-related attitudes, behaviour and risk factors, means that big data is likely to become part of the process of assessing the health of populations. The main study methods of epidemiology – cross-sectional or prevalence studies, cohort studies, case–control studies and randomized controlled trials – are described in the chapter. We place emphasis not just on the conceptual

bases of these important methods of investigation but also on their strengths and weaknesses and their applicability in particular situations. The final section of the chapter deals with the applications of epidemiology. In public health practice, results of investigations are required much more quickly than in an epidemiological research environment. The field of study is sometimes referred to as 'quick and dirty' investigation. We do not subscribe to this philosophy and place emphasis on the need for rigour even when a pragmatic approach is necessary in deciding the scope and urgency of a study.

Subjects that were only sections within chapters in the previous edition have increased greatly in importance over the past five years. We have created freestanding chapters to allow us to deal with them authoritatively and in depth. Quality and patient safety were previously a strand within the chapter on the National Health Service. A new chapter on the quality and safety of healthcare (Chapter 7) describes the principal schools of thought in quality, ranging from the original Donabedian triad of structure, process and outcome, through the Toyota Production System, to the idea of quality improvement collaboratives. Patient safety is also extensively dealt with in this chapter, as are the concepts of inspection and regulation. Previous editions of the book have covered health inequalities within chapters on health promotion and disease prevention. This subject has moved on a great deal and has been taken up as a global health concern with a major commission chaired by the British epidemiologist Sir Michael Marmot. There is now a chapter on the social determinants of health (Chapter 5). This still covers the ways in which social position and deprivation are delineated, but also discusses the main determinants of health: income, education, occupation, ethnicity, neighbourhood, social capital and social support. A new section in this chapter describes the growing understanding of the biological pathways that mediate the relationship beween social conditions and poor health.

Our feedback from readers over the years has shown how many enjoy, and are fascinated by, the historical material that has been part of several chapters. In reviewing the content prior to designing this new edition, we felt that the historical sections were rather fragmented and did not give a clear understanding of how today's public health has been shaped by the past. As a result, we have created a new chapter on the history of public health (Chapter 13). It covers developments in early civilizations, the great epidemics (including the Black Death and cholera), the people and events leading to the germ theory of disease causation, three of the classic investigations in public health (including John Snow and the Broad Street pump), the history of vaccination, the sanitary reform movement, the development of care services and other steps that helped to lay the foundations of public health.

'Non-communicable diseases' is another new chapter (Chapter 4) and a subject upon which international bodies like the United Nations have made forceful statements since the last edition of this book. This greater focus on diseases like cancer, cardiovascular disease, diabetes and chronic obstructive pulmonary disease, and on problems like obesity, recognizes that the burden of non-communicable diseases (also called chronic disease) no longer falls solely on richer countries. It is a rapidly emerging challenge for poorer parts of the world as well. The new chapter describes the pattern of non-communicable diseases in the United Kingdom and globally. It describes the main risk factors that create the greatest disease burden: poor diet, smoking, high blood pressure, obesity and overweight, physical inactivity and alcohol use. The public health aspects of unintentional injury (often called accidents) are also dealt with in this chapter. For most of the non-communicable diseases, and their main risk factors, the ways in which disease is initiated are complex. The policies and public health programmes that are most effective in reducing the burden of non-communicable diseases are discussed in the chapter. Single interventions are seldom the answer. The chapter describes the three levels of prevention: primary, secondary and tertiary. Each has a crucial part to play in a holistic view of public health action. The tertiary form of prevention (i.e. preventing the complications of established disease) used to be solely a clinical responsibility. Not any more. Clinical care is important, but the population perspective now sees slowing the progression of many chronic diseases as a core objective. Such an approach has the potential to improve quality of life, extend survival, empower those with long-standing conditions and save healthcare resources.

Three chapters deal with the health of important subgroups of the population: the disabled, mothers and children and older people. In each case, we have strengthened the relevant public health concepts since the previous edition, and instead of detailed service descriptions, we discuss the broader principles around which services should be designed.

Chapter 10, on disability, also looks fundamentally different to its forerunners. Physical disability and learning disability are both covered in the new chapter, whereas the latter used to reside in a mental health chapter. In 2015, the authors were crossing the street in Washington, DC, behind a disabled man in an electric-powered wheelchair. He had a sticker on the back that read, 'Attitudes are the real disabilities'. Many disability rights advocates hold that people are more disabled by environmental factors within society than by their impairments. They argue that illness and impairment need not disable people if society makes proper adjustments and allowances. These important themes are taken up in the chapter. The chapter is framed by two major reports produced by the World Health Organization in the early years of the twenty-first century. The first, *International Classification of Functioning, Disability and Health*, was developed over a long period of time, through discussion and consultation with a wide range of individuals and groups from the academic, policy-making and clinical worlds and, importantly, with disabled people and their representative organizations. It superseded a previous international classification. The second was the *World Report on Disability*.

Early life is the time when the foundations of health are laid and when some of the risks are greatest. Chapter 8 deals with the health of mothers and children. The main epidemiological features of health and disease in infancy and childhood are described, as are the risks to fetal and maternal health. The main measures of fertility in a population are described, along with the main trends in fertility over time and the factors that can influence it. The causes of death at different periods of infancy are discussed, and the various mortality rates in early life are defined. The range of approaches to promote health in pregnancy and childhood is described, as are the maternity and child health services themselves.

Chapter 11, 'Health in Later Life', has undergone major revision. With populations ageing steadily around the world, the main challenge for nations is to increase years of healthy life. The chapter discusses the various approaches to, and nomenclatures for, healthy ageing. It also describes the demography of population ageing, both globally and nationally. The implications of multimorbidity, frailty and other problems of later life are included, as are the characteristics of comprehensive, integrated care for older people.

Chapter 9, on mental health, has entirely new content. In previous editions, the comparable chapter had covered the detailed features of particular mental illnesses and the services provided for mentally ill people in the National Health Service. The content of the new chapter is built around the emerging, modern concept of public mental health. This is based on the principle that the tenets of public health can be applied to improving mental health in populations. Too often, a narrow focus to mental health is taken in which attention is only on improving the services available to those who have mental disorders. This is important, but a fuller approach to improving public mental health encompasses assessing the burden of poor mental health and of mental disorder; identifying risk factors and protective measures for poor mental well-being; taking appropriate interventions to promote well-being and prevent mental disorders and treat them early; assessing the intervention gap in a population for treatment, prevention and mental health promotion; tackling the health inequalities that are strongly related to the occurrence of poor mental health, and the extent to which disadvantaged people are unable to access the services that they need; understanding and reducing the extent to which mental ill health and physical ill health are interlinked; promoting mental well-being; and preventing mental disorder.

Chapter 3, on communicable disease, is the largest in the book. Such is the range of material to be covered, it could easily have become a mini-textbook masquerading as a chapter. In planning it, there was a need to be selective in the number of diseases to describe and in the amount of information on clinical features and microbiology to include. It is important to cover a wide range of individual diseases for a number of reasons. First, many diseases that used to be present in only a small part of the world, because of international travel, globalization of trade and mass migration, now have a global reach. Second, many communicable diseases can and do cause illness in the United Kingdom. Third, there are diseases that illustrate the principles of spread, surveillance, prevention and control. Specialist textbooks of communicable disease take different approaches to the classification of diseases. For example, some use categories based on the characteristics of the organisms themselves. Other textbooks organize the descriptions of disease by modes of transmission or clinical features. Still others use elements of both. In this chapter, we have grouped the communicable diseases into three broad categories: those that cause a major burden of mortality (HIV and AIDS, tuberculosis, malaria, diarrhoeal diseases and pneumonia), those that cause a major burden of morbidity and disability (e.g. neglected tropical diseases, blood-borne hepatitis viruses, dengue fever, measles, meningitis and healthcare infection) and new and emerging infections (e.g. Ebola fever, SARS, pandemic influenza and antimicrobial resistance). In each case, the key features of each disease are described. In some cases, there are also accounts of the challenges they can cause. The stories of SARS, the large outbreak of Ebola fever in Africa in 2014 and 2015 and the sudden emergence of cases of microcephaly linked to the Zika virus in 2016 all illustrate the practical difficulties of mounting a public health response in a major crisis. This chapter also covers the core concepts of spread, prevention and control, as well as surveillance. This essential knowledge includes reservoirs of infection, routes of entry into and exit from the body, modes of transmission, methods of investigation and protecting the susceptible host by vaccination and other measures.

The importance of the relationship between the quality of the environment and people's health has long been recognized. Moreover, there have been a number of major incidents around the world that have all too dramatically highlighted some of the contemporary threats and hazards, both to the well-being of individuals and to the planet itself. There is still an enormous amount to be learned about the influence of the environment on health. Rapidly rising concerns about climate change highlight many clear and direct links with health. In Chapter 12, 'Environment and Health', we describe the impact of the environment on health, as well as strategies for promoting health through the adoption of principles of sustainable development, and we discuss risk and its assessment.

In writing the chapters, we have tried to provide a clear, explanatory style with a single voice. Much of the material is derived from extensive synthesis of existing sources and from our own knowledge and experience. For this reason, the text is not underpinned point by point with detailed individual references. Specific studies are fully referenced where they have been drawn upon to devise or reproduce a table or figure. Much population data – both national and global – are now publicly available. We have referred to such data sources in general terms unless we have reproduced an analysis in a particular exact format. With this background, we have created a section towards the end of the book on references and further reading. The latter was not a feature of previous editions, and we hope that the sources we cite there will give readers a starting point to explore subjects that interest them in more depth. We have not provided individual web addresses for two reasons: (1) because some rapidly go out of date and (2) because we find that Internet search engines provide a wider range of sources and ensure that the reader is aware of contrasting perspectives on a subject.

In introducing this new edition of *Essential Public Health* to readers, both old and new, we believe we have built on the successful formula of its predecessor. However, looking at it afresh, and introducing much new material, we have been able to undertake a large-scale revision that encompasses the theory and practice of modern public health in a global and national context. We look forward to continuing to receive the views of readers in providing the kinds of constructive comments so valuable in the past.

We would like to acknowledge our special thanks to colleagues who have so generously provided their specialist expertise in the development of this book. We thank, in particular, Benedetta Allegranzi, Katherine Arbuthnott, Nicola Arroll, Mark Bellis, Jonathan Campion, Niall Fry, Antoneta Granic, Felix Greaves, Thomas Hone, Sarah Jonas, Clare Lemer, Hernan Montenegro, Oliver Mytton, Kristine Onarheim, Tom Shakespeare, Sally Sheard, Emma Stanton, Ester Villalonga and Leonora Weil.

Any omissions or errors of fact and interpretation are our own. Any opinions expressed are our own and not those of anyone we represent or may have represented in the past.

Liam J. Donaldson
Paul D. Rutter

Authors

Liam J. Donaldson was one of the two foundation authors of this book (which started life as Essential Community Medicine) when it was first published in 1983. The other author was his father Raymond "Paddy" Donaldson.

Liam Donaldson was the Chief Medical Officer for England, and the United Kingdom's Chief Medical Adviser, from 1998–2010. During this time he held critical responsibilities across the whole field of public health and health care. As the United Kingdom's chief adviser on health issues, he advised the Secretary of State for Health, the Prime Minister and other government ministers. He produced landmark reports set health policy and legislation in fields such as stem cell research, quality and safety of health care, infectious disease control, patient empowerment, poor clinical performance, smoke free public places, medical regulation, and organ and tissue retention.

Liam Donaldson has had a long and distinguished career in public health. He is recognised as an international champion of public health and patient safety. He was the foundation chair of the World Health Organisation, World Alliance for Patient Safety, launched in 2004. He is a past vice-chairman of the World Health Organisation Executive Board. He is now the World Health Organisation's Envoy for Patient Safety and Chairman of the Independent Monitoring for the Polio Eradication Programme. In the United Kingdom, he is Professor of Public Health at the London School of Hygiene and Tropical Medicine, Associate Fellow in the Centre on Global Health Security at Chatham House and Chancellor of Newcastle University.

Liam Donaldson initially trained as a surgeon in Birmingham and went on to hold teaching and research posts at the University of Leicester. In 1986, he was appointed Regional Medical Officer and Regional Director of Public Health for the Northern Regional Health Authority.

He has received many public honours: 16 honorary doctorates from universities, eight fellowships from medical Royal Colleges and Faculties, and the Gold Medal of the Royal College of Surgeons of Edinburgh. He was the Queen's Honorary Physician between 1996 and 1999. He was knighted in the 2002 New Year's Honours List.

Paul D. Rutter joins Liam Donaldson as co-author of *Essential Public Health*, for this substantially revised edition.

Paul Rutter's first public health role was as clinical adviser to England's Chief Medical Officer – at that time, Liam Donaldson. Over the subsequent decade, he has worked on a wide range of public health issues in the United Kingdom and globally. Most recently, he was the chief operations officer of the World Health Organization's programme to eradicate polio. The Global Polio Eradication Initiative is by several measures the world's largest public health programme, operating major surveillance and vaccination networks throughout the world. It is more than thirty years since smallpox became the first human pathogen ever to be eradicated. The programme's goal is to make polio the second. Paul Rutter's work at the World Health Organization also examined how the major global infrastructure that has been established to eradicate polio can be used to strengthen health systems and achieve other goals after polio is gone.

As this book goes to press, Paul Rutter will shortly join the United Nations Children's Fund (UNICEF) as Regional Health Adviser to its programmes in South Asia, which are working to improve maternal and child health in the diverse settings of India, Afghanistan, Bangladesh, Pakistan, Bhutan, Sri Lanka, Nepal and the Maldives.

Paul Rutter has also consulted on global health policy, global programme monitoring and clinical quality both globally and nationally. His research and published work has focused on polio eradication, influenza and patient safety.

Paul Rutter graduated in medicine from the University of Leeds and worked in London and York hospitals before becoming a public health physician. He is a member of the Faculty of Public Health. He holds a master's in public health from Harvard University and a master's in business administration (MBA) from London Business School.

CHAPTER 1

Health in a changing world

INTRODUCTION

Public health is about protecting and improving the health of whole populations and communities. Its motivation is to improve the health of individual people. But unlike clinical medicine, which focuses on people one at a time, public health takes a broader focus to understand and engage with the many factors (societal, behavioural and environmental) that promote or undermine health.

Public health emphasizes the promotion of health and the prevention of disease and disability; the collection and use of epidemiological data; population surveillance and other forms of empirical quantitative assessment; a recognition of the multidimensional nature of the determinants of health; and developing effective solutions to population health problems. Any list of activities and projects carried out by a department of public health would be lengthy and diverse and not necessarily consistent with a similar list produced by another department in the same country or in a different country. That is why perusing such lists or reading and talking about public health programmes often gives a better and clearer understanding of what public health is about than memorizing a formal definition.

Public health practice can involve tackling huge issues that affect the whole world, such as the health effects of climate change, as well as quite circumscribed and small-scale interventions, such as introducing new hygiene procedures at a local children's animal petting farm after an outbreak of serious illness caused by the bacterium *Escherichia coli* O157.

While most of the core concepts of public health have remained the same for many decades, there have been three big shifts of emphasis from the late twentieth century into the twenty-first century. First, the paradigm of public health is no longer national; it is global. Second, public health is no longer only the domain of professionals. Health system managers and political leaders have had to become engaged in order to address the challenges of new threats to health and the growing burden of potentially preventable, noncommunicable diseases. Third, pursuing effective solutions for problems that are mainly multifactorial in causation and influenced by broader environmental, social and economic conditions requires interdisciplinary practice and multiagency, multisector cooperative working. A simple medical model of intervention is not in keeping with a modern public health approach. This is emphasized throughout the book.

WHAT IS HEALTH?

The question 'What is health?' is not an easy one to answer. United Nations officials had to ponder it when, in 1948, they founded the World Health Organization (WHO). They came up with the following: 'Health is a complete state of physical, mental and social well-being and not merely the absence of disease or infirmity', a definition that has been widely cited ever since.

Many people do think of health, primarily, as the absence of disease. Diagnosing and treating disease is the central focus of most health systems, and at the core of traditional medical school curricula. Tackling disease is seen as the primary route to improving health – and there has been considerable success in doing so. In many parts of the world, including the United Kingdom, other government action to improve health has been far less convincing, and healthcare systems continue to focus on the absence of disease, rather than taking the more holistic view that the World Health Organization's definition suggests. For example, in the Conservative government's financial statement in the autumn of 2015, despite the need to find funds to pay down a deficit, a major increase was made in funding for the National Health Service (NHS), largely to address pressures in hospital services, while public health budgets were cut. In the late 1960s, the leading British public health thinker Thomas McKeown of Birmingham said, 'The disposal of society's investment in health is based on strange premises. It is assumed that we are ill and made well, whereas it is nearer to the truth that we are well and made ill'. Fifty years on, it is difficult to dispute the continuing validity of this telling observation when the policies of many health ministries are viewed in the cold light of day.

In the mid-1980s, the World Health Organization published the *Ottawa Charter for Health Promotion*. It followed the first major global conference to address the concept of health promotion, which is now a mainstream component of public health. The Ottawa Charter developed the idea of health as a fundamental human right, and identified a number of prerequisites for it, including:

- Peace
- Food
- Shelter
- Education
- Income
- Sustainable resources
- A sustainable ecosystem
- Social justice and equity

The Ottawa Charter saw it as more helpful to define the social and physical resources required for health and focus on improving those, rather than defining health at the individual level.

The original World Health Organization definition of health is more than half a century old. Some see its statement that health is a state of *complete* well-being as unhelpful. Very few people are completely well in every way, and on a pedantic view of the definition, most people are therefore unhealthy. As people age, many begin to accumulate chronic, non-communicable diseases. Arguably, a more helpful definition would not write them all off as failing to attain 'a complete state of physical, mental and social well-being'. The World Health Organization's original definition also says nothing about what physical, social or mental well-being means, simply stating that health requires each of these to be 'complete'. Some maintain that the definition has led to an ideal of perfect health, and that this utopian notion has fed an increasing medicalization of society's problems.

Today, while the World Health Organization still cites its original definition, it also discusses health in much broader terms. On a glance through its publications, the reader will see phrases linked to the concept of health like 'a resource for everyday living', 'a fundamental human right', and 'an essential component of development'.

There is a widespread consensus among international agencies, including the World Health Organization, that the concept of health, the influences on it and the language used to debate it should indeed be very broad, with strong links to economic and social development and – particularly in the poorer countries of the world – to gender and poverty.

Different cultures view health differently. For example, First Nation people in Australia and Canada think of well-being as more important than the absence of disease. Health is a balance of spiritual, emotional and physical factors, rooted in the traditions and culture of the community and connected to the spirit of the land and to nature. Traditional Chinese medicine focuses on maintaining harmony (between the two forces of yin and yang). People are healthy when there is harmony between body and mind, and the aim of healing is to restore this harmony when it has become disturbed.

In the West, the definition of health continues to be debated. This is not an esoteric activity, since one of the reasons for defining it is to move to the practical task of measuring it. Most so-called 'measures' of health are not explicitly linked to a definition of health, but rather describe an aspect of an *implied* definition. Some traditional measures are less valuable than they once were, for example, mortality rates in countries with prolonged expectation of life. At the end of the first decade of the twenty-first century, the Netherlands Organisation for Health Research and Development convened a conference of Dutch and international health experts, aiming to redefine health. The thrust of the meeting, to challenge the time-served World Health Organization definition, was captured in the title: *Health – A State or an Ability? Towards a Dynamic Concept of Health*. This conference did not conclude with an agreed, revised, new definition of health, but it did reveal the complexity of trying to do so and the multiple ways through which a definition could be arrived at. It was a deep and searching analysis of what health means and how it could be formally defined. Some of the key conclusions were:

- Health should not be considered a consistent 'state', but is dynamic, and is related both to the equilibrium of different aspects and to age.
- Characteristics of health include an inner resource, a capacity, an ability and a potential to cope with or adapt to internal and external challenges (resilience); to perform (relative to potential, aspirations and values); to achieve individual fulfilment; to live, function and participate in a social environment; and to reach a high level of well-being, even without nutritional abundance or physical comfort.
- Health should be considered in an individual and group context; social inequalities have a major influence on health.
- Operationalizing the concept of health is necessary for measurement purposes, to provide an evidence base for policies and interventions, and to enable appropriate evaluations.
- The individual's capacity for self-management, participation, empowerment and resilience is of major importance, and should be stimulated and trained.

Both the Ottawa Charter and the Netherlands expert meeting brought out a much rounder view of health than is currently the mainstream concept in much of the Western world. These, and other challenges to the established Western paradigm of health, emphasize two things in particular: health as a positive concept to be strived towards, not simply the absence of disease, and the importance of mental and social health, not just physical health.

Another strand of twenty-first century thinking on health encompasses the concepts of well-being, quality of life and happiness. Each of these is as complex and argued about as health itself. Happiness is the subject of a growing academic literature. The World Happiness Report, written by British social scientist Richard Layard and others, sets out the case for making population happiness the central aim of government. It argues that society's aim should be to maximize the happiness of its members. Judging the success of a country on factors other than economic prosperity is not a new idea. In 1968, Robert F. Kennedy (1925–1968), then a presidential candidate in the United States, raised the thought-provoking idea of an entirely differently constructed measure of nationhood. He said:

> The gross national product does not allow for the health of our children, the quality of their education or the joy of their play. It does not include the beauty of our poetry or the strength of our marriages, the intelligence of our public debate or the integrity of our public officials. It measures neither our wit nor our courage, neither our wisdom nor our learning, neither our compassion nor our devotion to our country, it measures everything in short, except that which makes life worthwhile.

This theme has been developed and recast in the twenty-first century. In Bhutan, the government's key measure of success is not gross national product but gross national happiness. Bhutan measures gross national happiness using a multipart index (psychological well-being, time use, community vitality, cultural diversity, ecological resilience, living standard, health, education and good governance). Just under half of its population is happy (8% are deeply happy and 33% extensively happy). The remainder is classed as 'not yet happy', and the government's aim is to understand and address the reasons why.

No country uses a direct measure of health as one of its central guiding measures.

Much of the political debate about health is rather superficial. Words like *behaviour* are bandied around to explain why some people develop conditions like obesity. There are several different determinants of behaviour, which are complex in their dimensions: an individual's level of understanding about risks to health, their beliefs, whether they hold the attainment of good health as a fundamental value, and self-control. In turn, all these strands, and the way that they interact, are shaped by the opportunities and the availability of the means to secure good health in the country, city, town and small community in which they live. They are also profoundly influenced by the culture and norms of their country and social group (Figure 1.1).

PUBLIC HEALTH

When a formal definition of public health is required, two tend to be quoted. The first was formulated in 1920 by Charles-Edward Amory Winslow (1877–1957), the founding chairman of the Department of Public Health at

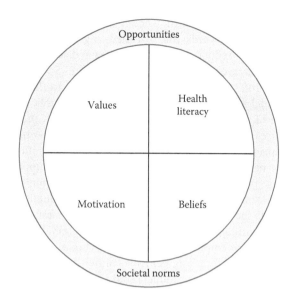

Figure 1.1 Determinants of health behaviour at the individual level.

Yale University. He defined public health as 'the science and art of preventing disease, prolonging life and promoting health through the organized efforts and informed choices of society, organizations, public and private, communities and individuals'.

Winslow was a bacteriologist by training, so his definition of public health seems remarkable in being so broad based and holistic. It was so modern in its orientation that when Sir Donald Acheson (1926–2010), England's chief medical officer, reviewed the public health function in 1988, he defined public health in a way that deviated little from Winslow's – although it was briefer. Acheson's definition tends to be the version more often cited in the United Kingdom: 'the science and art of preventing disease, prolonging life, and promoting health through the organized efforts of society'.

Since the 1970s, there has been an increasing emphasis on framing strategies aimed at promoting or improving public health. Governments of countries, international organizations like the World Health Organization and professional bodies like the Institute of Medicine in the United States and the Royal College of Physicians in the United Kingdom have all produced them. Many strategies have set goals and targets to be achieved over the life cycle of the plans.

In the United Kingdom, many public health White Papers have been produced over the last five decades. In earlier times, these were formulated for the United Kingdom as a whole, but more recently, Wales, Scotland, Northern Ireland and England have each produced their own. All have contained elements of an underpinning philosophy, a delivery system, legislative changes, targets, infrastructure, training needs, cross-government programmes and professional structures and functions. The mix and emphasis has differed from document to document. For example, much of the New Labour government's thinking on public health, when it came to power in 1997, was directed towards the so-called 'big killers'. Targets were set for reducing cancer and heart disease mortality, and interventions were aligned to them. Some public health professionals saw this as too oriented to the medical model and a step back from the modern public health theme of promoting positive health rather than preventing disease. Indeed, many viewed the term *prevention* as anachronistic and reflecting a narrow interpretation of public health. The approach was tolerated and supported because the incoming government gave great prominence to public health and the reduction of health inequalities. In contrast, the Coalition Government that was established in 2010, with a Conservative as health secretary, had fewer targets, more emphasis on individual choice and greater reliance on voluntary agreements (rather than legislation) with industries whose products could harm health. In contrast to England, the three other UK countries have consistently given greater emphasis to the social determinants of health in government policy discussions.

While governments' approaches to public health often vary according to political outlook, it is the role of the public health professions and the bodies that represent them to establish the concepts, principles and methods of public health and, to some extent, to be 'custodians of the flame'. In the United Kingdom, in the 1980s, this was particularly necessary during Margaret Thatcher's premiership. She opposed the idea of health having social determinants and stopped the use of the term *health inequalities*.

In the United Kingdom, the Faculty of Public Health of the Royal College of Physicians of London sets out the standards for public health practice and, in delivering that role, defines the scope of public health in practical terms. It identifies three domains of public health practice:

- Health improvement
- Health protection
- Improvement of services

There are many different areas within these broad domains (Table 1.1).

Public health does have an important role in improving health services – and this is discussed in later chapters – but in advancing population health, it operates in four broad strategic areas (Figure 1.2).

The term *health promotion* is used extensively internationally. Many of the descriptions of roles and functions within public health stem from considering the scope of health promotion in World Health Organization meetings and programmes. The Ottawa Charter defined health promotion as 'the process of enabling people to increase control over and improve their health'. In addition, it formulated five basic tools for health promotion:

- Build healthy public policy
- Create supportive environments for health
- Strengthen community action for health

Table 1.1 Key areas of public health practice

- Surveillance and assessment of the population's health and wellbeing
- Assessing the evidence of effectiveness of health and healthcare interventions, programmes and services
- Policy and strategy development and implementation
- Strategic leadership and collaborative working for health
- Health improvement
- Health protection
- Health and social service quality
- Public health intelligence
- Academic public health

Source: Faculty of Public Health.

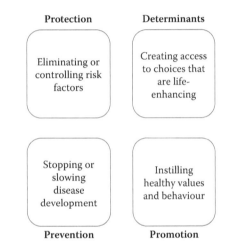

Figure 1.2 Public health: developing population health.

- Develop personal skills
- Reorient health services

The Ottawa Charter came out of the first international conference on health promotion. A later major conference on health promotion held in 1997 in Jakarta, Indonesia, revisited the concept and reviewed progress. It reaffirmed the earlier work, emphasized the importance of comprehensive approaches that use combinations of all the tools of health promotion, stressed the need to develop health literacy and drew attention to the potential of particular settings for advancing practical action. Over the years, the World Health Organization has fostered health promotion initiatives in a variety of settings, including healthy schools, healthy cities and health-promoting workplaces.

Most of the components in these expositions of health promotion are within the scope of public health in the United Kingdom. The term *health promotion* is less often used than it used to be (*health improvement* is the preferred term now).

National professional public health bodies around the world vary in their descriptions of the core roles and activities of public health services. The Pan American Health Organization has set out 11 essential public health functions that are fairly representative of many of the different approaches:

1. Monitoring, evaluation, and analysis of health status
2. Surveillance, research and control of the risks and threats to public health
3. Health promotion
4. Social participation in health
5. Development of policies and institutional capacity for public health planning and management
6. Strengthening of public health regulation and enforcement capacity
7. Evaluation and promotion of equitable access to necessary health services
8. Human resources development and training in public health
9. Quality assurance in personal and population-based health services
10. Research in public health
11. Reduction of the impact of emergencies and disasters on health

The way in which services are organized to deliver such functions again differs widely from country to country.

Public communication

In today's media-saturated, socially networked world, public communication is a more important element of public health practice than ever before.

Public health stories are frequently in the news. Sometimes these stories are of newly emergent diseases causing a threat to the public's health. Sometimes they are reports on an epidemiological research study that has suggested a new risk factor may cause cancer. Sometimes they express shock about the size of a particular health problem, such as childhood obesity. At other times, a public health story may attract media attention because of its curiosity value or because a public health investigation has provided the explanation to a medical whodunnit. An example of the latter came with the headline in *The Times* newspaper in Britain on 25 November 2015: 'Pheasant Trapped in Water Pipe Cost £25m'. This was the denouement of a public health mystery where the water supply in the northwest of England had become contaminated by *Cryptosporidium*, leading to 300,000 people having to boil their household water for two months. The media lambasted the water company for not being able to explain or resolve the problem. The total bill for the crisis, including compensation, was estimated as £25 million. The story generated huge public interest and some wry humour at the eventual explanation.

Such communications can act for good or for ill. High-quality journalism can provide valuable information to people, to inform their health-related decisions. Lesser-quality work can scaremonger and confuse. It is within the role of public health professionals to try to positively influence the balance.

Advertising is another communication form of intense relevance to public health. Over the last 30 years, advertising of tobacco products has been progressively curtailed in most high-income countries. The debate is now on the extent to which the same measures should apply to alcohol and sugar-laden foods. The techniques of advertising are highly effective in influencing behaviour, and the manufacturers of all these products have far deeper pockets than public health departments do. But the public health profession does now borrow some of the tools of advertising to influence health-related behaviours. This is so-called 'social marketing'.

Communication of risk is a particularly important, and difficult, element of public health communication. In the last decade of the twentieth century, there was a major growth in public concern about potential health hazards. This was reflected in widespread media coverage of scientific reports, government actions and human interest stories that appeared to suggest that a particular environmental or dietary agent carried a risk to human health. In Britain, the bovine spongiform encephalopathy (BSE) epidemic in cattle, the use of genetically modified crops and mobile telephones are all examples of issues that became the subject of media attention.

If a risk is claimed to exist, this is more likely to frighten people than other health stories (Table 1.2). While understanding what underlies the public perception of risk is important, the greatest difficulty for public health policymakers is to decide how a risk is assessed, when an intervention to reduce it should be made and what should be communicated to the public.

The most difficult areas to address are those in which an association is found (or claimed) between a risk factor and an adverse health outcome, yet it is not clear whether that association is causal. The question of establishing causality is a constantly recurring theme in this field of public health. Examples of issues that can be portrayed by the media as established cause and effect include a cluster of cases of childhood cancer around an industrial plant, people who take their stories to a tabloid newspaper with a claim that their illness is a result of exposure to a particular environmental hazard and people who believe they are at risk from industrial pollutants. The association may or may not be causal, or the evidence may not be available to prove the case one way or the other. Yet the public will usually expect an immediate response from the scientific community, the government and the public health authorities. There are no easy answers to these questions, but the scientific establishment of causality is discussed further in Chapter 2.

As a first step, a high-quality assessment of the scientific evidence is essential, sometimes coupled with a research investigation. At some point, a decision will have to be taken about whether it is appropriate to make an intervention to reduce the risk and what the nature of that intervention should be (e.g. legislation, providing public information or advice or altering a manufacturing or production process). Although it might be supposed that all the scientific evidence should be to hand before any intervention is contemplated, in practice, public concern or media pressure may be so great that early action has to be considered.

Table 1.2 Fright factors.

Risks are generally more worrying (and less acceptable) if perceived:
1. To be involuntary (e.g. exposure to pollution) rather than voluntary (e.g. dangerous sports or smoking)
2. As inequitably distributed (some benefit while others suffer the consequences)
3. As inescapable by taking personal precautions
4. To arise from an unfamiliar or novel source
5. To result from artificial, rather than natural, sources
6. To cause hidden and irreversible damage e.g. through onset of illness many years after exposure
7. To pose some particular danger to small children or pregnant women or more generally to future generations
8. To threaten a form of death (or illness/injury) arousing particular dread
9. To damage identifiable rather than anonymous victims
10. To be poorly understood by science
11. As subject to contradictory statements from responsible sources (or, even worse, from the same source)

Source: Department of Health (DH). Communicating About Risks to Public Health: Pointers to Good Practice. London: DH, 1997.

This particular aspect of risk – when and how to intervene – became the focus of a great deal of debate in the 1990s in Britain as a result of the BSE crisis. The concept of the 'precautionary principle' has emerged. This has been defined in various ways but essentially is a judgment that must be applied in situations of scientific uncertainty where the postulated risk is serious and where action is being contemplated before the results of further research or investigation are to hand. Thus, the precautionary principle holds that action to protect the public health should be taken to reduce or control the risk 'in the meantime'.

In the whole area of health and risk, it is essential that there is as much openness and transparency about the issues and the scientific evidence as possible. The guiding principles must be based not only on a rigorous approach to evaluating the risk but also on sharing information with the public. Without this, there will be a breakdown of trust and the value of public health advice will be weakened.

GLOBAL HEALTH

The terms global health and international health are often used interchangeably, but there are important differences. For most of the twentieth century, the richer countries of the world viewed the health problems of poorer countries as separate from, and different to, their own. International health was the predominant term. The dialogue was mainly framed as richer countries' concerns about poorer countries described, at the time, as 'developing countries'. International health was ascribed importance because of a humanitarian responsibility to provide support, funding and know-how to ameliorate the causes of disease, disability and premature death in the most impoverished parts of the world.

By the end of the twentieth century, the tendency to think about international health or tropical medicine as a specialist interest of a minority of health professionals and academics seemed a very narrow perspective. There were several reasons for this. First, the emergence of epidemics in the developing world – for example, AIDS and drug-resistant forms of tuberculosis – posed a direct threat to the populations in all countries, including the rich ones. Second, it was increasingly realized that supporting health in poorer countries enhances mutual respect and understanding in situations that could otherwise deteriorate into hostility and conflict. This motivation is sometimes referred to as 'health as a bridge to peace'. Third, there was clearly growing interdependence of nations in economic, social, political, communications and environmental terms: the emergence of globalization as both a beneficial and a malign influence.

With this shift in emphasis came a change in terminology – from international health, implying an interest in the health of other countries, to global health, implying an interest in the health of nations collectively. Other language was changing too. By the beginning of the twenty-first century, the terms developed and developing to classify the countries of the world sounded paternalistic and condescending, related to the colonial era and terms that did not fit the reality of fast-growing economies such as Brazil, India and China. Today, countries are characterized by their economic profile: low, middle and high income being the preferred prefixes attached to the word country.

The shift to a more collective mindset did not mean richer countries becoming disinterested in poorer countries. On the contrary, the poorer countries retain a high degree of focus in global health efforts that is disproportionate to their number but entirely appropriate to the burden of disease that they face. In the last 15 years, there have been substantial health gains in the poorer countries of the world, although very significant challenges remain.

Definitions of global health vary, but most emphasize that the health of populations must be seen in a way that transcends the concerns of individual nations, and is not limited by geographical borders. In understanding the current global health challenges, the international transfer of health risks is a key concept – that is, the way in which the movement across borders of people, products, resources and lifestyles can contribute to the spread of disease.

An often-used term, *globalization* is a complex phenomenon with several different aspects. It involves (1) an increasing degree of interaction between nations, (2) establishment of more formal agencies and structures that bridge nations and (3) growing integration between nations. The interactions, and integration, are political, economic, social, cultural, environmental, technological and more. In short, as a consequence of globalization, there is a closer interaction of human activity across a vast range of spheres. This is leading to faster production of knowledge and information and to changing expectations. The degree of integration varies. While 7 out of 10 Africans own a mobile phone, only one-quarter of HIV-infected children and one-third of HIV-infected adults are receiving antiretroviral treatment.

Globalization influences health in many different ways – particularly through its effects on the institutional, economic and social determinants of health. There are some positive aspects, such as dissemination of new knowledge about health and healthcare, allowing more people to benefit from successful treatment strategies. The benefit of other aspects is less clear, and there are detrimental impacts. In particular, the impact of international trade on health is controversial. Trade can contribute to economic growth and investments in population health, but some international trade agreements have had negative implications for health. Multinational companies promote smoking, sugary drinks and fast food all over the world now. An increase in travel and number of flights may be beneficial for cooperation, but has also enabled faster spread of infectious diseases.

The global health challenges are substantial. They require sharing of knowledge and information, and a high degree of global cooperation. Global health must involve a multidisciplinary approach – the challenges are multifaceted, and the most powerful determinants of health lie way beyond the bounds of healthcare. Trade, climate change, politics and economics are among the broader issues relevant to global health.

Populations in flux

In the middle of the twentieth century, two-thirds of the world's population lived in rural areas. Today, more than half of the world's population live in cities; an increasing proportion live in urban conurbations of more than 1 million people. Globally, the number of people living in large city slums is also rising.

In health terms, city dwelling has both pros and cons. It provides people with easier access to information and closer proximity to health facilities. However, living in densely populated areas – seen in slums in Mumbai, Rio de Janeiro and elsewhere – creates major health risks. Basic needs such as water access, toileting and shelter are often lacking. Educational status, child health and adult nutrition are common issues in these areas.

In the first decade of the twenty-first century, more than 200 million people were living outside their country of origin. There are many reasons for migration. Pull factors include better opportunities for work or living, while war, conflict and instability are push factors that drive people to leave their homes. This large-scale movement of people – as migrants, refugees and asylum seekers – has become a dominant consideration for health policymakers and global health professionals.

According to the United Nations High Commissioner for Refugees, there were more than 10 million refugees in the first decade of the twenty-first century, displaced mainly by conflict but also by other violence or intimidation, or by a natural disaster or famine. Half of all refugees are from just five countries – Afghanistan, Somalia, Iraq, Syria and Sudan. Half are children.

War and natural disasters can cause sudden migration, displacing very large numbers of people in a short period of time. As conflict took hold in Syria, for example, more than 250,000 fled the country in late 2012 and early 2013. As the conflict became more serious and prolonged, the number of refugees escalated. During 2015, the large-scale migration into Europe, through various routes and entry points, caused a massive humanitarian, economic and political crisis. By the end of 2015, there were more than 4 million Syrian refugees in the neighbouring countries: 1.2 million in Lebanon, more than 600,000 in Jordan, more than 2.5 million in Turkey, more than 250,000 in Iraq and more than 135,000 in Egypt. Many of these people have been displaced multiple times before reaching safety in neighbouring countries. An estimated 30% of them are living in extreme poverty.

Displaced people's safety, security and quality of life depend on the host country's resources and policies. Many face great risks living in refugee camps, rented houses or nomadic camps. With poor living conditions, food shortages, poor sanitation and no work, both physical and mental health can suffer immensely. Depending on the circumstances, refugees can face disease, starvation, homelessness, denial of healthcare, mental illness, violence and economic ruin. There may be widespread use of rape and other forms of sexual violence against women and girls. There are often epidemics of infection, including measles and other diseases that could be prevented by vaccination if strong systems were in place to provide it.

It is not only the refugees who suffer. Many of the host countries have serious problems of their own, and accepting refugees creates additional strain. The public services are challenged to offer basic services, such as health and education, to an increasing number of people. In 2012, the population of Lebanon was 4.7 million. With 1.2 million Syrian refugees, it grew to 5.9 million by the start of 2015. Lebanon and Jordan now have the highest per capita ratios of refugees worldwide. Both have used public funds to provide services for refugees, with negative knock-on effects for their established populations.

In 2015, the United Nations High Commission for Refugees was managing 50 refugee camps in different parts of the world, holding a total of 2 million people. Other refugee camps are run by the receiving country's government or by nongovernmental organizations, such as the International Red Cross. Many camps are intended to be time-limited facilities but operate for years, sometimes decades – as is the case for the camps of Palestinian refugees in the Middle East. The numbers seeking sanctuary in such camps are very fluid and can increase quickly. In some cases, many tens of thousands live on the periphery, unable to get into a camp that is already full beyond capacity. The combined population of a large refugee camp and town can easily overwhelm the municipal infrastructure. Not surprisingly, there are often tensions between the camp manager and the host country's government, especially when camps are expanded.

Many refugees do not live in refugee camps, are not registered and are therefore difficult to count. They face many of the same health challenges as those within camps, and are generally entitled to fewer rights.

Refugees within their own country are known as internally displaced persons. They often flee for similar reasons as refugees (armed conflict and other violence, or human rights violations) but are – according to the law – under the protection of their own government. In some cases, these governments are the cause of the refugees' flight. Natural disasters can also create internally displaced persons, such as the earthquakes in Haiti in 2010 and Nepal in 2015. As citizens, they retain all their rights and protection under both human rights and international humanitarian law, but in practice, there are few systems for holding governments accountable for fulfilling these rights.

Poverty

Poverty is inextricably linked to health through circumstances that include inadequate access to water, poor sanitation, lack of education and the unaffordability of healthy food. Poor people often have limited, or no, healthcare services. If care has a cost, they will delay seeking care until they are very sick. Unfortunately, the costs of care can be even higher when the disease has developed. Healthcare costs can become catastrophic, forcing families to sell belongings to afford them. This subject is discussed in more depth in Chapter 6. Countries with high rates of poverty usually have weak governments, and so are less likely to have good public healthcare systems to support people when they fall ill. If a person is sick and cannot go to school or work, this has implications for families, communities and the wider economy. Poor health therefore contributes to poverty and impedes development.

Poverty is most often measured by family or household income, but is increasingly being recognized in fuller terms, as described in Chapter 5. The Multidimensional Poverty Index, developed by the United Nations Development Programme, considers both monetary measures of poverty and deprivation in health, education and standard of living.

Worldwide, 2.5 billion people lack access to good sanitation, and more than 1 billion people practise open defecation. An estimated 1.8 billion people use a source of drinking water that is faecally contaminated. Such situations are strongly associated with severe poverty. Almost two-thirds of people without clean water live on less than $2 a day, while a third live on less than $1 a day. Clean water and safe disposal of sewage are a part of the basic infrastructure of health. There are many parts of the world in the twenty-first century where people are not afforded these fundamental protections to their health. A tenth of China's farmland is poisoned with chemicals and heavy metals, and some of China's urban water supplies are unfit to wash in, let alone drink. The main health consequence of poor water and sanitation conditions is exposure to a wide range of communicable diseases. Children are very vulnerable – almost 2 million die every year from diarrhoea. There is also physical hardship associated with collecting water: for millions of women, the central focus of the day is to collect water for drinking, cooking and personal hygiene.

The number of people living in poverty has decreased substantially over recent decades. Much of this has been due to development in India and China. Millennium Development Goal (MDG) 1A – cutting in half the proportion of people whose income is less than $1.25 a day – was met five years ahead of target, in 2010. Unfortunately, though, the number of people living in extreme poverty has increased. More than three-quarters live in rural areas, and children are at particular risk. Counterintuitively, most poor people now live in middle-income countries. When donors discuss not providing aid to middle-income countries, they often forget that many people are still poor, even though the country's average income is improving.

Development

In 1970, the United Nations General Assembly agreed on a target that countries should allocate 0.7% of their gross national income to development. Nearly 50 years on, only five countries do so. The United Kingdom is one of them, alongside four Nordic countries. The United Kingdom now gives approximately £12 billion a year in official development assistance.

Governments providing development assistance do so in a way that is consistent with their foreign policy objectives. For example, a number of governments view stability in Afghanistan as being a crucial part of reducing the risk of terrorism. In recent years, Afghanistan has received more development assistance than any other country.

Official development assistance is generally provided in two ways. *Bilateral aid* is provided directly from the donor government to the recipient country. Donor governments provide *multilateral aid* to intermediaries, such as the United Nations agencies. In general, the proportion of funds given as bilateral aid is decreasing, and multilateral aid increasing.

In recent years, consistent with the Millennium Development Goals, HIV/AIDS and maternal, newborn and child health have received much attention. Funding for non-communicable diseases is far less, even though these represent substantial and growing burdens of disease. The ways in which development agencies choose to spend their money change over time. In particular, disease-specific (vertical) programmes are now less in favour, with funds being shifted to horizontal systems-strengthening approaches instead.

The controversy about whether to focus on investing in health systems (horizontal) or specific programmes (vertical) has been going on for a long time. In an article published by the World Health Organization as a public health paper in 1955, Gonzales wrote,

> There are two apparently conflicting approaches to which countries should give careful consideration.... The first, generally known as the 'horizontal approach', seeks to tackle the overall health problems on a wide front and on a long-term basis through the creation of a system of permanent institutions commonly known as 'general health services'. The second, or 'vertical approach', calls for solution of a given health problem by means of single-purpose machinery.

In the 1978 International Conference on Primary Health Care held in Alma Ata, the capital of Kazakhstan, every country of the world was represented. The resulting declaration stated that primary care should be available to all. It defined primary care in broad terms. To some, this was a much-needed, inspirational step. To others, it was unrealistic to think that universal primary care, defined idealistically by the declaration, could possibly be funded. The years after the Alma Ata conference saw something of a backlash, and a move towards defining a more minimal set of interventions that could be funded, and that would improve population health in a cost-effective way. This was termed *selective primary care*. UNICEF took a lead in defining the list, in 1982, as growth monitoring, oral rehydration (to manage diarrhoeal illness), breastfeeding promotion and immunization, known by the acronym GOBI. Food supplementation, female literacy and family planning were subsequently added, making the acronym GOBI-FFF. Proponents saw this list as a set of cost-effective, practical interventions that it was feasible to implement and monitor. Opponents saw a lack of ambition: an acceptance that the poorer countries of the world would have to settle for a standard of healthcare of an entirely lower order than that available in the richer countries.

Providing GOBI-FFF required the implementation of a set of specific programmes, not the building of a healthcare system – in other words, a predominantly vertical, rather than horizontal, approach. The vertical approach to global health improvement has been furthered by a number of major disease-specific initiatives, including the Global Polio Eradication Initiative and the Measles and Rubella Initiative, and area-specific funding approaches, including through Gavi the Vaccine Alliance and the Global Fund to Fight AIDS, Tuberculosis and Malaria.

The vertical approach is epitomized by the 'mass campaign', which involves providing a single intervention to a large number of people in a short space of time. Large numbers of vaccinators can move from house to house vaccinating every child against polio, for example, or handing out oral rehydration solution (ORS) and providing education on how and when to use it. Mass campaigns are liked for the immediacy of their impact but disliked because they do little to build health systems for long-term benefit. An example of how targeted programmes can be effective is the use of oral rehydration solutions to prevent fatal dehydration in diarrhoea. Between 1980 and 1990, a collaboration between the government of Bangladesh, a nongovernmental organization formerly known as Bangladesh Rural Advancement Committee (BRAC) and a U.S. Agency for International Development–funded non-profit organization, the Social Marketing Company, scaled up a programme in which 12 million women were trained to provide oral rehydration solutions. Previously, this therapy had only been provided in hospital. The new campaign involved village workers visiting mothers at home, teaching them to make their own oral rehydration solution (using water, salt and sugar) when children developed diarrhoea. The workers' pay depended on whether the mother had learned properly how to make it, and could demonstrate this to an independent evaluator who visited a sample of women after the village worker had left.

Building a sustainable, resilient healthcare system involves taking a horizontal approach. It involves identifying the basic elements of a system and building them up. These include a healthcare workforce, governance systems, financing mechanisms, health facilities and training capacity. The set of activities directed towards doing so is known as *health system strengthening*. In some cases, 'strengthening' is a misnomer because it implies that there is some sort of functioning system already in place.

The attractions of a horizontal approach are clear. It involves constructing, in an ordered way, a healthcare system of the type that citizens of richer countries would recognize as true healthcare. A system that is able to deal with the range of ailments that people face, not simply to deliver a limited set of predefined interventions. Ideally, the system can be improved upon over time, in every element from buildings to people to processes.

The horizontal approach has problems, though. Strengthening a governance system is a far more difficult, nebulous activity than handing out sachets of oral rehydration solution and other such vertical interventions. It is challenging to monitor success, and this is off-putting to donors who want to be able to demonstrate impact and avoid money being lost to corruption. It takes time and patience.

The West Africa Ebola outbreak that started in 2014 re-energized the argument for building resilient healthcare systems. The countries affected had a series of vertical, disease-specific programmes in place to deliver vaccines, and HIV/AIDS treatments, but when Ebola emerged, these did not amount to a resilient healthcare system able to respond to this different need.

Mexico and Rwanda are two countries that have invested heavily in health and health systems. They have promoted an alternative – the *diagonal* approach. This tries to combine the best aspects of vertical and horizontal approaches. Rather than providing a set of priority interventions as separate vertical programmes, they are delivered through a single channel, which therefore forms the basis of a functioning healthcare system. Delivering a set of vertical programmes is expensive and requires duplicative work (e.g. each programme has to organize its own transport and storage logistics). In a diagonal approach, the funds that would have been spent on this are instead used to build a sustainable system that can deliver this set of priority interventions, and subsequently more too. Whereas a pure horizontal approach can take many years to yield tangible results, the diagonal approach aims to demonstrably deliver a set of priority interventions from the beginning.

Global health architecture

In most countries, it is relatively easy to describe how the health system is organized, how it is funded, who leads it and to whom it is answerable. In global health, this is not the case. A large number of organizations and individuals are involved, many of them with complex and ill-defined roles. Some have clear democratic authority – such as the World Health Organization. Some have no democratic authority, but huge power and the potential for great positive impact. Large philanthropic bodies such as the Bill and Melinda Gates Foundation, Bloomberg Philanthropies and the Clinton Global Initiative fall into this category. There is no overarching leadership or hierarchy in global health. Both state and non-state actors are involved. The power structures are difficult to grasp. Governance – that is, setting and monitoring direction – of the global health system is therefore a complex concept in theory, and problematic in reality. Indeed, the words *system* and *architecture* suggest something far more organized than is actually the case. Bringing some order to this tangle – as the Millennium Development Goals did and the Sustainable Development Goals (SDGs) are intended to do – is an important part of making the many different actors, agencies and institutions pull in the same direction.

The United Nations agencies are particularly important. The United Nations was established after the Second World War as the world, led by the victors, aspired to address challenges collectively, to promote peace and to avoid future conflict. Soon afterwards, specific United Nations bodies

were established – of which the World Health Organization was one. Established in 1948, its stated objective is to attain the highest possible level of health for all people. The World Health Organization is made up of 194 member states. It is headquartered in Geneva and has regional and country offices. It sets out to provide leadership on global health matters, shape the health research agenda, set norms and standards, articulate evidence-based policy options, provide technical support to countries and monitor and assess health trends. It can convene governments and others to discuss, negotiate and reach consensus.

On several occasions, most recently during the West African Ebola crisis of 2014, the World Health Organization has been criticized for slow decision-making, indecisiveness and a failure to show leadership. To some degree, the organization is constrained by its financing. Its budget comes from two sources. All member states make mandatory *assessed contributions*, calculated based on their economy and population. In addition, member states, intergovernmental bodies, private foundations and others can make *voluntary contributions*. For the first 30 years of the World Health Organization's existence, most of its budget came from assessed contributions. This has changed markedly over time. Now, assessed contributions represent just a quarter of its budget, and the vast majority comes from voluntary contributions. The importance of this is that voluntary contributions are almost always earmarked by their donors for particular projects and programmes, whereas assessed contributions are available to be spent on a broader strategic canvas. With three-quarters of the organization's budget earmarked, core functions that are of less interest to donors can suffer. This budgetary issue also has governance implications. In theory, the organization's priorities should be set by the annual World Health Assembly, at which each member state has an equal say. In practice, the countries and organizations that make significant voluntary contributions determine where the organization focuses its energies.

In contrast to the World Health Organization's broad focus, the newer global health organizations tend to concentrate on vertical programmes. Some of these have been very successful. Gavi the Vaccine Alliance involves cooperation between public and private bodies, aiming to improve childhood immunization coverage and access to new vaccines. The alliance was created to bring key United Nations agencies, governments, pharmaceutical companies, the private sector and civil society together. By 2015, Gavi the Vaccine Alliance, which was established in 2000, had reached 500 million children and prevented an estimated 7 million deaths.

Those who hold the purse strings have a loud voice in the global health landscape. They determine the countries, diseases and initiatives to which money is allocated. Spending on global health is really a subset of funding for development more generally. More than 80% of official development assistance (often simply known as foreign aid) comes from governments – the United Kingdom, through its Department for International Development, for example.

Donor governments – particularly those that provide large amounts – seek to do more than simply provide aid. They take an active interest in global health policy. They try to stimulate other countries to provide more funding. They monitor carefully how the funds are being spent, and try to understand and improve the effectiveness with which their funding enhances people's lives and countries' economic development.

More than 80% of official development assistance comes from governments. Most of the remainder of the development assistance comes from private foundations and other organizations. The Bill and Melinda Gates Foundation is the largest private foundation in the world. It differs from similar foundations in size, but is similar in its philanthropic mission of enhancing health and reducing extreme poverty globally. The Gates Foundation has much of its impact by funding specific programmes, but also contributes to global health in a number of other ways. Bill and Melinda Gates as individuals have powerful voices with which to shape the global policy agenda. Heads of state will take telephone calls from them. They have also been successful in interesting other very rich people in philanthropy. Many other foundations are prominently involved in global health, such as the Clinton Foundation, the Carter Center and the Rockefeller Foundation.

Collectively, representatives of the world's population are known as civil society. *Civil society organizations* primarily consist of individuals, rather than being allied to governments or other agencies. There are many thousands of civil society organizations. Medicins Sans Frontiers (also known as Doctors Without Borders) is among the best known. Since the early 1970s, it has delivered healthcare and assistance in humanitarian crises. Its principles are impartiality and neutrality, but when it witnesses human rights abuses or large-scale suffering that have been hidden from view, the leadership of the organization will surface them. It acted in this way in the 1994 genocide in Rwanda, and in the West African Ebola outbreak of 2014. It consistently advocates for humanitarian principles. The work of Medicins Sans Frontiers shows the three main ways in which civil society organizations are involved in global health – delivering direct services, advocacy and organizing a collective voice. Many civil society organizations concentrate their efforts in only one of these areas. Nongovernmental organizations and faith-based organizations are specific types of civil society organizations. Particularly through these organizations, civil society plays an important role in shaping the global health agenda. Unlike philanthropic bodies and individuals, civil society organizations do not primarily exert their influence through funding. Instead, their strength comes from representing the voice of the people; they communicate expectations and hold decision makers to account.

Regulatory mechanisms

Most regulations to safeguard and improve the health of populations are made at the national level. As the member states of the World Health Organization have increasingly recognized their shared risk, though, there has been increased interest in international and global law. The International Health Regulations, for example, are a legally binding agreement intended to improve global public health security. In the event of a public health emergency of international concern, the World Health Organization coordinates the management of events. The International Health Regulations also aim to improve all countries' capacity to detect, assess, notify and respond to public health threats. The International Health Regulations (also discussed in Chapter 3) create political pressure for countries to work collaboratively to deal with public health emergencies, but there is really no mechanism to actually enforce compliance where countries do not report the relevant data to the World Health Organization in a timely manner, or do not work together in the way that they should.

The World Health Organization has no legal system through which to establish enforceable global health law. In contrast, the World Trade Organization is a powerful entity with powers to make enforceable treaties. Its 'hard laws' force member states to adopt its regulations and treaties. The World Health Organization has only soft powers at its disposal, meaning that member states can largely select how, and to what extent, they follow up recommendations and action plans. The strongest international health law in place is the Framework Convention on Tobacco Control of 2002. But this, the first global health treaty, cannot be enforced as strongly as trade agreements can. Many countries comply, but others neglect at least some of their responsibilities.

Sometimes the hard laws made elsewhere can affect health detrimentally. For example, the Agreement on Trade Related Aspects of Intellectual Property Rights (TRIPS) is an international agreement governing the production of, and access to, health-related knowledge. Aiming to protect intellectual property, all member states of the World Trade Organization have agreed, among other things, to establish a minimum 20-year period for which patents on new technologies (including drugs) should apply. When new drugs enter the market, no manufacturer is able to copy them for 20 years. Pharmaceutical companies then have an incentive to invest heavily in research and development, knowing that financial returns will be protected by strong law. However, this limits the availability of generic medicines and results in high drug prices. In turn, poorer countries are hit. Countries have ratified the Human Rights Declaration establishing health as a fundamental human right, but the agreement makes this right difficult to fulfil when it comes to essential drugs. The World Health Organization and others have acknowledged the devastating effects that TRIPS has had on public health, but low- and middle-income countries tend to have a weak voice in trade negotiations.

Another example of the difficulties of global regulation is the health worker crisis. Populations with the poorest health invariably have least access to healthcare workers. This is made worse because healthcare workers can move between countries with increasing ease. When people move from lower- to higher-income countries, this is often described as *brain drain*. It is seen among other professionals with higher education, not just healthcare workers, whose qualifications enable them to attain a better standard of living abroad than they could at home. Brain drain is also seen within countries, when healthcare professionals trained in rural areas subsequently move to urban areas with similar economic motivations.

It has been repeatedly said – although it is probably a myth – that there are more Malawian doctors in Manchester, England, than in the whole of Malawi. Myth or not, it starkly illustrates the phenomenon of brain drain. When doctors educated in Malawi move to Manchester, healthcare delivery in Malawi becomes even more difficult, and the system does not get the return on its investment in the doctors' training.

Globalization has made migration of labour more common. An important part of strengthening healthcare systems involves addressing health workforce imbalances between, and within, countries. Several attempts have been made to tackle this, although doing so risks running counter to individuals' rights and expectations as global citizens. The World Health Organization has established a global code of practice on the international recruitment of health personnel, and the idea of more strongly regulating movement is under consideration. The Global Health Workforce Alliance has established a threshold of 59.4 skilled health professionals per 10,000 people, against which to measure progress. In 2013, 68 countries were above this threshold. Although far short of the 200 countries in the world, this is an improvement. It has been helped by the increase in skilled birth attendants prompted by the fifth Millennium

Development Goal. Estimates indicate that to reach a lower threshold of just 34.5 skilled health professionals per 10,000 population, an additional 7.2 million midwives, nurses and physicians are needed.

Changing patterns of disease

Globally, from 1970 to the beginning of the second decade of the twenty-first century, overall mortality has reduced markedly. The improvements have been proportionately greatest in low- and middle-income countries. The exceptions have been countries that have suffered the casualties of war and conflict and where there have been repeated natural disasters. The biggest decreases in mortality have been among the under-fives (Figure 1.3).

The Institute for Health Metrics and Evaluation, based in Seattle, is an organization that analyses and publishes data on disease levels, distributions and trends. The total burden of a disease is the sum of the mortality and disability that it causes. The term *burden of disease* is used to describe the work of this group. It is authoritative and almost universally cited when disease and mortality comparisons between countries are being made. The Institute's 488 researchers collect 1 billion data points to estimate the burden caused by 291 different diseases in 187 countries. Figure 1.4 shows the six leading causes of disease burden in the United Kingdom according to their data. Figure 1.5 shows the same for the world. Their Global Burden of Disease data are referred to throughout this book. Measures of health, mortality, disease and disability are described in later chapters.

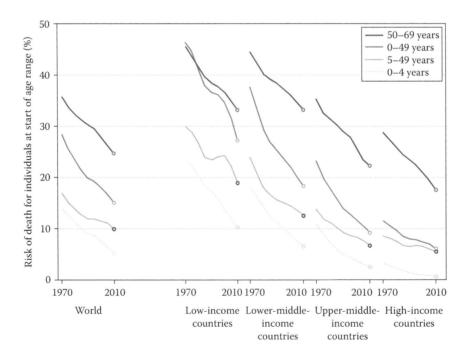

Figure 1.3 Forty-year trends in mortality worldwide.

Source: Norheim OF, Jha P, Admasu K, et al. Avoiding 40% of the premature deaths in each country, 2010–30: review of national mortality trends to help quantify the UN Sustainable Development Goal for health. *Lancet* 2015;385(9964):239–52. With permission.

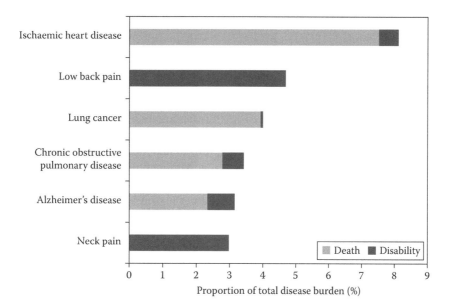

Figure 1.4 Leading diseases by total death and disability burden – United Kingdom, 2015.
Source: Institute for Health Metrics and Evaluation.

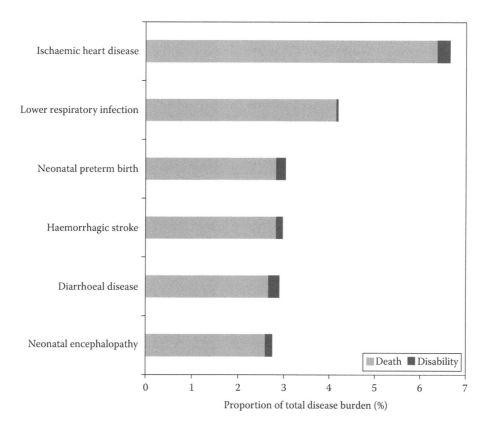

Figure 1.5 Leading diseases by total death and disability burden–worldwide, 2015.
Source: Institute for Health Metrics and Evaluation.

As well as quantifying the relative burden of diseases, the Global Burden of Disease project also assesses the adverse impact of each of the major disease risk factors. Almost 11% of all disease in the world is attributable to poor diet – that is, if everybody's diet was optimal, the amount of disease would be reduced by 11%. After diet, high blood pressure

and smoking are the main disease-causing culprits, both in the United Kingdom and globally. These themes are discussed in more depth in Chapter 4.

Worldwide, the patterns of disease burden are changing fast. Disability accounts for a growing proportion of the total burden of disease, reducing the relative contribution made by premature mortality. The relative importance of non-communicable disease is growing similarly (Figure 1.6).

Mental disorder is common. One in four people experience a significant mental health problem at some point in their lifetime. In England, almost half of all ill health affecting people under 65 years is mental illness. The World Health Organization estimates that mental disorder represents just under a quarter of the total disease burden worldwide (and 30% in the United Kingdom). This theme is picked up again in Chapter 9.

In the year 2000, the United Nations member states adopted eight Millennium Development Goals. These goals were the product of many years of discussion. They were founded on a consensus that there should be a global objective to end poverty. Expert discussions about goals that could address poverty led to the creation of 18 concrete targets and 48 indicators. One of the main proponents was the World Health Organization, the United Nations agency for health. With the aim of ending poverty, it was clear that efforts would require tackling key health issues – hunger, child survival, maternal mortality, reproductive health, HIV/AIDS, malaria, tuberculosis, neglected tropical diseases and access to essential medicines. Each of these was

the subject of a specific Millennium Development Goal, with an explicit health target.

In addition to the health-specific goals, many of the other goals (e.g. on education, sustainable environment and global partnership) were also important to health. This reflects the complexity of development, in which multiple issues are interlinked. For example, malnourished children who grow up without education will have increased risk of illness and limited economic opportunities.

Although many were positive about the goals when they were set, few expected the scale of effort and progress that the goals galvanized. Initial strong support came particularly from nongovernmental organizations and civil society. Very soon, global health and development became increasingly the focus of philanthropists and their foundations.

There has been a remarkable reduction in the under-five mortality rate (Figures 1.7 and 1.8), which was the target of Goal 4. The aim was to reduce this by two-thirds between 1990 and 2015, and many countries have achieved this. The annual rate of reduction particularly increased after 2003. The reduction in deaths has come notably from investment in vaccines (especially for measles), and treatments for diarrhoea and pneumonia. The leading causes of death among

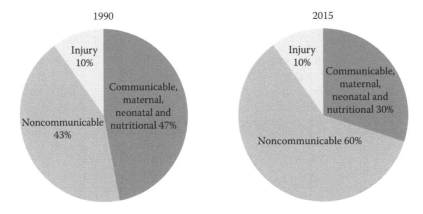

Figure 1.6 Global burden of disease by major category.

Source: Institute for Health Metrics and Evaluation.

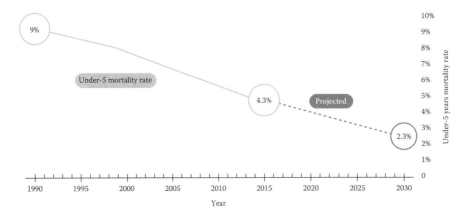

Figure 1.7 Under-five mortality rate worldwide.

Source: Historical data: United Nations Inter-agency Group for Child Mortality Estimation (IGME). Projected data: Bill & Melinda Gates Foundation (BMGF). Annual Letter 2015. Seattle: BMGF. With permission.

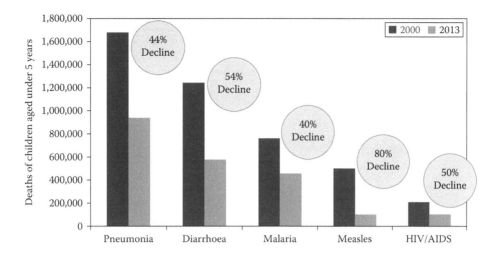

Figure 1.8 Global under-five deaths from five infectious diseases.

Source: Liu L, Oza S, Hogan D, et al. Global, regional, and national causes of child mortality in 2000–13, with projections to inform post-2015 priorities: an updated systematic analysis. *Lancet* 2015;385(9966):430–40. With permission.

children under five are now preterm birth complications (15%), pneumonia (15%) and intrapartum complications (11%). Newborn mortality is falling more slowly than later child mortality.

Despite impressive progress, the under-five mortality target has not been met in full and further progress is needed to avert more of the 6 million deaths of children under five years that occur every year. The highest mortality rates – and the highest numbers of deaths – occur in sub-Saharan Africa and in southern Asia. The large differences between regions and countries indicate that more can be done. In Singapore, the child mortality rate is 2 deaths per 1000 live births, while in Guinea-Bissau it is 153 deaths per 1000 live births.

Maternal mortality has also fallen impressively, although few regions have met the Millennium Development Goal of reducing it by three-quarters between 1990 and 2015 (Figure 1.9). Maternal and child health are closely linked in many ways, including that birth itself – the intrapartum period – is the most dangerous time for both mother and baby. This has therefore received particular focus. The Millennium Development Goals set a particular target for skilled birth attendants, which has been difficult to meet. Many also question the quality of care provided in health facilities. In particular, rural areas have low coverage of care.

More than 300,000 women die every year from maternal causes. The difference in maternal mortality rates between countries and regions is often highlighted as one of the widest disparities in public health. Sierra Leone has the highest maternal mortality rate in the world – 1,100 maternal deaths per 100,000 live births. In Belarus, by contrast, the rate is 1 maternal death per 100,000 live births – a 1000-fold difference. Reducing maternal mortality involves providing a continuum of care from conception to safe labour to post-natal follow-up. There is significant potential to make further progress, but it is not easy. In particular, strong systems

are required to identify high-risk cases in which assistance is required when complications occur.

New goals for the world

The year 2015 marked the end of the Millennium Development Goals. Heated debate about what should follow them started several years in advance of this. Most agreed that a successor to the Millennium Development Goals was needed – that there is value in setting a common framework to organize, at least to some degree, the action of the many countries and institutions wanting, and working, to improve the world. The successor is the Sustainable Development Goals, agreed on 25 September 2015 at the United Nations Sustainable Development Summit in New York. The United Nations document that sets out the goals is entitled *Transforming Our World: The 2030 Agenda for Sustainable Development.*

There were eight Millennium Development Goals. There are 17 Sustainable Development Goals (Figure 1.10) with 169 targets. There is some rationale for this expansion. Many felt that the Millennium Development Goals were too narrow – that they did not address the root causes of poverty, and they made no mention of economic development, human rights or sustaining the environment. The process of developing the Millennium Development Goals had been criticized for setting goals without consulting the people whom they most affected – those living in poverty. In response, the Sustainable Development Goals process aimed to be highly inclusive, through a series of 'global conversations'. Nevertheless, some comment that this process has created too many ideas, and that the Sustainable Development Goals are less focused than the Millennium Development Goals were. Most agree that the goals are ambitious, with many considering them aspirational and expressing concerns about whether the work to achieve them will be funded to the degree that is needed.

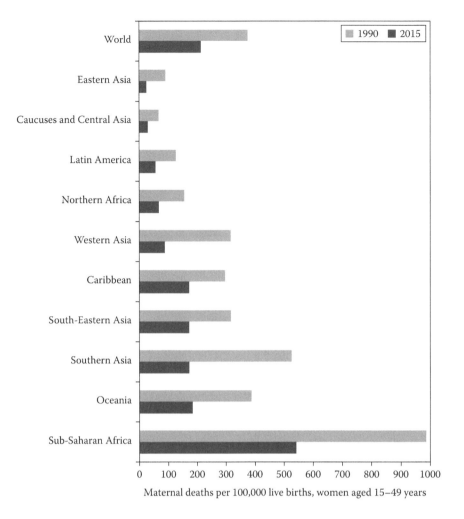

Figure 1.9 Maternal mortality by world region.

Source: United Nations (UN). *The Millennium Development Goals Report 2015.* New York: UN, 2015.

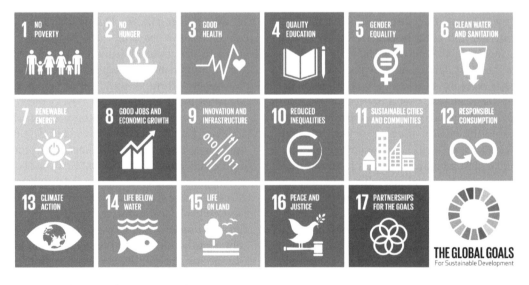

Figure 1.10 The Sustainable Development Goals.

Source: United Nations (UN). *Transforming Our World: the 2030 Agenda for Sustainable Development.* New York: UN, 2015.

The 2015–16 transition has thrown up two particular questions. First, what will happen to the programmes that were established in response to the Millennium Development Goals? If they receive less funding, many fear that the poorest countries' healthcare systems are not strong enough to take up the slack. Second, how will countries and the global community address the Millennium Development Goals that were not met; should they accelerate focus on this unfinished business, or simply move on to the new goals?

Many believe that the specificity and measurability of targets is important to their success, that this enables countries, donors and global organizations to work together with clear common purpose, rather than working in different directions. However, some argue that the targets narrow the approach, guiding action towards specific health problems rather than focusing on cross-cutting issues such as the health workforce crisis or health system strengthening.

CONCLUSIONS

Public health practice involves tackling issues that affect health for whole communities, whole societies and the whole world. In the last century, the world has experienced health improvements that few would have imagined.

People are living far longer than their grandparents did. Diseases are being eradicated and controlled, although new diseases as yet unknown are likely to emerge. Heavy investment in research and development has yielded valuable new knowledge and products – from diagnostic imaging to anti-retroviral treatment for HIV/AIDS. The success of some of the Millennium Development Goals shows that concerted, collective action can produce impressive results.

Today's public health practitioners face a different set of issues than their predecessors, and have an ever-expanding set of tools with which to understand and tackle them. The core principles of public health remain the same as ever, though – a holistic focus on health, not just disease; a grounding in data and evidence; and an emphasis on prevention, intervening early in the causal pathway.

The rest of this book addresses the considerable challenges that remain ahead – from the growing burden of non-communicable disease to the impact of the environment on health; from the potential for a new disease to emerge and rapidly spread worldwide, to the question of how people and societies cope with ageing. The book interweaves a UK and a global perspective. In a number of areas, the issues remain markedly different between the two. But in many, today's converging world is ever narrowing the distinction between them.

CHAPTER 2

Epidemiology and its uses

INTRODUCTION

One of the foundation stones of public health is epidemiology. The science of epidemiology is concerned with the states of health and disease in natural populations. In many fields of science, experiments can be carried out in laboratories where the researcher can control the conditions so as to examine the relationship between particular factors and an outcome. Many of the influences on health – the way that people behave, the social and economic conditions in which they live and work – cannot be controlled to create an experimental situation. Instead, the population and its milieu can be thought of as a living laboratory, in which the conditions are operating free of what the investigator might want to happen. This is not to say that epidemiology is not a science. It very much is, with its own concepts, rigour and discipline. At its heart lies a sophisticated set of methodologies, analytical techniques and rules of evidence through which carefully constructed observations of people, risk factors and events can be used to unravel the mysteries of health and disease in human populations.

Epidemiological methods can be used in diverse situations, for example, to investigate an outbreak of Ebola virus or food poisoning, to examine the claim that cases of a rare cancer are clustered around a waste incinerator plant, to explore differences in chronic disease occurrence among different ethnic groups within a country or to test the hypothesis that mobile telephone use increases the risk of cerebral tumours. Epidemiology can describe trends in disease over time, differences in disease between population groups or variation in levels of health and disease by place. Epidemiological data can be analysed to identify risk factors or suitable treatments for illnesses, and identify side effects of new medicines (pharmacoepidemiology) and other new treatments. Data analysis based on the principles of epidemiology can evaluate the effectiveness of policies and complex interventions. It can yield needs assessments to allow the planning of effective and accessible healthcare for a local population.

Epidemiology is the scientific approach to studying these questions. Formally put, epidemiology is the study of the distribution and determinants of disease in human populations. The key activities of epidemiology are careful, meticulous description; comparison of groups; investigation; interpretation; understanding the limitations of data and the sources of bias in observations; drawing causal inferences; and making and evaluating interventions.

ROUTINELY AVAILABLE DATA SOURCES

In public health, planned epidemiological studies are used to address specific questions about health and disease in populations and the factors that influence them. Generally, data are specially gathered to fulfil the study's purpose. The methods used in such studies are described later in this chapter. On the whole, they are used to *discover* and *analyse*.

The value of the epidemiological approach to public health is also through the ways in which so-called *routinely available data* are gathered, analysed and presented to assess a population's health status or investigate the pattern of disease occurrence. These methods are also described in the chapter. They are essentially used to *observe* and *describe*. This is not a passive activity because frequently what is observed is a trigger to either action or exploring a striking observation further using one of the formal epidemiological study designs.

There are many sources of routinely available data (the term is often shortened to *routine data*) that can be used for epidemiological purposes – mainly to describe, although less commonly such data can be the raw material for analytical research. Routine data are collected in different ways. For some data, there are continuous and systematic processes in place; other data are collected intermittently. Routine data sources may cover the whole population, part of it or a representative sample. When data are collected intermittently, this may involve taking repeat cross-sectional surveys or following the same group of people over time. The data may be collected to reflect the health experience of individuals over time, or may be based on episodes of ill health experienced by many people.

The term *routine* simply means that the data are collected as part of an ongoing data collection system, for example, for statutory, governmental purposes or in the health and social services, rather than as part of a predefined study to answer a particular question. This feature should be kept in mind when considering the uses of routine data: they are usually easy to access, the costs of obtaining them are low and they are often available over periods of years. This stability of collection and the consistency of methods mean that many sources of routine data facilitate comparisons of populations, countries or areas over time. On the downside, they have limitations that study data, especially collected to answer a question at hand, usually do not. Data may be missing and so introduce bias into results. For example, harder-to-reach groups, such as homeless or marginalized populations, will not be well represented, and their health status is likely to differ from the rest of the population. There may also be limited detail on the features of interest, data may be poorly presented and hard to interpret and use, and the base population may not be well defined or appropriate for the required use. This is not an exhaustive list, but illustrates some key questions that users of routine data should ask themselves: for example, who has collected the data and for what purpose? How complete are the data and has there been rigorous case identification? Can the population at risk be defined? How accurate are the data and are they up to date? How have matters of confidentiality been dealt with and how have the data been aggregated? Only when basic questions like these have been answered can it be determined if the data are fit for the intended use.

In practice, there are subtle or sometimes even substantial changes in how such data are collected, particularly over time. As the data are collected for 'routine' rather than 'study' purposes, these changes are not always given the scrutiny they should be.

The volume of data gathered about people – some official, some arising from their behaviour and transactions in a consumer society – is vast and ever expanding. This is driven by the capacity of modern technology to easily capture and analyse information. This type of data could be of great value to public health researchers, but when collected for commercial purposes (e.g. supermarket store card data), it is not readily available to them. The capability to know more about people as individuals, the social groups they fall into and their interactions, and to yield meaningful information (ideally in real time), is often referred to as *big data*. This combination of available data and large computer statistical power could change the potential to undertake large studies of populations without investigators having to collect any data themselves. It all depends on whether there are major barriers to access for the researcher. However, the exciting potential of big data should not be a shortcut for thoughtful timely analyses.

Traditionally, routine data have been described in four categories: *demographic* data, *mortality* data, *morbidity* data and *health facilities usage* data. The widening of the concept of health and of the range of influences on health and disease, as well as the growth in potential data sources to examine them, means that this classification is now outmoded. Today, the expectation of routine data sources is that they will enable a description of a population by the numbers and characteristics of people: being born, living, dying, falling ill, experiencing long-term illness and disability, living in particular social and economic conditions, and using health and social care services.

In this section, starting with the census (that counts and describes the population), the main sources and modes of collection of routine data are discussed.

Census data

The main source of demographic data within the United Kingdom is the census. It has taken place once every 10 years since 1801, except in 1941 during World War II. The original rationale for the census was the notion that the knowledge of a country must inform the basis of legislation and diplomacy. In times gone by, for example, knowing the number of seamen was important for national defence, while understanding the size of the population was essential to plan food supplies. Authority for the census is enshrined in an act of Parliament, the 1920 *Census Act*. Before each census, there is extensive public consultation on its proposed methods and content, as well as a programme of field testing. The very first census asked only five questions and counted 10 million people living in 2 million households. The 2011 census asked 56 questions and counted 63.2 million people living in 26.4 million households. Almost 25.4 million questionnaires were posted, and it required 35,000 staff to help people complete and return them.

The law requires that all people alive on the night of the census be enumerated, traditionally in the household or establishment where they spent that night. A household is defined as one person living alone or a group of people, not necessarily related, living at the same address, with common housekeeping – sharing at least one meal a day or a living room, temporary residents being included. For example, university students are counted at their term-time address.

The census in England and Wales is planned and carried out by the Office for National Statistics (ONS). It collates and processes all census data under conditions of strict confidentiality. Names are not entered into computers for processing but used only for internal checking of completeness and accuracy of forms. The quality of the census data depends on the enumerator filling out the form, and also whether those surveyed trust the census. Generally, censuses are not suited to asking complex questions. In analysis, great care is taken not to differentiate very small communities in which an individual person might be identified.

Completeness of a census is important if the data are to be reliable. The response rate is essential to this – in 2011, the response rate was 94% in England and Wales. The response rate varied with age and sex, with the lowest response rate in 2011 among men aged 25–29 years. The rate also varied geographically. For example, it was 78%

in Inner London, 10 percentage points lower than in 1991. In contrast, 17 local authority areas had response rates of more than 99%.

The census provides an incredibly detailed amount of information on the inhabitants of the United Kingdom. The high response rate and coverage are an asset, although some subgroups of the population are underrepresented (analytical techniques can now adjust for this). Census data are valuable in providing information at the local level for the allocation of resources. Given the comprehensive coverage, the data are good for examining subgroups within the population and between areas, while the regular periodicity enables trends over time to be compared. The comprehensive coverage does mean that census data are very expensive to collect.

Census results are publicly available through the Internet. They are usually made available in tabular form. Three main standard sets are produced: key statistics, standard tables and census area statistics.

Many other countries also have a census system, each with its own strengths and weaknesses. In some, there is a high level of migration of nomadic or farming communities between seasons, so the results of the census may be heavily influenced by whether data are recorded for the normal (*de facto*) residents or residents on the day of the census (*de jure*).

Many censuses run on 10-year cycles. There is often a delay in publishing the data from the census, so between the years of the census, most countries' census offices give population estimates, based on projections derived from the census data (taking into account births, deaths and migration) and information from interim surveys. This can be especially challenging in areas with high or unpredictable migration rates.

Civil registration and vital statistics

In the United Kingdom, it is compulsory to register births and deaths. These registrations are an important routine data source for planning, policymaking and describing the health of the population. The information on births is usually supplied to the registration system by one of the parents. In the United Kingdom, the baby's name, date of birth and sex, and the mother's and father's (where included) date of birth, are entered on the certificate, along with information on economic status of the parents and whether the birth was part of a multiple birth.

The compulsory registration of deaths is by death certification. This is a process by which the main cause of death and those conditions that have contributed to the death are recorded. Once a certificate has been issued, the death is registered with a registrar. The date of registration and the date of death are not the same – often when data are processed, there is a lag time between the date of death and registration. This is especially true if the death is reported to a coroner. Data on deaths are made available by date of death, but this requires time. Real-time

surveillance on death counts makes statistical corrections for this lag period.

A UK death certificate (more fully known as the medical certificate of cause of death) has two parts. Part 1 of the certificate allows the doctor to record diseases or conditions that led directly to death, in a causal chain of up to three elements: 1a is the disease or condition that led directly to death, 1b is a disease or condition that led to 1a and 1c is a disease or condition that led by 1b. Part 2 of the certificate records other relevant diseases that contributed to the death but were not related to the disease that caused it. From this information, expert coders determine which element to record as the underlying cause of death, following a fairly complex set of rules set out in the *International Classification of Diseases*.

The quality of mortality statistics therefore depends on the quality of death certification. In reality, the doctor completing the death certificate may have incomplete information about the cause of death, or may record a simplification in complex cases. For example, bronchopneumonia is often recorded in part 1a of the death certificate in elderly patients who in reality had multiple comorbidities, and for whom pneumonia was the last in a string of related illnesses and age-related decline. Postmortem examination is the gold standard for determining cause of death, but is undertaken in less than 20% of deaths – a proportion that has decreased over time. The broader issue is that systems of ascribing deaths to a single disease do not work very well in old age, which is when most people die.

Internationally, the process of registering all births and deaths (together with recording cause of death) is usually referred to as a *civil registration and vital statistics* (CRVS) system. Having such a process in place in every country is important, for example, to enable international comparisons of patterns of fertility and mortality. Evaluations have shown that only a third of deaths are recorded in civil registries that include cause of death information.

Data on occurrence of disease and disability

While mortality data are vital for public health use, they give an incomplete picture of disease within the population. This is because not all diseases cause death, and most of those that cause death do not do so in a consistent way. For this reason, mortality and various other sources of data provide a proxy for the true amount of a disease in the population. The extent to which the proxy reflects reality varies greatly, depending on which disease is being studied and the characteristics of the source of data.

Data on disease and disability are derived from a range of sources. Generally, these fall into four categories: hospital databases, primary care records, case or disease registers and official household and population surveys. Within any of those routine data sources, no single one can give a complete picture of the amount and distribution of disease and disability within a population. If they are based on the collection of information about patients who have made contact with services (as many are), they will not provide comprehensive information about all cases of the disease that exist in the population (Figure 2.1). Traditionally, many countries have used hospital inpatient data as an indicator of disease in the wider population. However, such data can only take account of those conditions for which inpatient care is required. There are many important health problems (e.g. upper respiratory illnesses, headache and backache) that affect a significant proportion of the population and create substantial economic impact through working days lost, yet seldom lead their sufferers to require hospital care. For other conditions, such as asthma or rheumatoid arthritis, a proportion of people afflicted will not make the decision to seek healthcare (even though they may recognize themselves as ill). A further proportion will visit their general practitioners only. Others will come to the attention of hospital services as outpatients or inpatients. Only the very last group will be recorded in a system of morbidity data based on hospital data. In some disorders where hospitalization is virtually mandatory, such as a fractured neck of femur, hospital rates may approximate to the total size of the disease problem in the population. These situations are so few that conclusions about incidence of disease based on hospital inpatient data should be interpreted with great caution.

Hospital Episode Statistics (HES) is the system of data recording of every episode of inpatient care in English National Health Service (NHS) hospitals and also all care given to NHS patients by the independent sector in treatment centres. An *episode* is defined as a period of treatment under the care of a particular hospital consultant. The data broadly cover administrative and demographic, diagnostic and procedural matters. The items of data collected include hospital of treatment, area of residence, patient administrative details (e.g. birth date, sex, postcode of usual address and ethnicity), admission details (e.g. referring general practitioner, admission or discharge details and method or source of admission), consultant episode details (e.g. consultant code and specialty) and clinical details (primary and subsidiary diagnoses and operations and procedures undertaken). For maternity admissions, details of the delivery record are entered, as are details about the baby itself. For people with mental illness, additional information is collected.

In theory, deriving information on disease and disability from records of patients in primary care is a better option since it is likely to cover a greater part of the spectrum of conditions (minor as well as major) than hospital-based systems. To some extent this is so, but in practice, making and recording diagnoses in primary care settings is very different to hospitals; many conditions are undifferentiated (i.e. they are clusters of symptoms) and the use of clinical investigations to reach a formal diagnosis is much less. Therefore, establishing a diagnostic label for morbidity recording is not straightforward. Using primary care records to determine the amount of disease and disability at the population level (its proxy value) is helpful but has its own strengths and weaknesses as a data source.

In the past, the NHS gathered data from samples of general practices around the country that agreed to participate and supply clinical and management information; often, they have been managed by academic or professional bodies. Some continue to operate. For example, the Royal College of General Practitioners established a network of *sentinel practices* in 1957, across England and Wales; this national Research and Surveillance Centre has provided invaluable morbidity data from some 100 practices on

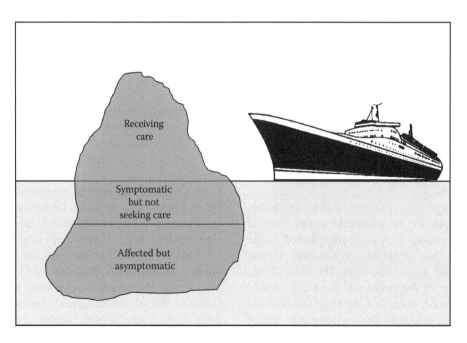

Figure 2.1 The iceberg concept of healthcare.

influenza, other diseases and vaccine effectiveness over time. The Clinical Practice Research Datalink (CPRD) also covers general practices in England. Jointly funded by the NHS National Institute for Health Research (NIHR) and the Medicines and Healthcare products Regulatory Agency (MHRA), it provides anonymized NHS clinical data that can be linked to facilitate many types of observational research. The Quality and Outcomes Framework (QOF), which is part of an incentive-based payment system for general practices to achieve quality standards, records data on a range of chronic diseases and therefore provides a picture, although incomplete, of their prevalence and distribution in the population (Figure 2.2).

Access to, and availability of, morbidity and other data in primary care is increasing greatly as a result of the spread of electronic records. Official and academic bodies have developed, and continue to develop, systems to extract such data in anonymized form. With these are coming better estimates of the level and pattern of different diseases and other health problems in the population, and more timely data.

Over recent years, the proportion of healthcare that is provided outside of hospitals and beyond the walls of general practice has grown. As community-based services have expanded, so has the need for data to describe their activity. The Health and Social Care Information Centre has established a Community Information Data Set that providers of NHS-funded community services share annually, but this system is currently less sophisticated than those that have existed for hospitals and general practice for some years.

As a source of population-level data on the frequency of disease and disability, *disease registers* (also called *case registers*) are greatly valued because they usually come closer to an accurate estimate of disease frequency, gather in-depth information on people who have a disease and are based on a properly defined population.

The National Cancer Registration Service has been operating since the end of World War II, although a system was in operation in some parts of the country in the 1920s, when radium treatment commenced. Public Health England, through notification by each region, assembles a minimum data set. Each regional cancer registry collects data on the identity and type of neoplasm of each person resident or treated in the region who has been diagnosed as having cancer (certain premalignant tumours are also included). An effective cancer registry will have a very low proportion of cases where the first notification comes after the patient's death. Such data enable the incidence of cancer to be examined geographically, within subgroups of the population and over time. They also allow survival to be compared for cancer at different anatomical sites. A registry is necessary to compute survival statistics. Survival statistics have many purposes, for example, to discuss clinical management plans with patients and families; to make international, or between-hospital, comparisons; and to monitor quality of treatment over time.

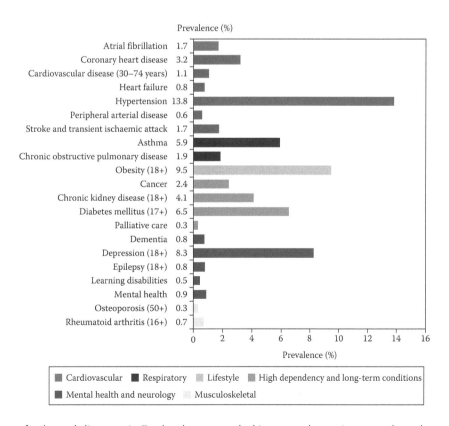

Figure 2.2 Prevalence of selected diseases in England, as recorded in general practice records and extracted as part of the Quality and Outcomes Framework, 2015–16.

Source: NHS Digital.

A good disease register has six key characteristics:

1. It sets out clear criteria for the disease that will then determine which people will be included in the register.
2. It registers individuals with the requisite disease criteria and records them in the register.
3. It is longitudinal, in that the information held about individuals is updated in a defined systematic manner.
4. It is based on a geographically defined population.
5. It is assiduously curated, often with a team that works on it over many years.
6. It maintains high standards of information governance.

Registers have been established to study many conditions in the United Kingdom and around the world. Cancer registries are probably the most widespread, but registers also cover mental illness, child abuse, ischaemic heart disease, stroke, trauma, diabetes and many other diseases and conditions. There is also a varied pattern of registers collecting data on the incidence of congenital abnormalities. While, in practice, many disease registers have a single disease focus, they also have the potential for multiple uses. In addition, they can monitor temporal trends, enable comparisons of treatment outcomes and health behaviours, be used for studies of disease causation and provide information for planning and organizing services for patients.

Government-run surveys provide further useful information about health and disease within the population. The Health Survey for England, described later, does not record specific diagnoses, but captures information on the prevalence of long-standing illness, including whether that illness limits daily life and whether participants need, and receive, help with their activities of daily living. This is helpful in understanding the overall patterns of disability, and related need, within the population.

Data on health-related behaviour and risk factors

Information about people's health-related behaviours and risk factors is generally not well recorded within routine data systems. Research studies and population surveys therefore play a vital role in supplementing this information, and are described in more detail later in this chapter.

Routine data systems do record at least some information on health-related behaviours and risk factors, though. General practice records provide a fairly complete picture of height and weight, and therefore body mass index, although it is not always up to date. They also record smoking status, blood pressure and, for those who have had the blood tests, information such as serum cholesterol. In children, vaccination coverage is well recorded, as is whether mothers are breastfeeding their infants.

The volumes of alcohol and cigarettes being consumed within the country form part of the routine data tracked carefully by Her Majesty's Revenue and Customs (HMRC), to ensure that the appropriate taxes are paid. These data can be of some secondary use to public health professionals. This illustrates that routine data need not come from within the healthcare sector to be of value to health.

The Health Survey for England (described as an example of a cross-sectional study later in the chapter) records physical activity, smoking, alcohol and diet (although the information on diet is very limited). For alcohol, the survey asks what the respondent drinks, as well as frequency and binge drinking. These data can be explored by age, socioeconomic status and ethnicity since social and economic demographic questions are asked of each respondent.

Other official surveys also provide health-related data, for example, the National Food Survey and the National Diet and Nutrition Survey. Surveys collecting travel data can be relevant to public health if they ask about walking and cycling journeys.

Data on social and economic determinants of health

The social and economic determinants of health are even less well captured within individuals' healthcare system records than risk factor information is. Such systems do not routinely record income, occupation or education level, for example.

In the United Kingdom, the census remains centrally important in providing routine information about the social and economic determinants of health. For each household, it records income, occupation, education, household composition and more. Data on individual households are not made available until a century later, when it can be assumed that they are no longer sensitive. But the data are made available in aggregate, to describe the socio-economic profile of small geographical areas, each numbering approximately 1000 households. These are termed Lower Layer Super Output Areas (LSOAs). There are 32,482 of them in England. Additional statistics to describe each of these areas – such as on crime and safety, housing and the physical environment – are published regularly by the Office for National Statistics. These data have many uses, including the construction of an Index of Multiple Deprivation. This is described in Chapter 5, on the social determinants of health, and provides an overall measure of an area's deprivation.

The techniques of data linkage are important in using these routine sources to shed light on how social and economic conditions are related to health outcomes. For example, data from the census can be linked with data from general practice records to map out how deprivation is related to the incidence of a given disease by Lower Layer Super Output Area.

Data to evaluate the performance of health services

A very substantial, ever-growing amount of data is collected by health services as they operate day-to-day, and is potentially useful to evaluate their performance. The challenge is in selecting appropriate data from the masses available, and using them in the appropriate way. This is both difficult and controversial because inappropriate data, or appropriate data used in the wrong way, can easily provide a misleading picture of health service performance. The challenges of evaluating health service performance are described in more detail in Chapter 6, on health systems.

The Hospital Episode Statistics database was described in the section above. This database provides detailed information about each hospital's activity, which is one part of its performance – how many patients it sees and treats with different diseases. Of more interest than the number of patients seen, though, is those patients' outcomes. The same database records if a patient dies, and this is the basis for calculation of the hospital standardized mortality ratio (SMR) for each hospital or group of hospitals. It can also be used to calculate the mortality rate associated with individual doctors, or individual services, within a hospital. The inherent difficulty in calculating and using these figures, though, lies with their standardization. It is not fair to simply judge one hospital as performing more poorly than another because a greater proportion of its patients die. It may be located in an area with an older population, or it may be providing highly specialist services to which patients with the poorest prognosis are referred. Measures such as the hospital SMR must therefore include adjustment to reflect this, so that they indicate how the actual mortality compared with the mortality that would be expected given the characteristics of the patient population.

In the United Kingdom, more routine data are available for primary care than for hospitals. This is largely because of the Quality and Outcomes Framework, which has been requiring general practices to provide a standard set of data since 2004, and because primary care is further ahead in the move from paper-based to electronic health records. Administration of the Quality and Outcomes Framework involves extracting data that are held within the electronic primary care record. From these, it is straightforward to see disease-specific

measures of health service performance – for example, the proportion of hypertensive patients whose hypertension is controlled, or the proportion of asthmatic patients who have had an annual asthma review. It is also possible to compare the number of patients in the practice's population who are known to have hypertension with the number who would be expected to have hypertension, which indicates the practice's performance in identifying such cases. However, because it is a performance tool rather than a data recording tool, the information is more prone to bias. For example, general practitioners have the option of discounting some patients from being included in the denominator. Also, there can be a ceiling effect: when a practice reaches a performance target, recording of data may become less complete.

Disease nomenclatures and classifications

For accurate reporting of causes of death or diseases, it is essential to have a nomenclature. This is an agreed listing of approved names and terms. Strictly, if it stays as a list, it is a nomenclature. If the causes and diseases are organized into topics, subject areas or categories, it is termed a classification. The value of a nomenclature or classification depends on the extent to which it is internationally agreed, adopted and consistently applied using accepted rules and conventions. This determines the reliability of routine and descriptive epidemiological data for making comparisons in mortality and disease patterns over time and between populations. Classifications, groupings and terminologies are all somewhat different in scope and in how they are used (Figure 2.3).

The World Health Organization produces the *International Statistical Classification of Diseases and Related Health Problems* (ICD). Its principal use is to classify cause of death information from death certification. It is increasingly also used in systems that gather data on illness, disease and disability. It has gone through many revisions over the decades since the Second World War. Each time there is a new edition, countries have to agree to adopt it,

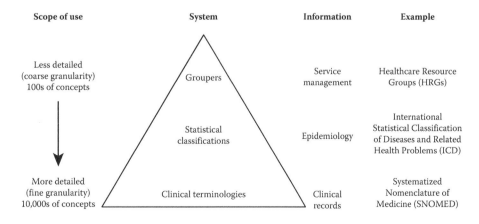

Figure 2.3 The relationship between terminologies, classifications and groupings.

Source: Read JD, Sanderson HF, Sutton YM. Terming, Encoding, Grouping, The Language of Health. In: *Proceedings International Medical Information Association's 8th World Congress on Medical Informatics.* Vancouver, 1995.

and introduce it into their statutory death certification and other processes of gathering statistics. This is a slow business. Some countries adopt the new version relatively quickly, but many countries lag behind, using older versions for years or even decades afterwards. This hinders international disease comparisons, although statistical adjustments can be made. The most recent revision is the 10th, known as ICD-10, published by the World Health Organization in the early 1990s. This groups diagnoses, signs and symptoms, causes and other factors into 21 chapters, starting with those relating to infectious diseases and ending with codes for factors influencing health status and contact with health services. An 11th ICD is being worked on. Through the years, the classification has moved from being disease-orientated, and primarily a means of assigning causes of death, to include a wider framework of illness and other health problems. There are some further classifications that have evolved to fulfil more specific purposes. For example, the *International Classification of Diseases for Oncology* was developed by the World Health Organization and is used extensively by cancer registries around the world.

With the growing importance of data in healthcare, it is essential to have systems of nomenclature and classification that enable aggregation of clinical data on patients. Terms are needed to describe concepts that are then arranged formally to produce an electronic thesaurus. These terminologies cover most of the information in a medical record (symptoms, physical signs, diagnoses, treatments and clinical procedures). Two such systems are prominent: Systematized Nomenclature of Medicine (SNOMED) and Clinical Terms Version 3 (Read Codes). Collaboration between the College of American Pathologists and the NHS has led to the development of SNOMED Clinical Terms, which has been adopted as the standard nomenclature and is replacing the Read Codes from 2016. These clinical terminologies are intended to allow doctors to use their preferred clinical terms, which can then be converted automatically by computer software into codes. In this way, the detailed clinical information required to support patient care and the electronic healthcare record can also be aggregated into statistical classification and groupings.

In the United Kingdom, the primary classification of operative procedures and other interventions is the fourth revision of the *Classification of Surgical Operations and Procedures* (OPCS-4). The codes use a similar format to those in ICD-10 and cover procedures within anatomical systems, as well as subsidiary codes for methods (e.g. laser therapy) and specific sites of operation (such as upper inner quadrant of the breast). The classification was designed specifically for operating theatre–based surgery. Continuing advances in the provision of treatment means that the classification requires annual review, with substantial new codes being added to keep pace with clinical practice.

Healthcare Resource Groups (HRGs) aggregate treatment data into larger categories for the purpose of higher-level analysis, for example, resource management needs assessment, commissioning and performance monitoring.

They are grouped to reflect a similar level of resource, and so can be a fair basis for reimbursing hospitals for the costs of care.

Surveillance data

Surveillance is a system of using descriptive epidemiological data to maintain an overview of a population's health or to monitor a disease, syndrome, or other health variable or event of interest. It involves the continuous analysis, assessment and feedback of systematically gathered data. Surveillance systems are of most value if they are comprehensive and if they supply data on health events soon after they happen, rather than weeks or months afterwards. The longest established are communicable disease surveillance systems based on notification of infectious diseases (see also Chapter 3, on communicable disease), but there are many others. For example, pharmacosurveillance systems monitor adverse effects of medication and enable early detection of problems. Had this form of surveillance been in existence at the time of the widespread use of the drug thalidomide to treat morning sickness in pregnancy, the tragedy in which 10,000 babies were born (and 5,000 survived and grew up) with missing limbs might have turned out very differently.

Indicators

Routine data can be used to construct indicators. An indicator is a measure chosen to highlight an aspect of the health of the population or the performance of the healthcare system. They can be drawn from any of the sources of routine data described earlier. They are selected purposefully. They are usually chosen for use on a regular basis, for example, to track aspects of the health of the population, to measure progress against policy objectives, to compare between and within populations, to support commissioning, to trigger action and for accountability purposes.

The health department of a government will often create a framework to group indicators into monitoring categories when there is an expectation of progress. An example is the *Public Health Outcomes Framework* in England (Table 2.1). Indicators can be released with commentary and interpretation in press releases or special reports addressing a theme of public, professional, media or political interest.

Access and transparency

With so much data now stored electronically about almost every aspect of health and social care, the question of who should be able to access those data, and for what purposes, has come increasingly to the fore. In many countries, including the United Kingdom, there is a major drive towards improving data transparency. Some politicians argue that openness and transparency about public services can save money, strengthen people's trust in government and encourage greater public participation in decision-making. In short, data comparing performance between different

Table 2.1 The Public Health Outcomes Framework for England

Objective	Included indicators (examples)
Increased healthy life expectancy	• Healthy life expectancy at birth
Reduced differences in life expectancy and healthy life expectancy between communities	• Gap in life expectancy between each local authority and England as a whole
Improving the wider determinants of health	• Percentage of children in poverty • 16- to 18-year olds not in education, employment or training
Health improvement	• Smoking prevalence at age 15 • Average portions of fruit eaten
Health protection	• Population vaccination coverage with meningitis C vaccine • Incidence of tuberculosis
Healthcare public health and preventing premature mortality	• Mortality rate from causes considered preventable • Infant mortality rate

Source: Public Health England (PHE). Healthy lives, healthy people: Improving outcomes and supporting transparency. London: PHE, 2016.

health services, surgeons or medical devices should be available to the public who fund and use them.

There is also a strong argument for making data collected within health services available for research purposes – that if researchers are readily able to access rich data about health services and their patients, they can study these to provide useful insights that can in turn improve care. Linkage of different records of individuals from separate sources can be particularly valuable for answering important research questions. It needs identifiable information, to ensure that the records relate to the same person, but the researcher often does not need to see the identifiable information, he or she just needs to know that the record linkage has been carried out reliably.

The balance between transparency and confidentiality is a difficult one. Medical information must be treated with particular care. Data often have greater value to researchers and analysts if they paint a full picture of each individual patient, for example, their age, geographical location, full medical history and drug history. The more data available on an individual, the more potentially identifiable he or she becomes. Finding the right balance is essential.

There is a degree of public scepticism and distrust about data transparency. There have been high-profile incidents in which discs or computers containing large amounts of confidential information have been stolen or left on a train. These have not helped public confidence. The issues are complex, so it is not easy to have a proper public dialogue about the benefits of data transparency, and the appropriate safeguards required to maintain confidentiality.

NHS data are generally considered in three categories – anonymous or aggregated data, pseudoanonymized data and personal confidential data. Anonymous, aggregated data can be published openly for all to see. These compare sizeable geographic areas. They should be published in such a way that no individual could be identified. Pseudoanonymized data contain information on individual patients, but their personal identifiers, such as name and date of birth, are removed, and each patient is instead referred to by a unique code. Such databases do not allow any patient to be directly identified, but they could potentially be linked with other databases to build up a fuller picture of individual patients in a way that could compromise anonymity. For that reason, they are not made publicly available. Pseudoanonymized data are only made available to approved researchers and analysts, under a particular contract for a particular purpose. Finally, personal confidential data are only shared rarely, in circumstances such as a public health emergency, if a patient gives explicit consent or if a research proposal meets very tight criteria and it is impossible to ask patients' consent.

The practicalities of dealing with vast amounts of data are difficult, particularly when they are being made openly available. Most existing systems for collecting, storing and sharing data have not been developed in a coordinated way, but have arisen and evolved separately over time. Many thousands of different spreadsheets circulate around the NHS, for example. Making them more widely available, and of greater value, requires that they are collated, linked, curated and appropriately anonymized.

DISTRIBUTION OF DISEASE IN POPULATIONS

The essence of epidemiology lies in measures that are essentially of two main kinds: (1) those that assess how common or uncommon a disease, risk factor or other variable is, and (2) those that allow comparisons to be made. These measures can be constructed from data that are readily available on the health or demographic characteristics of a population (i.e. the kind of routine data sources described in the previous section) or from planned studies where new data are collected to answer specific questions.

Counting events in populations

The starting point to a population perspective on health and disease (which is what distinguishes epidemiology from clinical medicine) is the ability to identify and express, in a simple statistic, health-related events that occur in populations. An *event* in this context can be many things, for example, a case of disease, a death, a birth, a risk factor, an unhealthy behaviour or an admission to hospital. The use of these terms is not intended to depersonalize. Events happen to people and people make up populations, but in studying groups of people, it is necessary to aggregate all the individual experiences of health and disease.

Constructing statistical measures to describe these events in populations is the basic building block in understanding the health of a population. To simply state the number of events (e.g. cases or deaths) is seldom enough. That number needs to be related to the size of the population in which the events occurred. This brings in the need for a *numerator* (number of events) and a *denominator* (the size of the group of people in which the events occurred). A statement of absolute numbers, such as '100 deaths from coronary heart disease occurred last year in District A compared with 700 in District B', may be of value to the local undertakers in helping to assess their likely workload, but it does not establish whether mortality from coronary heart disease is a greater health problem among the inhabitants of District A or District B, nor does it enable the study of trends or the evaluation of prevention programmes. A denominator is needed because the relative sizes of the two populations must be taken into account.

The measures used in epidemiology are calculated differently, and the differences relate to what quantity is used as the numerator and what quantity is used as the denominator.

A *proportion* is a fraction in which the numerator is a subgroup of the denominator. For example, the number of deaths from prostate cancer (numerator) divided by the total number of deaths from all cancer causes in the population (denominator) is a proportion: the proportion of all deaths from cancer that are due to prostate cancer.

A *ratio* uses data in which the numerator is not part of the denominator. This distinguishes it from a proportion. The number of deaths from prostate cancer in high-income groups in a country (numerator) divided by the number of deaths in low-income groups (denominator) is a ratio since the figures in the numerator do not also appear in the denominator.

A *rate* consists of three components: the numerator, for example, the number of people in the population who

have died; the denominator, for example, the total number of people in the population; and the time period (in this case, during which deaths took place). A rate allows a comparison between different populations, between different subgroups within the same population and between different time periods for one population. These terms are not used consistently in everyday epidemiology and public health practice. This can be confusing. For example, metrics that are quite clearly ratios with no inclusion of a time factor are often referred to as 'rates'. The person who pedantically interrupts a colleague's presentation on a disease problem to point out that the term *rate* is being misapplied is not likely to be popular. In practice, provided that the construction of such indices is understood by everyone, it is better to accept the reality that only a subset of how epidemiological terms are used would satisfy the purist; other usage employs terms flexibly, but their meaning is still clear, while still other usage is potentially misleading.

Measures of morbidity

Incidence and prevalence are the two main statistics traditionally used in epidemiology to answer the question 'How common is this disease?' (Table 2.2).

INCIDENCE

Incidence is the occurrence of new cases of a disease arising in a population at risk. Incidence can be stated in two main ways – as an incidence rate or as a cumulative incidence. Incidence rate is typically stated as x cases per 100,000 people per year. It is the rate at which new cases occur. Cumulative incidence counts the cases that arise during a specified time period. If in a population of 100,000 women, over five years, 100 develop breast cancer, the five-year cumulative incidence of the disease would be 100 per 100,000 women. This could also be stated as an incidence rate, which would be 20 cases per 100,000 women per year.

Because cumulative incidence refers to the cases that occur over a whole time period, time does not form part of the equation to calculate it. Incidence rate, by contrast, refers to the cases that occur per year (or other unit of time). Time is therefore included in the equation to calculate it. This explains why the denominator for cumulative incidence is

Table 2.2 Measures of morbidity

Cumulative incidence	$= \dfrac{\text{Number of new cases of disease during a time period}}{\text{Number of individuals at-risk during the time period}}$
Incidence rate	$= \dfrac{\text{Number of new cases of disease during a time period}}{\text{Number of individuals at-risk} \times \text{length of time period}}$
Point prevalence	$= \dfrac{\text{Number of individuals with disease at a point in time}}{\text{Total population}}$
Period prevalence	$= \dfrac{\text{Number of individuals with disease during a time period}}{\text{Total population (at mid-point of time period)}}$

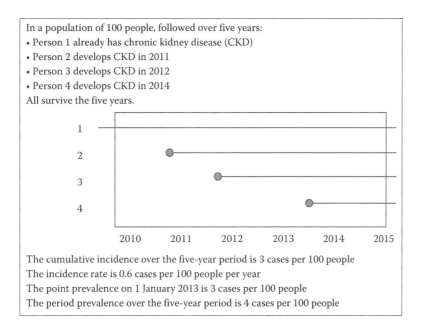

In a population of 100 people, followed over five years:
- Person 1 already has chronic kidney disease (CKD)
- Person 2 develops CKD in 2011
- Person 3 develops CKD in 2012
- Person 4 develops CKD in 2014

All survive the five years.

The cumulative incidence over the five-year period is 3 cases per 100 people
The incidence rate is 0.6 cases per 100 people per year
The point prevalence on 1 January 2013 is 3 cases per 100 people
The period prevalence over the five-year period is 4 cases per 100 people

Figure 2.4 Illustrative example of incidence and prevalence measures.

the number of individuals at risk, while for incidence rate, it is the number of individuals at risk multiplied by the length of time each individual is at risk (i.e. person-years at risk).

PREVALENCE

This measures *all* cases of the disease (both recent and long-standing) either at a point in time (point prevalence) or over a period of time (period prevalence). Point prevalence is best used for a disease whose clinical features are relatively stable, for example, diabetes. Period prevalence is a better measure when they fluctuate, for example, arthritis. Point prevalence is often described as a snapshot of the population. Whereas incidence counts new cases, prevalence includes people within the whole spectrum of that disease, from those who have newly developed the disease to those in its late stages. Prevalence depends on two factors: a disease's incidence and its duration from onset to its conclusion (either recovery or death).

Many non-communicable diseases are not immediately fatal; indeed, people survive for years or decades. In such circumstances, the number of cases is added to each year as new people develop the disease, and reduced by people dying. Today, with treatments ever improving and people living longer, the pool of prevalent cases is expanding, creating a substantial burden of care for health services.

Even diseases that are uncommon (i.e. have a low incidence) may still be important health problems if people with the disease are kept alive for a long time (producing a high prevalence). End-stage renal failure illustrates the difference between incidence and prevalence very well. New cases are not common, but because dialysis and transplantation can keep sufferers alive for many years, the prevalence of the disease is high and can easily outstrip available local resources.

Figure 2.4 provides an illustrative example of the main two incidence and two prevalence measures. The only rate among the four measures is the incidence rate. It includes time within its equation.

Measures of mortality

The simplest mortality measure is the crude death rate. It takes the number of deaths in a period, usually a year, and expresses that number per 1000 population at risk of dying. The crude death rate has the advantage of simplicity. Its disadvantage is that it does not make any correction for the age and sex structure of the population. A new town, for example, is likely to have a lower crude death rate than a seaside retirement resort. This is simply because the former has a younger population. Invariably, it is essential to use measures of mortality that allow comparisons of mortality between populations, free of the effects of differences in age structures.

SPECIFIC MORTALITY RATES

The need to look beyond crude death rates leads to the use of *specific mortality rates*. A specific mortality rate is restricted to a particular subgroup of the population, for example, people in an age range. The specific mortality rate is arrived at by dividing the number of deaths in that subgroup by the number of people in it. The annual age-specific mortality rate for males aged 15–24 years would be expressed as number of deaths in the year among men aged 15–24 years divided by the number of men of that age in the population. Multiplied by 1000, this gives the rate per 1000. A specific mortality rate can be constructed for any subgroup of the population (provided that data are available); commonly used subgroups are age, sex, occupation, socio-economic status and ethnicity.

Specific mortality rates can be calculated for all causes of death (as in the previous example) or for individual causes of death (e.g. mortality rate for acute leukaemia in 15- to 19-year-old males). Many health problems are more frequent at some ages than others, and the age structure of populations can be very different, so crude death rates are of little value in comparing population mortality experience. In contrast, studying age- and sex-specific mortality rate differences in a particular disease between (say) countries, regions or towns can be very valuable.

Specific mortality rates have one major drawback compared with crude death rates. It is very cumbersome to compare, say, 20 different age- and sex-specific death rates for 10 different areas. By contrast, crude death rates describe a population's mortality in a single figure.

STANDARDIZED MORTALITY RATES

The requirement for a statistic that makes comparison easier, but still allows features of the population (e.g. age structure) to be taken into account, leads to the concept of *standardization*. In age standardization, a single mortality rate is calculated in which allowance has been made for the age (and usually also sex) structure of the population in question.

There are two methods of standardization: indirect and direct. Both involve choosing a standard population (e.g. the population of England in 2016 or the European standard population), which is broken down into specific age (and usually sex) groups.

In *indirect standardization*, the mortality rates of each age group of the standard population (e.g. females aged 15–24 years in England and Wales) are applied to the population of the same age groups in the study area. This shows how many females aged 15–24 years in the study area would have died if the standard population's death rate had prevailed. After the calculation has been performed for all age groups, the resulting total number of deaths is added up. These deaths did not actually occur, but are those that *would* have occurred if the study population had experienced the same mortality as the standard population, and hence they are referred to as *expected deaths*.

The expected number of deaths can then be compared with the number of deaths that *did* actually occur – the *observed deaths*. The most commonly used statistic derived from the process of standardization is the *standardized mortality ratio*. This is the ratio of observed deaths to expected deaths and is usually expressed as a percentage. By definition, the standard population has an SMR of 100% (i.e. observed and expected deaths are the same). SMRs over 100 (the percent sign is usually not used) represent unfavourable mortality experience, and SMRs below 100 show relatively favourable mortality experience, the effect of differences in the age and sex profile of each population having been taken into account.

Table 2.3 illustrates the process of calculating the SMR for deaths in females aged 15–64 years in one part of the country, compared with the standard female population of England and Wales. The SMR of 106 for the area in question indicates that the mortality rate was 6% higher than if the specific rates for the England and Wales population had been observed in the area.

In indirect standardization, the mortality rates occurring in the standard population are applied to the study population. In *direct standardization*, the reverse process is used (Table 2.4). The age-specific mortality rates of the study population are applied in turn to the numbers in each corresponding age group of the standard population to give the number of deaths that would have occurred in the standard population if the death rates in each study population had been applied. This number of deaths is then divided by the total standard population to give an age-standardized death rate for the population.

In these examples, standardization has been used to examine mortality in different areas. The process can be applied to any subgroup of the population for which suitable data are available – for example, social deprivation level or occupational group. Although most commonly used to take account of age and sex, standardization can also be used to adjust for differences in other characteristics. For example, perinatal mortality rates may be standardized for birthweight.

The essence of standardization is that it holds constant, and therefore eliminates, the effect of the characteristic being standardized (e.g. age or sex) so that the effect of other factors can be examined. Once a factor has been used in standardization, it cannot be used to explain variation between rates. Figure 2.5 shows variation in standardized mortality rates for prostate cancer between different populations. The pattern of variation cannot be explained by different places having different age structures, since age has been standardized. The significant variation seen is likely due to genetic differences; differences in the prevalence of risk factors such as physical inactivity, diet and obesity; and the accessibility and quality of healthcare services to diagnose and treat prostate cancer effectively.

CASE FATALITY AND SURVIVAL

The *case fatality rate* is the proportion of people who, having developed a disease, die from it. In practice, it is used in different ways according to the disease being studied. In severe communicable diseases with an acute onset, the outcome can be survival or death. The case fatality rate is then a clear marker of the severity of the disease, and information made public about it can be dramatic and alarming. Case fatality rates for Ebola fever when it emerged in West Africa were 66% among healthcare workers and 70% in non-healthcare workers. These may not be the true figures because data were incomplete in the affected countries, but the visibly high proportion of deaths among people who fell ill struck fear into local communities. Case fatality rates in most communicable disease outbreaks need to be interpreted with caution. Much depends on the accuracy of the denominator. If there are many mild and subclinical cases that are not known about and counted, then the numbers

Table 2.3 Indirect standardization: worked example of the calculation of a standardized mortality ratio (SMR)

The aim is to compare the mortality experience of women (aged 15–64 years) in one part of the country (the study population) with that of all women of the same age group in England and Wales (the standard population)	
Age-specific death rates for all females in England and Wales (standard population)	
	Deaths per 100,000 population
15–24 years	29.7
25–34 years	44.2
35–44 years	110.7
45–54 years	290.2
55–64 years	855.4
Population of females in the study population	
	Population
15–24 years	70,100
25–34 years	72,000
35–44 years	65,000
45–54 years	57,200
55–64 years	59,400
'Expected' number of deaths of females living in the study population if their experience was the same as all females in England and Wales	
	'Expected' deaths
15–24 years	$29.7 \times (70,000 / 100,000) = 21$
25–34 years	$44.2 \times (72,000 / 100,000) = 32$
35–44 years	$110.7 \times (65,000 / 100,000) = 72$
45–54 years	$290.2 \times (57,200 / 100,000) = 166$
55–64 years	$855.4 \times (59,400 / 100,000) = 508$
Total 'expected' deaths	799
'Observed' (actual) deaths of study population females aged 15–64 years	849
SMR (as a percentage) (England and Wales = 100)	

$$SMR = \frac{observed\ deaths}{expected\ deaths} \times 100$$

$$= \frac{849}{799} \times 100$$

$$= 106$$

of cases in the denominator will be too small and the case fatality rate will be inflated.

In non-communicable diseases, with acute onset, the case fatality rate can also be useful in understanding the course of the disease. Examining the proportion of suicidal actions that result in death will show differences between the sexes, age groups and methods chosen, and will help in planning preventive strategies and mental health service responses.

In non-communicable diseases with a longer course, the relationship between survival rates and time is key (Figure 2.6). In diseases like cancer and conditions such as heart failure, it is important to calculate the proportion still alive at different points after diagnosis. This can serve multiple purposes from comparing the performance of services,

to seeking and testing improved treatments, to motivating people at risk to change their behaviour.

As described earlier in this chapter, epidemiological terms are not always accurately used. The case fatality rate is an example of this. It is actually a proportion, not a rate, since it does not include a time dimension.

Measures of healthy and unhealthy ageing

A few decades ago, mortality and morbidity rates sufficed as measures of the ill health in a population. With the increasing importance of non-communicable diseases, with which people live in a state of incapacity for many years, more

Table 2.4 Direct standardization: worked example of the calculation of a standardized death rate

The aim is to produce an age-standardized death rate for females (aged 15–64 years) in one part of the country (the study population) standardized to the England and Wales population.	
Age-specific death rates for females in study population	
	Deaths per 100,000 population
15–24 years	25.7
25–34 years	36.1
35–44 years	103.1
45–54 years	304.2
55–64 years	949.5
Population of females in England and Wales (standard population)	
	Population
15–24 years	3,631,600
25–34 years	3,852,300
35–44 years	3,500,400
45–54 years	2,873,200
55–64 years	2,631,500
Total population	16,489,000
'Expected' number of deaths of England and Wales females if their experience was the same as females in the study population	
	'Expected' deaths
15–24 years	$25.7 \times (36,316,000 / 100,000) = 933$
25–34 years	$36.1 \times (3,852,300 / 100,000) = 1391$
35–44 years	$103.1 \times (3,500,400 / 100,000) = 3609$
45–54 years	$304.2 \times (2,873,200 / 100,000) = 8740$
55–64 years	$949.5 \times (2,631,500 / 100,000) = 24,986$
Total expected deaths	39,659
Age standardized death rate of the study population	

Deaths per 100,000 population

$$= \frac{\text{expected deaths}}{\text{standard population}} \times 100,000$$

$$= \frac{39,659}{16,489,000} \times 100,000$$

$$= 241 \text{ per } 100,000$$

sophisticated measures have been developed and paint a richer picture of a population's health. Some of the most commonly used indices are described in this section.

HEALTHY LIFE EXPECTANCY AND DISABILITY-FREE LIFE EXPECTANCY

Whereas *life expectancy* describes the number of years that an individual can expect to live, *healthy life expectancy* describes the number of these years that an individual can expect to live in good health, and *disability-free life expectancy* the number that an individual can expect to live without disability. Measuring healthy life expectancy requires 'good health' to be defined, and this definition varies

somewhat between jurisdictions. It is often self-reported. The measure allows a number of questions to be answered: Are those who live an exceptionally long life burdened with disease and disability? Does longer life necessarily lead to a prolonged period of dependency? Is disability more prevalent in women than in men? What are the trends in poor health and disabilities in developed versus developing countries with population ageing? Understanding these processes is essential for planning of healthcare and social care.

YEARS LIVED WITH DISABILITY

This measure is not simply a count of the number of years lived with disability, but incorporates a weighting

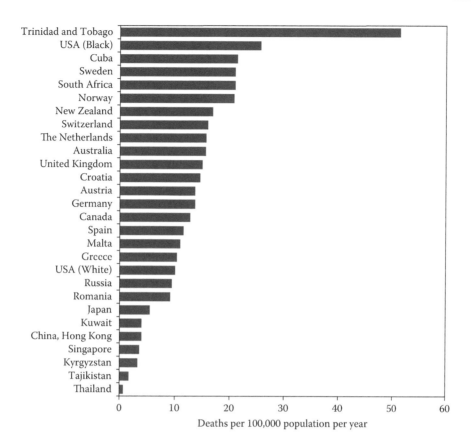

Figure 2.5 Prostate cancer mortality rate by country.

Source: Jemal A, Center MM, DeSantis C, Ward EM. Global patterns of cancer incidence and mortality rates and trends. *Cancer Epidemiology and Prevention Biomarkers* 2010;19(8):1893–907.

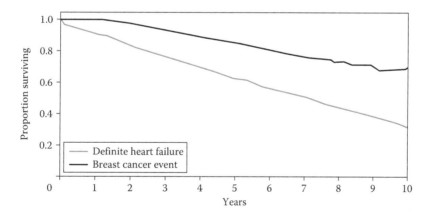

Figure 2.6 Survival curves for breast cancer and heart failure.

Source: Copson E, Eccles B, Maishman T, et al. Prospective observational study of breast cancer treatment outcomes for UK women aged 18–40 years at diagnosis: the POSH study. *Journal of the National Cancer Institute* 2013;105(13):978–88; Taylor CJ, Roalfe AK, Iles R, Hobbs FD. Ten-year prognosis of heart failure in the community: follow-up data from the Echocardiographic Heart of England Screening (ECHOES) study. *European Journal of Heart Failure* 2012;14(2):176–84.

to take account of how severe that disability is. The four biggest causes of disability in the world are sensory impairments (visual impairment and hearing loss), osteoarthritis, ischaemic heart disease and dementia. In low- and middle-income countries, visual impairments due to cataract, refractive errors and neglected tropical diseases are major causes of moderate to severe disability, as well as years of life lost due to disability. On the other hand, in high-income countries dementia has a higher impact.

DISABILITY-ADJUSTED LIFE YEARS

The disability-adjusted life year (DALY) measures the combined effect of premature death (years of life lost) and disability. One DALY represents one year lost of healthy (active) life. The greatest number of years lost within this index in later life is due to ischaemic heart disease, visual impairment, dementia, cancer and stroke. The majority of causes of healthy life years lost globally are non-communicable diseases.

Some variations in disease burden observed across countries and regions of the world are methodological (e.g. definitions of disability and disease diagnosis). Others are due to differences in behaviours, metabolic risk factors (e.g. smoking and hypertension), environmental conditions and access to healthcare.

Making comparisons: Describing population patterns of health and disease

Having assembled the necessary information to examine a given indicator of disease – such as mortality under the age of 65 years from coronary heart disease, or the incidence rate of fractured neck of femur – further questions inevitably arise: How does the population under study compare with other populations? How does the occurrence of the problem in the population currently compare with earlier time periods? Are different subgroups within the population affected by the health problem to a greater or lesser degree?

Descriptive epidemiology traditionally examines disease patterns across three main dimensions: in relation to time, in relation to place and in relation to person.

The occurrence of disease varies with *time*. Changes can occur over a short period of time, such as when a new communicable disease emerges. Changes can occur over a long period of time. And there are changes of a cyclical nature, classically seen when the occurrence of disease varies with the season – influenza or hay fever, for example.

Changes over the long term are known as *secular trends*. Studying the pattern of diseases over long periods of time (years, decades or even centuries) highlights many changes. Major diseases of the past have faded from importance, while others have become increasingly prominent. There are many pitfalls in interpreting secular trends in the incidence or prevalence of a disease. Its true frequency may not have changed over time, but improvements in methods of detection and diagnosis, fashions in diagnosis and changes in the criteria used to define or classify it may suggest that it has. Prevalence can also change without a change in age-specific incidence, if a population ages.

Figure 2.7 shows how a disease appears to be becoming more common when this is not in fact the case. In Sweden, registered cases of autistic spectrum disorder arising from routine clinical diagnosis steadily increased over the course of a decade. But the prevalence of autism as measured by strict diagnostic criteria hardly changed over the same period.

There has been a spectacular secular change in the pattern of disease in high-income countries over recent decades, as communicable diseases have declined as major health problems and causes of death.

Examining time trends in health service usage can also provide important insights. In the 1960s, there was no major intervention for someone who had a heart attack. Their pain could be relieved and bed rest, usually in hospital, was the preferred treatment. It was a question of waiting to see who would die and who would survive. By the 1980s, an option became possible for revascularization of obstructed

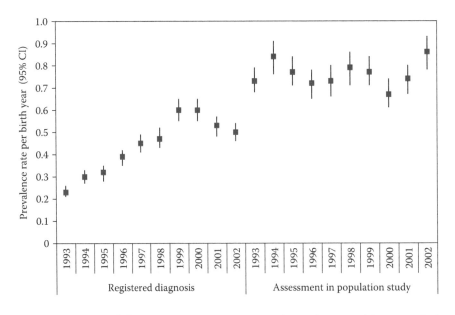

Figure 2.7 Autism prevalence: registered diagnoses versus assessment (as autism score) in a population study.

Source: Lundström S, Reichenberg A, Anckarsäter H, Lichtenstein P, Gillberg C. Autism phenotype versus registered diagnosis in Swedish children: prevalence trends over 10 years in general population samples. *BMJ* 2015;350:h1961. With permission.

coronary arteries through a coronary artery bypass graft, a surgical operation in which blood vessels taken from other parts of the body are used to bypass diseased coronary segments. This was not usually undertaken after a heart attack but for people who had advanced coronary disease. In the United Kingdom, through the late 1980s and early 1990s, this operation was not available to everyone who would have benefitted from it, with access varying around the country. An alternative to this major surgery emerged with the advent of angioplasty – a procedure in which a balloon is inflated within the vessel so as to widen it. With stents (cylindrical meshes to hold open a vessel once it has been widened), angioplasty became a true alternative to bypass surgery in many (but not all) cases of coronary artery disease. The treatment of heart attacks also changed from the late 1990s into the first decades of the twenty-first century, first with the use of thrombolysis so that myocardial damage could be limited. The therapeutic approach then changed again so that for most patients experiencing a heart attack, the treatment of choice became immediate, or primary, angioplasty. The switch from one therapeutic approach to another happened over a relatively short period of time (Figure 2.8), although there are still problems of access for patients in some parts of the United Kingdom.

So, describing these health events over time yields an understanding of the disease and how the health service has responded to it. The data tell a number of stories. There is a story of rapid advances in beneficial medical technology. There is a story of improved patient outcome. There is a story of falling death rates from coronary heart disease.

Many diseases have another relationship with time – they show *seasonal variations* in their occurrence, with peaks in the frequency of these diseases at particular times of the year. Respiratory infections, for example, are more common in the colder months.

Several studies have shown apparent seasonal variation in the onset of insulin-dependent diabetes mellitus in children, with peak occurrence in the autumn and winter. This has led to the idea that this disease may be caused or precipitated in genetically susceptible individuals by an infectious agent, possibly a virus. Such findings must be interpreted cautiously because they raise questions about the extent of detection of cases and the way in which the onset of the disease is determined. Even if such a seasonal pattern is established, it is not proof of a causal link. However, it is an example of how examination of the pattern of disease can provide a clue that may prompt further investigation of the relationship between genetic and environmental factors, which in turn may lead to a greater understanding of the causal mechanism.

Finally, changes in the frequency of disease can sometimes be seen over a short period of time. This is commonly the case, for example, in outbreaks of communicable disease. Epidemic curves are used to plot such changes, and are very useful in providing clues about the disease and its spread.

Description of the pattern of disease by *place*, that is, in geographical terms, can be undertaken in a number of ways. Many diseases vary in incidence between countries (Figure 2.9). Difficulties arise in comparing the incidence of disease between countries. This is because countries can use different definitions for the same disease (although the existence of an International Classification of Diseases – see earlier – helps to minimize this effect); whether affected individuals become known depends to some extent on the country's healthcare system; and countries have different systems for recording the incidence of disease (some of which have considerable limitations).

In the United Kingdom, as in many other countries, there is variation in both disease and the determinants

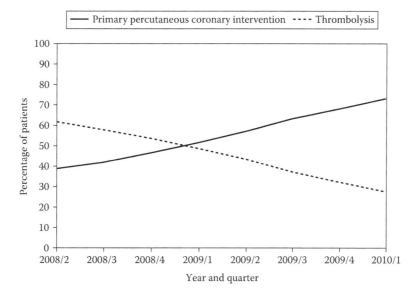

Figure 2.8 Treatment for patients with ST segment elevation myocardial infarction, England.

Source: NHS England. With permission.

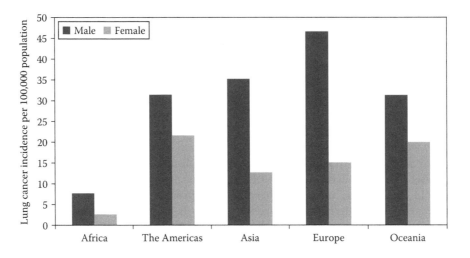

Figure 2.9 Incidence of lung cancer by world region.

Source: Ferlay J, Soerjomataram I, Dikshit R, et al. Cancer incidence and mortality worldwide: sources, methods and major patterns in GLOBOCAN 2012. *International Journal of Cancer* 2015;136(5):E359-86.

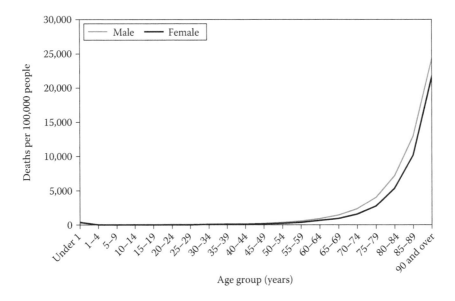

Figure 2.10 Mortality rates in England and Wales, 2015.

Source: Office for National Statistics.

of disease between areas of the country. This is classically described as the 'north–south divide'; general mortality within Britain is lower for the population of southern and eastern England and higher for northern England, Wales and Scotland. While true, this is a generalization. There are parts of the north in which health is better than parts of the south, and health can vary at a much smaller level – for example, between London boroughs or wards.

There are many ways of examining the pattern of disease by *person*. Variation by age and sex is the most commonly described. Almost all diseases show a marked variation with age. Indeed, mortality rates from all causes show a distinctive pattern (Figure 2.10). Once the first few years of life have been passed, there are relatively few deaths per unit of population

until the age of about 35 years, when death rates begin to increase sharply with each successively higher age group.

There are differences, too, in the importance of various causes of death at each age. Figure 2.11 shows that in the younger age groups, accidents and violence are a more important cause of death than diseases, while in the older age group, cancer and diseases of the respiratory and circulatory systems come to the fore.

Figure 2.12 shows that within the disease category, there can be marked age and sex patterns. In a study of fracture incidence, the risk increased rapidly with age among males until age 15–24 years, after which it declined until there was a second peak at 85 years and older. This reflects a higher participation in sports, other activities and violence among

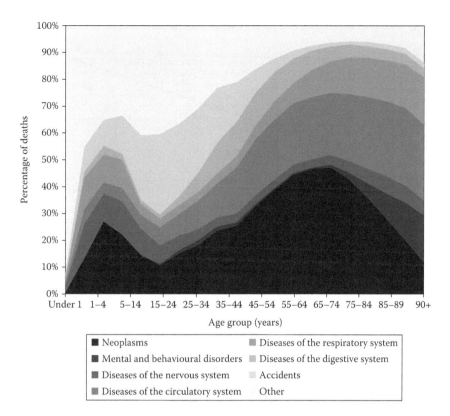

Figure 2.11 Selected causes of death by age, England and Wales, 2015.

Source: Office for National Statistics.

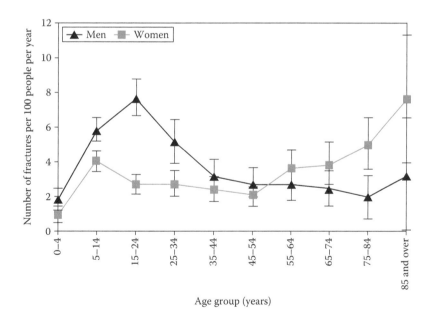

Figure 2.12 Annual fracture incidence by age and sex, England, 2002–04.

Source: Donaldson LJ, Reckless IP, Scholes S, Mindell JS, Shelton NJ. The epidemiology of fractures in England. *Journal of Epidemiology and Community Health* 2008; 62(2):174-80. With permission.

boys, teenagers and young adult males than among their female counterparts. For girls and women, there is a peak in early childhood but no early adult peak, and there is a sustained earlier rise in incidence from 55 years onwards. As with any descriptive epidemiological data, these interesting age and sex differences do not provide direct evidence of causal association, but they do point the way for further epidemiological studies aimed at elucidating causation and possibly provide scope for prevention of an important public health problem.

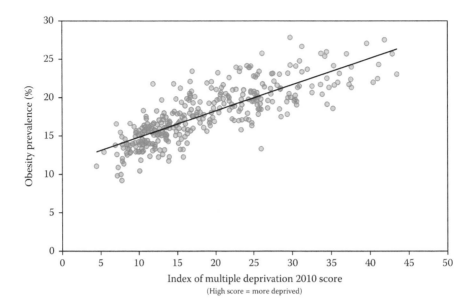

Figure 2.13 Obesity prevalence in children aged 10 years by deprivation of local authority area, England, 2015.

Source: Public Health England.

It is also common to see variation between ethnic groups and populations living in varying degrees of deprivation. Figure 2.13 shows the striking relationship between childhood obesity and deprivation; this analysis explores a *person* measure against a *place* measure.

Pitfalls in interpreting health and disease patterns

Before drawing conclusions about any variation in the pattern of health and disease in different geographical areas, between subgroups of the population or over time, it is essential to be sure that the differences are real and not due to aspects of the data. It is important to pose three main questions.

WHAT ARE THE CRITERIA FOR DEFINING THE DISEASE?

There are variations in medical practice (between different time periods, different places and even individual doctors on different occasions) that influence the way in which a particular diagnostic label is applied to a particular condition.

Table 2.5 shows the results of an analysis of two samples of patients in psychiatric hospitals in London and New York. There appeared to be a much higher percentage of people with schizophrenia and alcohol dependency in the New York sample than in the London sample. In contrast, patients with depression and mania were much more common in the London sample. If such differences were real, then valuable clues to the causes of certain psychiatric illnesses might have been available. An investigation was therefore carried out, to examine these findings more closely.

Table 2.5 The hospital diagnoses of the London and New York samples

	New York percentage (n = 192)	London percentage (n = 174)
Schizophrenia	61.5	33.9**
Depressive psychoses	4.7	24.1**
Mania	50.0	6.9**
Depressive neuroses	1.6	8.0**
Other neuroses	2.6	6
Personality disorders	1.0	4.6*
Alcoholic disorders	19.8	3.4**
Drug dependence	0.0	0.6
Organic psychoses	5.2	1.7
Other diagnoses	3.1	10.9**

Source: Cooper JE. *Psychiatric Diagnosis in New York and London: A Comparative Study of Mental Hospital Admissions.* Oxford: Oxford University Press, 1972.
*Difference significant at 5% level; **Difference significant at 1% level.

Using a standardized interviewing technique, each patient in the sample was examined by a member of a team of project psychiatrists as soon as possible after admission and independently of the hospital staff. Table 2.6 shows the results of comparing the original hospital diagnoses with the subsequent project diagnoses in the two samples. Once alcoholics and drug addicts had been excluded, the comparison of the two sets of project diagnoses showed no significant difference for schizophrenia, personality disorders, neurosis (other than depressive) and organic psychosis.

Table 2.6 The diagnoses of the London and New York samples after the exclusion of alcoholics and drug addicts

	New York percentage	London percentage
Schizophrenia	39.4	37.0
Depressive psychoses	26.8	24.2
Mania	7.7	6.7
Depressive neuroses	9.2	15.2
Other neuroses	2.1	4.2
Personality disorders	5.6	3.6
Organic psychoses	3.5	3.6
Other diagnoses	5.6	5.5

Source: Cooper JE. *Psychiatric Diagnosis in New York and London: A Comparative Study of Mental Hospital Admissions.* Oxford: Oxford University Press, 1972.

This suggests that the original differences – in the hospital diagnoses – between the two centres were largely the result of variation in the diagnostic criteria used by the psychiatrists at the time.

The report concluded that the most important of these differences was that the New York concept of schizophrenia, at that time, was much broader than that used in London, and it included cases that many British psychiatrists would have called depressive illnesses, neurotic illnesses or personality disorders (Figure 2.14).

This study illustrates a principle that can be a pitfall for any comparison of disease frequency. Variation among doctors in the choice of labels for particular clinical problems or causes of death is quite commonplace, as with the example of autistic spectrum disorder in Sweden shown earlier.

While it may not be of paramount importance as far as the individual doctor and patient are concerned, it becomes central when data are aggregated for the purpose of producing a population count of the number of cases of a disease or the number of deaths from a particular cause. It is important to establish the diagnostic criteria that have been used to count cases of the disease when comparisons are made between different populations or when a disease trend over time is observed. Otherwise, spurious conclusions about apparently major differences may be made (just as in the mental health example described above). This potential problem is applicable to all diseases, no matter how objectively the diagnosis is made.

HAVE ALL CASES OF THE DISEASE BEEN IDENTIFIED?

False conclusions about the amount of disease in one population compared with another may be drawn if the efficiency of case detection is not known. For example, the observation that a particular cancer is more common in a high-income country than in a low-income country may lead to speculation about risk factors in the two countries. Such a line of thought would be unwise without first examining the efficiency of the two cancer registration systems. The apparently higher occurrence of the cancer in the high-income country may simply reflect the fact that it has an efficient, well-maintained cancer registry that detects and records most cases of cancer that occur. The cancer registry of a low-income country, perhaps covering a rural population that does not readily have access to medical services, may not be so efficient at detecting cases of the cancer. This does not necessarily mean that they are not occurring as often as in the high-income country, but merely that they are not being recorded.

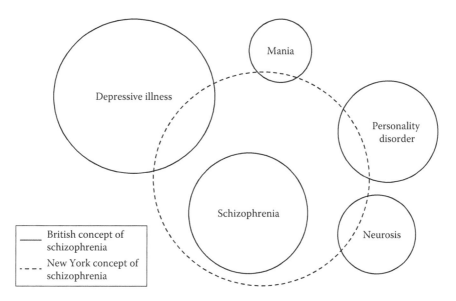

Figure 2.14 The difference between the New York and British concepts of schizophrenia.

Source: Cooper JE. *Psychiatric Diagnosis in New York and London: A Comparative Study of Mental Hospital Admissions.* Oxford: Oxford University Press, 1972.

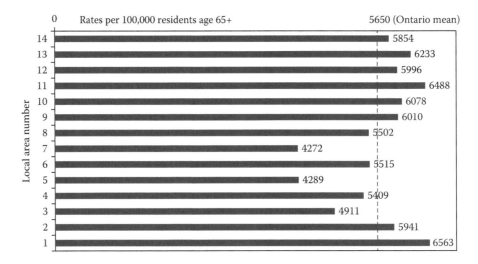

Figure 2.15 Age- and sex-adjusted rates of cataract surgery per 100,000 residents aged 65 and older in Ontario by local area.

Source: Hatch WV, Cernat G, Singer S, Bell CM. A 10-year population-based cohort analysis of cataract surgery rates in Ontario. *Canadian Journal of Ophthalmology* 2007;42(4):552-6. With permission.

This is a rather obvious example to illustrate the importance of being aware of possible differences in disease detection rates when making comparisons. This pitfall can be encountered when comparing disease frequency from region to region, city to city and hospital to hospital, not just between two countries with contrasting levels of healthcare resources.

An example is the analysis depicted in Figure 2.15. This shows the rate of cataract surgery in different parts of Ontario, Canada. Thus, it is describing the treatment of patients who have a disease of the eye causing impaired vision. The figure shows marked geographical variation between services in the different localities of Ontario: the service with the highest rate (area 1) performed surgery 50% more often than the service with the lowest rate (area 7). The incidence of cataract is strongly age related, so the data in Figure 2.15 have been age and sex standardized. The error in interpreting this variation would be to assume that these data show a variation in the occurrence of cataract between different parts of Ontario. They do not – they simply show variation in operation rates, which may or may not be a proxy for disease incidence. The variation may exist for any number of reasons (Table 2.7). There may indeed be genuine geographical variation in the incidence of cataracts, but a study based on surgical treatment rates is not the way to establish it.

IS THE POPULATION AT RISK ACCURATELY DEFINED?

It is important to be sure that all cases of a disease (or all deaths) under study are related to a defined population, for which accurate estimates of size and structure are available. Mistakes in doing this are often seen when hospital data are involved, because people do not necessarily receive hospital

Table 2.7 Possible reasons for variations in surgical operation rates between populations

Demographic difference
Different rates of underlying illness
Random fluctuation
Availability of resources or supply
Clinical judgment varies
Different patient expectation of demand
Prevailing clinical traditions vary
Inaccuracies in data sources

Source: McPherson K. *The Challenges of Medical Practice Variations.* London: Pallgrave Macmillan, 1990.

treatment in the area in which they live. If hospital data are used to identity deaths from a particular cause, those deaths need to be ascribed to the place where the patient lived, rather than the place where the hospital is. Otherwise, the population in areas such as London with a high concentration of hospitals, or with particular specialist facilities, will appear to have higher rates of mortality from particular diseases than is actually the case.

MAKING COMPARISONS BETWEEN GROUPS THROUGH PLANNED STUDIES

Many epidemiological studies have one of two main purposes. The first is to establish the causes or risks of developing a particular disease. The second is to test the ability of particular activities or technologies to stop diseases from developing or to slow their progression. The overall goal of both is to generate the evidence and knowledge to make disease more amenable to prevention or treatment, or to promote health.

In this field of epidemiology, the studies carried out are based on making comparisons between groups who are exposed or not exposed to risk factors (or beneficial interventions) and those who are affected or not affected by particular diseases or other health outcomes.

An ideal study to compare the disease experience of two groups for purposes of drawing conclusions about whether specific exposures increase the risk of the particular disease can be imagined as follows: One group of people goes through two parallel existences simultaneously. In one existence, they remain unexposed to the risk under investigation. In the other, they are exposed. All other conditions in the two universes are identical. The outcomes of the two experiences could then be compared, in the certain knowledge that any differences were due only to the exposure, because the people and everything else would have remained the same. In real life, parallel universes cannot be invoked. However, it is useful to keep this thought experiment in mind when carrying out epidemiological work involving group comparison. This concept is called the *counterfactual ideal*. All real-life comparisons fall short of the ideal. Understanding how and why they fall short is the essence of both good study design and meticulous interpretation of findings.

One of the principal reasons for the existence of the epidemiological study methods described in the sections that follow, and their complexity, is that the investigator of causal relationships in human populations is denied the experimental approach. If a laboratory scientist wishes to investigate whether a suspected cause results in a particular outcome or effect, he frequently does have the experimental approach at his disposal. Suppose, for example, that a particular chemical is suspected of causing breast cancer in white mice. The investigator could take a strain of white mice and allocate them at random into two groups. One group would receive the presumed causal chemical, and the other group would not receive the chemical, but otherwise be treated identically. The investigator would then observe the occurrence of breast cancer in the two groups of animals and draw conclusions. In the laboratory experiment, the investigator is in control of the events and, as a result, has an extremely powerful and direct method at his disposal.

Similar experiments to test the effect of a suspected causal factor in groups of humans are usually quite unacceptable. Thus, if the same chemical that caused breast cancer in the white mice was suspected of causing breast cancer in human females, an experiment could not be carried out in which one group of women was given the chemical and the other was not. The most usual experiment carried out in human subjects is the randomized controlled trial (RCT). This is discussed later in this chapter, and can be used to test potentially beneficial interventions.

Sometimes, fortuitously for the investigator but often to the great misfortune of the population concerned, *natural experiments* take place that allow conclusions to be drawn about causation. Examples of this are the observations on the incidence of cancer following the exposure to radiation from the Hiroshima bomb and the Chernobyl nuclear accident, as well as the observation of the incidence of vaginal tumours in the female offspring of women treated during pregnancy with diethylstilboestrol.

Usually, the experimental approach is ruled out for ethical reasons when investigating the effects of causes in human populations. Instead, the search concentrates on associations between the factor, or set of factors, and a disease. This observational approach (to distinguish it from the experimental) involves comparing the disease experience of two or more groups of people in relation to their possession of certain characteristics of exposure to a suspected factor or factors.

Four main types of study design account for the vast majority of published epidemiological research: the cross-sectional study, the cohort study, the case–control study and the randomized controlled trial. Within each, the role of chance, bias and confounding must be thought about before firm conclusions are drawn.

Of the four described designs, the randomized controlled trial stands alone. It is the only study that is actually an experiment and gets closest to the counterfactual ideal described. The researchers usually divide the people who have agreed to participate in the trial into two groups. They take a particular action, say a preventive intervention, in one group, and do not take this action in the other group. They then measure how well the two groups fare, comparing the health outcomes in the intervention group and the control group, and so draw conclusions about how beneficial (or otherwise) the intervention is.

The other three types of study are observational rather than experimental. The researchers do not intervene. They define the groups and observe to see what happens–or, in some cases, what has already happened. Observational studies can answer some questions that experimental studies cannot. What is the health impact of smoking? An observational study can compare those who smoke with those who do not, whereas no reasonable human study could examine the impact of smoking using an experimental design, for example, making half the participants smoke throughout their lives and the other half not. Many major public health studies have been observational rather than experimental.

Example: Epidemiological study leading to successful prevention

Thousands of babies' lives have been saved around the world by a series of studies: an observational (case–control) study of cot death, followed by an intervention to reduce the risk factor, followed by a descriptive epidemiological study to monitor the fall in deaths.

Researchers at the University of Bristol carried out a case–control study during 1989, in the west of England, into *sudden infant death syndrome*. From the first set of analyses, it became clear that a prone (face-down) sleeping position was an important risk factor. Traditionally, putting babies face down in their cots seemed a sensible precaution to avoid choking if the child were to regurgitate milk while asleep. However, time-honoured common sense was now emerging, counterintuitively, as a dangerous thing for parents to do. The preliminary findings were presented that summer to local healthcare professionals (health visitors, general practitioners and midwives) as part of the study protocol.

A follow-up study was planned for the autumn to get more information on how and why prone sleeping appeared to be such a risk. Part of this study was to recruit infants whose parents planned to put them down prone, supine or on the side, and to look at the effects on the developmental physiology of thermoregulation and respiratory control in the three groups.

By October 1989, however, it became clear that very few parents in the area were now putting their babies down prone. The health visitors and midwives had decided to strongly advise them not to do so in the light of the results of the previous study.

The data from Avon then showed a remarkable temporal fall in sudden infant death rates, in line with the reduction in prone sleeping. The results of this study were published in the *British Medical Journal* in February 1992. Because of the importance of the findings, the editor agreed that, ahead of the paper being published, the UK government should be informed of the potentially life-saving effect of reducing prone sleeping among infants.

The lead researcher took part in television programmes, including a high-profile BBC Panorama documentary called *Every Mother's Nightmare*. The involvement of a major television celebrity, Ann Diamond, whose own child had suffered a cot death, meant that the subject attracted massive public interest. A national public information campaign,

Back to Sleep, started almost immediately, and the effect on sudden infant death rates was remarkable (Figure 2.16).

Similar changes have been seen in every country in which there has been a Back to Sleep–type campaign – with an average fall of between 60% and 80% in sudden infant deaths in the years that followed it.

With the fall in the number of sudden infant deaths after the Back to Sleep campaigns, the proportion of deaths associated with babies sharing a sleep surface has increased. The same University of Bristol researchers have reviewed the factors involved in so-called *cosleeping*. It can be a harmless activity, is common and varies between cultures. In some circumstances, it increases the risk of sudden infant death. The evidence points to cigarette smoking and alcohol or drug use by a mother or her partner being important risk factors, as are low birthweight, prematurity and cosleeping on a bed rather than a sofa.

This study shows how a rigorous approach by a research team that maintains its interest in the subject over the long term can yield great benefits.

Cross-sectional studies

OUTLINE OF METHODOLOGY

Cross-sectional or prevalence studies (also known as population surveys) describe the population at a point in time, like a snapshot. They are mainly used to answer descriptive questions about disease prevalence, but can be used to compare risk factors between the groups that make up the study population. In this latter respect, they can be used as a starting point to examine analytical questions about causation. Apparent findings about causation can be misleading, however, and so associations found in cross-sectional studies are more often used to generate hypotheses to then be tested through a more robust study design.

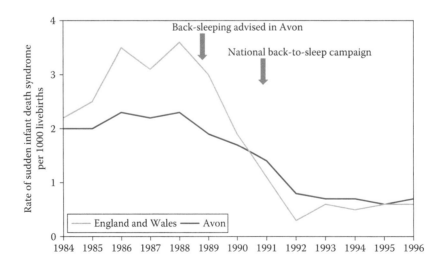

Figure 2.16 Rate of sudden infant death syndrome in Avon versus England and Wales.

Source: Blair PS, Sidebotham P, Berry PJ, Evans M, Fleming PJ. Major epidemiological changes in sudden infant death syndrome: a 20-year population-based study in the UK. *Lancet* 2006;367(9507):314-9. With permission.

Many of the elements in design described here (such as defining outcomes and background information to be measured) are applicable to other study designs and are therefore described in some detail.

The fact that cross-sectional studies describe the population at a point in time can make this study design problematic for answering analytic epidemiological questions. For example, in a cross-sectional study examining the link between diet and irritable bowel syndrome, the information on diet and the medical condition are collected simultaneously. Any sequence of causation is then difficult to disentangle – did those with irritable bowel syndrome change their diet because of bowel symptoms, or were the bowel symptoms brought on by their diet?

In some instances, though, where the order of exposure and outcome are distinguishable or unlikely to be affected by one another, a cross-sectional study can be used to examine causation. For example, a classic study in 1979 examined the neurotoxicity of low-dose lead exposure. Researchers studied a group of six- to eight-year-old students in and around Boston. They measured lead levels in the students' teeth (which indicates cumulative body burden). They asked teachers to rate the students' behaviour, which was also corroborated by neuropsychological testing. The findings were striking: bad behaviour increased in proportion to lead concentration. Since antiquity, it had been known that high doses of lead exposure could cause neurotoxicity. This important study illustrated that much lower, subclinical levels of lead exposure could also impair children's functioning and school performance.

CHOOSING A STUDY POPULATION

The cross-sectional study gathers data on one or more characteristics of individuals in a population at a particular point in time. It will seldom be feasible or necessary to gather such data about every member of the population; usually, a sample is chosen. On the basis of the findings within the sample, general conclusions are drawn about the population as a whole. The process involves gaining access to a representative list of members of the population and then applying the technique of sampling.

SAMPLING

Uppermost in the choice of a sample is the capacity to make true statements about the population itself. The technique of drawing a sample has an important bearing on this. There are two main ways of obtaining a sample of people: (1) by the quota method and (2) randomly.

Quota sampling involves the interviewer seeking a specified number of people to fit into a preagreed sample configuration. Men or women of particular ages or social backgrounds may be sought out, for example, by approaching people in the street. This type of sampling is generally unsatisfactory because it is unlikely to result in a sample that is representative of the whole population. For instance, a sample of middle-aged men drawn by quota sampling in a shopping centre on a Thursday midmorning would be unlikely to be truly representative of all middle-aged men in the particular town. Groups such as the unemployed and shift workers would tend to be overrepresented.

Random sampling is the most commonly used sampling method in survey research. If the sample is random, the results can more easily be generalized to the total population from which the random sample was drawn, and the precision of the estimate derived from the sample can be calculated statistically.

The first step in drawing a random sample is to construct a suitable sampling frame. A sampling frame is merely a list (actual or notional) of the population. The nature of the sampling frame will vary according to the purposes of the survey. A sample for a survey of infant feeding practices might be drawn from all birth registrations in a particular area. In a survey of occupational diseases, the sampling frame might be the employment records in particular companies.

Many population surveys in public health aim to conduct an investigation in a sample of the population of a geographically defined area, say within a local government boundary. In obtaining a suitable sampling frame (i.e. a list of the residents of that authority) from which to draw a suitably sized sample, a traditional approach is to use the electoral roll – a list of people qualified to vote listed by the street within the different electoral wards of a town or city. As a sampling frame representative of the general population, however, this has limitations. The most obvious is that people below voting age are excluded. In addition, the rolls often become out of date as people move into or out of the area.

Having obtained a suitable sampling frame, there are a number of different approaches to obtaining the random sample. The most direct is to choose people at random from the sampling frame until the required sample size is achieved. This is termed a *simple random sample*.

A simple 10% random sample of a population of 1000 people would involve picking at random 100 names from among the 1000 listed. It is absolutely essential that each time a name is chosen, every individual has an equal chance of being picked. Traditionally, a technique for ensuring this is through the use of a table of random numbers: people in the population are numbered from 000 to 999. Using a special table of random numbers, 100 numbers are then picked, and the people corresponding to the numbers listed become the sample. Today, a random sample can be generated by computer if the sampling frame is held on an appropriate database.

Another approach is to draw a *systematic random sample* in which individuals are picked from the sampling frame in sequence. A 10% random sample drawn in this way would involve choosing every 10th name on the list (a 1 in 10 sample), only the first selection being made from the table of random numbers. This is often a much more convenient way of drawing a sample. Systematic sampling is usually a perfectly satisfactory method, but it depends on people or items listed on a sampling frame being arranged in a way that does not introduce bias. For example, a 1 in 10 systematic sample drawn from a list of married people in which the husband's name always came first would result in either every person chosen being female or every person being male.

Stratification may be used to ensure adequate representation of different sections of the population. The population is divided into sections or strata, such as age groups or places of residence. A random sample is then drawn from within each stratum. Stratified sampling has the additional advantage that it allows a different size of sample to be taken from each stratum to reflect the varying size or importance of the different strata.

Multistage sampling is often a convenient technique in large surveys. For example, a survey of lung disease in steel workers might take as its first-stage sampling frame a list of all towns with steelworks. Having chosen an appropriate number of towns randomly, a second-stage sampling frame consisting of the names of employees could be drawn from the towns that had initially been chosen. The workers for examination would then be drawn at random from the second frame. The advantage of having adopted a two-stage sampling technique is that the need to draw up a named list of steel workers in the whole country was bypassed, thus saving time and avoiding difficulty and cost to the investigators.

DATA SPECIFICATION

At the outset, decisions need to be taken about what information is required to address the aims of the study, and how it is to be collected. There will be some types of information that address the central research question (e.g. a person's blood pressure in a population survey of hypertension), while other information will be gathered because it provides important background on the characteristics of the sample or because it may be relevant to the analysis of the main factors under study. To return to the earlier example, a prevalence study of the extent of dementia in the population would be unlikely to limit itself to assessing elderly people for the presence or absence of dementia. It would also gather data on factors such as their domestic circumstances, their capacity for self-care and their physical status. It might also gather information on previous exposures (occupation, alcohol or drug use and medical conditions), although in this instance, recall bias may present a particular challenge. If the study is analytical, data may be gathered on both cases and noncases for comparison.

Consideration must next be given as to how best to obtain the required information. This may sound like a simple matter, but it seldom is. Consider a seemingly straightforward variable such as socio-economic status, which might be collected as important information in a population survey of mothers' infant feeding practice. Interviewers questioning members of the sample could not simply ask, 'What is your socio-economic status?' The responses to such a general question by a population with varying perceptions of what was meant would yield data from which no valid conclusions could be drawn. A rigorous approach would involve the construction of a question that would provide the elements

necessary to categorize the respondent by, for example, the National Statistics Socio-economic Classification. Ideally, such a question should be derived from established survey work and be of proven validity.

Even for simple information, such as age, it is important to establish whether respondents should be asked their precise age, to place their age in a banding or age group, or be asked their precise date of birth. This needs to be discussed in the planning stage of the survey, and be consistent with the aims of the study and method of data collection. For more complex information, established and validated measures or questions should be used wherever possible.

Special and more difficult judgements have to be made when gathering data to provide information about the prevalence of a disease. The first step is to agree on an operational definition of the disease under study and the method by which it is to be measured or detected. Even a formally stated definition of a disease may be of little practical value in conducting a survey to determine its prevalence. It is necessary to agree on strict criteria that must be fulfilled in order for a person to be counted as having the disease.

In planning a population study to determine the prevalence of a disease, it is essential to resolve and adhere to a working definition, or the results collected will have no meaning outside the context in which they are collected.

DATA COLLECTION

Another important decision in planning a population survey is choosing the method through which the necessary data will be derived. To a certain extent, this will also depend on the aims of the investigation.

The survey instrument

The term used to describe the method of data collection is the *survey instrument*. This is usually the document in which survey data are recorded – for example, a questionnaire to be administered by trained interviewers or a pro forma used to extract data in a standardized format from various clinical records. Questionnaire design is a complex process, and a number of important aspects should be considered, such as the structuring of questions (including the relative merits of closed vs. open), the order in which questions should be asked, the avoidance of questions likely to lead to ambiguous or biased answers, the layout of the questionnaire and the coding of responses to facilitate analysis.

Questionnaires are of two broad kinds: postal questionnaires and those that are administered face to face by an interviewer. Although postal questionnaires have the advantage that they allow a much larger sample size, they can have serious disadvantages because of the restricted range of topics that can be covered and the generally higher levels of nonresponse.

Whatever survey instrument is chosen, it is important that before the full-scale survey is undertaken, a pilot study is carried out on a small number of people within the sample. This allows difficulties with the questionnaire or other aspects of the survey to be ironed out or corrected before the survey proper is commenced.

Standardization of measurement and interview technique

Variation between measurements is another important consideration in a population survey. The main concern is with systematic variation or bias. Standardizing the procedures in the study when, for example, physical examinations are being carried out will reduce variation. Training examiners and checking their technique at intervals during the conduct of the study will help to achieve this. Similarly, if interviewers are being used to elicit information from members of the study population by questionnaire, they must be trained. This training may include how to phrase questions, agreeing on rules to be adopted when the respondents are reluctant to answer the questions posed, what to do when other family members seek to participate in answering questions on the respondent's behalf and the extent to which interviewers should react to (or make observations on) responses made to the questions. A lack of clarity on these and many other aspects of interviewing can risk the results obtained being invalid or biased in ways that may be impossible to detect or eliminate from the analysis.

Variation in scientific instruments can be reduced by strict quality control. In studies using laboratory measurements, test solutions or reagents can be employed to ensure standardization.

The problem of nonresponse

A major difficulty when gathering data in population surveys is the problem of nonresponse or noncooperation.

The planning and organization of the study should be geared to obtaining the highest possible recruitment of the sample under investigation. Key factors for success in minimizing nonresponse include the nature of the initial approach made to members of the sample, the wording of a letter of introduction and the perception of the institution carrying out the research. These are factors that can make the difference between a very high rate of participation in the subsequent interview and a disastrous level of refusals or nonresponse.

It is inevitable, however, that some degree of nonresponse will remain, even after the most careful planning efforts to reduce it. The main concern is that the nonresponders are unlikely to be typical of the remainder of the sample. Depending on the circumstances, they may be more (or less) likely to suffer the disease or other subject of the investigation, and therefore their omission can lead to difficulties in drawing generalizable conclusions from a sample that is biased or unrepresentative. If nonresponse does occur, the first approach is to make extra efforts to gain the nonresponding group's cooperation. Where this fails, a second strategy is to obtain as much indirect evidence as possible about the nonresponders to understand the kind of bias that may be introduced by their omission.

Some degree of nonresponse is a feature of nearly all population surveys. While there is no specific minimum response rate, most investigators would be happy to achieve a response rate in the 80%–100% range. It is more common, however, to see reports of surveys with response rates in the mid to upper 70% range. This can still yield valuable findings, particularly if some data are available on the nonresponders and if conclusions are drawn more cautiously than would be the case with higher response rates.

A further problem in interpreting data from population surveys to establish disease prevalence is the need to be fully aware that the population being dealt with is a *survivor population*. If the disease has an appreciable mortality, the most severe cases will have died and any cross-sectional study will not include the entire spectrum of disease.

EXAMPLE OF A CROSS-SECTIONAL STUDY: HEALTH SURVEY FOR ENGLAND

Cross-sectional surveys that are repeated regularly are of particular value – because they generate data that can be studied for temporal trends, and because they allow methodologies to be refined and improved on successive occasions (although doing so can hinder the study of temporal trends). Such a study is the Health Survey for England. This is a government-funded annual health survey of private households in England. It includes interviews and some examinations and tests of children (over two years old) and adults in each household surveyed.

The sampling frame for the Health Survey for England is the Postcode Address File (PAF), which contains 720 postcode sectors. The method of sampling is a multistage stratified technique – a number of stratification factors are used to ensure that the eventual sample is broadly representative of the whole population of England. Sampled addresses are sent an introductory letter, which is then followed by initial contact with an interviewer. At each household that agrees to cooperate, an interviewer-administered questionnaire is first completed with the head of household or partner, and then an individual questionnaire interview is carried out with each household member. Height and weight are also recorded at this first interview. Interviewees are then asked to agree to a second-stage visit at which further measurements and a blood sample are taken.

Detailed sampling rules govern which members of the household (particularly children) are to be included. Explanatory leaflets describe the purpose of the survey and help to gain compliance. Quality control measures include training of interviewers and nurses, checking of interview and measurement quality, and protocols for interviewing and measuring children. There are rules to govern what to tell people if abnormalities are found and what action needs to be taken. Some information is gathered on nonresponders and reasons for nonresponse.

Valuable information about the health of the population has been derived from it, including general health, long-standing and acute illness, limitation of function,

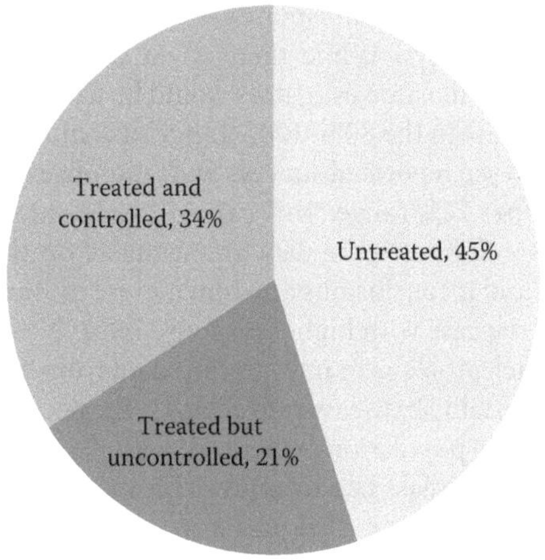

Figure 2.17 Treatment and control amongst people with high blood pressure in England.

Source: Health Survey for England, 2015.

respiratory disease and certain other specific illnesses, experience of major and minor accidents, smoking and drinking, physical activity, obesity, blood pressure, lung function, blood haemoglobin and use of health services.

An example of the kind of information that is yielded by this cross-sectional study is shown in Figure 2.17. The public health importance of this finding was striking: high blood pressure is a risk factor for coronary heart disease and stroke. Yet just under half of the people with high blood pressure were not being treated, and 40% of those who were being treated did not have their blood pressure under control.

Cohort studies

OUTLINE OF METHODOLOGY

The cohort study is a type of epidemiological investigation in which a population apparently free of the disease under study is assembled and each individual is categorized according to whether he or she has been exposed to the risk factor(s) of interest. The cohort is then followed up to see whether individual members of it develop the disease under study (or other diseases, in some cases). Comparisons are then made between the occurrence of the disease in the *exposed* and the *nonexposed* groups within the cohort. If the intention is to test the hypothesis that smoking causes lung cancer, the initial step is to classify the study cohort into smokers and nonsmokers. The cohort is then followed up over time, and cases of lung cancer are detected as they occur. The results are analysed to show what proportion of the smokers developed lung cancer compared with the proportion of nonsmokers.

A cohort study may be conducted prospectively or retrospectively. In a *prospective cohort study*, the initial exposure data are collected on the members of the cohort and the investigators then wait for cases of the disease to crop up over time. This is the most common type of cohort study.

A *retrospective cohort study* is conducted where data on both the cohort's exposure and its disease experience are already available. This can only really be contemplated where good past records exist to define a historical cohort. For example, suppose that a very large general practice had maintained very comprehensive records on medications prescribed to the practice population over a long period of time. If, in the present day, a particular drug became suspected of causing a type of cancer, the records of such a practice may allow a retrospective cohort study to be carried out. In such a study, a cohort would be assembled at some notional past date from the old practice population records, and the people within it would be classified according to whether they had been prescribed the drug of interest. Their past and present medical records would then also be examined to record their disease history and particularly whether they developed the cancer that was under study. This is a simplified description of a complex methodology, but in the relatively unusual situation where past data are available comprehensively on a large population, the retrospective cohort study has advantages of speed and lower cost compared with the more common prospective approach.

CHOICE OF STUDY POPULATION

A cohort is a group of people who share a similar experience at a point in time. A birth cohort is people born on a particular day or in a particular year, and a marriage cohort those married in a given year. People residing in a particular geographical area or workers in an industry at a certain time also constitute a cohort.

In a cohort study investigating a causal hypothesis, the precise choice of cohort will depend on the nature of the disease or exposure under investigation. The cohort might be a group of people who have been exposed to a particular hazard (e.g. a serious water pollution incident), a large workforce in a particular industry (e.g. asbestos workers) or the population of a geographically defined area (e.g. a small town). These cohorts are of course only half the picture, and it is important to have a control cohort where possible.

CHARACTERIZING THE COHORT

The way in which data are assembled to characterize the initial cohort of people to be followed up depends very much on the aims of the study. In a cohort study examining the risk of cancer arising from an industrial hazard, it is likely that quite detailed information would be gathered on the employment history of the workers concerned and their likely exposure in the workplace to quantified levels of the presumed risk factor, as well as whether they had other habits or characteristics that might influence the possibility of them developing the disease (such as cigarette smoking). In a cohort study examining the risk of development of heart disease in a population, a sample of the population might form the study cohort and each member be assessed by questionnaire, and by clinical and biochemical examination, to determine their baseline status in terms of the risk factors under investigation.

FOLLOW-UP PHASE

The follow-up phase of a cohort study, conducted prospectively, requires very careful planning and preparation. Particularly in studies where a long period is required, the difficulties in keeping track of members of the cohort who move away from the area can be very great and the process can be expensive. Considerable stability is also required in the investigative team, particularly among its leaders, if the study is to be brought to a successful conclusion.

A number of decisions need to be made when this follow-up phase of the cohort study is being designed. One important decision is how, and at what intervals, reassessments of the original members of the cohort will be made. This decision is somewhat easier when the outcome under study is a clear endpoint, such as death. In such circumstances, sources of mortality data can be kept under constant review, and the records of members of the original cohort can be flagged as the deaths occur to denote the outcome. Where the study is examining less dramatic outcomes, such as the progress of children whose mothers were exposed (and not exposed) to a particular hazard in pregnancy, it would be necessary to decide on the time periods at which the children in the original cohort would be given further developmental assessments. Clearly, it would be quite impractical to undertake this with great regularity on the very large numbers of children who would be involved.

EXAMPLE OF A COHORT STUDY: THE NURSES' HEALTH STUDY

In 1976, researchers at Harvard University started a major cohort study that continues to this day and has become a classic. All members of the cohort were married, female nurses living in 11 states of the United States. They were 121,000 in number. Initially, the researchers' main goal was to study the health effects of oral contraceptives, but the Nurses' Health Study has since expanded to examine many different risk factors for a range of important diseases.

Each participant is sent a questionnaire every two years. The early questionnaires asked about oral contraceptive use, smoking and menopause. Questions about additional exposures have been added over time. In particular, dietary habits have been recorded in detail since 1980. The researchers also find out any diseases that the participants develop – both from their questionnaires and from their doctors.

The decision to study nurses was carefully thought out. The researchers judged that because of their profession, the participants would be able to accurately answer the questionnaires. They also thought that nurses would feel motivated to take part in such a study, and to continue answering questionnaires for many years. They were correct. When each questionnaire is sent out, only about 10% of the participants fail to return it.

The same research group has since established two further cohorts. Nurses' Health Study II started in 1989, recruiting 116,000 nurses. It has collected similar information on diet, oral contraceptive pill use and lifestyle – but in a younger cohort. Nurses' Health Study III started recruiting participants in 2010. It is entirely web based, asking participants to complete a questionnaire every six months.

The Nurses' Health Study was initially set up to examine the health effects of oral contraceptive pills, and has successfully done so. Its results have helped to inform decisions about which oral contraceptive pills are safest. But the study has collected information on many more exposures than this, and on a large number of outcomes. This has enabled many different research questions to be answered using a single cohort. A single example of this – the relationship between whole-grain consumption and the risk of coronary heart disease – is shown in Figure 2.18 (those with the highest whole-grain consumption had a risk 30% lower than

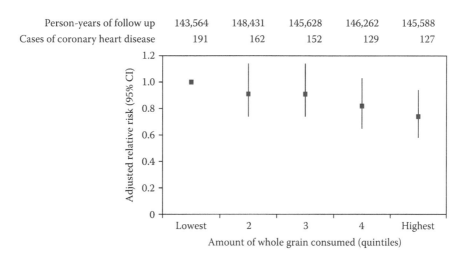

Figure 2.18 Whole-grain consumption and risk of coronary heart disease in 75,521 female nurses aged 38–63 years.

Source: Liu S, Stampfer MJ, Hu FB, et al. Whole-grain consumption and risk of coronary heart disease: results from the Nurses' Health Study. *The American Journal of Clinical Nutrition* 1999;70(3):412-9.

Table 2.8 Main findings about breast cancer risk from the Nurses Health Studies

Exposure	Risk of breast cancer
Smoking	No relation with past or current smoking
Oral contraceptives	Current use increases risk. Past use no association
Postmenopausal hormones	More than 5 years of estrogen plus progestins increases risk. More than 10 years of estrogen alone increases risk
Obesity	Increases risk among postmenopausal women. Weight loss after menopause is associated with reduced risk
Alcohol	One or more drinks per day increases risk
Diet	Higher intake of red meat increases risk of premenopausal breast cancer
Physical activity	Physical activity (>3 hours/week) reduces risk
Other exposures	Family history of breast cancer, high breast density, high circulating hormone levels, and shift work all increase risk

Source: Nurses' Health Study. *Key Contributions to Scientific Knowledge.* Available from: www.nurseshealthstudy.org/about-nhs/key-contributions-scientific-knowledge (accessed 26 May 2017).

those with the lowest). Conducting multiple such analyses using a single cohort is a far more cost-effective way of doing research than establishing a different cohort for each individual question. The Nurses' Health Study has been vital in establishing the health effects of different diets, and therefore what dietary advice should be given to the population. It has also helped to quantify how much physical activity (and of what kind) is needed to reduce the risk of different diseases. Table 2.8 summarizes the insight that the Nurses' Health Studies have provided about breast cancer – just one of the many diseases that it has studied.

Case–control studies

The main attraction of a case–control study, especially when compared with a cohort study, is that it is relatively quick and cheap to undertake. Gathering data does not involve a long period of follow-up of the study population. It is particularly useful when investigating possible causes of rare or uncommon disorders, where it would take decades to assemble enough cases for a cohort study to be statistically meaningful. On the other hand, case–control studies are more prone to bias and have other adverse features associated with the study design.

OUTLINE OF METHODOLOGY

The case–control study is a type of epidemiological investigation in which an assessment is made of the extent to which people with an established disease (*cases*) and a comparable group who do not have the disease (*controls*) have been exposed to a risk factor believed to be responsible for causing the disease.

For example, if the intention is to investigate the hypothesis that smoking causes lung cancer, the investigation begins by taking people with lung cancer and suitable controls who do not have lung cancer. Enquiries are then made to discover how many of the lung cancer patients were smokers and how many of the control patients were smokers. The method of investigation in a case–control study is almost always retrospective. The investigator looks back in time on the exposure history of present-day cases of the disease and of the controls. This contrasts with a cohort study (Figure 2.19). A variant on the conventional case–control study design is to conduct a nested case–control study within a cohort study. Cases of a particular disease that occur within the cohort can be matched against controls – people also within the cohort, who have not developed the disease. The cases and controls can then be compared. The nested case–control study approach does not consider all the disease-free members of the cohort to be controls, only a sample of them. The advantage of a nested case–control study over the traditional case–control study design is that a consistent set of information is available for both cases and controls from the time before disease onset (because they were enrolled in a cohort study). This may well include blood samples and other physical measures, which are rarely available with any consistency in a standard case–control design. The reason for limiting the number of controls, rather than including all cohort members, is chiefly that this limits the extent to which previously collected samples need to be analysed, and therefore the cost.

CHOICE OF A STUDY POPULATION

In practice, the design of a case–control study is much more difficult than this broad outline of the methodology implies. One of the key initial decisions for the investigator is the way in which the cases and controls that make up the study population will be chosen. If wrong decisions are made at this stage of the investigation, the sources of bias that are introduced could render the results of the study invalid and useless.

Selection of cases

The choice of cases must start with the formulation of a clear operational definition of what constitutes a case of the disease under study. Decisions will need to be taken on whether to study a broad diagnostic category (e.g. adult acute leukaemia) or a more homogenous diagnostic grouping (e.g. adult acute myeloid leukaemia). This decision depends on the nature of the investigation, but in general, the more heterogeneity in the diagnostic group, the less likelihood of being able to link a specific risk factor to the disease causation.

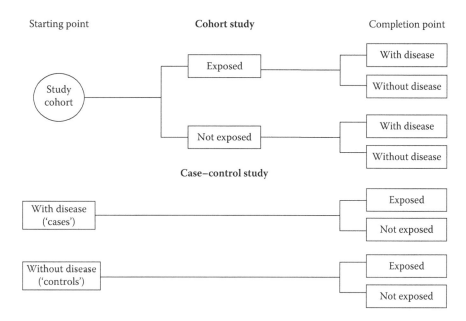

Figure 2.19 The main features of cohort and case–control studies.

On the other hand, the narrower the category of disease for inclusion of cases in the study, the less general applicability the findings will have. For example, a case–control study to investigate possible risk factors in osteoarthrosis that took, as cases, people with disease of the metacarpal joints and yielded a finding of an apparently new risk factor for the disease would throw light on the causation of osteoarthrosis. However, general conclusions could not necessarily be drawn about osteoarthrosis of other joints in the body, because the cases were limited to people with disease at one particular site.

Having established a case definition, it is most important to identify a source of all cases so that all eligible cases can be recruited into the study.

Selection of controls

The choice of an appropriate control group will usually cause the greatest discussion when planning a case–control study. While the issues involved in selecting controls are complex, and often particular to the circumstances of the study, it is important to keep in mind the central purpose of the control group. This is to provide an indication of the level of exposure to the risk factor in the population, to which the exposure experienced by the people who have developed the disease can then be compared.

Put in the simplest terms, suppose that a case–control study was carried out to test the hypothesis that regular consumption of a particular kind of herbal tea led to the occurrence of pancreatic cancer. If 40% of cases were found to be drinkers of the herbal tea, such a finding would be of much less interest if 40% of the general population were regular herbal tea drinkers than if only 2% were. In this example, the controls are there to represent the same types of people as the cases and allow an estimate to be made of the normal pattern of herbal tea drinking.

In practice, to find controls that are representative of the population from which the cases have arisen can be extremely difficult. For example, some case–control studies using hospital cases take as their control group patients who attended the hospital for the treatment of diseases other than the one that is the subject of the study. This approach has advantages in that access to controls is usually relatively easy and information can be gathered in a fashion similar to that of the cases. It is also open to a number of potential sources of bias. For example, the hospital may have different catchment populations for the disease that is the subject of the study (the cases) and for the disease from which the control group patients were suffering. In such circumstances, the controls may not be representative of the general population from which the cases were drawn, so the degree of their exposure to the risk factor may be an unreliable basis for comparison with the cases.

Controls that are drawn from the general population do not suffer from this drawback but are less easy to identify and gain cooperation from. The way in which they provide information may also be different to the cases in ways that may introduce bias.

The relative advantages and disadvantages of different numbers and types of controls require the most careful consideration before final decisions are taken. It is possible to choose more controls than cases. This can be done to boost the statistical power of the analysis, particularly if there are few cases; another reason is to ensure that there is more than one type of control group (e.g. drawn from the community and from hospital).

MATCHING CASES AND CONTROLS

Matching in case–control studies is the process whereby controls are set alongside cases to ensure that they have similar characteristics. The purpose of matching is to eliminate the effect of so-called *confounding* variables. Confounding can occur in other types of epidemiological investigation and is a term used to describe circumstances where there are factors, in addition to the risk factor being studied, that may influence whether the disease occurs. If such confounding factors are unevenly distributed between study groups, they can distort the comparisons that are being made (and hence the conclusions that are drawn). One of the most common confounding variables is age. The occurrence of many diseases is strongly associated with age. If, in a case–control study, there are major differences in the age structure of cases and controls, this may distort other more important comparisons between the two groups. In descriptive epidemiological studies, standardization is the method through which the confounding effect of age is reduced. Confounding is discussed further later in this section.

The technique of matching should be used very sparingly because there are serious problems that can result from overmatching. With statistical analytical techniques, the matching of characteristics of cases and controls can also be undertaken during the analysis stage. The tendency in case–control studies now is to take account of confounding variables (except age and sex) in the analysis of results rather than to eliminate them at the study design stage of matching.

ASSEMBLING DATA ON THE EXPOSURE

Data on the exposure of cases and controls are usually obtained by three main methods: (1) by extracting information from medical or other records, (2) by interviewing cases and controls (or where there have been deaths, their relatives) and (3) by conducting physical examinations, scans and laboratory tests.

Further potential sources of bias are inherent in these approaches. Records may not provide comprehensive or detailed enough information to fully satisfy the requirements of the investigation. This is hardly surprising, because such records seldom will have been created in the knowledge that they would be needed for a study. For example, when retrospectively obtaining data on exposure from medical records of lung cancer patients and hospital patients with other diseases (used as controls), it would be more likely that a smoking history would be recorded in the lung cancer patients because of the known association between that disease and cigarette smoking.

When exposure data are obtained retrospectively by interview, a person with the disease may be more likely to remember or report an exposure (perhaps because he or she is trying to rationalize the presence of the disease) than would be a disease-free person serving as a control. For example, imagine that a surgeon notices that many female patients presenting at his outpatient clinic with breast lumps give a history of localized trauma. To investigate this further, he takes two groups of women: one group comprises those who have presented to the outpatient clinic with a breast lump; the other comprises a sample of healthy women of similar ages. Each group of women is asked if they can recall having any bang, knock or bruise of the breast during the previous 12 months.

A much higher occurrence of such trauma is found in the group with breast lumps than in the control group of healthy women. Should it then be concluded that localized trauma predisposes to the formation of breast lumps? This is possible, but rather biologically implausible. Women who have developed a breast lump are often in a very anxious state, and their principal fear is that the lump is malignant. They will often cling to any alternative explanation of the origin of the lump. Hence, when such women are questioned about a history of trauma, they are far more likely to remember and volunteer some trivial occurrence than are those women without breast lumps. This is *recall bias*.

Since data are obtained retrospectively on the exposure, whether by abstraction of case notes or by interview survey, serious problems arise when there are differences in the completeness of information or selectivity between the two groups (cases and controls). The investigator may not be aware of it and may draw misleading conclusions – such as in the examples given above. It is not possible to fully guard against this, but an additional measure that may help is to ensure that the person gathering the data (whether abstracting it from records or questioning patients) relies on a structured format and is blind to whether the individuals are cases or controls. There is less risk of these sources of bias when examinations or tests are carried out.

There is evidence to show that recall bias can be influenced by the seriousness of the condition being studied (cancer vs. an infection), the perceived importance of the event in the life of the individual (childbirth vs. drug exposure), the respondent (patient vs. proxy), the length of time since the event and the phraseology used either in the questionnaire or by the interviewer.

EXAMPLE OF A CASE–CONTROL STUDY: THE INTERSTROKE PROJECT

An international study set out to assess the risk factors for stroke (ischaemic and haemorrhagic). Few studies have examined this question in low- and middle-income countries. The methodology was case control. The study populations were recruited from 22 countries. Cases were people who were admitted to hospital acutely with a first stroke. Very strict diagnostic criteria were used. Controls were people with no history of stroke, matched for age and sex. All those with stroke had routine neuroimaging. Data were gathered by questionnaire, physical examination, clinical assessment and laboratory testing. The investigators concluded that 80% of global stroke was accounted for by five risk factors: hypertension, current smoking, diet, abdominal obesity and physical inactivity. Figure 2.20 shows one of the analyses. This study is different to many of the case–control studies that are described in traditional textbooks of epidemiology. It is ambitious in its scope. It spans 22 countries but, nevertheless, gathers extensive data in a standardized way. By incorporating populations from low- and middle-income countries, it fills an important gap in epidemiological knowledge about the risk of stroke.

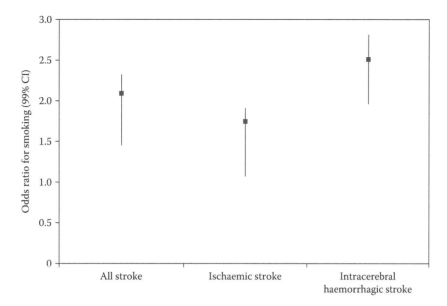

Figure 2.20 Smoking and risk of stroke.

Source: O'Donnell MJ, Xavier D, Liu L, et al. Risk factors for ischaemic and intracerebral haemorrhagic stroke in 22 countries (the INTERSTROKE study): a case-control study. *Lancet* 2010;376(9735):112-23. With permission.

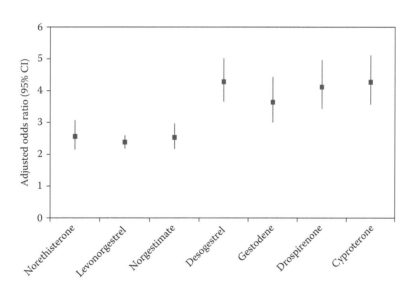

Figure 2.21 Use of combined oral contraceptives and risk of venous thromboembolism.

Source: Vinogradova Y, Coupland C, Hippisley-Cox J. Use of combined oral contraceptives and risk of venous thromboembolism: nested case-control studies using the QResearch and CPRD databases. *BMJ* 2015;350:h2135. With permission.

EXAMPLE OF A NESTED CASE–CONTROL STUDY: RISKS OF ORAL CONTRACEPTIVES

A case–control study with a *nested* design was used to investigate the risks of oral contraceptives. It used the existing UK Clinical Practice Research Datalink and Q Research databases that contribute information from 618 and 722 general practices, respectively. More than 5000 cases were identified in each database for the study period. The databases contained prospective information on all prescriptions issued and also information on diagnoses made in primary and secondary care, test results and standard demographic data. Up to five controls were matched for each case by age, general practice and calendar year. Statistical adjustment was carried out in the analysis to try to eliminate the influence of certain confounding factors. The risks of venous thromboembolism compared with no exposure varied between the various types of oral contraceptive, with certain progestogen-containing contraceptives showing a strong association with the adverse outcome (Figure 2.21).

This study highlights some key concepts of case–control design, and ways in which a nested case–control study can overcome some of the possible biases in its traditional design.

Nesting the cases and controls within a cohort means that the selection of controls is less prone to bias. They represent the population from which the cases arose, as both were taken from the same cohort. The study design is also less prone to recall bias, as the exposure was recorded prospectively and obtained from an objective source – practice prescription data (although this has the limitation that it is not known whether the drugs were taken after prescription). One limitation with using nested case–control studies, however, is that relevant data on all confounding variables may not have been collected as part of the cohort study.

Measures of association

A key activity in analytical epidemiological studies (particularly those using the cohort and case–control designs) is making comparisons of the occurrence of disease or other outcome in groups exposed or not exposed to a hypothesized source of risk (usually simply called the *exposure*), or vice versa. The first step is to assess whether there is an association between the exposure and the disease and, if so, how strong it is. Measures derived from the data collected in such studies enable assessment of the importance of the exposure to disease occurrence.

One such measure is the *relative risk* (RR). In a cohort study, the relative risk of the disease or outcome is calculated from the ratio of incidence rates in the exposed group and the nonexposed group. In a case–control study, incidence rates cannot be calculated; this is because the subjects do not properly represent the population as a whole.

However, an estimate of the relative risk is produced by the *odds ratio*. This ratio is constructed by dividing the odds of the case group having been exposed to the risk factor by the odds of the control group having been exposed. The statistical theory underlying these indices is beyond the scope of this book, but they have been introduced in outline to give an insight into the way in which the results of cohort and case–control studies may be presented and interpreted.

Relative risk and the odds ratio are measures based on *relative* differences in disease between two study groups. They address the question, how many times more common is the disease (or exposure) in one group than in the other group? Thus, they measure the strength of an association.

An alternative approach is to take the data that have been gathered and calculate the difference in disease occurrence between the exposed and unexposed groups. Rather than create a ratio of the two incidence figures, instead the difference in incidence can be calculated. This is an *absolute* measure of risk rather than a relative one. The attributable risk is such a statistic. It is useful in examining the absolute additional risk that individuals experience as a result of their exposure.

Measures of population disease impact

A further elaboration on the principle of absolute risk is to calculate it scaled up to population level. The *population attributable fraction* (also called *population attributable risk*) is a measure of the extent to which the disease that occurs in the whole population is due, or attributable, to the risk

	Smokers (exposed)	Nonsmokers (nonexposed)
Lung cancer	100	20
No lung cancer	900	980
	1000	1000

$$\text{Risk} = \frac{\text{Number developing outcome}}{\text{Number at risk}} = \frac{100}{1000} = 0.1, \text{ or } 10\%$$

$$\text{Risk among smokers} = \frac{100}{1000} = 0.1, \text{ or } 10\%$$

$$\text{Risk among nonsmokers} = \frac{20}{1000} = 0.02, \text{ or } 2\%$$

$$\text{Risk among population} = \frac{120}{1000} = 0.06, \text{ or } 6\%$$

$$\text{Attributable fraction} = \frac{\text{Risk among exposed} - \text{Risk among unexposed}}{\text{Risk among exposed}} = \frac{0.1 - 0.02}{0.1} = 0.8, \text{ or } 80\%$$

$$\text{Population attributable fraction} = \frac{\text{Risk among population} - \text{Risk among nonexposed}}{\text{Risk among population}} = \frac{0.06 - 0.02}{0.06} = 0.67, \text{ or } 67\%$$

Figure 2.22 Ten-year cumulative incidence of lung cancer in a population of 2000 people (illustrative data).

factor. The population attributable fraction is valuable in assessing the public health impact of a risk factor, and hence the benefits that could be obtained by preventive action.

It is usually calculated by multiplying the attributable risk by the prevalence of the risk factor in the population (it can also be calculated from relative risk). A relatively small excess (i.e. attributable) risk of developing a disease where a large number of people are exposed to the risk factor would yield many additional cases. The benefits of preventive action could be great.

A good example of the relative merits of relative, absolute and population measures of risk is to think about the causative effect of cigarette smoking. Figure 2.22 shows illustrative data from a hypothetical 10-year study of lung cancer incidence among a population of 2000 people, half of whom smoke and half of whom do not. As the calculations show, the absolute risk of lung cancer among smokers was 10% over the period. Among nonsmokers, it was 2%. Calculating the attributable fraction shows that 80% of lung cancer among smokers was due to smoking. The other 20% of cases would have happened even if they were not smokers.

The population attributable fraction shows that smoking is associated with 67% of lung cancer cases within the population as a whole. The population attributable risk is useful in assessing the public health impact of a risk factor, and hence the benefits that could be obtained by preventive action.

The simple 2 × 2 table from this hypothetical study therefore provides a great deal of information about smoking and lung cancer. It illustrates that the average smoker has a 10% chance of developing lung cancer within the next 10 years. It shows that smokers are five times more likely to develop lung cancer than nonsmokers are. It shows that 80% of lung cancer among smokers is due to smoking. The population attributable fraction shows that 67% of lung cancer could be prevented if nobody smoked.

Analysis of data from cohort and case–control studies

This section goes further into analysis than the examples of cohort and case–control studies described in the previous sections. It uses different examples of published studies.

Table 2.9 shows data from a cohort study that compares incidence. The risk calculation is added to the table. The data are from a large study in which married women using different forms of contraception were followed up and information was gathered on a range of health outcomes. The aspect of the study shown in the table explores the relationship between use of oral contraceptives and the subsequent development of two inflammatory bowel diseases (ulcerative colitis and Crohn's disease). There was a higher incidence of both ulcerative colitis and Crohn's disease in current oral contraceptive users than in women who had never used the pill or had given up using it. While the difference did not achieve statistical significance for Crohn's disease, it did for ulcerative colitis. Incidences in those who had stopped using oral contraceptives were similar to those who had never used them. The authors concluded that while the associations between oral contraceptive use and chronic inflammatory bowel disease could not be regarded as established, they provided important clues to its causation.

Table 2.10 shows data from one of the earliest case–control studies ever carried out – an investigation in the 1950s into the possible causes of childhood cancer. One of the factors investigated was whether irradiation of the fetus by abdominal X-ray examinations of the mother during pregnancy was associated with childhood cancer.

The data are shown to illustrate the way in which such an analysis can be presented (not to describe the study in detail). As Table 2.10 shows, there was a significantly elevated odds ratio of childhood cancer in children who were irradiated in utero. The authors concluded that fetal irradiation by diagnostic X-raying of the pregnant mother was a risk factor for childhood cancer.

To repeat an important point made earlier, the only outcome measures that can be assessed by case–control studies are odds – that is, the odds of exposure in cases and controls (which is equivalent to the odds of disease occurring in those exposed) and corresponding odds ratios. If information has been collected on confounding factors, then these can be adjusted for in a multivariate analysis (to give the *adjusted* odds ratio).

Table 2.9 Analysis of data from a cohort study investigating the association between oral contraceptive usage and the occurrence of chronic inflammatory bowel disease

Use of oral contraceptives	Woman-years of observation	Ulcerative colitis		Crohn's disease	
		Number of cases	Incidence/1000 woman-years	Number of cases	Incidence/1000 woman-years
Never used	75 950	8	0.11	6	0.08
Ex-user	67 319	8	0.10	4	0.06
Current user	61 116	16	0.26	8	0.13
Total	204 385	31	0.15	18	0.09

Source: Vessey M, Jewell D, Smith A, et al. Chronic inflammatory bowel disease, cigarette smoking, and use of oral contraceptives: findings in a large cohort study of women of child-bearing age. *British Medical Journal* 1986;292: 1101-3. With permission.

Table 2.10 Analysis of data from a case–control study

	Cases	Controls
Abdominal X-ray of pregnant mother (exposed)	141	81
No abdominal X-ray of pregnant mother (unexposed)	1125	1204
Total	1266	1285
Odds ratio 1.86; 95% confidence interval 1.40–2.47		

Source: Stewart A, Webb J, Hewitt D. A survey of childhood malignancies. *British Medical Journal* 1958;1(5086):1495. With permission.

Making causal inferences

Cohort and case–control studies are the principal ways to explore hypotheses involving factors that may cause disease. If such links can be established, there may be scope for prevention by intervening against causal agents. A causal hypothesis may spring from clinical impression, from laboratory observations, or from examining descriptive data in populations in relation to time, place or person, as described earlier in this chapter. Table 2.11 gives some ways in which ideas about causation emerge.

When an epidemiological study (cross-sectional, cohort or case–control) comparing groups finds that a risk factor (or exposure) occurs more frequently in a group of people with a disease (or other adverse outcome) than in groups without the disease (using statistics such as relative risk and odds ratios), an association between the risk factor and the disease has been established. The next step is to understand what this association means.

This first goes back to the counterfactual ideal, discussed previously. Studies that yield data are by their nature imperfect. The explanation for the association could be spurious due to poor study design or explained by factors not taken account of. In other words, could the observed association be due to anything else? Examples of the problems encountered in cohort and case–control studies have been given in the previous sections, and the roles of confounding and bias were briefly discussed. Here, the triad of factors that must be considered when scrutinizing an association between a potential risk factor and an adverse outcome are set out.

CHANCE

When more disease occurs in a group of people exposed to a risk factor than in those unexposed, this may simply be due

Table 2.11 Common ways in which ideas about causation emerge

Laboratory study
Clinical impression
Clusters of rare diseases
Descriptive epidemiological studies
Cohort and case–control studies

to chance. Statistical tests can help to indicate the likelihood that this is the case.

By chance alone, groups differ in certain characteristics. This can result in outcomes that are different between the groups, simply due to the random variation between samples (so-called sampling variation). As the size of the groups increases, the degree of chance variation between them tends to decrease.

When an association is found, statistical tests can be used that take into account the size of the study groups and the size of the association, to help determine how likely it is that the observed values could have occurred by chance. A *p* value gives the probability of a result as extreme as that seen occurring by chance alone. For example, a *p* value of 0.05 can be interpreted as there being a 5% chance that the association *could* have occurred by chance alone. The smaller the *p* value, the more confidence that can be placed on random chance not being the reason for a difference between the groups. By convention, if *p* values are less than 0.05, the conclusion is that the difference did not occur by chance alone. In other words, there is a real difference between the groups. This is *statistical significance*.

Confidence intervals also give information about the role of chance. They are more useful than a *p* value, because they assess both the size of the effect and the precision of that estimate. It is common to use 95% confidence intervals, that is, the range of values that can be said with 95% confidence to contain the true estimate (which would have been obtained by analysing data from the whole population).

If the 95% confidence interval does not include the *null effect* (no difference between the groups under comparison), then the results are at least equivalent to a *p* value of 0.05. The value that indicates a null effect depends on what estimate of risk is used. For a risk or odds ratio, it is 1. For example, if a relative risk for a given disease between exposed groups compared with nonexposed groups is reported as 2.7 (95% confidence interval 1.5–3.9), this indicates 95% confidence that the true relative risk lies between 1.5 and 3.9. Since this value does not contain 1, researchers can be at least 95% confident that the difference between groups has not occurred by chance alone. If interpreting a confidence interval for an absolute difference, the *null value* is zero. For example, if the difference in prevalence of all cancers between two geographical areas is 8% (95% confidence interval 3%-13%), this difference would be significant at the 95% level.

BIAS

Bias is nonrandom error (literally, 'deviation from the truth'). In order to make valid comparisons between groups, researchers need to be as sure as possible that those being compared only differ in either their exposure or their outcome. If there are other important differences between the groups, the validity of the results is questionable. Statistical tests cannot help to eliminate the effect of bias from study results. A very large study can still be a very biased study. It is always important to consider whether biases have influenced a study's results.

Many forms of bias can generate spurious results. Consider an investigation of the influence of birthplace on newborn outcomes, which finds a higher incidence of perinatal mortality in consultant-led obstetric units than in general practitioner–led maternity units. So, is it safer to have a baby in a general practitioner–led unit? It is much more likely that, because of their special expertise and facilities, obstetrician-led units select higher-risk cases to deliver. This is an example of *selection bias*, and it can affect many study designs, but is most problematic for case–control designs. It occurs when groups are selected to take part in a study (or different parts of a study) in a systematically different manner.

The other main form of bias is *information* or *observation bias*. This occurs when there is inaccurate recording of information. For example, it may occur as a result of participants' recall of past disease exposures (*recall bias*), or if those carrying out the study record or measure information inaccurately.

CONFOUNDING

Confounding describes the situation in which an association between two variables is observed, but a third factor is also related to both. For example, consider a study showing an association between coffee intake and lung cancer. Taken at face value, this may seem to indicate that coffee causes lung cancer. In fact, the result is explained by a third variable – smoking. Smoking is associated both with increased coffee consumption (people who smoke drink more coffee) and with lung cancer. In this example, smoking is a *confounding factor*, otherwise known as a *confounder*.

In randomized controlled studies (described fully later), confounders are unlikely to play a part in the results, as they should be randomly and evenly distributed between groups. In observational studies, it may not be possible to do this. Instead, known confounders can be *controlled for* using various different design and analytical techniques. This simply means taking account of, or adjusting for, confounders in the analysis. Results may be presented as a simple relative risk or odds ratio, or these may be converted into an *adjusted* measure of association, which presents the measure of association adjusted for confounding factors. Age and gender almost always confound associations between exposures and health outcomes, and almost every study controls for these. Randomized controlled trials have the considerable advantage that they control for both known and unknown confounding factors, whereas observational studies can generally only control for confounding factors that are known about.

Even when an association is brought to light by a well-designed study, free of bias and confounding factors, it cannot be simply concluded that the relationship between exposure and disease is one of cause and effect.

The next question is, how likely is it that this exposure has caused the disease? Is the association in fact causal? A decision on this is not a snap judgement; it is a process

as rigorous as the study that made the finding in the first place. The best established set of criteria are those set out by the British statistician Sir Austin Bradford-Hill (1897–1991). These, in modified form, are

1. *Plausibility*: It fits the known pathology of the disease.
2. *Consistency*: It persists when studies carried out by different investigators, in different populations and at different times find the same.
3. *Temporal relationship*: The factor precedes in time the development of the disease.
4. *Strength of association*: There is a much higher frequency of disease in those who have the risk factor than in those who do not.
5. *Dose–response relationship*: An additional piece of evidence that is strongly indicative of causality is the presence of a dose–response relationship: with increasingly greater exposure to the risk factor, the incidence of the disease rises.
6. *Specificity*: The postulated causal factor is related to the disease being studied and no other. This cannot be a deciding matter since a factor may be causally related to more than one disease.
7. *Change in risk factor*: If the factor is removed or reduced, then the incidence of the disease falls.
8. *Alternative explanations*: Other explanations have been thoroughly considered and excluded.
9. *Coherence*: The association is consistent with existing scientific knowledge in this field.

Intervention studies (including randomized controlled trials)

OUTLINE OF METHODOLOGY

The randomized controlled trial is very different to the other epidemiological study designs. It has an *experimental* design. It is not based on analysing *observed* events that happen to people or populations. Instead, it involves analysing the impact of a planned *action* on particular health outcomes in groups of people or populations. In public health studies, the action is usually a preventive intervention – intended to stop a disease occurring, slow a disease's progression, detect a disease in its early stage, modify a risk factor or alter behaviour, for example. In clinical studies, most randomized controlled trials evaluate the effect of a treatment. Whether used in public health or clinical research, the principles involved in planning and conducting this type of study are very similar.

The main study design feature is that those carrying out the investigation do not decide who will be offered the intervention and who will not. This is done by a process of random allocation within a selected study population, in such a way that each participant has an equal chance of receiving the intervention or not receiving it. The latter is termed the *control group*. The outcomes between these groups are compared, to assess effectiveness of the intervention.

If this random allocation is preserved and combined with other features, such as *blinding* (maintaining the lack of knowledge of which group a participant belongs to – the intervention or control group), then the study design should avoid the biases and risks of confounding that cannot always be adequately controlled in observational studies.

SELECTION AND DEFINITION OF THE INTERVENTION, CONTROL AND STUDY OUTCOMES

In most cases, the intervention being tested by a randomized controlled trial is clear. However, when such studies are used to assess more complex interventions – such as educational or community-based interventions – specifying the exact nature of the intervention can be quite difficult. It is essential to do so if it is to be replicated accurately both within and after the study.

The outcomes being assessed must also be defined and measurable, with as little inter- or intra-observer variation as possible, and with the same level of accuracy between control and intervention groups. The aim of many trials in public health is to reduce mortality or morbidity, or to modify a risk factor or health-related behaviour. Most trials do not have mortality as an endpoint. To be a useful endpoint, it needs to occur with sufficient frequency within the experimental population to generate enough events to analyse. Often, shorter-term outcomes are used in trials, even when the ultimate study aim is to discover whether the intervention reduces mortality.

The simplest trial design involves two groups: those who receive the intervention and those who do not. The intervention that the control group will receive must also be determined. It is often standard current practice. In clinical trials of therapies, it can be a dummy treatment (*placebo*). Ideally, to reduce bias, the investigator assessing the outcome should not know whether the subject of the assessment was in the intervention or control group. This is easier to achieve in a clinical trial where one group of patients receives a tablet with the active ingredient being studied and the control group receives a look-alike tablet with no active ingredient (placebo). This approach is called *blinding*. Using a placebo also controls for the *placebo effect*: the change in a patient's outcome or health status achieved simply by being given an inactive therapy or through being a participant in a study. Designing these features into a randomized controlled trial of a public health intervention is much more difficult. It helps, though, if the outcome is something that can be objectively measured, rather than being a judgement by a human observer.

SELECTION OF THE STUDY POPULATION

The study or experimental population is derived from a *base population*. This is the group of people to whom the investigators expect the results of the trial to be applicable. The population could be unrestricted or restricted. For example, it could be restricted to boys between 5 and 10 years. The extent of restriction determines the generalizability of the results. For example, the effectiveness of an obesity reduction programme in boys of that age could not be assumed to achieve the same outcome in other age groups or in girls.

RANDOMIZATION

Consent and eligibility must be established before study participants are randomized to the intervention or control group. Failure to do so may introduce bias, because people with certain characteristics may only consent to take part, or be deemed eligible by staff, if they were due to receive the intervention. In such circumstances, the results of the trial may not completely reflect those that would have been obtained from a complete sample of the base population. Collecting data on those who were eligible but did not consent to participate may give information on how generalizable the findings are.

Once eligibility and consent are obtained, those who are taking part are randomized to treatment or control groups. A well-designed study gives everyone an equal chance of ending up in either of the groups. The statistical tests to evaluate the role of chance in producing the study results can then be interpreted to assess the effect size of a given intervention.

Randomization involves generating a random sequence, which must be concealed from those enrolling participants into the trial. The random sequence can be carried out using random number tables or through computer-generated random sequences. Some studies use block randomization, in which the randomization takes place within blocks of specified sizes, so that the numbers in each block are the same. There are other more complex approaches to randomization.

The intervention decisions are usually put in sealed, opaque envelopes. It is known that some practitioners may try to discern what is in the envelope by shining a light on it, perhaps because they feel that the person with them should receive the intervention rather than be a control. An alternative process of allocation is to require the person applying the intervention to telephone through to a trial centre to be told which group that the participant must be placed in.

FOLLOW-UP AND ANALYSIS

Clear study rules must govern how the outcomes for the patients in the two groups of the trial are defined, assessed and recorded. The outcomes (or endpoints) that are the subject of the investigation will vary according to its aims but might include (in a preventive trial) the onset of disease; death; change in physical or physiological characteristics, such as weight, serum cholesterol or fitness; or (in a trial of a new therapy) improvement or worsening in a patient's condition or length of survival.

In addition to blinding those assessing outcomes, it is important to try to minimize dropout rates and noncompliance. Both may introduce biases in results. There is a difference between people dropping out of the intervention and still being followed up and people pulling out of the study completely (or being lost to follow-up) so that there are no follow-up data. In the former group, the preferred approach is to do an intention-to-treat analysis, according to the randomized group to which they were originally allocated; in the latter, this is not possible.

Most measures reported in randomized controlled trials are the same as those reported for the study types already described. One additional measure that arises particularly in randomized controlled trials is the *number needed to treat* (NNT). This reports the number of people who must be given the intervention under study in order for one life to be saved. The calculation is made by comparing mortality in the intervention and control groups. For example, aspirin is an effective treatment for myocardial infarction. But not everybody who is treated with aspirin lives, and neither does everybody who is not given aspirin die. The studies have shown that for every 25 people treated with aspirin, 1 more person survives. This is the number needed to treat. When an intervention causes harm, rather than benefit, an equivalent calculation can be made of the *number needed to harm* (NNH).

In order to justify carrying out a randomized controlled trial, which is both time-consuming and expensive, it is necessary to establish that it will answer a useful and valid question and that it is ethical. There are many dimensions to this, but a starting point is that there must be genuine *equipoise*, a real uncertainty about the effectiveness of an intervention that justifies exposing people to it or depriving them of it. In the conduct of a study involving human populations, a strict ethical code must be obeyed. A number of organizations have laid down codes of practice or guidelines for the conduct of research investigations involving people. Of particular importance are those that have been produced by the Helsinki Declaration (1964), the World Health Organization and the Royal College of Physicians of London.

Within the NHS is a network of research ethics committees (RECs) to which application must be made for approval of research to be undertaken on NHS patients or for use of their records or NHS premises in the area. The National Research Ethics Service manages these committees, training their members, providing ethical guidance and promoting consistency of approach across England. It also provides information on the relevant national and European legislation, most recently the European Clinical Trials Regulation of 2014.

The committees satisfy themselves that due regard has been taken for the safety of the participants in a study, that proper arrangements for consent are in place, that appropriate information on the trial and its aims is available for participants and that the trial is scientifically valid – capable of coming to conclusions and likely to yield important information that could not be obtained by other means.

EXAMPLE OF A RANDOMIZED CONTROLLED TRIAL IN PUBLIC HEALTH: ABDOMINAL AORTIC ANEURYSM SCREENING

The United Kingdom now has a population screening programme using ultrasound examination to detect abdominal aortic aneurysm in older men. A number of randomized controlled trials in North America, the United Kingdom and other countries have been carried out to assess whether such a programme saves sufficient lives to be justifiable (the full criteria for justifying screening are described in Chapter 4, on non-communicable diseases).

One population-based study involved a sample of men aged 65–74 years recruited from four centres in the United Kingdom and randomized to receive an invitation to screening (invited group) or not (control group). Randomization was conducted centrally using computer-generated random numbers, stratified by centre and general practice. Aortic diameter was measured using ultrasonography. Men with an aortic diameter of 3 cm or greater were diagnosed with abdominal aortic aneurysm. Among this group, those with smaller increases in diameter were followed up and regularly reassessed. Those with larger diameter, evidence of expansion or symptoms were considered for surgery. The occurrences of rupture, deaths due to the aneurysm and deaths due to other causes were identified in as many people in the sample as possible. Overall, the risk of abdominal aortic aneurysm–related mortality and rupture was almost halved (Table 2.12). There was also a small reduction in all-cause mortality. The authors of the study estimated that the number needed to be invited to screening to save one abdominal aortic aneurysm–related death over 13 years was 216; they noted that this was better than for breast cancer.

Some variations of the design, such as cluster randomized controlled trials, also exist. Cluster trials entail individuals being randomized in groups (e.g. whole villages or whole schools may be randomized to a treatment group – the unit of randomization is the village or school) and can be used for a variety of reasons (including cost limitations). The types of intervention assessed by clustered trials include public health campaigns (in which exposure cannot be limited to some people but not others within an area). They can also help with issues of 'contamination' – where participants may be affected by the intervention even if they do not receive it directly themselves. For example, whole villages may be randomized to receive vaccination for an infectious disease. The statistical analysis must take account of this clustering.

QUALITATIVE RESEARCH AND MIXED METHODS

Epidemiology is largely concerned with numbers and their interpretation. It is a quantitative science. Among its many strands of activity, public health is concerned with the way

Table 2.12 Results of a randomized controlled trial of abdominal aortic aneurysm (AAA) screening

	Control group (n = 33,887)	Invited-to-screening group (n = 33,883)
Person-years of follow-up	350,800	353,100
AAA-related deaths	381	224
Hazard ratio (95% CI)	1.00 (reference)	0.58 (0.49–0.69)
Ruptured AAA	476	273
Hazard ratio (95% CI)	1.00 (reference)	0.57 (0.49–0.66)

Source: Thompson SG, Ashton HA, Gao L, Buxton MJ, Scott RA. Final follow-up of the Multicentre Aneurysm Screening Study (MASS) randomized trial of abdominal aortic aneurysm screening. British Journal of Surgery 2012;99(12):1649-56.

that people behave as individuals; the way that people in groups behave, interact and respond to social and economic influences; and the way that people's attitudes, beliefs and values relating to health and disease are formed in childhood and play out in adult life. These are important questions for public health policymaking and practice, but they cannot be explored satisfactorily by analysing routine data or conducting epidemiological studies. The disciplines necessary to address them are in fields like the social sciences, behavioural sciences and anthropology. Their methods are qualitative rather than quantitative.

More and more studies that appear in journals reporting on the health of groups and populations have used what has become known as *mixed methods*. This simply means that the study design has used both qualitative and quantitative approaches.

SYSTEMATIC REVIEW AND META-ANALYSIS

The epidemiological study methods described in the previous sections mostly involve analysing routine data or collecting data for a study from scratch and, for that reason, can be thought of as *primary research*. Studies that use data that other investigators have collected and analysed are usually regarded as *secondary research*. This approach is used *par excellence* in the field of public health history, for example, examining different published accounts of epidemic disease at various points in the past.

A particular type of secondary research is a vital analytical tool of modern public health. Systematic reviews are a rigorous and balanced assessment of evidence from individual studies. They are essentially a 'study of studies'. The topics and study types included in systematic reviews are varied, but the fundamental building blocks of the process are the same. Essentially, published studies are brought together in a systematic manner to present a comprehensive and nonbiased view of research in a particular field. These reviews are the basis of much of the evidence-based

guidelines for practice or the evidential underpinning of policymaking. This is certainly the case in clinical medicine, where evidence-based medicine is regarded as a core component of good practice. It is not so straightforward in public health, where published systematic reviews based on randomized controlled trials (the gold standard for clinical evidence) are fewer in number. Systematic reviews are also available for more social interventions from the Campbell systematic review database.

The Cochrane Collaboration, founded in 1992, is the main global digital repository for high-quality systematic reviews undertaken by experts in a wide range of fields. Many systematic reviews are also published in peer-reviewed journals. There are thousands of systematic reviews of many diverse areas and interventions.

Systematic reviews are now a study type in their own right. They can be done well or badly, they can be biased and they can be flawed in other methodological ways. There are guidelines for ensuring high-quality methods covering literature search strategies, how to decide which studies to include, rules for combining results from different studies and procedure for presenting and reporting results.

The results from the studies can be presented by either a narrative analysis or a statistical meta-analysis. A narrative analysis describes effect size of the studies, but does not make an attempt to estimate an average effect size because this is either not possible (e.g. because of how the data are presented) or not appropriate because the interventions or study populations are too different, such that an 'average' effect does not make sense.

A meta-analysis statistically pools data from all the studies. It generates a weighted average of the study results (giving more weight to larger studies) to estimate a single result.

The benefit of a meta-analysis is not simply that it generates an average from several different study results. It can also often provide a more precise result (i.e. with a small confidence interval) than any of the individual studies can. This is because it uses information from a greater number of people, therefore reducing the impact of chance variation.

Meta-analysis has two major difficulties. First, its validity depends on the similarity (homogeneity) of the studies that it combines. If the studies involve different interventions or different populations from one another, the result is less meaningful and can even be meaningless. Second, it can only include studies that the researchers are aware of. The phenomenon of *publication bias* means that studies with positive results are more likely to be published in a journal – and therefore found by such researchers – than those that do not find a positive result. When published studies are combined in a meta-analysis, this can therefore erroneously indicate a more positive finding than is actually the case.

GENETIC EPIDEMIOLOGY

The burgeoning field of genetic epidemiology applies the techniques of epidemiology to study the role of genes, and genetics, in health and disease. Sequencing a person's entire genome – some 3 billion DNA base pairs, containing more than 20,000 protein-encoding genes – is becoming quicker and more affordable with every passing year. In genetic-based studies, a person's genes are effectively his or her exposure to the risk of disease, and the traits or diseases that he or she is known to have are the outcome. Such studies therefore examine the association between these exposures and outcomes within families, or across entire population groups.

Although genetic sequencing is a modern technology, the fundamentals of epidemiology that were developed well before its inception are being successfully applied to analyse the data that it yields. Genome-wide association studies, for example, are essentially retrospective case–control studies. In their simplest form, they compare the frequency with which certain genetic markers (single-nucleotide polymorphisms) are found among people known to have a particular disease (the cases) with the frequency in which the same genetic markers are found among those without the disease (the controls). These studies can therefore suggest which genes, and which variants of those genes, are associated with the disease.

So-called *biobanks* have been set up in a number of different countries, including the United Kingdom, Iceland, Canada, Estonia, and the Kingdom of Tonga. These studies take baseline tissue and blood samples that can be used later for genetic analysis. Further data on medical history, lifestyle and environment are gathered on each individual. Over time, as diseases occur the details are recorded. This rich source of information then allows the exploration of individual susceptibility to disease and the interplay of genetic factors, behaviour and environment.

APPLICATION OF EPIDEMIOLOGY

In 1957, Professor Jerry Morris (1910–2009), of the London School of Hygiene and Tropical Medicine, published what was to become a classic in public health. His book, *Uses of Epidemiology*, went through four editions. It was groundbreaking because, for the first time, it showed how the rigour of epidemiology as a science could be harnessed for practical benefit in explaining population health, in understanding what the data were showing and in searching for ways to achieve beneficial health change.

Not all of Morris's seven uses are widely deployed today, but they still bear serious attention as the founding principles of applied epidemiology. They are:

1. To study the history of the health of a population
2. To diagnose the health of a community and the condition of the people
3. To estimate from group experience individual risks and ways to avoid them
4. To identify syndromes
5. To complete the clinical picture of chronic diseases and describe their natural history
6. To search for causes
7. To study the working of health services

The major epidemiological methodologies (randomized controlled trials, cohort studies and case–control studies) are infrequently used in day-to-day public health practice (aside from the use of the case–control method in the investigation of infectious disease outbreaks). However, the classical designs must be understood in order to evaluate the published work of others. This is especially important if decisions about healthcare priorities and programmes are to be based on such studies.

In everyday public health practice, there are many questions that arise that need data or analysis to answer them. The results are often required quickly to inform a decision, to enable a policy to be formulated or to help design a public health programme. It is seldom feasible or affordable to initiate a formal epidemiological study. There is a great deal of misunderstanding about this area of public health practice. First, this field of investigation is not really debated and certainly is not the subject of texts, such as those written about case–control and cohort studies, which deal with methodologies in depth. Second, health service problem investigation is sometimes seen as flawed or unscientific, particularly by epidemiological researchers. Third, the investigation of a health service problem usually leads to a report that is presented to a health service policymaking board or used as an aid to decision-making at an operational level. All energies are usually deployed to this end, and it is less common for the investigator to set aside the time to write up a study separately for submission to a journal. This process works against practical investigations gaining the respectability that they often deserve.

The approach of investigators based in academic institutions is very different. A report will always be produced (or internally published) for the funding body, but major emphasis will also be placed on identifying those aspects of the study that can be submitted to journals. This will often result in a publication in a peer-reviewed journal, all of which adds to the standing of this type of investigative work.

This debate is epitomized by the phrase used to describe investigations within the public health service: 'quick and dirty'. As with any catchphrase, it is easy to see why it has gained widespread usage, but the juxtaposition of the terms 'quick and dirty' when applied to any form of *bona fide* public health investigation is both inappropriate and unfortunate. The term 'dirty' is intended to convey the impression of crudeness or unreliability in either the study methods used or the findings. It is only necessary to think of a cohort study of disease causation, taking many years to carry out, with consequent consumption of resources, having had a seriously flawed design at the outset to realize that 'dirtiness' can equally apply to large-scale investigation using methods traditionally associated with scientific purity.

The importance of this issue cannot be overemphasized, because it draws attention to fundamental principles that should apply equally to the investigation of a circumscribed and urgent problem in a health service as to the study of possible risk factors for the genesis of a disease that poses a large-scale public health problem.

Whether using routinely available data on an *ad hoc* and limited data-gathering exercise, conducting a population survey or conducting a case–control or cohort study, the investigator should have a clear view of the aims of the investigation and the questions that need to be answered by it. He or she should choose the appropriate method to carry out the investigation (bearing in mind the prevailing constraints, including time and money). He or she should be aware of the strengths and weaknesses of the approach chosen and, most importantly, should present the findings of the study in a way that makes clear the extent of the conclusions that can be drawn from them. Thus, some studies are more limited in scope than others because of time constraints, the availability of resources or the quality of available data. Even in such circumstances, good investigations can still be carried out, provided that it is made clear precisely what conclusions can be drawn from them (bearing in mind the limitations of the data). This does not make them dirty.

Table 2.13 Some reasons for carrying out a public health investigation

Assessing health needs
Describing a problem
Searching for causes
Identifying areas for improvement
Evaluating new and existing services
Planning service responses
Pointing to scope for prevention
Assisting resource allocation decisions
Defining characteristics of a population

Decisions about health service priorities and the allocation of resources are being made on a daily basis and, sadly, too often on purely subjective grounds. Even a limited investigation, if carefully carried out, potentially can improve the quality of decision-making. Some practical pointers to the use of public health investigations are shown in Table 2.13.

CONCLUSIONS

This chapter has described important building blocks of public health practice, namely, the study methodologies and investigative approaches used for classical epidemiological studies and how these approaches can be modified to solve everyday public health problems. It has also described sources of routine data that may be used to throw light on these problems. The practice of clinical medicine is often compared to a series of detective stories in which the clues to the diagnosis of a patient's clinical problem are investigated. In population medicine, the mysteries of health and disease in entire populations, some extremely complex, are also very challenging. The benefits of solving these problems in delaying death, preventing disease and improving the quality of healthcare are enormous. To develop the analogy, while the clinical detective is pursuing the ordinary criminal, the public health investigator is on the trail of the godfathers of syndicated crime.

CHAPTER 3

Communicable diseases

INTRODUCTION

Ask a group of people in a high-income country today what disease they most fear, and they are likely to say cancer, dementia or perhaps stroke. They are unlikely to name an infection. This is a very modern phenomenon. From the dawn of human existence until the twentieth century, infectious disease was what people rightly feared.

Schoolchildren learn about the Black Death (plague) that swept across medieval England killing millions of people. This terrifying disease is thought to have cut the global population from 450 million to 375 million. Historical accounts of the Great War often cover what followed it – an influenza virus that spread globally in 1918–19. The Spanish flu infected 20% of the world's population and killed 40 million to 50 million people (more than died during the war itself). The threat of death from consumption (tuberculosis) was never far from mind throughout the nineteenth century and well into the twentieth. As recently as the 1980s, polio paralyzed a quarter of a million children every year worldwide.

Down the centuries, public health interventions have improved human health in many ways, but two stand out: sanitation and vaccination. In comparison with modern medical technologies, each is remarkably simple. Yet, each has been highly effective in reducing the harm that communicable disease brings to the human population, and each is more cost-effective than any other health intervention. Many would add a third to the list, although its impact is more curative than preventive: the advent of antibiotics, from the time of the Second World War.

In 1901, communicable diseases in England killed 369 people in every 100,000. By 2000, that figure was 2 per 100,000. The Global Burden of Disease study has estimated that, in 1990, 47% of all ill health globally (measured in disability-adjusted life years) was caused by communicable disease. By 2010, this had been reduced to 35%. Over the same period, the under-five mortality rate fell by 70% – again, mostly because of reductions in communicable disease.

But the story of infectious disease is not yet at an end – far from it. It remains a story of inequity between the richest countries of the world and the poorest. Globally, the top three causes of death at the beginning of the second decade of the twenty-first century were heart disease, stroke and chronic respiratory disease. In sub-Saharan Africa, the top four causes were malaria, pneumonia, human immunodeficiency virus (HIV)/acquired immune deficiency syndrome (AIDS) and diarrhoeal disease. In the world's poorest countries, tuberculosis kills more than 1 million people in a year. There are also many so-called neglected tropical diseases – infections that cause serious illness, disability and sometimes death to people living in poor, tropical countries. Their access to treatment is often weak or absent.

In the 1960s and 1970s, improvement had been so rapid that some started to believe that the threat from infectious disease would indeed be gone. In the 1960s, U.S. Surgeon General William Stewart was so buoyed by optimism that he commented, 'It is time to close the book on infectious diseases, and declare the war against pestilence won'. This has been quoted extensively in the decades that followed. Recently, the attribution to Stewart has been challenged, as no one can find the primary source in a publication or a speech. Nevertheless, there is no doubt that the late 1960s and early 1970s was an era of great confidence about the conquest of communicable disease. This was misplaced. The battle between humankind and microbes – organisms that have survived and evolved over billions of years – continues to rage. Dozens of new infections have emerged – including HIV, severe acute respiratory syndrome (SARS), Lassa fever and the influenza A (H1N1) virus that caused a pandemic in 2009. In 2014, the Ebola virus, which causes an infection with a particularly high fatality rate, threatened whole countries in Africa and thousands died. Previous outbreaks of the disease had affected only villages in that continent and been controlled relatively quickly. As international travel becomes ever more commonplace, so the spread of infectious disease hastens. In early 2016, the director general of the World Health Organization invoked the International Health Regulations to declare the emergence of *Zika virus* in the Americas, with associated clusters of

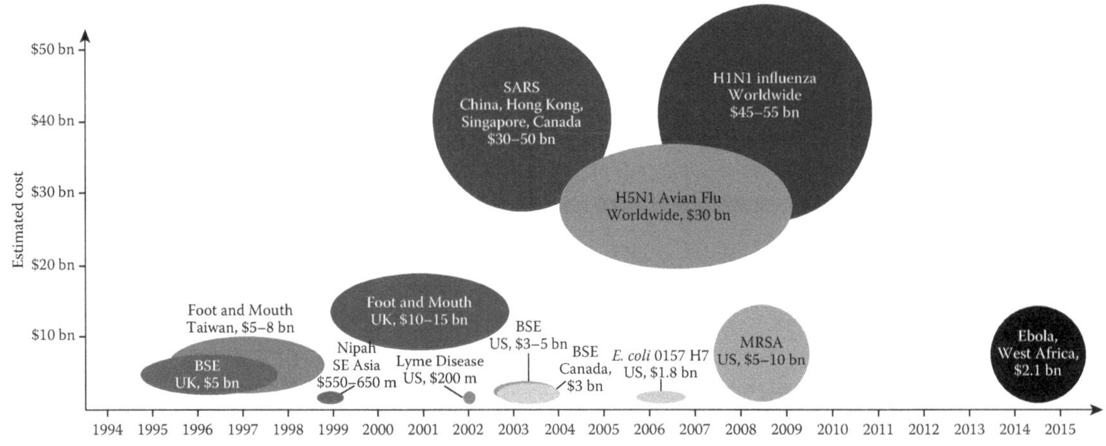

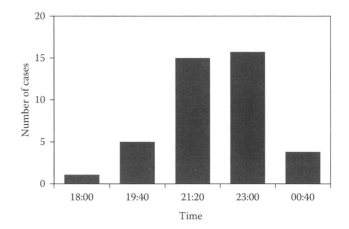

Figure 3.1 Recent communicable disease outbreaks and their economic cost.

Source: World Bank (Ebola); Newcomb J. *SARS and the New Economics of Biosecurity.* Cambridge: Bio Economic Research Associates, 2009.

neurological disease and babies born with microcephaly, as a public health emergency of international concern.

As some infections are conquered, others emerge. Some go into abeyance only to later pose a new threat in drug-resistant forms. Barely a year passes without some major outbreak making the headlines (Figure 3.1). Mother nature has the recipe book, and the world can be certain that there will be new and unexpected threats when she starts to cook.

ESSENTIALS OF COMMUNICABLE DISEASE

Knowledge and skills in observing the passage of infections through populations, and ways to control their spread, have been a feature of public health practice since late Victorian times. The fundamental concepts are largely unchanged.

An *endemic* infection is one that is constantly present in a given geographical area. It circulates in a continuous and steady manner. If it increases rapidly, it is no longer endemic and can be termed an outbreak or an epidemic.

An *outbreak* of infectious disease occurs when the incidence of the infection is greater than would be expected at that time in that place. It is a relative term. Ten cases of measles in a population with high vaccine coverage and no recent cases of measles would be an outbreak, whereas 300 cases of the common cold would not. Similarly, hundreds of cases of influenza in a town in the winter would be at about the expected level, and so would be thought of as endemic rather than an outbreak. In contrast, that number of influenza cases in the same place over the summer months would be an outbreak. Dozens of cases of malaria in a city in West Africa is likely to be endemic, but the same number of cases in a village near Heathrow airport in London would certainly be an outbreak. It would lead to an investigation into whether airport employees had been infected (perhaps by a mosquito from an endemic area surviving on a long-haul flight).

Figure 3.2 Point source outbreak.

The term *epidemic* is also used to describe numbers of cases of a communicable disease that are in excess of the endemic level in the population concerned. An epidemic is a rise over time in cases of a particular illness, clearly above the endemic level, in a defined area or region. It can take different forms that are usually evident if a graph is plotted of cases of the illness against time. A *point source epidemic* is when everyone who is infected catches the infection at the same time from a common source. The cases peak and then fall as there is no further exposure. This typically occurs with outbreaks of food poisoning (Figure 3.2). Sometimes, though, the source stays broadly the same and people continue to be exposed to it over time. This is a *continuous epidemic.* Figure 3.3 shows the number of confirmed cases of hepatitis E in England and Wales increasing with most infections coming from pork sausages or other pork foodstuffs. It was estimated that 1 in 10 sausages contained the virus, and people were advised that they should be cooked until caramelized. This is an example of a continuous, rather than a point source, epidemic because the source of infection was not eliminated and continued to cause

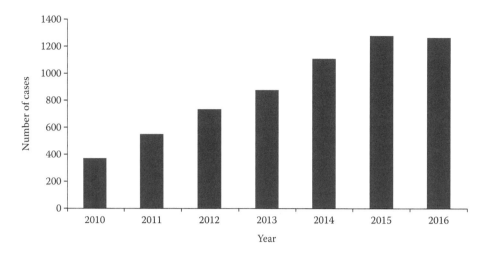

Figure 3.3 Confirmed cases of Hepatitis E in England and Wales.

Source: Public Health England.

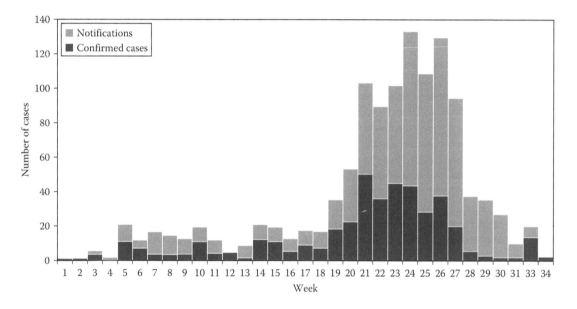

Figure 3.4 Epidemic curve of a propagated measles epidemic in Wales, November 2012 to June 2013.

Source: Public Health Wales. *Outbreak of Measles in Wales Nov 2012 – July 2013.* Cardiff: Public Health Wales; 2013.

infection. Hepatitis E can cause very serious liver damage but usually causes an unpleasant, prolonged flu-like illness with jaundice. Ultimately, the solution lies mainly with better animal husbandry. A third pattern is the *propagated epidemic* where transmission is prolonged by person-to-person spread. Many communicable diseases can produce this kind of epidemic. It stops when there are no more susceptible people, or when it is stopped by targeted vaccination or other control measures. An example is the upsurge of measles in Wales that occurred because too many children were left susceptible by not having their scheduled course of MMR vaccinations in early childhood. This situation was created by the parents' belief in the now discredited research that linked the vaccine to autism. The lowest MMR coverage was in Swansea and the surrounding region where, at

the time, one in six children aged 11 years were unprotected. The propagated epidemic of measles (Figure 3.4) was slowly brought under control by a catch-up vaccination programme.

The term *epidemic* is much less commonly used than it used to be. The pattern of disease it describes could usually just as easily be called an outbreak. In fact, the former surgeon general of the United States, David Satcher, reflecting on his time as director of the Centers for Disease Control and Prevention (CDC), used the two terms synonymously (emphasis added): 'I was called upon to send a team of public health workers to Zaire to fight an Ebola *outbreak*. We along with colleagues from WHO were successful in ending that *epidemic*'.

The exact reason that the historically established term *epidemic* has largely been replaced in day-to-day parlance by *outbreak* is not clear. It does seem, though, that the use of *epidemic* is more likely to generate newspaper headlines and cause public alarm, and this may be why modern public health authorities seldom use it.

The fear factor arising from the term *pandemic* is much more clear-cut. Technically, a pandemic is an epidemic that rapidly spreads to infect people in most parts of the world. However, the first mention of a pandemic will hit the 24-hour news bulletins, and tends to be seen in the public mind as something severe that threatens them and their families directly. Recent pandemics – SARS and influenza A(H1N1) pdm09 virus – have been controversial because the timing and tone of the World Health Organization's announcements that a pandemic state existed created drama and anticipation. There was a political dimension too, as the declaration of a pandemic had positive financial implications for vaccine and antiviral drug manufacturers, and a negative financial impact on some countries' tourist industry.

This all goes to show that, having once been a quiet professional backwater, communicable disease control is now firmly in the public and political arena.

Eradication is the penultimate goal of infectious disease control: a situation when an infection's global incidence is reduced to zero, and no prevention and control measures are necessary to keep it that way. Only one human infection has so far been eradicated – smallpox, in 1980. However, it is not *extinct* because the governments of Russia and the United States retain samples of the virus under secure conditions. Current eradication campaigns are aimed at polio and Guinea worm disease. The ultimate goal is *extinction*, when the infectious agent would no longer exist in the environment, in any living host or in a laboratory. However, these ideal states currently are in the realm of futurology. For very few communicable diseases can eradication even be contemplated, and therefore a varying state of disease control exists (Table 3.1).

Infectious agents

Bacteria, viruses, protozoa, helminthes and fungi cause most of the communicable diseases. These infectious agents generally have two parts to their proper name. The first is the *genus* of the organism and is written with an upper-case letter at the start; the second is the name of its *species* and starts with a lower-case letter. By convention, these proper names are italicized.

Bacteria are single, living cells, able to replicate themselves. Many are beneficial and essential to life. They are present everywhere on the planet and predate human life by billions of years. Some cause illness, for example, cholera (caused by the bacterium *Vibrio cholera*), typhoid (*Salmonella typhi*), tuberculosis (*Mycobacterium tuberculosis*) and whooping cough (*Bordetella pertussis*). *Viruses* are simpler and smaller in structure. A virus is a not living cell but a piece of genetic material, protected by a protein coat. Viruses invade human (or other host) cells and commandeer those cells' genetic machinery to replicate. Viral illnesses include the common cold, measles, mumps, rubella, chickenpox, polio and AIDS. In contrast, *protozoa* are single-celled organisms but are more complex in structure than bacteria and usually replicate through clearly defined life cycles. Amoebic dysentery is a protozoal illness caused by *Entamoeba histolytica*. Others include malaria and *Giardia*. *Helminthes* are multicellular organisms that cause illness. This group of infectious organisms, roundworms and flatworms, affects more than 2 billion people worldwide. Most fungal infections, such as *Candida* (thrush), are mild and not life threatening except in circumstances where immunity is impaired, but some, such as aspergillosis (caused by an opportunistic fungus, with 40 species of the *Aspergillus* genus), cause disease, mainly of the lungs, that can be much more serious. *Prions* are the most recently discovered of all the infectious agents, and the least well understood. They appear to initiate abnormal protein folding within cells. The best-known prion disease is bovine spongiform encephalopathy (BSE), a fatal illness of cattle (known colloquially as Mad Cow Disease) that crossed the species barrier in the mid-1990s to cause variant Creutzfeldt–Jakob disease, a devastating new human disease.

Classifications

There are three traditional ways of classifying communicable diseases. The first is *clinical*, in which the symptoms, signs or body system is the basis for grouping the

Table 3.1 States of disease control

Control: The reduction of disease incidence, prevalence, morbidity or mortality to a locally acceptable level as a result of deliberate efforts; continued intervention measures are required to maintain the reduction. Example: diarrhoeal diseases.

Elimination of disease: Reduction to zero of the incidence of a specified disease in a defined geographical area as a result of deliberate efforts; continued intervention measures are required. Example: neonatal tetanus.

Elimination of infections: Reduction to zero of the incidence of infection caused by a specific agent in a defined geographical area as a result of deliberate efforts; continued measures to prevent re-establishment of transmission are required. Example: measles, poliomyelitis.

Eradication: Permanent reduction to zero of the worldwide incidence of infection caused by a specific agent as a result of deliberate efforts; intervention measures are no longer needed. Example: smallpox.

Extinction: The specific infectious agent no longer exists in nature or in the laboratory. Example: none.

Source: Dowdle WR, Hopkins DR. *The eradication of infectious diseases: report of the Dahlem Workshop on the Eradication of Infectious Diseases.* Chichester: John Wiley & Sons, 1998.

diseases together. Clinical classifications vary somewhat, but they use either general terminology, such as febrile illness, or categories referring to anatomical sites affected by the infection, such as respiratory infection, diarrhoeal disease and meningitis. The second approach is *microbiological*. This groups infections by the type of organism that causes them. Again, the precise categories vary, but a broad classification of diseases in this way would be bacterial, viral, protozoan, rickettsial, chlamydial, mycoplasmal, spirochaetal, helminthic and fungal. The third form of classification is *epidemiological*. This allocates infection to categories by mode of transmission: waterborne, foodborne, airborne and vector-borne.

Each of these approaches to classification serves a different purpose. The clinical classifications are concerned with understanding the impact of the disease on patients and establishing the approach to diagnosis and treatment. The microbiological classifications are very much about how the organism looks and behaves, what similarities and differences it has to other infective agents and how its pathogenic effects could be disabled. The epidemiological classifications direct attention to how the pathogen spreads, and therefore how the disease could be prevented or its transmission interrupted.

There are also taxonomies for microorganisms. A taxonomy is a little different to a classification system. It is a scientific process that looks for the common characteristics of the organisms and gives them names. For example, the International Committee on Taxonomy of Viruses has a very rigorous process, involving experts around the world, for naming and categorizing viruses in a way that is internationally agreed.

Developments in modern genetics are enabling the gene sequences of more and more microorganisms to be mapped. This will increase as more, better and cheaper techniques are found. Genomics allows the spread of infectious agents to be followed and analysed in a more sophisticated way, enables changes and mutations (and the mechanisms behind them) to be studied and opens up opportunities for vaccines and treatments.

The three frameworks described above (clinical, microbiological and epidemiological) are each comprehensive, in the sense that every infection has a particular place within each of them. There are many other ways of grouping communicable diseases that do not purport to be part of comprehensive classifications, but are still useful. For example, a commonly used category is the *new and emerging diseases*: the previously unrecognized bacteria, viruses, fungi or parasites that cause illness, outbreaks and even deaths. For the public, such events are often alarming because news of them initially brings uncertainty as to how the new infection could affect them or their community. Zika virus illustrates very well how a communicable disease with apparently stable clinical features and geographical distribution can suddenly develop into a perceived global threat. The infection, first described in the late 1940s, is not usually a severe illness; symptoms include fever, rash,

joint pain and conjunctivitis. For more than 50 years, it was largely confined to an area around the equator encompassing African and Asian countries. The virus belongs to the same family as the one that causes dengue fever and is carried by the same species of mosquitoes. In 2015, the infection was detected in South America and the Caribbean. In early 2016, there was great international concern when clusters of the birth abnormality microcephaly were apparently associated with maternal infection by Zika virus in Brazil. This led to the World Health Organization declaring an international public health emergency, and some countries issued advice to pregnant women not to travel to affected areas. Another adverse feature of the emergence of the virus was the occurrence of cases of the rare neurological condition Guillain–Barre syndrome. Zika virus is usually transmitted by mosquito bite but can also be acquired by sexual and blood-borne routes.

Many other communicable diseases are classified as *re-emerging*. They are diseases that have previously been controlled, but have then become re-established. Scarlet fever is a disease characterized by a severe sore throat infection and a prominent sunburn-like rash. It is caused by a particular group A *Streptococcus* (*Streptococcus pyogenes*). In the pre-antibiotic era, it affected a large number of children in the United Kingdom each year. Some died, and it caused serious illness in others (rheumatic fever and kidney disease are among its complications). It was much feared in earlier times. Two of Charles Darwin's children died of scarlet fever. Its pathogenicity reduced, and with the advent of penicillin, it all but disappeared as a serious threat to children's health in the twentieth century. It has re-emerged to cause some large outbreaks (Figure 3.5), and although generally mild, it is still capable of producing serious outcomes if not effectively treated.

There is no hard and fast rule about when an emerging disease ceases to be labelled as such. HIV was a classic example of an emerging disease when it was first recognized in the mid-1980s. It is still a major killer globally, but with the widespread use of effective antiretroviral treatment, it has increasingly become a chronic disease. For these reasons, we have not classified HIV as an emerging disease because we believe it is now endemic and established.

Some earlier texts contained classifications that were specific to the United Kingdom. They distinguished between diseases that could be acquired in the country and those that were imported. This approach has little meaning today because travel across international borders is so common that exposure to infectious agents is on a much greater scale. Moreover, a working knowledge of the global pattern of communicable disease is essential to understanding the way that organisms transmit and mutate, as well as the illnesses they cause.

In this chapter, specific communicable diseases are described in three broad categories: those that cause the greatest burden of mortality, those that cause large amounts of illness and disability (sometimes also death), and emerging and re-emerging diseases. Although we have chosen a

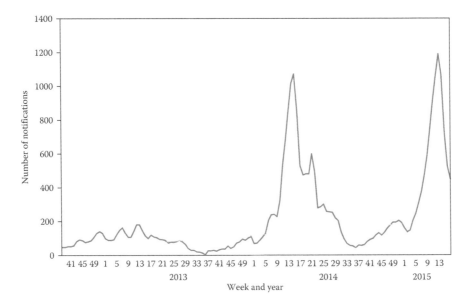

Figure 3.5 Notified cases of scarlet fever in England.

Source: Public Health England.

free-form classification in three parts, other communicable diseases are described throughout the chapter where they best illustrate key principles and concepts.

Reservoirs

A reservoir for a communicable disease is any person, animal, substance, plant, soil, arthropod or combination of these where the organism lives, multiplies and relies upon for survival, and from where it can infect a person, animal or arthropod vector. Reservoirs are essential for communicable diseases to persist. People or animals that are reservoirs are known as *infective hosts*. They harbour the organism, and from them, it is transmitted to another susceptible host, for example, animal to human or person to person. Some pathogens have human beings as their sole host (e.g. polio). Many, though, have reservoirs in animals and other sources. The *Salmonella* group of organisms is found in many domestic and wild animals. Brucellosis occurs in cattle, while leptospirosis is found in rats and other species. Many protozoa have reservoirs in wild or domestic animals, sometimes with insect vectors and complex life cycles involving several hosts. The rabies virus has its reservoir in wild dogs, cats, bats and other animals. The largest reservoir is in bats, but this is seldom the direct source of a human infection. Instead, the human infection usually comes from an intermediate host (dogs), which bites a human after having been bitten by a bat.

Routes of entry into and exit from the body

Each organism that infects a person must enter the body through one or more routes. It must later exit, again via one or more routes, in order to reach a new host. Entry to the body can be through the mouth into the gut, the mouth or nose into the bronchi and lungs, mucous membranes, eyes, genitals or a breach in the skin barrier (e.g. a mosquito bite or a contaminated needle). Exit can be by breathing out; coughing; sneezing; vomiting; defaecating; urinating; exuding fluid or serum from the gut, sexual organs, open wounds, pustules or other lesions; release of blood; or donation of organs or tissue.

When a disease agent infects someone, symptoms do not immediately follow. The interval between infection and onset of symptoms is the *incubation period*. Depending on the infectious agent, it can be as short as 30 minutes or, in extreme circumstances, as long as a few decades (e.g. kuru, a prion disease). For most infections, it is between 4 and 30 days. An individual infected with a particular organism does not necessarily pass the infection on to others. The period during which they are able to do so is known as the *infectious period*, and the period before this is the *latent period*.

Figure 3.6 shows an example of how these periods interrelate. They vary considerably between infectious agents, and between people infected with the same agent. They vary in duration and in the extent to which they overlap. One important characteristic of an infectious agent is whether the infectious period overlaps with the incubation period. If so, an individual can unwittingly transmit the infection to others before they are aware of being infected themselves. If all infectious agents produced recognizable symptoms before they became infectious, disease control would be more straightforward. In reality, most agents have an infectious period that starts before their symptomatic period – and so are unknowingly spread by their hosts.

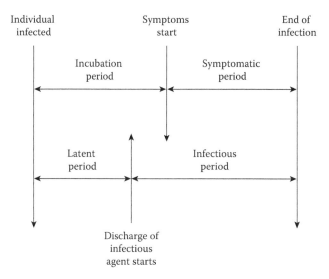

Figure 3.6 An example of an infectious course.

Modes of transmission

There are four main ways that infection transmits from one person to another.

Direct transmission involves transfer of microorganisms to the skin or mucous membranes by touching, biting, kissing or sexual intercourse. Diseases that spread in this way include scabies (touching), rabies (animal bites), glandular fever (kissing) and syphilis or HIV infection (sexual intercourse). Some infections spread directly from pregnant mothers to their babies (so-called vertical transmission), such as rubella and HIV infection.

Indirect transmission involves an intermediate stage between the source of infection and the individual. The infection may be vehicle-borne (e.g. in infected food or water), in soil (e.g. tetanus) or vector-borne (such as by insects). Malaria is an example of a vector-borne infection. The vector is a mosquito. Vehicle-borne infections include *Salmonella* and other organisms that cause food poisoning. Food is the vehicle here, but it can be many other things, such as children's toys in a nursery where there is a rotavirus outbreak, or a surface in a hospital that is colonized by methicillin-resistant *Staphylococcus aureus* (MRSA).

Droplet transmission occurs primarily when an infected person coughs or sneezes, spreading droplets to other people's noses, mouths or eyes. Measles is one such example.

Airborne transmission involves inhaling aerosols containing microorganisms. Smaller droplets can penetrate deep into the lungs. Whereas droplets are too large to be airborne for long, microorganisms in aerosols can remain suspended in the air for a substantial amount of time. Legionnaires' disease and tuberculosis are examples of infections spread by airborne transmission.

Organisms that infect people have evolved over long periods of time, over which period many have developed highly effective mechanisms for their ongoing propagation.

Viruses that make us cough cause themselves to be spread by airborne transmission. Viruses that cause diarrhoea give themselves more chance of being passed on to others in food or water. Malaria causes its hosts extreme fatigue. They lie still, lacking the energy to fight mosquitoes off from biting them, and so assisting in the vector-borne spread of the malaria parasite that has multiplied within their bloodstream.

Susceptible recipient

Not all people who come into contact with an infectious agent will become infected by it. Recipients of an infectious agent vary in their response. Some will quickly fight off the infection, while others will not and will become unwell. Whether a person develops an infectious disease after contact with any given causal agent is governed by many factors. These include:

- The virulence of the organism
- The dose of the organism on exposure
- Whether previously exposed or vaccinated
- Age
- Nutritional state
- The presence of other diseases
- Whether immunosuppressed (due to illness or therapy)
- Genetic factors

The spread of an infectious agent within a population, and its likely further transmission, can be estimated by mathematical modelling techniques that are growing in sophistication with the greater power of computing. A simple metric that is widely used in communicable disease control is the *basic reproductive number*, or R_0. It is the number of secondary cases that would occur in an entirely susceptible population in response to a single typical case of that particular infection. An R_0 of less than 1 means that transmission of the disease will eventually burn out. If it is greater than 1, then the disease is still spreading and more susceptible people will come down with it. A high value of the R_0 means, all else being equal, that the disease will spread more quickly. The main factors that influence the size of the basic reproductive number are the *infectivity* of the organism, that is, how likely it is that a susceptible person will become infected if exposed to a person who is infected; the *duration* of infectiveness; and the *number of susceptible people* that an infective case has contact with.

Investigation

Many situations can be triggers for a public health investigation: a sudden upsurge in the incidence of a particular disease, the clustering of several cases in a certain geographical area, the emergence of one or two cases of a very rare disease or unusual strain type or a call for help from a hotel after a large number of guests have developed diarrhoea and vomiting, for example. Broadly, such investigations involve five tasks:

1. To identify the infective agent
2. To identify the source and mode of transmission
3. To establish control measures to interrupt the chain of transmission
4. To prevent secondary spread
5. To give public health advice

The logical sequence of action in investigating an outbreak or epidemic is outlined in Figure 3.7. The first requirement is to collect as much information as possible about the disease and its characteristics. It is important to involve epidemiologists, public health professionals and microbiology, infectious disease and infection control experts at a very early stage. A microbiologist can ensure that the most appropriate arrangements are made for the collection and rapid processing of clinical and environmental specimens. The next crucial step requires the identification of the number of people affected and what they have been exposed to. In order to do this, a working case definition must be created. A case definition will usually contain personal (clinical and demographic), temporal and geographical characteristics. When an outbreak presents, the investigators might have a shrewd idea about the causative organism from a combination of the event that took place and the average incubation period. When constructing the case definition, the incubation period range should be used in order to take account of what might appear to be unusually swift or late presentations.

It is surprising how often constructing a case definition is overlooked, but without it, highly misleading conclusions can be drawn from an investigation. For example, in an outbreak of food-borne illness in which people have presented with symptoms of vomiting, are people who report feelings of nausea to be counted as cases? In outbreaks of illnesses with ill-defined symptoms, several case definitions may be used to test an association between illness and exposure, but great care must be taken to ensure that whichever case definition is used is rigorously adhered to.

Case-finding methods will vary according to the severity or importance of the suspected disease and the setting in which the outbreak or epidemic has occurred. In a hospital outbreak, there is likely to be a clearly identifiable risk group. However, in a community outbreak this is likely to be far more complex because people are widely dispersed.

Cases are usually found either by locating other people who were exposed to the probable risk factor (e.g. people on an affected aeroplane flight) or by contacting local doctors or hospitals. For diseases that do not have a clear presentation (e.g. atypical pneumonia), extensive checking of possible cases, which may be recorded under a different diagnosis, on a local surveillance system or in clinical notes will need to be undertaken. This ensures that case ascertainment is as comprehensive as possible.

Once data have been collected, they are analysed by time, place and person. When graphs are plotted, it is often possible to distinguish the different types of epidemic discussed earlier in this section of the chapter. Plotting data geographically can often provide a clue to the source of an infectious agent or the nature of exposure; for example, it can prove useful in determining the source of *Legionella pneumophila* in outbreaks of Legionnaires' disease. Arranging data by patient characteristics, such as age, sex or occupation, may point to a particular risk group or mode of spread.

By this time, the investigators may have a very good idea about the organism responsible and its source and mode of spread. It is still necessary, however, to determine the most likely exposure that caused disease. It is at this stage that hypotheses are formulated, and those concerning causation

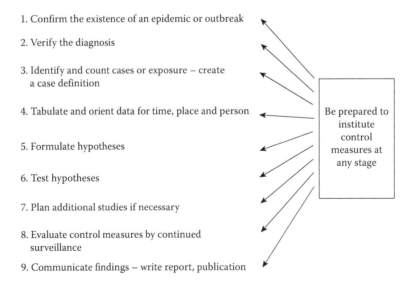

1. Confirm the existence of an epidemic or outbreak

2. Verify the diagnosis

3. Identify and count cases or exposure – create a case definition

4. Tabulate and orient data for time, place and person

5. Formulate hypotheses

6. Test hypotheses

7. Plan additional studies if necessary

8. Evaluate control measures by continued surveillance

9. Communicate findings – write report, publication

Be prepared to institute control measures at any stage

Figure 3.7 Actions investigating an outbreak.

Source: Goodman RA, Buehler JW, Koplan JP. The epidemiologic field investigation: science and judgment in public health practice. *American Journal of Epidemiology* 1990;132(1):9-16.

are then tested by using appropriate analytical epidemiological techniques.

Care is required in choosing appropriate controls if either a case-control or a cohort study is undertaken. This reduces the risk of inadvertent biases. There is a discussion of the use of controls in studies of chronic diseases in Chapter 2.

The precise method of gathering information from cases and controls depends on the incident being investigated. With a group of tourists who are leaving shortly for their next travel destination, the chosen method may be a simple listing of case details along one side of a grid and exposures down the other side. Where there is less urgency, the chosen method may be administration of a detailed, carefully constructed questionnaire. Whichever method is chosen, it is important that the interviewers ask questions in the same way so that one group of people is not prompted to remember more details than the other. Investigations establish associations; deciding whether the association is causal or otherwise is a separate process. The same rules of attributing causality apply in communicable disease investigation as in chronic disease investigation.

In outbreak investigation generally, having identified the probable source, it is important to revisit the facts and ask the following question: Does the hypothesis fit with the natural history of the disease in question? The clinical, laboratory and epidemiological results, together with those of any environmental investigations, should provide a logical, biologically plausible explanation of the events that have taken place.

At this stage, the investigation may be complete or the decision may be taken to conduct additional systematic studies. In any event, communicating the findings of an outbreak investigation is extremely important, and the final report should contain details of the investigation, the findings and any recommendations.

Once control measures have been implemented, continuing surveillance must be put in place to monitor their effects. If the surveillance data suggest that the outbreak is continuing despite the control measures implemented, the facts must be revisited and some, or all, of the steps described above must be repeated.

The question of when to instigate control measures during a communicable disease investigation can be very difficult. However, it is important both to investigate quickly using sound methodologies and to have the best possible information available when taking such decisions. The main elements for deciding which prevention and protection measures to use, and when, are patients' clinical symptoms and potential routes of transmission. When in doubt, the balance should always lie with the highest protection possible of both the public and health professionals involved in the outbreak investigation and clinical management.

Good communication, both within the outbreak control team and between the team and others, is vitally important. Investigations flounder when communication is poor, and this may have a detrimental impact on public confidence. An important point to bear in mind, particularly when dealing with a larger outbreak, is the relationship with the media. Possibly because of a fear of sensationalism by the

local press, radio and television, many health professionals are apprehensive about having contact with the media. A single spokesperson who is acceptable to both health and local authorities should be appointed, and he or she should be available to the media at appointed times only. If either organization has a press officer, he or she might be the right person to act as a spokesperson, although members of the press often prefer to discuss such matters with someone who is medically qualified. In any case, it is essential that factual information is reported in an unbiased way. Reporters are quick to realize when relevant information is being withheld. They will not expect personal details about patients to be divulged. Experience shows that a more accurate report is much more likely to result when the fullest possible information is released to the media. It is wrong to regard the media as a nuisance. Indeed, if good relations are established, particularly with local press, radio and television, this contact can be a great asset – helping, for example, to trace contacts or give health education advice to the population.

The following story of a communicable disease outbreak illustrates the realities of investigating in the public eye.

On 19 May 2011, a paediatrician at the University Hospital of Hamburg, Germany, developed an uneasy feeling. He had seen three children admitted to his hospital that day with haemolytic uraemic syndrome (HUS). People affected by haemolytic uraemic syndrome develop anaemia, acute kidney injury and impaired blood clotting. It is a serious illness – fatal, despite treatment, in around 1 in 50 cases. Most cases are caused by *Escherichia coli* infection, with bloody diarrhoea that starts a few days before the full-blown syndrome. The hospital normally has just one such case every year or so – why now three in a single day?

The paediatrician quickly shared his concerns with the Hamburg Public Health Department. In turn, the public health department informed the National Public Health Organization in Germany. By the next day, it was clear that several adults in Hamburg had also developed the illness. Cases in adults are rare. A team of 30 public health professionals was quickly established to investigate and manage the outbreak. By 25 May 2011, five days later,

- There were 214 known cases of haemolytic uraemic syndrome in Germany. More than half were in four northern states: Hamburg, Bremen, Lower Saxony and Schleswig-Holstein.
- Two people in Germany had died of it – a woman in her 80s and a woman in her 20s.
- Four other European countries had reported cases in people who had recently travelled to Germany.

Microbiological tests of stool and blood samples isolated *E. coli* O104. This was a surprise. The strain responsible for most previous cases of the syndrome worldwide is *E. coli* O157. In these five days, the public health team knew that the cause was likely to be contaminated food. *E. coli* can be contracted from contaminated water, but the people who were unwell lived in many different parts of Hamburg; they did not share a water supply. To identify the food responsible, the team established a case-control study. The cases were 25 people hospitalized with haemolytic uraemic syndrome or with bloody diarrhoea caused by *E. coli*. Each was asked what food they had eaten during the week before their symptoms started. The controls were 96 people, matched to the cases by age, sex and residence. Each was asked what they had eaten during the past week. When these data were analysed, they pointed to a cause. The cases were significantly more likely to have eaten raw tomatoes, cucumbers or lettuce than the controls. This association suggested that one or more of these foods was the likely source of the infection. The public health team held a press conference. They reported what they had found. They advised the public not to eat any raw tomatoes, cucumbers or lettuce until further notice.

Just as the paediatrician was becoming concerned in Hamburg, so something strange was happening 300 miles away in Frankfurt. Between 9 and 17 May 2011, 60 people who worked at a consultancy firm in Frankfurt had developed bloody diarrhoea. Eighteen of these had developed haemolytic uraemic syndrome. A public health team in Frankfurt investigated. The 60 affected people had eaten at one or other of the company's two canteens. The canteens had an electronic billing system. The investigators accessed these records for 23 of the cases and for 30 healthy controls. As in Hamburg, they did a case-control study. Their study showed that the cases were six times more likely to have eaten salad than were the controls. Twenty of the 23 cases investigated had eaten salad. No other food was significantly associated with the illness. These results seemed consistent with findings in Hamburg.

As the days passed, concern grew and more people died. By 3rd June, there had been 570 cases of haemolytic uraemic syndrome in Germany (Figure 3.8) and 12 deaths.

There were also 31 cases in 11 other European countries and one death. Major questions remained unanswered: Exactly which salad item was causing this? Where had it come from, and how had it become infected? The case-control study in Hamburg had asked people to recall what they had eaten. There are limits to how well people can remember this, particularly for meals that they did not cook for themselves. The study in Frankfurt had implicated salad, but the canteen's billing system had not recorded exactly what was in each salad. The team needed a more precise answer.

A particular restaurant was associated with many cases. Between 12 and 16 May 2011, 10 sizeable groups had eaten at the restaurant, numbering 176 people in total. Of these, 31 had now developed bloody diarrhoea. The existence of these 31 cases and 145 controls from a single restaurant allowed for detailed investigation. Each one was asked what dishes they had eaten. Many of them had pre-ordered, so their answers could be confirmed with the restaurant's booking records. The chef then provided an exact ingredient list for every dish. The team therefore knew precisely which ingredients each case and each control had eaten. This provided the breakthrough. It found that people who had eaten sprouts were at 14 times the risk of becoming unwell than those who had not. Every one of the cases had eaten a dish containing sprouts. The chef reported that the restaurant used just one sprout mix in its dishes – a mix of fenugreek sprouts, alfalfa sprouts, adzuki bean sprouts and lentil sprouts. This mix came from a single supplier, and this supplier got all of its sprouts from a farm in the German state of Lower Saxony. This single, well-designed study led right to the source.

On 10 June 2011, the German authorities announced that sprouts were the cause. They had previously advised people to avoid eating raw tomatoes, lettuce or cucumbers. They now withdrew this advice. In retrospect, it is clear how the earlier conclusion had erroneously been reached. Dishes that contain sprouts often contain tomatoes, lettuce

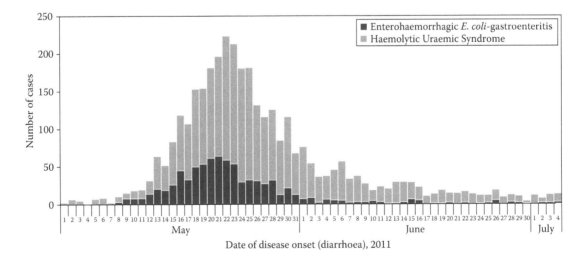

Figure 3.8 Epidemiological curve of the 2011 *E. Coli* outbreak in Germany.

Source: Robert Koch Institute. *Final Presentation and Evaluation of Epidemiological Findings in the EHEC 0104:H4 Outbreak, Germany.* Berlin: Robert Koch Institute, 2011. With permission.

or cucumbers. People remember, and therefore report, eating the tomatoes, lettuce or cucumbers, but not the sprouts. So the case-control study results implicated the wrong food items. This is an example of confounding.

Just as the German investigation was entering its final stages, similar events started to unfold in France. On 8 June 2011, a children's community centre in Bordeaux, France, was holding an open day. Those attending were treated to a cold buffet – of vegetables, soups and cheese. The soups were served with fenugreek sprouts, which were also sprinkled decoratively on the vegetables. Between 15 and 20 June, 15 of the attendees became unwell. They had all eaten the fenugreek sprouts. But these sprouts had not come from the farm in Lower Saxony, but from a farm in Bordeaux. Further investigation revealed that the Lower Saxony and the Bordeaux farm had something in common – they were both supplied with sprout seeds by the same supplier, in Egypt.

In retrospect, then, there were three key findings in this investigation. First, there was a case-control study that implicated salad, but not a particular ingredient. Second, there was a recipe-based cohort study that provided a more specific answer – sprouts. Third, there was a link between the German outbreak and an outbreak in France, in that both shared the same supplier in Egypt. The source was therefore determined – both the foodstuff and where it had become infected.

This description in retrospect makes the process sound neat, even simple. In reality, the investigation was difficult and highly charged. As every day passed, more people were becoming infected and more people were dying (by the end, there had been 3950 cases and 53 deaths). The outbreak quickly became international news. The team got to the right answer quickly, but not before they had publicly released the wrong answer – tomatoes, cucumbers and lettuce. Doing so caused havoc. Across Europe, many people stopped eating salad. Some countries banned the import of salad items from the European Union. Statements from the German Ministry of Health pointed the finger more specifically (but incorrectly) at Spanish cucumbers, which investigations at that stage suggested were the most likely source. Obviously, everybody stopped eating Spanish cucumbers. There was major political fallout from this. Farmers were stuck with millions of pounds' worth of stock that was not sellable and simply rotted. In the aftermath, the European Commission provided €200 million in compensation. Many were angry at the German authorities for releasing what turned out to be incorrect information. But from a public health perspective, it is difficult to criticize their approach. They took a precautionary approach and were transparent, releasing information as it became available.

The outbreak demonstrated the havoc that bacteria can cause, particularly now that people, and our food, so frequently cross international borders. It is a classic public health detective story. The investigation demonstrated, in very difficult circumstances, the value of getting the basics right – of using high-quality methods in investigating an outbreak, to come to a reliable answer quickly.

Prevention and control

A wide range of public health measures is used to prevent communicable diseases and to control their spread. Many of the same kinds of action are applicable to different diseases, such as a good sanitation system; the widespread availability of a safe, potable, public water supply; and high standards of personal hygiene. These are all conditions that will help to prevent or reduce the risk of a long list of illnesses spread by the faecal–oral route. The well-established process of contact tracing is applicable to many diseases, despite their different modes of transmission and clinical features, for example, sexually transmitted diseases and meningitis. Control measures for a particular disease can be different in an endemic, compared with an epidemic situation, although the difference may be mainly in their speed and scale of deployment; for example, the reduction of endemic, sporadic Legionnaires' disease (a form of bacterial pneumonia spread through water droplets) depends on measures such as good maintenance of cooling towers, of fountains in public space and of air conditioning in domestic, municipal, healthcare and commercial buildings. In an outbreak of Legionnaires' disease, attention would also be directed at those types of installation in a locality, but the focus would be on quickly discovering which was the reservoir of infection.

The main strategies for the prevention and control of communicable diseases are covered in this section. They encompass action to protect the potential recipients in a population, interrupting routes of transmission, eliminating or mitigating reservoirs of infection, early diagnosis of disease, identifying risk groups and targeting intermediate hosts. In combating many communicable diseases, more than one of these strategies must be used.

PROTECTING THE SUSCEPTIBLE HOST: VACCINATION AND OTHER MEASURES

Vaccination is the most definitive way of reducing the risk of contracting a particular communicable disease for people exposed to the infective agent. For many communicable diseases, no vaccine exists or it is not accessible. Also, no vaccine is 100% effective.

Other measures can be taken to protect a potential host against infection, in the presence or absence of vaccination. Some, although very general, address the fundamentals of maintaining a healthy immune system and avoiding exposure. These include good levels of childhood nutrition, adequate dwellings and proper sanitation. All these factors, and more, are important in reducing someone's vulnerability to infection. Fundamentally, the single factor common to all these is poverty, so addressing poverty and its causes is crucial.

Smaller-scale measures can also make a big difference. Some of these create physical barriers. For example, condoms (if properly used) give a high degree of protection against sexually transmitted infection; sleeping under a bed net can create an impenetrable barrier against insect bites (essential in malaria endemic areas); and wearing clothing that fully covers body, arms and legs can also protect against daytime mosquitoes (such as those that carry dengue fever). Chemoprophylaxis can help reduce risk of some diseases – for example, antimalarial tablets for travellers to endemic areas, or antibiotics for someone who has been in close contact with a case of meningitis.

Vaccines save millions of lives and are highly cost-effective, but one in five children worldwide still does not receive even the simplest course of vaccination. Some children do not receive any vaccines; many others are not reliably provided with a full course. This is because they do not have access to healthcare facilities where vaccines are available, or the public health system in their country is not sufficiently well organized. Vaccination is so cost-effective that its provision is a key health goal even in countries that have virtually no organized healthcare system. In such places, the aim is to deliver vaccines even where there are no accurate birth registers, few health centres, few doctors in primary care and an unreliable cold chain for transporting vaccines across the country. Much of the challenge of tackling vaccine-preventable disease is therefore in dealing with these kinds of practical and logistic difficulties, at scale. Vaccines themselves are impressively simple to give, but getting them reliably to the children in need of them is far from simple.

A country's basic vaccination coverage is reported as the percentage of children who have received three doses of the diphtheria, tetanus and pertussis vaccine. The abbreviation for this is DTP3. In many countries, DTP3 coverage is 99%. But in others, it is far lower. Equatorial Guinea is at the bottom of the current official table, with 24% DTP3 coverage. In Central African Republic, coverage is 28%, and in Somalia, 34%. Such figures are notoriously unreliable. A healthcare system that is only able to vaccinate one-fifth of its children is unlikely to accurately report the number of births and the proportion that are subsequently vaccinated. In the 1980s, the Expanded Program on Immunization (led by the World Health Organization and UNICEF) set out to increase DTP3 coverage in the world's poorest countries. At the start of the decade, DTP3 coverage in the lowest-income countries was 20%. Ten years on, it had been increased to 62%. But this momentum was not sustained, as focus and funding shifted to other global health endeavours, such as HIV/AIDS. The twenty-first century brought a revival, with the launch of the Global Alliance for Vaccines and Immunization (now known as Gavi, the Vaccine Alliance) to fund vaccine procurement and campaigns for the world's poorest 70 countries (Figure 3.9).

Bill Gates, the founder of Microsoft, and now the cochair of the Bill and Melinda Gates Foundation, is devoting much of his fortune to improve health in the poorest countries of the world. He has described vaccines as magic. The 2010s were declared the Decade of Vaccines and *a Global Vaccine Action Plan* agreed on by 200 countries. This initiative aims to extend vaccination to all people worldwide by 2020, and so save 20 million lives.

Vaccines are remarkable for their simplicity as a public health intervention. Somebody who has received very basic

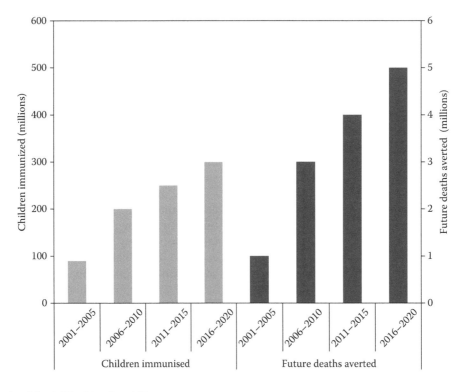

Figure 3.9 The work of Gavi, The Vaccine Alliance.

Source: GAVI Alliance. *Investing Together for a Healthy Future: The 2016–2020 GAVI Alliance Investment Opportunity.* Geneva: GAVI Alliance, 2014.

training can give a vaccine effectively. It cannot be assumed, though, that once a vaccine has been developed, the world's population will readily be protected from that disease. Where routine immunization systems are weak, or where there is a particular need to boost population immunity fast, supplementary immunization activities (SIAs, often referred to as campaigns) are used in addition or instead. Run over a short period (typically three to five days), vaccines are given to children by vaccinators who circulate around an area moving from one house to the next, or who establish fixed posts (perhaps in the community's central market place) to which parents are encouraged to bring their children. The organization and delivery of these campaigns is no mean feat. Vaccines must reach every part of a country in sufficient quantities, and trained personnel must be in place to work simultaneously to deliver the vaccines to children. In India, for example, a nationwide campaign to deliver polio vaccine involves 2.5 million vaccinators, overseen by 150,000 supervisors, working in 700,000 vaccination booths to immunize 175 million children over just five days.

In the United Kingdom, and many other high-income countries, the situation is very different. Delivering vaccines in a well-developed healthcare system such as the National Health Service (NHS) is relatively straightforward. Every newborn baby is registered with a general practitioner. A call and recall system prompts the baby's parents to bring him or her to a clinic at the correct times for the various childhood vaccines to be given. There are established systems to transport vaccine around the country. Children are vaccinated against eight different infections before their first birthday, and a further three before they start school (Table 3.2).

The early vaccines were given against one type of infection (monovalent). Today, more vaccines are given as a combined dose, giving protection against more than one infection in a single injection.

Surprisingly, even some high-income countries do not use the call–recall system, in which every child is registered with a local healthcare practitioner, and an automated system ensures that every vaccine dose is received at the correct time. Instead, they put the onus on parents to keep track of the vaccines that their child receives. In such systems, parents are typically provided with a card for each newborn baby. This system is also common in lower-income countries. On this card are listed the vaccines that the child needs to receive. It is then the parents' responsibility to take the child to the healthcare facility at the appropriate times. Although they vary somewhat, these approaches are generally referred to as routine immunization, since the delivery of vaccination to children on a continuous basis is determined by their age.

Although challenging, it is somewhat more straightforward to organize campaigns than it is to make routine immunization systems work well on an ongoing basis. For this reason, when poorer countries want to improve population immunity rapidly, they often rely on campaigns. This is controversial, because strengthened routine immunization systems can benefit the population over a longer term.

In a minority of countries, childhood vaccination is legally required. In the United States and France, children must prove their vaccination status before starting school.

The terms *vaccination* and *immunization* are frequently used interchangeably, but they actually have

Table 3.2 United Kingdom routine childhood immunization schedule: protecting against 12 infections

Age	Vaccine
Two months	• Diphtheria, tetanus, pertussis, polio, *Haemophilus influenzae* B • Pneumococcal • Rotavirus
Three months	• Diphtheria, tetanus, pertussis, polio, *Haemophilus influenzae* B • Meningococcal C • Rotavirus
Four months	• Diphtheria, tetanus, pertussis, polio, *Haemophilus influenzae* B • Pneumococcal
12–13 months	• *Haemophilus influenzae* B, Meningococcal C • Pneumococcal • Measles, mumps, rubella
Between three years, four months, and five years	• Diphtheria, tetanus, pertussis, polio • Measles, mumps, rubella
Girls aged 12–13 years	• Human papillomavirus
13–18 years	• Tetanus, diphtheria, polio • Meningococcal C

Source: Public Health England (PHE). *Immunisation Against Infectious Disease.* London: PHE, 2013

different meanings. 'Vaccination' is the giving of a vaccine. 'Immunisation' is the act of making a person immune to an infection – the intended result of vaccination. Vaccination does not always result in immunization. The Bacillus Calmette–Guérin (BCG) vaccine against tuberculosis, for example, creates immunity in approximately 70% of cases.

Vaccines are produced in different ways. The key concept is that the components of the vaccine must be similar enough to the infectious agent to provoke an immune response and generate an effective immune memory, but sufficiently altered that the vaccine cannot cause the disease that it is intended to protect against. Live attenuated vaccines (e.g. MMR) contain the infectious agents themselves, but in a weakened form. Inactivated vaccines (e.g. Salk polio vaccine) contain a killed version of the infectious agent. Toxoid-based vaccines (e.g. diphtheria and tetanus) contain a version of the toxin produced by the infectious agent. Acellular vaccines (e.g. pertussis) contain some parts of the infectious agent's cells – enough that the immune system would recognize the whole cell later, but not enough to cause active infection.

The design of the vaccine is very important, affecting both its efficacy and its side effects. For example, the polysaccharide vaccine used against meningococcal A and C meningitis is not very effective in creating an immune response, particularly in young children. By contrast, the conjugate form of the C vaccine (made by attaching a protein to the polysaccharide) provokes a better reaction in children and provides long-term immune memory. Techniques to design and make vaccines are advancing within the rapidly developing biotechnology field. Also, genome mapping is allowing the genetic sequences of microbiological agents to be elucidated, providing novel vaccine candidates.

Whether a population is protected from vaccine-preventable diseases depends on the extent of so-called herd immunity. This concept relies on the principle that if there are 1000 children in a population and 999 of them have been successfully vaccinated against measles, the unvaccinated 1000th child is unlikely to catch measles because there is nobody for him or her to catch it from. In more general terms, when a sufficient proportion of the population (herd) is vaccinated against an infection, this provides protection for even those who have not been vaccinated. The proportion that must be immunized in order to generate herd immunity differs between infectious agents. It depends on how readily transmitted the infection is. For the highly transmissible measles virus, for example, coverage of 92%–94% is required. For mumps and rubella, less than 90% is sufficient.

Most vaccines are given in childhood, but they are also used in other circumstances, including the seasonal influenza vaccine. Before and during every winter flu season, many countries offer vaccination to individuals in at-risk groups – for whom infection with influenza carries a higher risk of serious illness – and to individuals who have frequent contact with at-risk groups. In the United Kingdom, the at-risk groups are people aged 65 years or older, people

aged less than 65 years who are pregnant or have a particular chronic disease (including diabetes, chronic respiratory, heart, kidney and neurological disease; splenic insufficiency; and immunodeficiency) and people who live in a residential care home or other long-stay facility. Others offered vaccination are front-line health and social care workers, and carers.

Because every country has different infectious diseases in circulation, anybody travelling outside of their own country should be advised to determine what additional travel vaccination they may require.

Mass vaccination may be offered in the event of a new infectious disease emerging, such as the 2009 influenza A(H1N1)pdm09 virus pandemic. There is a currently a significant lag between the emergence of a new disease and the mass production of a vaccine, though.

Many thousands of children are alive who would have died from the infectious disease scourges of the past, were it not for vaccination. Many others would have suffered the misery of these illnesses or sustained disability as a result. The folk memory of many of these diseases now rests in the mind of older grandparents and great-grandparents. For example, three generations ago, polio was much feared. Parents would have given anything to protect their child from the risk of this cruel disease. It struck seemingly at random, maiming and killing. Now, people in much of the world do not know what polio is. As the fear fades, what was once demand for the vaccine retreats into mere acceptance. Some people start questioning the need for vaccines or even refusing them. With the fear factor missing, some parents worry more about the possible complications of vaccines than about the diseases themselves. In such a climate, unfounded claims about adverse effects of vaccines can too easily cause real harm.

Decisions about vaccination policy need to be based on sound assessment of the best available science. Committees often assist with this. In England and Wales, the government is advised by an independent group of scientific experts – the Joint Committee on Vaccination and Immunisation (JCVI). The World Health Organization is advised by the Strategic Advisory Group of Experts (SAGE) on Immunization.

Vaccination is now a highly complex field. New vaccines are being developed, and scientific advances are also changing the ways in which vaccinations are being given. The newer vaccines include human papillomavirus (HPV) vaccine, which is given to teenagers and protects girls against cervical cancer. Varicella zoster virus (VZV) vaccine protects against both chickenpox and shingles. New rotavirus and pneumococcal vaccines offer enormous promise in lower-income countries. Rotavirus causes diarrhoea, which in turn leads to dehydration. Pneumococcus causes respiratory infections. Both cause childhood illness and death on a wide scale.

Among the many candidate vaccines currently under development, the most exciting prospects include vaccines against HIV and malaria. There is also potential for a universal flu vaccine that would protect against seasonal flu without the need for annual revaccination and also against newly emerging flu viruses that could otherwise cause pandemics. None of these vaccines are imminent, but in each case, a number of candidate vaccines are progressing through trials.

INTERRUPTING TRANSMISSION

Identifying the modes of transmission of individual diseases creates important opportunities to stop epidemics, to prevent cases of the disease, to reduce risk to a population and sometimes to eliminate spread entirely.

Throughout history, up to the present day, establishing and maintaining high standards of hygiene – both in environments of human habitation and in personal behaviour – has been the most important way of preventing or interrupting the transmission of communicable diseases. Quarter of the world's population (1.8 billion people) use a source of drinking water that is faecally contaminated. More than a third (2.5 billion people) do not have access to good sanitation. One billion people practice open defacation. Clean water and safe disposal of sewage are taken for granted in the richer parts of the world, but are far from universally available. Absence of clean water, sanitation and hygiene greatly elevates the risk of communicable disease. Children are particularly vulnerable – almost 2 million die every year from diarrhoea. Water, sanitation and hygiene are distinct but inter-related public health issues: clean water is required for good hygiene; without toilets, water sources become contaminated. The three issues are often therefore tackled together, through widespread Water, Sanitation and Hygiene (WASH) programmes that seek to both improve infrastructure and change behaviour. Good personal hygiene encompasses many different infection prevention measures – from hand washing, to sneezing into tissues, to careful food preparation and to healthy sexual practices. For most of the communicable diseases, there is some hygiene measure that will limit their spread.

A wide range of measures is important in preventing and controlling the spread of infection. Some are general. Some are specific to particular diseases, or routes of transmission. Some examples are early diagnosis and prompt treatment (e.g. tuberculosis), screening of blood and blood products (e.g. HIV), pasteurization of milk (e.g. brucellosis), use of alcohol hand-rubs in hospitals (e.g. MRSA), rodent control (e.g. Weil's disease), inspection of food outlets (e.g. *Salmonella*), training of catering staff (e.g. many food-borne illnesses), use of disposable instruments in tattoo parlours (e.g. hepatitis B), education of pet owners and banning dogs from children's outdoor play areas (e.g. *Toxocara canis*), tracing and treatment of contacts (e.g. syphilis) and public education on recognition and prevention of transmission (e.g. scabies).

TARGETING RESERVOIRS OF INFECTION

Eliminating reservoirs of infection – or reducing their potential to initiate disease transmission – is the main control measure for some diseases, and one part of a wider strategy for others. The precise action taken depends on the nature of the reservoir and having a full understanding of it. This is not always easy because the true reservoir may be part of a complex ecological system in which there are multiple hosts for the infection.

Where the reservoir is a single animal host, a solution may be to cull. This was the approach taken in Hong Kong in 1997 when an outbreak of bird flu, due to the influenza A virus H5N1, jumped the species barrier and spread to the human population, causing deaths. Millions of chickens and ducks were slaughtered. This appeared to stop the outbreak at the time, although H5N1 continued to affect bird populations over the next two decades and, occasionally, to infect people who were in close contact with infected birds or poultry. In the United Kingdom, during the Bovine Spongiform Encephalopathy epidemic in the 1990s and early 2000s, millions of cattle were slaughtered to stop it from entering the human food chain. In Malaysia, in 1999, a million pigs were destroyed to attempt to stop the transmission of Nipah virus. Generally, such action is only taken where the threat to human health is immediate and particularly high, or where an infective agent has emerged whose properties are not understood. It may also be taken when a problem is due to a circumscribed and very localized animal reservoir. It would not be logistically possible, or even desirable, to slaughter potential animal hosts on a large scale in most situations. For example, no one would contemplate the destruction of large bat populations. If a disease reservoir is in a mosquito population, treating breeding grounds with insecticide can help, but seldom clears the source of the infective agent completely.

In epidemics of food-borne infection, identifying the foodstuff that is the reservoir and removing it from the food chain is a vital piece of targeted action. For communicable diseases in which the reservoir is a human host, possible measures include quarantine, isolation and screening to detect people who are carriers.

Surveillance

If a country hopes to have effective communicable disease control, a strong surveillance system is an absolute must. Surveillance systems provide information on communicable diseases and their spread through the population. Such systems must provide information in a timely manner, and in a way that allows the appropriate action to be taken.

There are many ways in which information can guide public health action; for example,

- A young boy is admitted to hospital in London, very unwell with bloody diarrhoea. Fifty miles away in Reading, a girl is admitted to a different hospital with the same problem. Both children are found to have *E. coli* O157 – a dangerous infection that can cause kidney failure and death. Their doctors do not know it yet, but both caught the infection at a busy tourist attraction. The facility remains open, with more children at risk of catching the infection as every hour passes. A good surveillance system will recognize that these two cases, apparently separated in time and space, might be connected, and then trace them back to the tourist attraction. This use of surveillance data can enable action to be taken to prevent more people from catching the same infection, and so potentially save lives.

- Hospital doctors admit a young girl whom they diagnose as having meningococcal meningitis. This is a life-threatening infectious disease. With a surveillance system in place, the local public health team will quickly be made aware of this, and can trace contacts of the girl to give them information and, in some cases, prophylactic antibiotics that significantly reduce the risk of spread.
- Reports of fatality rates of 40% among people in China admitted to hospital after contracting H7N9 influenza virus infection from pigs caused great concern. Enhanced surveillance identified many more cases that had not been hospitalized because they had milder illness. In situations like this, a comprehensive surveillance system allows a further spectrum of disease to be understood, and so gives a more balanced estimate of risk than the narrow hospital-based information provided.
- Every winter, thousands of people develop minor coughs and colds. But many thousands also catch influenza, a more serious illness. A particular surveillance method extracts information automatically from the electronic records of people consulting their general practitioners with flu-like illness. This can provide an estimate of how much influenza there is, who is most affected and how it is spreading. Plans to deal with the additional burden of illness for the healthcare system, and to encourage uptake of vaccine, can then be made.

A strong surveillance system underpins effective prevention and control of communicable diseases. It also triggers the investigation of outbreaks, and the tracking of disease trends and spread. Good surveillance is essential to evaluate the impact of vaccination programmes and other control measures. Over the years, within-country and global communicable disease surveillance has allowed many new and emerging threats to the public health to be identified and dealt with.

There are a number of basic differences between surveillance systems. First, they can be *universal*, covering an entire population, or *sentinel*, collecting data from just certain locations. Second, they may be *active*, relying on reporting, or *passive*, extracting data from sources such as general practitioners' records. Third, they may be *disease specific* or *syndromic*.

Active, routine surveillance systems have two key elements at their core: First, there is a system of notification of clinical conditions, which requires doctors to inform the public health authorities when they encounter an infectious disease. If information remains in the clinical arena and is not appropriately shared in this way, population surveillance is seriously weakened and public health interventions necessary to protect the public may not be taken. Second, there is an equivalent notification duty for laboratories, when a patient tests positive for an infectious agent. Surveillance systems are not currently able to track every possible infectious disease, but legislation requires specified illnesses, diseases or clinical signs to be notified. The law sets out a list of diseases that the health protection system needs to be made aware of.

In England and Wales, every medical practitioner has a legal duty to notify a local proper officer if they suspect a patient has one of the infectious diseases listed in Table 3.3. A proper officer is a professional person (usually a

Table 3.3 Diseases notifiable to local authority proper officers under the Health Protection (Notification) Regulations 2010

Acute encephalitis	Malaria
Acute infectious hepatitis	Measles
Acute meningitis	Meningococcal septicaemia
Acute poliomyelitis	Mumps
Anthrax	Plague
Botulism	Rabies
Brucellosis	Rubella
Cholera	Severe Acute Respiratory Syndrome (SARS)
Diphtheria	Scarlet fever
Enteric fever (typhoid or paratyphoid fever)	Smallpox
Food poisoning	Tetanus
Haemolytic uraemic syndrome	Tuberculosis
Infectious bloody diarrhoea	Typhus
Invasive group A streptococcal disease	Viral haemorrhagic fever
Legionnaires' disease	Whooping cough
Leprosy	Yellow fever

Source: Public Health England. *Notifications of Infectious Diseases (NOIDs)*. Available from: https://www.gov.uk/government/collections/notifications-of-infectious-diseases-noids [accessed 4 May 2017].

consultant in communicable disease control) appointed by a local authority to oversee the notification process. He or she shares each notification with Public Health England. The legal basis for this is the Health Protection (Notification) Regulations 2010.

Doctors are expected to make their notifications on clinical suspicion, not waiting for a definitive laboratory-confirmed diagnosis. This makes sense because the purpose of notification is to allow early public health action to control the spread of disease. Waiting even a few days for laboratory confirmation might mean that onward transmission has already taken place. For many notifiable diseases, there is serious underreporting, low levels of laboratory testing and inaccuracy of clinical diagnosis. Nevertheless, notification remains a key source of information about the occurrence of infectious diseases in the population, as long as it is not claimed to produce data on the true incidence of a disease.

In most areas of England, the local authority delegates its proper officer duties to Public Health England. Public Health England therefore receives disease notifications and takes the appropriate action. Individual notifications are also collated, to produce weekly, quarterly and annual reports. They are published by Public Health England, and monitor infectious disease trends.

Second, there must be a system of laboratory reporting. In England, a range of different laboratories report many different microbiology results to Public Health England's Centre for Infections, and to local and regional health protection teams. As with disease notifications from medical practitioners, such reports serve two broad purposes: individual reports (or a cluster of reports) may stimulate further public health investigation and action, and reports are collated to produce weekly data that describe communicable disease trends by area and across the country as a whole. In England, the laboratory reporting system is part statutory and part voluntary.

Disease-based surveillance provides only a small slice of the overall picture of communicable disease in a population. The vast majority of cases are never seen by a doctor.

Many are seen by a doctor but (usually appropriately) not reported to a surveillance system (Figure 3.10).

Syndromic surveillance gathers information about particular sets of symptoms (e.g. diarrhoea and vomiting), not about infectious agents or diseases directly. It can use active or passive methods. The requirement for doctors to report particular symptom patterns can be added to their reporting responsibilities. This can be especially valuable following the emergence of a new threat, when the disease entity and the infective agent are not known or understood. The passive approach seeks to recognize symptom patterns within record or information systems. The existence of electronic medical records makes syndromic surveillance far more practical than when records were paper based. This surveillance method is therefore becoming increasingly common. England, for example, has a number of separate such surveillance systems – monitoring general practices, hospital emergency departments and telephone health helplines. Syndromic surveillance also proves useful during mass gatherings, such as the London 2012 Olympic and Paralympic Games, as it provides real-time information.

In many of the poorer countries of the world, places that are often the locus of serious outbreaks of communicable diseases or newly emergent infectious threats, surveillance mechanisms are virtually non-existent. There are few laboratories to identify organisms, care is not organized to enable clinical reporting and information technology infrastructure is poor. As a result, there is growing interest in more novel methods of acquiring surveillance data. Internet-trawling tools can detect unusual occurrences in local media websites, blogs and social media. The challenges in mining big data like these are formidable, but they have significant potential and, unlike traditional surveillance systems, can potentially provide real-time warning of symptom clusters even when the disease entity is not yet known.

There are three main global aspects to surveillance. First, specific global surveillance networks have been established for some individual infections, most notably influenza. The Global Influenza Surveillance Network involves 151 laboratories in 106 countries. By sharing information, they are

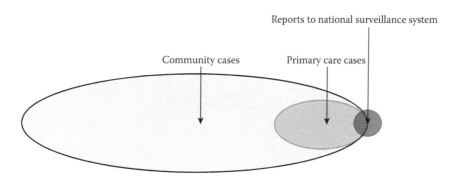

Figure 3.10 Surveillance of gastrointestinal disease: a narrow window.

Source: Food Standards Agency (FSA). *The Second Study of Infectious Intestinal Disease in the Community (IID2 Study).* London: FSA, 2012.

able to create a far more comprehensive picture of influenza circulation and evolution globally than any could hope to do individually.

Second, the International Health Regulations (which are discussed more fully later) require each country to have a surveillance system that is capable of detecting a serious disease threat, and to report any such detection to the World Health Organization. Many countries do not yet have such a system, and the World Health Organization and others are working with them to help remedy this.

Third, surveillance is only of value if there is an effective response. The Global Outbreak Alert and Response Network, also run by the World Health Organization, aims to help organize this response. In the aftermath of the West African Ebola outbreak that started in 2014, however, the World Health Organization's capacity to lead the appropriate response has been criticized. In response, it is establishing a sizeable new Emergencies Programme.

INFECTIOUS DISEASES CAUSING A MAJOR BURDEN OF MORTALITY: THE BIG KILLERS

While deaths from communicable diseases do occur in high-income countries, they are relatively uncommon compared with deaths from noncommunicable diseases. In contrast, in the poorest countries of the world and some middle-income countries, the communicable diseases cause many deaths, a substantial proportion of which would not occur in circumstances with better prevention and treatment measures. Five conditions lead the league table of causes of this burden of mortality. They are described in this section.

HIV and AIDS

AIDS emerged as an apparently new disease in the 1980s when, in the United States, increasing numbers of cases of opportunistic infection (particularly *Pneumocystis*

carinii pneumonia) and unusual tumours (e.g. Kaposi's sarcoma) were reported in previously healthy men who had sex with men.

The presenting clinical features of HIV infection are often general: weight loss, fever, malaise and lymphadenopathy. The fully developed AIDS syndrome involves opportunistic infections or patterns of malignancy infrequently seen in people with normal immune systems, although any one of a wide range of infections or malignancies can occur. HIV belongs to the retrovirus group. By infecting a subset of the T-lymphocyte population (CD4 cells), it gradually destroys the normal immune response mechanism. Groups at highest risk are men who have sex with men (particularly in the big cities), sex workers and their clients, intravenous drug users and children born to infected mothers.

Although in the public mind HIV infection is often associated with homosexual transmission, the biggest group of people living with HIV is those who caught it through heterosexual transmission.

The number of people living with HIV was estimated as 37 million in 2015. There were 2.1 million new infections that year – almost half of them in sub-Saharan Africa (Figure 3.11). This represents a 34% decrease since 2000. There were 1.1 million deaths. The greatest improvements have been in sub-Saharan Africa, among young people aged 15–24 years, and in maternal–child transmission.

Despite the gains of the latter half of the first decade of the twenty-first century, the disease remains devastating in its scale and impact in human, societal and economic terms. The twin challenges of HIV prevention and improving access to treatment are formidable. In some parts of the world, there are profound cultural barriers – fear, superstition, stigma and denial – which seriously restrict the scope for preventive action. It is vital to address these. Strong, enlightened commitment from the most senior levels of government, and from local community and civic leaders, is the key to successful action. Like successful treatment

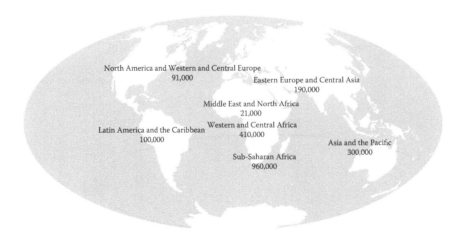

Figure 3.11 Estimated number of children and adults newly infected with HIV in 2015 – 2.1 million worldwide.

Source: UNAIDS. With permission.

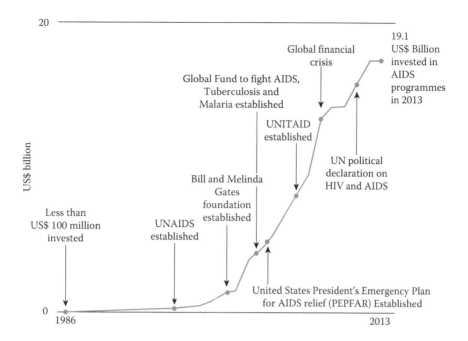

Figure 3.12 Funds invested in AIDS programmes in low- and middle-income countries, 1986–2013.

Source: UNAIDS. With permission.

programmes, good prevention cannot be easily delivered without a strong health system in the country concerned. This is a problem in many of the worst-affected parts of the world; a great deal of resources have been invested in strengthening healthcare systems in low-and middle-income countries (Figure 3.12), but there is still a long way to go.

Basic health education programmes are important for modifying people's (especially young people's) attitudes and behaviour towards issues such as condom use and avoiding multiple partners. A particularly difficult problem is communicating with and influencing the harder-to-reach groups – injecting drug users and sex workers. The evidence base for the effectiveness of different preventive strategies has expanded in the last decade. For example, voluntary male circumcision has been shown to reduce transmission, and is now recommended by the Joint United Nations Programme on HIV and AIDS (UNAIDS) and the World Health Organization. There are many good examples around the world of successful local programmes based on health education and community engagement.

The development of antiretroviral drugs revolutionized the treatment of HIV infection and AIDS. They have prolonged survival for those infected by many decades, so that HIV has in effect become a chronic disease. In the poorer parts of the world, the challenges are funding the drugs required, distributing them effectively and then achieving long-term compliance with therapy. Stories of successful treatment in sub-Saharan Africa are truly inspiring, as people have been rescued from death's door. However, the challenge is to reach the very substantial numbers who still lack access to life-saving therapy (Figure 3.13).

Many international organizations are important in combatting the HIV pandemic:

- UNAIDS started work in 1996, pooling functions among a variety of United Nations agencies. It sets policies and priorities and implements action plans, and increasingly guides governments of affected countries in the best strategies to use limited resources most effectively. UNAIDS annual reports give an unrivalled picture of all aspects of HIV/AIDS worldwide.
- The World Health Organization, as part of its wide range of functions, assesses progress in the fight against HIV and AIDS, sets standards and coordinates action within its regions and member states.
- The Global Fund to Fight AIDS, Tuberculosis and Malaria was created in 2002 as a vehicle to attract, manage and distribute funds to fight the three diseases of its name. It works closely with other multilateral and bilateral international organizations, individual countries and other donors. It channels some 20% of global funding for AIDS.

Other bodies, such as the World Bank, are important. So too are the international development departments within governments (e.g. the Department for International Development [DFID] in the United Kingdom) and nongovernmental organizations (such as the Bill and Melinda Gates Foundation). Spending by governments is very important, but so too is the significant donor aid that goes to low- and middle-income countries. There has been massive concerted global action and resources to try to tackle the HIV and AIDS pandemic.

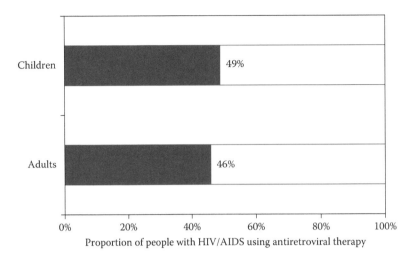

Figure 3.13 Antiretroviral therapy coverage worldwide, 2015.

Source: UNAIDS. With permission.

The UK government ran a major public education campaign between 1986 and 1987, relatively early in the occurrence of the HIV epidemic. The campaign made heavy use of mass media: television, radio, cinema and posters. A leaflet was delivered to every household in the country giving information about HIV infection and AIDS. A telephone line, the National AIDS Helpline, was also established.

The AIDS: Don't Die of Ignorance campaign was judged to be remarkably successful. Many consider it, along with the early introduction of needle exchange schemes for injecting drug users, responsible for initially keeping the prevalence of HIV infection in the United Kingdom relatively low. However, the position is not now reassuring. The number of people with HIV infection was estimated at 100,000 at the end of 2014, of whom 22% were unaware of their infection. Three-quarters of all infections were in either black African heterosexuals or men who have sex with men. Around 47% of diagnoses are made late – this group is 10 times more likely to die within a year. The highest proportion of new diagnoses is in people aged 35–49 years. HIV diagnoses in intravenous drug users have remained low and relatively stable in recent years, while a small number of cases occur among children by vertical (from an infected mother) transmission and in past recipients of blood transfusion.

In the early 1990s, most people who were diagnosed as HIV positive lived (or received services) in London. By the late 2000s, 50% were receiving their care outside London.

There are a number of strands to HIV surveillance in the United Kingdom: data on new diagnoses confidentially reported by clinicians, data on HIV testing reported from laboratories, data on CD4 T-cell levels (this gives an indication of the stage of disease at the time of diagnosis) and an annual statement of all patients seen for HIV-related treatment and care – the Survey of Prevalent HIV Infections Diagnosed (SOPHID).

Early diagnosis of HIV infection is crucial because it reduces the risk of transmission to others and because it allows the infected individual to start treatment early, giving him or her a much better prognosis. Failure to provide HIV testing to someone who attends a genitourinary medicine (GUM) clinic with another sexually transmitted disease is a major lost opportunity for HIV control.

In England, the National AIDS Trust has identified three broad themes in a comprehensive strategy:

1. HIV as a sexual health condition and the prevention and testing needs associated with this
2. HIV as a long-term condition and the health, social care and welfare needs this brings
3. HIV as an equality and human rights issue, including the steps needed to end stigma and discrimination

The network of genitourinary medicine clinics is a key element of HIV services. Ensuring open access and very short waiting times is important. Unless resources are invested in this area, the risk of an explosive increase in HIV infection in the United Kingdom is ever present.

One of the problems for public education programmes for HIV infection in a country like Britain is that a number of target groups are being addressed simultaneously. Thus, the health education initiative must continue to target the sexual behaviour of men who have sex with men, but this emphasis must not lead the heterosexual population to believe that HIV infection is not a risk for them. Campaigns and programmes must be appropriately targeted for men who have sex with men, intravenous drug abusers, sex workers and travellers to high-risk areas of the world.

Public education, while a vital element of programmes to prevent and control HIV infection in the population, is only one part of a comprehensive range of measures that have been adopted. For example, well-organized needle exchange schemes are particularly important in reducing risk among intravenous drug abusers. Free, open-access genitourinary clinics provide the main entry point for most HIV patients. Other key elements of the overall programme include training of staff in the care of infected people and in the risks of transmission during the process of patient care.

Tuberculosis

Tuberculosis is the second most common cause of death from infectious disease worldwide. Tuberculosis has retained its dominance as a threat to human health for several reasons. It is predominantly a disease of poverty, still prevalent in many countries. Although treatable, the treatment regimen is complex and lengthy compared with that of many other infections and is too costly for people in countries with poor access to healthcare. With the advent of HIV infection, affecting tens of millions of people, tuberculosis has become a common co-infection.

Tuberculosis, caused by *M. tuberculosis*, in its most common form is a respiratory disease caught when someone inhales *M. tuberculosis* from an infected person. A short period of exposure to infection does not usually result in the disease if the person was previously healthy. Someone living in poor environmental, social and living conditions is much more likely to contract it. People who have HIV infection and thus impaired immune systems are particularly vulnerable. Non-respiratory tuberculosis is also important, particularly among immigrants to the United Kingdom. It accounts for just under half the cases where a site has been identified. It can affect any part of the body – particularly the lymph nodes, genitourinary tract and bone – and is becoming more common.

The burden of disease caused by tuberculosis can be assessed in a number of ways but most commonly by incidence (the number of new or relapsed cases arising in a population in a year, or other period), prevalence (the number of cases in a population at a point in time) and mortality (the number of deaths attributable to the disease in a year, or other time period). Viewed against these measures, the global burden of tuberculosis is huge. The World Health Organization estimates that in 2015 there were 10 million incident cases, 11 million people were alive with tuberculosis (i.e. prevalent cases) and there were 1.4 million deaths from the disease, of whom 400,000 were HIV positive. Tuberculosis is not evenly distributed around the world: a quarter of cases are in Africa, and the incidence and deaths per thousand population are higher there than in other parts of the world. In purely numerical terms, 60% of cases are in the Southeast Asia region (mainly India) and western Pacific region (mainly China). In the European Union, 60,000 people a year contract tuberculosis. Six countries have much higher incidence rates than the rest: Bulgaria, Estonia, Latvia, Lithuania, Portugal and Romania.

The drug resistance that has developed against the tubercle bacterium is a major threat to the control of the disease globally. It is categorized into two main types: multi-drug-resistant tuberculosis (MDR-TB) and extensively drug-resistant tuberculosis (XDR-TB).

Despite this, control programmes have been making an impact. The global prevalence of tuberculosis has fallen by 40% since 1990, due largely to the *STOP TB* strategy that, although multifaceted, has a strong emphasis on directly observed therapy - short course (DOTS).

In the United Kingdom in 2015, there were 6240 new cases of tuberculosis reported to the authorities – a figure that had decreased over the previous five years (Figure 3.14). Its highest occurrence is in areas of the country classified as being the most deprived. A substantial proportion of the disease burden – 36% – is concentrated in London. The city has one of the highest levels of tuberculosis in western Europe (Figure 3.15).

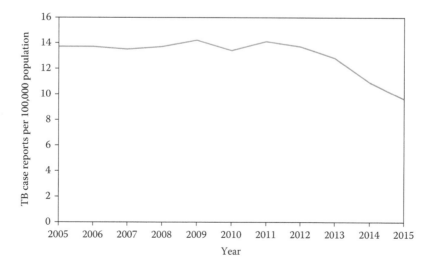

Figure 3.14 Tuberculosis case report rates, United Kingdom.

Source: Public Health England.

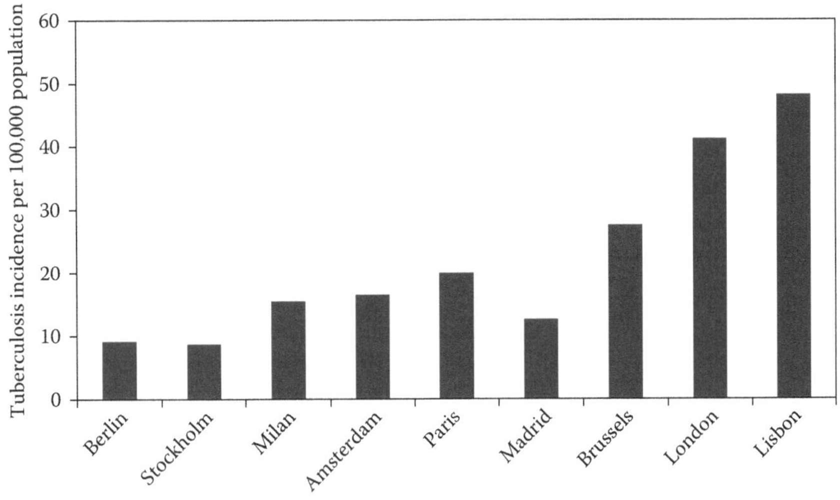

Figure 3.15 Tuberculosis incidence in major Western European cities, 2012.

Source: Public Health England (PHE). *Collaborative Tuberculosis Strategy for England 2015 to 2020.* London: PHE, 2015.

The four UK countries have comprehensive approaches to tackling tuberculosis; for example, the strategy for England has 10 action areas:

1. Improve access to services and ensure early diagnosis
2. Provide universal access to high-quality diagnostics
3. Improve treatment and care services
4. Ensure comprehensive contact tracing
5. Improve BCG vaccination uptake
6. Reduce drug-resistant tuberculosis
7. Tackle tuberculosis in underserved populations
8. Systematically implement new entrant latent tuberculosis screening
9. Strengthen surveillance and monitoring
10. Ensure an appropriate workforce to deliver tuberculosis control

Mycobacterium bovis, closely related to *M. tuberculosis*, has a reservoir in animals, particularly cattle. It used to be a source of transmissible disease in the United Kingdom, but since the advent of pasteurized milk and dairy products, it is very rare. It has been controversial in recent years because of the re-emergence of tuberculosis in cattle. The prime route of transmission is badgers. The use of badger culls to curb the infection has pitted cattle farmers against animal rights and environmental campaigners, as well as the latent public sentiment in favour of badgers.

Malaria

Despite the Nobel Prize being awarded on four separate occasions during the twentieth century for scientific work on malaria, the disease remains one of the major challenges in global health. It imposes a high burden of illness and death. The economic and social impact on countries and their government is major (estimated at US$12 billion annually). Its association with poverty is strong.

An estimated 3 billion people in the world are at risk of malaria. The disease is actively circulating in 97 countries. There were 212 million cases in 2015 and an estimated 430 thousand deaths. More than 90% of these deaths were in sub-Saharan Africa, and more than 70% were in the under-fives. Malaria kills one child every 60 seconds in Africa. Countries' surveillance systems do not give an accurate picture of the numbers, so the World Health Organization uses statistical modelling to make annual estimates of the number of cases and deaths.

Malaria is caused by a protozoan parasite of the *Plasmodium* genus. Four species cause human malaria. Two are common: *Plasmodium vivax*, the cause of benign tertian malaria, and *Plasmodium falciparum*, which causes malignant tertian malaria, a nonrelapsing and serious disease with a high fatality rate. The other two are uncommon: *Plasmodium malariae* and *Plasmodium ovale*. *Plasmodium knowelsi* causes malaria in nonhuman primates and can rarely cause human malaria.

Transmission of malaria is by the bite of an infected female anopheline mosquito. The mosquito ingests human blood containing gametocytes (the sexual stages of the parasite). In the mosquito's stomach, these male and female stages join together to form sporozoites. These concentrate in the salivary glands of the mosquito and are injected into the next person that the mosquito bites. They pass in the bloodstream to the liver, where they develop into merozoites (*pre-erythrocytic cycle*). The clinical attack begins when they invade the red cells, and undergo a complete cycle of development (*erythrocytic cycle*), resulting in further release of merozoites into the bloodstream and another clinical attack. Some also develop into male and female gametocytes, which can then be taken up by another mosquito. The life cycle in the mosquito spans 8–35 days, depending on the infecting species. The duration of the erythrocytic cycle also varies with the species of parasite and is between 36 and 72 hours.

Globally, and in affected countries, malaria control is a priority with a wide range of governments, specialist agencies, nongovernmental organizations and foundations involved in active programmes, initiatives and research. At the population level, in endemic areas, insecticide-impregnated bed nets have been successful not just in protecting individuals but also in reducing transmission, because they kill mosquitoes. Many charities in the West have focused their fund raising on nets. Personal protective measures such as covering the body and limbs, particularly at dawn and dusk, and spraying with strong insect repellent are also effective in reducing risk. Spraying of the walls of dwellings with long-lasting insecticides and spraying areas of the environment where larvae are present are also important control measures. Early diagnosis with accurate tests and prompt effective treatments are life saving, particularly among children, but are difficult to achieve in areas where health systems are poorly developed and resourced.

While eradication of malaria is a theoretical goal, achieving it is a highly complex challenge that amounts to much more than interrupting transmission. Current research is directed at areas such as developing a vaccine; creating a single-dose cure; combatting drug resistance; designing new, rapid diagnostic tests; and disabling the life cycle of the parasite.

Malaria was almost certainly endemic in the low-lying, marshy areas of the United Kingdom centuries ago, but there has been no transmission in the country since the late nineteenth century. Today, malaria in the United Kingdom is a disease of returning travellers. Since 1990, there have been between 1300 and 2500 cases a year and between 4 and 16 deaths. Over half the cases were acquired in West Africa. Very rarely there have been small outbreaks when a mosquito from an affected area has survived a flight (so-called *airport malaria*). Although malaria is not normally transmitted from person to person, it has done so rarely where there have been lapses in infection control procedures in hospitals. From a UK perspective, action is directed at raising awareness among travellers out of the country, making sure they take all necessary precautions, as well as maintaining high levels of vigilance to detect the disease among returning travellers and visitors and immigrants from endemic areas of the world. It is important that travellers are aware of the risks and adopt such protective measures, as well as taking prophylaxis when advised to do so. Taking the correct dose for the necessary period of time and ensuring that the prescriber of the medication is aware of the latest information on drug resistance in the areas to be visited are vital to risk reduction.

Diarrhoeal disease

On a global scale, diarrhoeal disease is common: the World Health Organization estimates that it affects 1.7 billion people each year. A very wide range of infectious agents – viruses, bacteria and parasites – produce diarrhoeal illness.

It can occur in three main forms: an acute watery form when a great deal of fluid can be lost over a short space of time, bloody diarrhoea and persistent diarrhoea (defined as longer than 14 days). It can lead to electrolyte depletion and loss of protein. Worldwide, a high proportion of diarrhoeal disease is associated with poor sanitation, impure drinking water and living conditions that do not allow the rudiments of personal hygiene. Many infectious agents, most spread by the faeco-oral route, cause diarrhoeal disease, some with more serious consequences than others. Sometimes, contaminated food can be the vehicle for infection – the food-borne illnesses are covered separately later in this chapter.

Diarrhoeal disease can be viewed from three main perspectives:

1. Its impact on young children in low- and middle-income countries.
2. Its occurrence among adults in the poorer parts of the world.
3. The range of infective causes that are endemic in high-income countries or are contracted by returning travellers.

The first of these categories, diarrhoeal disease in the under-fives, has received the greatest public health attention because it is common and life threatening. Childhood mortality reduction was one of the Millennium Development Goals set by the United Nations, and addressing it meant acknowledging that diarrhoeal disease was responsible for as many as 700,000 deaths among the under-fives, almost three-quarters of whom are children under two years old.

To tackle diarrhoeal disease in children, the cornerstone is addressing the key underlying risk factors: water, sanitation and hygiene – all of which are linked to poverty. Achieving good levels of nutrition, and particularly prolonged breastfeeding, reduces risk. About a quarter of cases are due to rotavirus, and a small but important proportion are cholera related. Vaccines against both of these infective agents are strong interventions that can save lives. The main reason for death is the rapid deterioration that occurs in young children when they lose fluid from vomiting, diarrhoea and fever. The profuse watery diarrhoea, typical of illnesses in the under-fives, is particularly lethal, with severe dehydration rapidly followed by death. A revolution in the approach to this problem has been the work in many low-income countries to get oral rehydration solutions into people (particularly children) early in their illness. It is a particularly effective population-level strategy when parents are educated in the therapy and can use it themselves for their children.

Consideration of the wider problem of diarrhoeal disease in all age groups means recognizing that the long-term aim, just as with the approach in children, must also be to address underlying determinants like poverty, poor sanitation and access to healthcare. The root causes of these are very diverse and include serious failures of governance, preventing the development of a country's infrastructure. In their most dramatic manifestations, they are associated with displaced populations due to conflict or natural disaster.

Evidence of the devastating effects that epidemics of the disease can still have in many parts of the world is seen from time to time on the television screens of the West when there are floods or earthquakes or war. In such circumstances, sanitation can break down as people are displaced from their houses into makeshift and overcrowded camps. Many diseases flourish, but one in particular is a marker of extreme circumstances: cholera. It can be associated with huge loss of life. For example, in Iraq in 2007, 3300 cases of cholera were reported. In that country, sewage works had been targeted by insurgents and water supplies were polluted. Similarly, late in 2008, an outbreak initially affecting more than 10,000 people began in Zimbabwe, triggered by the breakdown of the country's infrastructure (poor governance was the reason). When the 2010 earthquake in Haiti laid waste to the country's sanitation systems and displaced millions from their homes, this started a cholera outbreak that has since affected more than 1 in 20 of the population. Over the next two years, it hospitalized hundreds of thousands of people and killed more than 5000. Infection with *Vibrio cholera* causes the characteristic clinical features of cholera: very severe diarrhoea with copious watery stools ('rice water') accompanied by vomiting and rapid dehydration. Acutely ill patients require hospital treatment with careful management to replace lost fluids and electrolytes. If patients are able to drink, prompt administration of oral rehydration solutions can play a crucial life-saving role. Surveillance of contacts is an important control measure. Vaccination gives low protection and short-lived immunity and is therefore of limited value. The main environmental control measures are the protection of water supplies and the supervision of disposal of sewage. In a country with modern water supply and sewage disposal systems, cholera is of almost no public health importance (aside from occasional imported cases).

A case of cholera in a high-income country is extremely rare, but most of the organisms that cause diarrhoeal disease have no such geographical restriction. Those of greatest relevance to high-income countries – causing illness at home and among returning travellers from abroad – are *E. coli*, which takes several forms; *Shigella*; amoebic dysentery; typhoid; cryptosporidium; and *Giardia*. Each is discussed below. Two of the most common causes of diarrhoea – Salmonella and Campylobacter – are discussed in the section on food-borne illness. Many of these organisms can be food-borne, of course – but Salmonella and Campylobacter are considered in that section because food is their major medium of transmission. In high-income countries, waterborne diarrhoeal disease is far less common than in low-income countries, and so food-borne disease is relatively more important.

Enterotoxigenic E. coli (ETEC) produces toxins and watery diarrhoea rather like that which occurs in cholera. It is a common cause of diarrhoeal illness among infants in tropical countries and in adults visiting tropical countries. It is one of the causes of traveller's diarrhoea and is acquired by contaminated water or sometimes food.

Enteroinvasive E. coli (EIEC) is the other major cause of bacillary dysentery, usually in a less severe form but also characterized by bloody diarrhoea. It is very similar in its modes of infection to *Shigella* and occurs in sporadic cases and outbreaks in similar circumstances.

Another group of *E. coli* causing potentially serious illness is *verocytotoxin-producing E. coli* (VTEC). This organism can cause just mild symptoms, but severe disease – in particular, haemolytic uraemic syndrome and thrombotic thrombocytopaenicpurpura (TTP). These can be fatal, particularly in young children and the elderly. The most common subtype is *E. coli* O157.

Of the infective causes of bloody diarrhoea worldwide, Shigella dysentery is the most common. The *Shigella* bacillus has four species: *S. sonnei*, *S. flexneri*, *S. boydii* and *S. dysenteriae*. *S. sonnei* is the most common organism involved and results in an infection known as bacillary dysentery. When the full clinical picture occurs, it is typified by diarrhoea of acute onset (with mucus, blood and pus in more severe cases), abdominal pain and fever. The reservoir for infection is the human gastrointestinal tract, and transmission is by the faecal–oral route, either directly or indirectly. Indirect transmission by ingestion of contaminated food or drink is also quite common.

The classical clinical presentation of amoebic dysentery is also recurrent attacks of abdominal pain and bloody diarrhoea. It is caused by *Entamoeba histolytica*, a protozoan that can become a cyst with a tough, resistant membrane. In the human intestine, it emerges from the cyst in its active form and causes symptoms. It is most common in the tropics and subtropics. If there are periods of remission, the cycle may continue for years with cysts in the faeces. The sole reservoir is human, either as symptomless excreters or with the chronic disease. The usual vehicle for transmission is contaminated water or food – especially salads and raw fruit.

Typhoid symptoms can include pyrexia, headache, anorexia and diarrhoea (occasionally constipation). A classical rose-spot rash may appear on the trunk, and enlargement of the spleen may also occur. Rarely, there is intestinal ulceration and perforation. Paratyphoid fever has similar but milder symptomatology, with a lower fatality rate. Typhoid vaccine gives around 50%–70% protection and is recommended for travellers to areas where typhoid is endemic, but it is important that travellers are aware of the risks.

Parasitic causes of diarrhoea are also important both globally and in the United Kingdom. *Cryptosporidium* is a protozoan organism with a number of species, the most common being *C. parvum* and *C. hominis*. It has a parasitic life cycle. It is a relatively commonly reported cause of diarrhoeal illness (there are between 3000 and 5000 cases in England and Wales per year), and it usually produces watery diarrhoea that can last up to a month. In immunocompromised individuals, it can last much longer. It is transmitted by the faecal–oral route: either person to person, animal to person, by water or by food. Outbreaks have happened when treatment of the public mains' water supply has failed. A large outbreak in England occurred after drinking water from a borehole supply became contaminated. Contact with farm animals, along with poor personal hygiene, is a cause.

Giardia is another parasitic cause of diarrhoea. It produces a cyst, which lodges in the duodenum after ingestion and releases trophozoites that multiply and occupy the small bowel. There are a number of *Giardia* species that infect people. It causes acute and chronic symptoms (particularly diarrhoea, abdominal pain and bloating). The organism is found in the faeces of wild and domestic animals (sometimes pets), and its cyst is quite environmentally resistant. It can be water- or food-borne or contracted because of poor personal hygiene when in contact with animals or animal pastures. Although the classic occurrence is among backpackers drinking from mountain streams, in some parts of the world it can be contracted from public water supplies. Notably, the cysts are resistant to chlorine disinfection (a method of water purification in some jurisdictions). The initial bout of diarrhoea may subside and be passed off as traveller's diarrhoea. Then chronic symptoms can become insidious – malaise, weight loss, flatulence and abdominal pain – and the diagnosis may not be suspected. Moreover, it is notoriously difficult to detect in stool samples. In such cases, the affected person may soldier on for a long period of time being investigated for persistent and vague bowel symptoms or even for more sinister causes, such as malignancy. Treatment with high doses of appropriate antibiotics is usually effective but may need more than one course. The key is to have a high awareness of the possible diagnosis in returning travellers, even from developed countries where it may be thought that public water supplies are safe.

Pneumonia

Pneumonia is estimated to cause 2.8 million deaths every year worldwide – more than any other communicable disease. In 1990, it caused a greater burden than any other disease at all – although by 2010 it had fallen to second, replaced by ischaemic heart disease.

By definition, pneumonia is inflammation of the alveoli of one or both lungs. In the vast majority of cases, this inflammation is caused by infection. A wide range of infectious agents can cause it – bacteria (including *Streptococcus pneumoniae*), viruses (including influenza) and fungi (such as the *Pneumocystis* pneumonia that can affect people with suppressed immunity, particularly due to HIV).

Pneumonia affects all age groups, but is both more common and more serious in children (particularly infants) and the elderly, smokers and people with preexisting lung conditions or immunodeficiency. Its classic triad of symptoms is cough (which may be purulent or bloody), fever and shortness of breath. In the elderly, it can often cause acute confusion. Antibiotics are the mainstay of treatment for bacterial pneumonia.

The bacterium *S. pneumoniae* is the most common cause of pneumonia, although its incidence is declining substantially since the introduction of pneumococcal vaccine. In the United Kingdom, this has been part of the childhood immunization programme since 2006, and is also given to adults aged 65 years and over.

While pneumonia does represent a very major and real disease burden, in one sense its impact appears exaggerated. Burden of disease data rely on death certification. It is common for pneumonia to be the final illness of somebody who has multimorbidity and is increasingly frail. In such cases, it is technically correct to record pneumonia as the cause of death, but this belies a more complex picture. This phenomenon is well known, but does not negate the importance of pneumonia.

In the United Kingdom, pneumonia affects approximately 1 in every 1000 adults every year – mainly during autumn and winter. It requires hospitalization in a subset of cases, mainly when it leads to respiratory failure, septicaemia or acute confusion.

Globally, the impact of pneumonia falls particularly heavily on children aged under five years. Diarrhoeal disease is often considered together with pneumonia since their combined effect represents a major loss of productive life and a global target for public health action, and because there are common features to their prevention and control. The *Integrated Global Action Plan for Pneumonia and Diarrhoea* (GAPPD) aims to end preventable deaths from childhood pneumonia and diarrhoea by 2025. It focuses on establishing general protective measures, specific disease-preventing measures and appropriate treatment (Figure 3.16).

INFECTIOUS DISEASES CAUSING A MAJOR BURDEN OF MORBIDITY AND DISABILITY

The World Health Organization has prioritized 17 specific infections in the poorest parts of the world caused by *protozoa* (Chagas disease, human African trypanosomiasis and leishmaniasis), *bacteria* (Buruli ulcer, leprosy, trachoma and yaws), *helminths* (cysticercosis or taeniasis, dracunculiasis, echinococcosis, food-borne trematodiases, lymphatic filariasis, onchocerciasis, schistosomiasis and soil-transmitted helminthiasis) and *viruses* (dengue, chikungunya and rabies).

As a group, they have been designated as *neglected tropical diseases*. They are endemic in 149 countries and

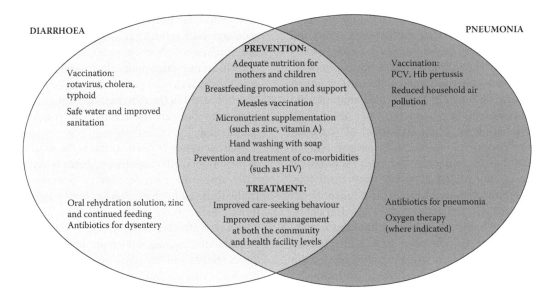

Figure 3.16 Prevention and treatment strategies for diarrhoea and pneumonia: substantial overlap.

Source: UNICEF. *Pneumonia and Diarrhoea: Tackling the Deadliest Diseases for the World's Poorest Children.* New York: UNICEF, 2012. With permission.

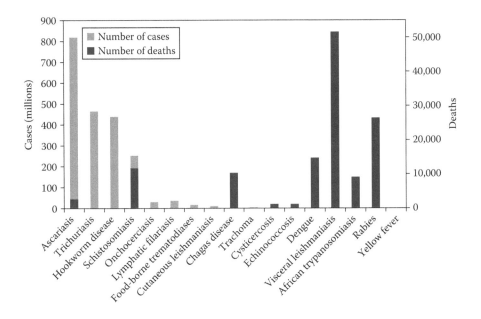

Figure 3.17 Mortality burden of neglected tropical diseases: number of cases and the total number of deaths.

Source: Hotez PJ, Alvarado M, Basáñez MG, et al. The global burden of disease study 2010: interpretation and implications for the neglected tropical diseases. *PLoS Neglected Tropical Diseases* 2014; 8(7):e2865.

affect 1.4 billion people. Many can and do cause death (Figure 3.17). Many affected children and adults live with these diseases untreated (or inadequately treated) and, as a result, suffer varying degrees of permanent impairment and disability, as well as severely reduced quality of life.

This section of the chapter deals with this group of disabling diseases, as well as a range of other conditions that can also cause death but are mainly a challenge because of the relatively high burden of illness that they produce.

Neglected tropical diseases

Almost all of the neglected tropical diseases can be cured and, in some cases, actually eradicated. The standard treatments and vaccines remain very effective with little sign of drug resistance emerging. The key step is to create access to these treatments and vaccines.

The main diseases and their features are described in the following.

Onchocerciasis (river blindness) is caused by a parasitic worm (*Onchocerca volvulus*), transmitted by the bites of black flies. Some 18 million people are infected world-wide. A high proportion (90%+) of cases are in African countries near fast-moving rivers. Once infected, people experience intolerable itching due to the parasite burrowing under the skin, visual impairment and then blindness. Treatment with an antimicrobial drug only stops the disease progressing and must be taken regularly for up to 15 years. Aerial spraying with larvicides in affected areas is also an important control measure.

Schistosomiasis (bilharzia) is caused by a parasite of the genus *Schistoma* (*S. mekongi*, *S. mansoni*, *S. haematobium*, *S. intercalatum* and *S. japanicum*) that enters the body through the skin and migrates through the blood system (and continues its life cycle) to target organs such as the bowel and bladder. The vector, which also forms part of the parasite's life cycle, is a freshwater snail. An estimated 200 million cases occur worldwide affecting some 70 countries. The disease can be successfully treated with antimicrobial drugs. Control measures include health education (on the dangers of swimming in natural water and drinking contaminated water) and elimination of the relevant snail population.

Trachoma is caused by a bacterium, *Chlamydia trachomatis*, that is transmitted by close contact between people or vectors, such as clothing. It can, if untreated, eventually lead to blindness, because chronic infection produces scarring of the conjunctiva so that the eyelashes turn inwards. It is intensely painful. The disease is endemic in more than 50 countries, and some 40 million people are affected. The prevention and control strategy is based on the acronym SAFE (surgery of the eyelids in 'late' cases, antibiotics to treat community infection, facial cleanliness and environmental improvements to improve sanitation and access to clean water so as to reduce transmission).

Chagas disease is caused by a protozoan parasite, *Trypanosoma cruzi*. It largely occurs in Latin America, where around 7 million people are affected. It is starting to appear in some other countries. Its main route of infection is via the faeces of triatomine bugs, but it can result from blood transfusion or transplantation of organs. In the early stages of infection, symptoms are mild and nonspecific, although in a proportion of people there is a characteristic unilateral purple swelling of the eyelid. If the infection is not treated, it progresses so that parasites enter the heart, bowel or nervous system. It can then become life threatening. In the early stage of infection, antimicrobial drugs are highly effective but therapeutic benefit wanes the longer the person has the disease. Insecticide spraying in and around homes (the vector bug lives in the cracks and crevices within houses) can be very effective in destroying this vector.

Leprosy has been documented up to 4000 years ago by examination of skeletons from that time. DNA sequencing of the leprosy bacterium, *Mycobaterium leprae*, from medieval human bones has found that some of the strains are identical to those still infecting people today. The bacterium infects skin, mucous membranes and peripheral nerves. If untreated, it causes scarring, deformity and loss of function

and sensation of the hands and fingers in particular. It can be treated with multidrug therapy, but the sequence of advanced disease cannot be reversed. It is strongly associated with poverty. It is not highly contagious, but the precise mode of transmission is not clear.

New cases of leprosy are recorded each year; it is now mainly concentrated in 17 countries. In Florida, recent growth in the incidence of leprosy has been blamed on the armadillo population. Armadillos are one of the few animals that carry *M. leprae*. The building of retirement communities in Florida has encroached onto armadillos' land, and a small number of people have developed leprosy after contact with armadillos and their saliva.

Lymphatic filariasis (elephantiasis) is caused by a nematode, *Wuchereria bancrofti* (or other strains), in a life cycle that involves mosquito vectors transmitting infective larvae. Once bitten by such a mosquito, a person becomes the host to numerous thread-like worms that invade the lymphatic system, in effect clogging it up. Not everyone is symptomatic, but severe symptoms include gross swelling of the legs, arms and scrotum. There is an effective drug therapy, but it will not reverse this gross lymphoedema. Strategies to eliminate transmission involve mass drug administration and insect vector control.

Buruli ulcer is caused by the bacterium *Mycobacterium ulcerans*. Its precise mode of transmission is unknown. It starts with a painless skin nodule that leads to large ulcers on the arms and legs. Early treatment with antimicrobial drugs is often successful, but if untreated, serious complications, including deformities of the limb and serious secondary infections, occur. Early diagnosis and treatment is the main control strategy.

Dracunculiasis (Guinea worm disease) is caused by a nematode roundworm parasite, *Dracunculus medinensis*, that is mainly found in static water sources where water fleas harbour Guinea worm larvae. The life cycle of the parasite continues within the human body after someone drinks infested water. Larvae turn into worms that then form blisters on the skin. People tend to bathe these excruciatingly painful areas, which releases larvae back into the water and the cycle continues. Infected people become sick, listless and unproductive but do not usually die. There is no drug treatment, and the worm must be gradually (a few centimetres a day) and painfully extracted through the skin (it can be up to a metre long) by wrapping it around a stick and ensuring that it does not break off, leaving a part of the worm behind. Elimination of this disease – that in 2016 affected just 25 people in five countries – requires supplying clean water, early diagnosis and treatment, health education of communities, and spraying affected areas with larvicides.

African trypanosomiasis (sleeping sickness) is caused by a parasite (*Trypanosoma brucei gambiense* or *Trypanosoma brucei rhodesiense*) spread by the bite of infected tsetse flies. The parasite invades the central nervous system, causing a range of unusual and debilitating symptoms, including alteration of the biological clock (hence the term *sleeping sickness*). These symptoms develop over a period of months to years. Trypanosomiasis is fatal if untreated. The *gambiense* form accounts for 98% of cases, and affects 24 countries in western and central Africa. The *rhodesiene* form is more rapidly progressive and affects 13 countries, in eastern and southern Africa. Oral antiparasitic drugs are effective treatment. The mainstays of control are prompt diagnosis and treatment of cases, and measures to reduce the presence of the tsetse fly.

Leishmaniasis is caused by protozoan parasites of more than 20 *Leishmania* species, transmitted by female sand-flies. The cutaneous and mucocutaneous forms affect the skin and superficial tissues, the former causing scarring and the latter destruction. The visceral form is also known as kala azar and affects internal organs – usually the spleen, liver and bone marrow. The visceral form is usually fatal if not treated. Early diagnosis and effective treatment is the mainstay of control, and insecticides also play an important role.

Yaws is a chronic bacterial infection (*Treponema pallidum pertenue*) found in humid tropical areas of Africa, Asia, Latin America and western Pacific. It is spread directly between humans, and mainly infects children. The initial infection is seen as a single skin lesion. If not treated with antibiotics, multiple lesions develop, affecting skin, bone and cartilage, often causing disfigurement and disability. In 2012, it was discovered that a single dose of oral azithromycin is effective treatment. Because of this, and because it is spread directly between humans, yaws is a strong candidate for global eradication. It has already been eliminated in many countries, most recently India.

Cysticercosis is caused by larvae of the tapeworm *Taenia solium*, spread in contaminated food (classically under-cooked pork and beef) or water. The larvae pass from the bowel throughout the body, where they can develop in the muscles, eyes and central nervous system. Those that develop in the central nervous system can cause epilepsy. This is thought to be responsible for 50 million cases of preventable epilepsy (termed neurocysticercosis) world-wide. A series of control measures are required, including ensuring effective prompt treatment, vaccinating pigs and improving pig husbandry. The related infection tae-niasis is caused by adult tapeworms that have developed from the same larvae. It causes only mild illness, but is important in public health terms because it continues transmission of the tapeworm, which subsequently pro-duce larvae.

Alongside dengue, which is discussed elsewhere, *rabies* is the neglected tropical disease best known in the richer parts of the world. In part, this is because of the fear factor – the idea that a dog bite can cause death. International travellers are aware of rabies as a threat. In fact, rabies remains geo-graphically widespread. Half the world's population lives in countries where rabies is endemic. But more than 90% of human cases occur in Asia and Africa. The vast majority of cases worldwide come from dog bites, but the last non-imported case in the United Kingdom was in 2002 in a bat handler. There is a vaccine for rabies, but it is not wholly efficacious. Prompt medical treatment is essential in the event of a bite or scratch from a high-risk animal in a rabies-endemic country. This should consist of wound irrigation and consideration of vaccine and/or immunoglobulin use, based on a risk assessment that considers the animal, the nature of the bite or injury and the geographical location. However, there is no specific antiviral drug to treat rabies.

Blood-borne hepatitis viruses

There are six types of hepatitis virus that cause infection, known by their letters, A, B, C, D, E and G (there is no hepa-titis F).

Hepatitis A and E are mainly transmitted by contami-nated food or water. Hepatitis D virus is blood-borne but requires the presence of hepatitis B virus for replication; it is therefore always associated with coexisting hepatitis B infection. Infection is usually more severe and fatality rates higher than with simple hepatitis B infection.

Most public health attention is given to hepatitis B and C.

Hepatitis B occurs throughout the world, particularly in Africa, the Far East, Southeast Asia and parts of Europe. In some individuals, hepatitis B virus persists, resulting in chronic infection. The risks of this declines with age – from around 80%–90% in neonates to around just 5% in immune-competent adults.

Chronic carriers of hepatitis B, defined as those with the presence of hepatitis B surface antigen (HBsAg) in the serum for six months or longer, are at increased risk of developing progressive liver disease, including cirrhosis and hepatocel-lular carcinoma. In the United Kingdom, seroprevalence is low but varies geographically. For example, the prevalence among antenatal women varies between 0.05% in areas such as East Anglia and 1% in some parts of London. In southern Europe, the carrier rate is up to 5%, and in parts of the Far East, some 10%–15% of people may have serum that is posi-tive for HBsAg. Although notifications of acute hepatitis B are low, seroprevalence varies within population subgroups, such as men who have sex with men and immigrant com-munities. Most of the carriers in the United Kingdom have no previous history of jaundice.

The reservoir of infection is humans and possibly other primates. Hepatitis B can be transmitted from another case, or more often from a carrier, either parenterally or sexu-ally, via intravenous drug misuse, tattooing, acupuncture, ear piercing and medical and dental instrumentation. It is an occupational risk for healthcare workers and those involved in handling blood products and dialysis equip-ment. Hepatitis B can be transmitted from infected moth-ers to their babies at or around the time of birth (perinatal transmission). Blood transfusion is a less likely method of transmission in the United Kingdom, because of strict screening of donated blood.

Close household and sexual contacts of a case of acute hepatitis B or a chronic carrier of the virus should be screened for hepatitis B markers, and immunization offered where necessary.

General preventive measures include strict precautions in all settings where needles or instrumentation is used. Adequate sterilization of instruments should be undertaken, and wherever possible, disposable needles and instruments should be employed and used once only for each patient. There is a clear need for close supervision of tattooing, body piercing and acupuncture. Special risks apply to patients and staff of renal units, where vigilance should be especially high.

Health education is vital among special and high-risk groups, such as drug takers and men who have sex with men. Patients who are HBsAg positive must be made aware of the mode of spread of the disease and the behaviour necessary to protect others. Perinatal transmission of hepatitis B infection can be prevented by immunization from birth of infants of infected mothers. Specific hepatitis B immunoglobulin is available for passive protection and is normally used in combination with hepatitis B vaccine to confer active as well as passive immunity after exposure (e.g. after being pricked by a needle from an infected person), or when immediate protection is required. Chronic hepatitis B can now be treated with antiviral agents, with the aim of preventing progression to cirrhosis or hepatocellular carcinoma.

Hepatitis C virus is a blood-borne virus that is a leading cause of liver disease worldwide. Globally, an estimated 170 million people have antibodies to hepatitis C. Around 300,000 die from the infection each year. When symptoms do occur, they include fatigue, loss of appetite, weight loss, abdominal pain or discomfort, poor memory or concentration and depression. However, most acute hepatitis C infections produce no symptoms or produce a mild illness. Moreover, many of those with chronic infection, which develops in about 60%–80% of those infected, will not have symptoms. Chronic hepatitis C infection progresses over about 20–30 years to liver cirrhosis and liver cancer in a proportion of people affected. In some cases, liver transplantation is required.

In the United Kingdom, the majority of hepatitis C infections have arisen among current or previous injecting drug users; some may have experimented with drugs many years ago, and have never been habitual users. Hippie era recreational drug users are often unaware of their potential exposure to risk and may have undiagnosed chronic infection. The late Anita Roddick, founder of The Body Shop, tested positive for hepatitis C and then played a public role in raising public awareness of the infection. She was diagnosed with hepatitis C in 2005, but caught it from a blood transfusion during childbirth in 1971. She harboured the infection silently for many years, as do many chronically infected people. The prevalence of hepatitis C antibodies among people who inject drugs in the United Kingdom is around 50%, with variation in this figure for different parts of the country, for example, northeast England (37%), northwest England (68%), Scotland (57%), Northern Ireland (32%) and Wales (47%).

The true prevalence of hepatitis C infection within the population of the United Kingdom is unknown, but it is estimated that around 214,000 have chronic infection, the majority of whom have probably not been formally diagnosed. Of those with chronic infection in England, just 3% are receiving treatment.

Infection is twice as common in men. High-risk sexual behaviour among men who have sex with men is an area of concern in which co-infection (HIV and hepatitis C) is increasing. Those who received blood products before 1986 and blood transfusions before 1991 are also at increased risk. A small proportion of cases arise through mother-to-baby transmission. There is also a risk from medical or dental treatment abroad in countries where infection control is inadequate and infection is common. Tattooing and body piercing using unsterile equipment is another risk factor.

Deaths from liver failure or cancer caused by hepatitis C have been rising since the mid-1990s, and there have been similar increases in the numbers scheduled for liver transplants because of the infection (Figure 3.18). The future burden of disease from chronic liver damage or cancer in the United Kingdom is likely to be considerable, and worldwide even more so.

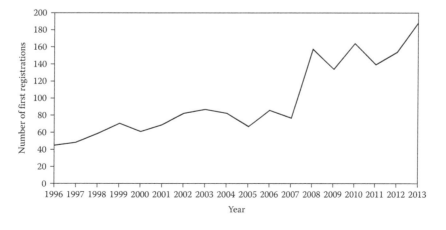

Figure 3.18 Registrations for a liver transplant due to post-hepatitis C cirrhosis, United Kingdom.

Source: Public Health England (PHE). *Hepatitis C in the UK: 2014 Report.* London: PHE, 2014.

The public health strategy to combat hepatitis C must address four key elements:

1. Preventing new infections
2. Raising awareness among the public and risk groups
3. Ensuring widespread access to diagnostic and testing facilities
4. Effective treatment of those with a positive diagnosis

In England, three in five people with hepatitis C infection may be unaware of it. This necessitates strong public awareness–raising campaigns, coupled with the offer of testing to reduce the number of undiagnosed infections. In addition, it is important to increase testing among high-risk populations, such as those in specialist drug treatment centres, in prisons and attending genitourinary medicine clinics.

Preventive measures aim to reduce ongoing transmission of hepatitis C, particularly among injecting drug users and other at-risk populations. Key activities include increased drug education (particularly in schools), drug intervention programmes, provision of needle exchange schemes, safe disposal of drug-injecting equipment, distribution of disinfection tablets in prisons and sex education programmes.

Special control measures are needed to ensure that the small number of healthcare workers who are infected with hepatitis C do not pass the infection on to their patients. In the United Kingdom, there is detailed guidance to the NHS with particular emphasis on restricting infected healthcare workers from carrying out exposure-prone procedures (such as surgical operations).

Advances in therapy mean that treatment has an average success rate of 55%, varying from 40% to 80%, depending on the virus genotype. Not everyone is suitable for treatment, and there may be unpleasant side effects that are intolerable for some. The aim of treatment is to reduce the viral load in the body to undetectable levels and so prevent progression to serious liver disease.

Dengue fever

Some of the older communicable disease classifications categorize dengue fever as a neglected tropical disease. It is in fact one of the viral haemorrhagic fevers; however, given its importance as a rapidly emerging disease, we describe it here in its own right. The pattern of dengue in the twenty-first century has been of surges in parts of the world that have seen little of it in earlier decades. It is one of the fastest-growing communicable disease problems in the world; it is now present in 150 countries. Researchers using the most up-to-date scientific modelling techniques have produced estimates for the burden of disease that are much higher than those that the World Health Organization is working with. The estimated number of new infections producing illness in a year is 96 million, while the number of very mild or unapparent infections is about 390 million, the highest incidence being in Asia and the Americas (Table 3.4).

Table 3.4 Estimated burden of dengue by continent

	Apparent	Inapparent
Africa	16 million	48 million
Asia	67 million	204 million
Americas	13 million	41 million
Oceania	180 thousand	0.5 million
Global	96 million	294 million

Source: Bhatt S, Gething PW, Brady OJ, et al. The global distribution and burden of dengue. Nature 2013;496(7446):504-7.

A *flavivirus* comprising four types causes dengue fever. When it produces symptoms, they can range in severity from mild to severe flu-like illness to the most serious forms: dengue haemorrhagic fever and dengue shock syndrome; they may cause death. The key to the epidemiology of dengue is the mosquito *Aedes aegypti*. This arthropod is endemic in many tropical and subtropical regions of the world. It lays eggs in pools of water both big (e.g. ponds) and very small (e.g. the base of plant pots standing on balconies). It only really needs a teaspoonful of water in which to breed. A ubiquitous breeding ground for the mosquito, and one that is blamed for being a major factor in the transmission of dengue fever, is discarded tyres. They retain heat from the sun and have multiple crevices for rainwater to collect. *A. aegypti* is a daytime mosquito and so poses risks in the waking hours rather than the classic dawn and dusk pattern of many mosquitoes. It flies only short distances and close to the ground, so bites on the ankle and feet are common.

There have been outbreaks in France and Croatia in recent years, but dengue has not become established in Europe, although many experts believe this will happen given global warming and the spread of the disease globally. There was a very large outbreak in Madeira, Portugal, in 2012–13, with more than 2000 probable cases and around 1000 confirmed cases (Figure 3.19). Madeira is a subtropical island with no history of dengue transmission for a hundred years. However, a population of *A. aegypti* mosquitoes became established and the tourist-based economy sustains strong links with endemic parts of the world, particularly South America.

There is no specific treatment or vaccine for dengue fever, and actions targeted at the mosquito vector have limited success because it breeds in such small pools of water in many locations in a neighbourhood. For these reasons, it is very difficult to eradicate from endemic areas, with no night-time frosts. However, outbreaks in nonendemic areas can usually be brought under control by good surveillance, mosquito spraying and trying hard to eliminate domestic, industrial and municipal sources of standing water, no matter how seemingly insignificant. Individuals can protect themselves by covering up, using insect sprays containing DEET and, again, eliminating standing water from terraces, balconies and gardens.

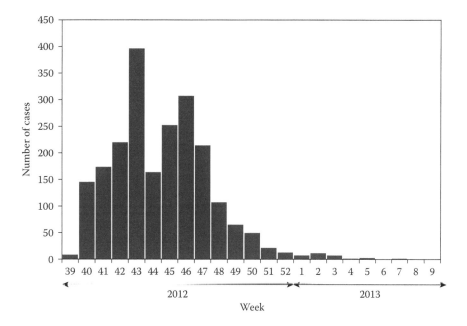

Figure 3.19 Dengue cases (probable and confirmed) by week, Madeira.

Source: European Centre for Disease Prevention and Control (ECDC). *Epidemiological Update: Outbreak of Dengue in Madeira, Portugal.* Solna: ECDC, 2013. With permission.

The most recent developments involve research and field studies to release genetically modified male mosquitoes that pass on a mutation when reproducing so that the resulting eggs are fatally flawed. This has caused concerns about unforeseen circumstances, but trials are underway. Another novel approach involves introducing a bacterium *Wolbachia* that is found within the cells of a high proportion of insects, including mosquitoes (although not those that transmit malaria or dengue fever). The relationship between the bacterium and the insect is not fully understood but is symbiotic or parasitic rather than pathogenic. It appears to influence the host's reproductive processes and to protect against viral infection. Scientists are seeking to introduce *Wolbachia* into the bodies of *A. aegypti* mosquitoes in ways that will make them resist the dengue virus.

Measles

Measles is an extremely contagious infection, caused by a paramyxovirus. Transmission is via droplet spread and via objects freshly contaminated by secretions from the nasopharynx. It is so contagious that transmission is sometimes reported from entering a room that an infected individual has recently left.

Cases of measles are almost always in unvaccinated children. Infection with the virus produces a prodromal illness with upper respiratory symptoms, pyrexia and spots (Koplik spots) on the buccal mucosa. Classically, a maculopapular rash appears on the fourth day of the illness, but this is variable. This blotchy rash starts on the face and neck and spreads over the body. Secondary bacterial infection of the respiratory tract and otitis media are common complications, and encephalitis is rare. Such complications occur in approximately 10% of cases. A very rare complication is subacute sclerosing panencephalitis, which develops late (approximately seven years after infection) and results in death within a few months. Three groups of people are at particular risk of severe illness if they contract measles: pregnant women (measles can cause preterm labour or intrauterine death), infants and people who are immunocompromised.

Melinda Gates said, 'Women in the developing world know the power of vaccines. They will walk 10 km in the heat with their child and line up to get a vaccine, because they have seen death. Americans have forgotten what measles deaths look like'. It is true that measles vaccine has saved, and is continuing to save, millions of children's lives worldwide, yet the World Health Organization estimates that the disease still kills around 145,000 children a year. This makes it an important cause of global child mortality. The Measles and Rubella Initiative is a major global partnership, which aims to eliminate measles and rubella from most of the world by 2020. At the time of writing, this goal was highly unlikely to be met, although it may receive a surge of funding and political attention when polio is successfully eradicated. Reducing the number of measles cases to zero presents quite different challenges in different parts of the world. In the poorest countries, it is a case of improving the reliable provision of vaccines to children. In the richest countries (including the United Kingdom), it is a case of overcoming the apathy – and antipathy – associated with vaccination.

Meningitis

Meningitis is an infection involving the meninges, which line the brain and spinal cord. It often has very serious consequences. The infectious agents that cause meningitis are viral, bacterial or fungal. The viral forms of meningitis generally cause less serious illness. The majority of cases of bacterial meningitis are caused by one of three organisms: *Neisseria meningitidis* (this forms 12 serogroups, but 6 are important in causing illness: A, B, C, W-135, X and Y); *S. pneumoniae* and *Haemophilus influenzae* type B (Hib). Between them, they cause 9 in 10 cases of meningitis in children worldwide and 3 in 4 among adults.

The most important form of meningitis that produces cluster outbreaks and epidemics is meningococcal meningitis caused by one or another of the six serogroups of *N. meningitidis*. Taking a global view, one of the most seriously affected areas is the so-called meningitis belt of sub-Saharan Africa, stretching from Senegal in the west to Ethiopia in the east, and covering 26 countries. In the dry season, dust, cold and upper respiratory infections increase the likelihood of transmission of *N. meningitidis*. Overcrowded dwellings, population churning in movements due to conflict, pilgrimages and trade accentuate the conditions for transmission. The predominant organism in the meningitis belt has been the A subtype of meningococcus.

The precise subtype of meningococcus causing disease varies by country, and this makes the epidemiology very different. This also depends on the vaccine programmes in operation. Several vaccines are available to control the disease. Polysaccharide vaccines to protect against A, C, Y and W-135 subtypes have been available for nearly 30 years. This type of vaccine is not as effective as a conjugate vaccine; it provides protection for a relatively short time (three to five years). Nor is it effective in very young children. Over time, the more effective conjugate versions have been introduced into the meningitis vaccine portfolio. There is now a quadrivalent (serogroups A, C, Y and W-135) vaccine, while the creation of a meningococcal A conjugate vaccine has opened up a cheaper and better option for targeting the high-risk areas of Africa. By the beginning of 2015, more than 200 million people had been vaccinated with it and the incidence of meningitis was falling rapidly.

In the United Kingdom during the 1980s and 1990s, there were clusters of deaths from meningococcal infection in schools and universities. This caused much public anxiety, extensive media coverage and the formation of pressure groups that called for more action and research to combat the disease. A persistent pocket of high incidence of meningococcal infection with fatalities occurred in Stroud, Gloucestershire. The reason for the higher frequency in this area was not shown conclusively. The major breakthrough in meningitis in the United Kingdom was the introduction of a conjugate vaccine against meningococcal C disease. This was introduced into the childhood vaccination programme in 1999 and has brought about a big reduction in the incidence of, and deaths from, meningococcal C disease. In the

early 2000s, Hib vaccine was introduced into the childhood routine vaccination programme and has reduced, to a very small number, the cases of meningitis due to *H. influenzae* (less than 1% of the total). As a result of these additions to the vaccination programme, on average, there are approximately 3200 cases of bacterial meningitis and septicaemia annually in the United Kingdom. Three in every five are due to meningococcus, mainly serogroup B; the remainder are caused by pneumococcus (12%), *Streptococcus* B in the neonatal period (9%) and tubercle bacillus (6%). A conjugate vaccine against serogroup B meningococcus has been approved for use in the United Kingdom but not yet implemented, while a special campaign to vaccinate all 14- to 18-year-olds was introduced in the summer of 2015 to combat a rapid rise in the previously uncommon W serogroup using the conjugate quadrivalent vaccine.

Nasopharyngeal carriage of the organism in asymptomatic individuals can be surprisingly high, with up to 15%–20% of individuals being carriers in some age groups. The overall prevalence lies somewhere between 2% and 4% of the population. Most people catch the disease from an asymptomatic carrier, not from an infected person. Only capsulated strains have the capacity to cause invasive disease. Carriage of noncapsulated strains and other commensal *Neisseria* species can help to boost natural immunity. Long-term carriers of pathogenic strains rarely become cases themselves. Their natural defences have learned to cope with the organism.

The incubation period ranges from 2 to 10 days. The patient is infective for as long as the organism is present in the nasopharynx. Penicillin (the antibiotic of choice in the treatment of meningococcal disease) suppresses the organism but does not eradicate it. This is important, since it means that people who have recovered from meningitis should receive a second antibiotic to eliminate nasopharyngeal carriage of the pathogen.

In cases where meningitis does develop, symptoms are fever, headache, neck stiffness and photophobia. A haemorrhagic rash that does not blanch under pressure (e.g. if a glass is rolled over it) often accompanies this. Septacaemia can occur with or without the typical signs of meningitis; it causes flu-like symptoms and general malaise and can rapidly lead to deterioration and death. A very high level of clinical suspicion is necessary and skill in the recognition of septicaemia and shock in primary care. So too is parental education to ensure that the dangers of rapid deterioration in a sick child or teenager are a reason to seek urgent medical help; awareness of the significance of the rash and the glass test is also important.

With the presence of the characteristic rash, the administration of antibiotics, even before admission to hospital, is vital to reduce mortality from this disease. The organism can be identified by nonculture techniques, so administration of antibiotics should not be delayed in order that it can be grown in culture. Action rests largely with the general practitioner or accident and emergency unit in early treatment. National Institute for Health and Care Excellence

(NICE) guidance is in place for the diagnosis and management of suspected or established meningococcal disease both in hospital and in the prehospital phase. Deafness and limb and digit gangrene are among the most serious complications. Children who recover from meningococcal disease must be carefully assessed and receive the necessary support and further specialist clinical care.

Household contacts and other intimate contacts (e.g. kissing contacts) should be traced and offered antibiotic prophylaxis as soon as possible after the diagnosis has been made, preferably within 24 hours.

Healthcare-associated infection

Modern healthcare has brought untold benefits to millions of patients and their families. Against this the risks must be set. Even now in the twenty-first century, and even in high-income countries with well-funded healthcare systems, the risk of infection in hospitals and other facilities is a matter of serious concern for patients, the public, politicians and healthcare professionals.

Healthcare infection is a feature of health services in every country of the world to a greater or lesser extent, but in low- and some middle-income countries, weak infrastructure, poor standards of sanitation and lack of availability of clean, running water make it especially difficult to prevent (Figure 3.20).

In a country like the United Kingdom, with its system of comprehensive care driven by national standards and regimes of inspection, it might be expected that the rate of healthcare infection would be very low. Although there were improvements during the 2000s, the levels of infection

are still higher than they should be and there is marked variation across the country (Figure 3.21). There is no single reason for the growth of healthcare-associated infections. The factors that drive this are multiple. They include:

- *Patient-related factors*: The increase in people with serious illness (e.g. cancer) or treatments (e.g. transplants and cytotoxic drugs) that weaken their immune systems; the mixing of large numbers of patients from different referral sources.
- *Organizational factors*: High bed occupancy levels; poor staff–patient ratio; increased movement of patients within the hospital.
- *Healthcare staff factors*: Poor hand hygiene compliance; poor aseptic techniques when carrying out procedures such as insertion of tubes and intravascular lines and cleaning wounds; inadequate skills and training.
- *Environmental factors*: Defective environmental cleaning, contamination of frequently touched surfaces in clinical areas, inadequate decontamination and sterilization of instruments and equipment.
- *Structural factors*: Lack of easy access to essential preventive equipment such as hand sanitizers and sinks; low numbers of single rooms, isolation cubicles, hand basins and toilets; inadequate waste disposal facilities.
- *High antibiotic usage*: The emergence of drug-resistant bacteria. This is discussed more fully in a separate section of this chapter.

Intensive care units of hospitals are important hot spots for healthcare infections. They contain many patients who are seriously ill and who have compromised immune systems.

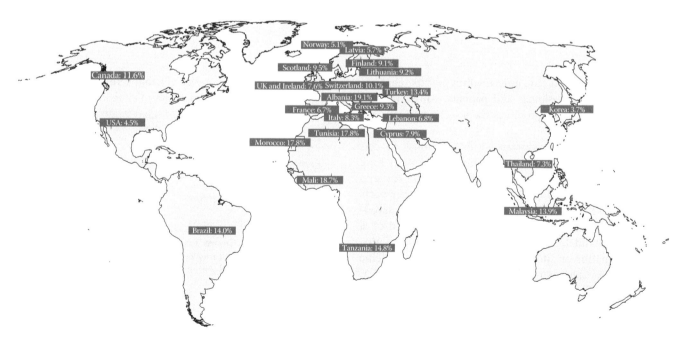

Figure 3.20 Prevalence of healthcare infection by country, 2010.

Source: World Health Organization (WHO). *The Burden of Health Care-Associated Infection Worldwide: A Summary.* Geneva: WHO, 2010. With permission.

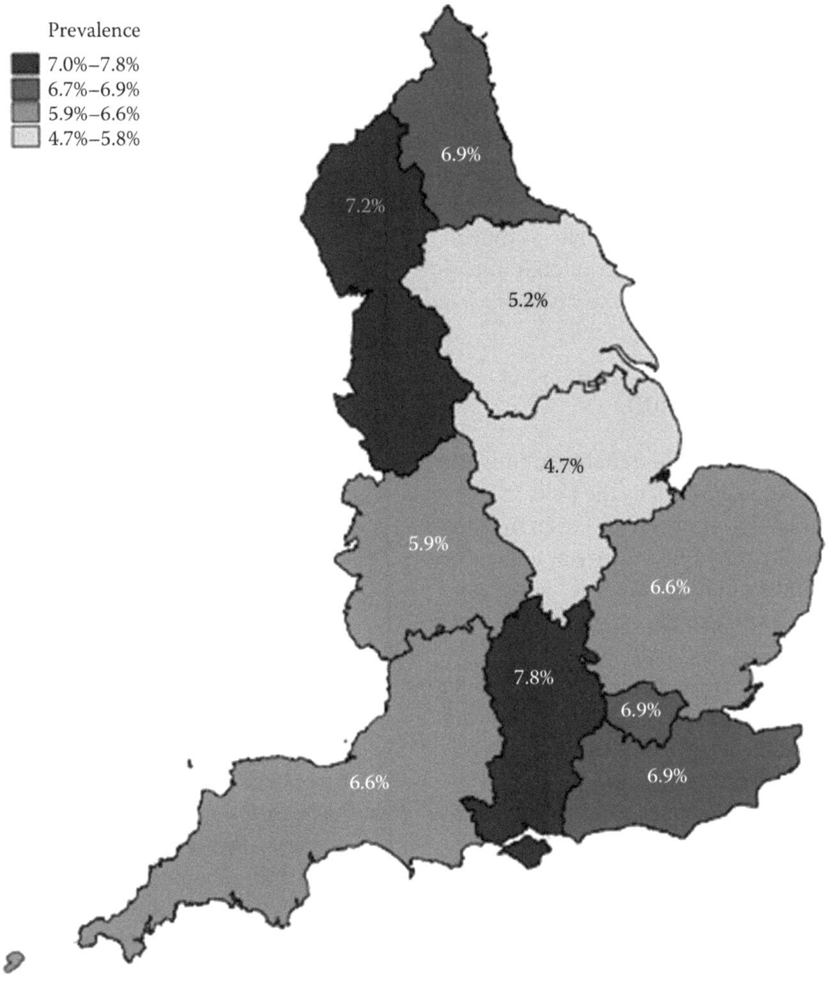

Prevalence
- 7.0%–7.8%
- 6.7%–6.9%
- 5.9%–6.6%
- 4.7%–5.8%

Figure 3.21 Prevalence of healthcare infection in England, 2011.

Source: Public Health England (PHE). *English National Point Prevalence Survey on Healthcare-Associated Infections and Antimicrobial Use,* 2011. London: PHE, 2012.

Patient care in intensive care units involves multiple contacts between health professionals and patients. Antibiotics are extensively used, which promotes the selection of resistant organisms.

Data on healthcare-associated infection must be collected by surveillance systems, and not all countries have adequate ones in place. The alternative is special surveys. Public Health England (and similar bodies in other parts of the United Kingdom) plays an important role in surveillance of healthcare infections. Surveillance is based on a mixture of mandatory and voluntary reporting and provides information on sites of infection as well as on specific organisms (e.g. bloodstream infections caused by MRSA, *Clostridium difficile*, glycopetide-resistant *Enterococcus* and other antibiotic-resistant microorganisms).

The most common types of healthcare infections are respiratory, urinary tract, surgical site, bloodstream and gastrointestinal (Table 3.5). The UK overall level of healthcare-associated infection is towards the middle of the range of other western European countries. International

Table 3.5 Estimated number of healthcare infections in acute care hospitals by major site of infection, Europe

Site	Estimated number of patients
Surgical site	15,700
Pneumonia	15,500
Urinary tract	15,200
Bloodstream	8,600
Gastro-intestinal	6,200

Source: European Centre for Disease Prevention and Control (ECDC). *Point Prevalence Survey of Healthcare-Associated Infections and Antimicrobial Use in European Hospitals 2011–2012.* Solna: ECDC, 2013.

comparisons are not straightforward, because definitions, surveillance systems and laboratories all vary. Studies in developed countries show a range of healthcare-associated infection prevalence between 3.5% and 12%, with the prevalence in England at 6.4% in 2011. The European

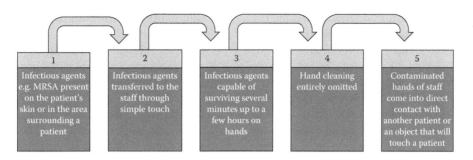

Figure 3.22 Spread of healthcare infection.

Centre for Disease Prevention and Control reported that on any given day, 80,000 people have an infection acquired in healthcare in Europe. Overall, an estimated 4 million cases of healthcare infection occur in Europe annually, causing 37,000 deaths. There is a considerable economic burden arising from the costs of care, loss of productivity and reduced quality of life.

METHICILLIN-RESISTANT *STAPHYLOCOCCUS AUREUS*

S. aureus can be naturally found on human skin or hair or in the nasal cavity and throat. However, it is also an important cause of infection, both in the community and in healthcare settings. The organism has become resistant to many antibiotics, notably methicillin (and other beta-lactam antibiotics), hence the term *methicillin-resistant* Staphylococcus aureus.

MRSA can also be carried harmlessly on the skin and nasal mucosa of patients and healthcare workers. About 3% of the general population carries an MRSA strain (i.e. 10% of all *S. aureus* carriers), but the carriage rate is 6%–7% among patients screened on admission to hospital. However, it can result in serious infections that are very difficult to treat effectively. These infections prolong hospital stay and can lead to major complications (such as necessitating limb amputation) and death. MRSA spreads rapidly in

Table 3.6 Risk factors associated with MRSA colonization

Recent hospitalization
Recent (3–6 months) antimicrobial use
Invasive lines or tube
Recent surgery
Nursing home resident
Advanced age
Underlying severe disease
Exposure to colonized or infected patient
Morbid obesity
Orthopaedic implant surgery

Source: Marwick CA, Ziglam HM, Nathwani D. Your patient has a blood culture positive for Staphylococcus aureus-what do you do? *Journal of the Royal College of Physicians of Edinburgh* 2006; 36(4):349.

hospitals and other healthcare settings. Colonized patients who are admitted but whose carrier status remains unrecognized can act as a reservoir of infection. Healthcare workers' hands act as mediators of transmission from one patient to another, and this is the main method of transmission of MRSA (Figure 3.22). Contaminated clinical environments contribute to the likelihood of hand-to-patient transfer of MRSA. Inadequately decontaminated equipment is another important factor, as are a lack of proper isolation or cohorting facilities and poor antibiotic prescribing policy and practice (Table 3.6).

As with any infection, MRSA infections that show up within 48 hours of hospital admission are usually classified as community acquired (although many of the patients will have had prior contact with a healthcare facility). Those occurring later than 48 hours are regarded as hospital acquired. In recent years, there has been a growth in community-acquired MRSA infections. Where there is no prior healthcare link, they are often different strains to the MRSA that occurs in hospital.

CLOSTRIDIUM DIFFICILE

C. difficile is an anaerobic, spore-forming bacterium that is the most common cause of diarrhoea acquired by patients in healthcare facilities. It is present in the gut of a small proportion (about 3%) of healthy people, but the spores are also readily acquired from contaminated surfaces or via the hands of healthcare workers. They can then grow and produce toxins that cause diarrhoea and colitis when the normal gut flora are disturbed – for example, by the use of antibiotics or by the immune system being suppressed.

C. difficile became an increasing cause of concern in the United Kingdom and other developed countries because of its rising incidence in the early 2000s. There were a number of serious outbreaks in NHS hospitals in the mid-2000s; for example, in Stoke Mandeville, in 2003–4, 174 people contracted *C. difficile* and 19 died, and then in the same hospital, a year later, 160 further cases and another 19 deaths occurred. Around the same time, in Maidstone and Tunbridge Wells, 500 hospital patients caught the infection and 60 of them died. But it began to fall towards the end of the decade, as it was made a priority for the NHS. It is more common amongst older patients, causing serious and, in some cases, life-threatening infections.

A number of different strains of *C. difficile* exist. Ribotype 001 predominated in the United Kingdom from 1990, but since 2004–5, this country and some other parts of western Europe and North America have been affected by more virulent strains (particularly ribotypes 027 and 106).

C. difficile produces spores that can survive in the hospital environment for weeks or months and that are resistant to most non-chlorine-based cleaning agents and disinfectants.

The control of healthcare infection requires a comprehensive and consistent approach in the hospital or other institution, as well as at the level of the healthcare system as a whole, emphasizing:

- An organizational culture and leadership and accountability that view healthcare-associated infection as a patient safety issue and a priority for action
- Clear, agreed evidence-based policies and procedures to reduce risk of infection in all care settings
- High-quality information to assess the problem, track progress and act as an early warning system

Table 3.7 Control measures effective against the spread of *C. difficile*

Isolation or cohorting of infected patients
Use of gowns and gloves for contact with *C. difficile* patients
Hand washing with soap and water after contact with patients with *C. difficile* infection
Rigorous environmental cleaning with chlorine-based products in adequate dosage of rooms occupied by *C. difficile* patients
Antibiotic stewardship, avoiding broad-spectrum antibiotics, particularly third generation cephalosporins and fluoroquinolones

- Commitment of front-line staff to the highest standards of hand hygiene
- Competent practitioners supported by robust pre- and postregistration education and in-service training in infection control

Infection control policies within institutions are directed at healthcare workers' hand hygiene, clinical procedures and practices, decontamination of high-risk equipment and design and maintenance of a supportive physical environment and infrastructure. Control of *C. difficile* has some additional special features (Table 3.7).

In the United Kingdom, the Care Quality Commission requires all health organizations registered with it to have management and governance systems in place to prevent and control infection in their institutions and facilities.

Hand hygiene improvement is central to ensuring a clean and safe environment for patients and reducing healthcare infection (Figure 3.23). Hand-mediated transmission of microbes from one patient to another via healthcare workers can be interrupted through use of hand sanitizers or hand washing at the sink. Since the late 1990s, there has been a growing emphasis on hand hygiene at the point of care, and hand sanitizers (alcohol gels and rubs) have revolutionized hand hygiene improvement methodology, making it possible for healthcare workers to adhere more easily and effectively to the demands of hand hygiene policies. Hand sanitizers are not a panacea and should not be used on soiled hands or with certain microorganisms (including *C. difficile*). They act as a safety net for the myriad microbes that threaten patients in the hospital and have been demonstrated to dramatically increase the likelihood of maximum compliance and to reduce risk.

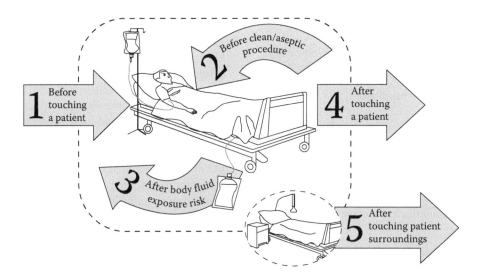

Figure 3.23 Five moments for hand hygiene.

Source: World Alliance for Patient Safety. *Your 5 Moments for Hand Hygiene.* Geneva: World Health Organization, 2006. With permission.

Food-borne infection

The causal agents that are responsible for food-borne illness are bacterial, viral, parasitic, fungal and other substances (e.g. heavy metals, mushroom toxins, shellfish toxins, chemicals and biotoxins). It is not currently possible to produce a reliable global estimate of the burden of food-borne illness because surveillance and investigative data are not good enough. Also, in many countries, attributing a food source to the causation of a gastrointestinal illness is very difficult. The World Health Organization is conducting a lengthy exercise with international experts to try to come up with scientifically based estimates, but the process is extremely complex.

The whole question of food safety and security (including infectious causes) has grown in importance in the last two decades. The advent of globalization has played a big part, as the process of manufacturing and transport of foodstuffs (for human consumption, but also animal feed that has an eventual bearing on the food chain) covers huge distances. New food industries like aquaculture have emerged. Regulation of food standards and safety is poorly developed in many parts of the world. As Professor Chris Elliott, director of the Institute for Global Food Security at Queen's University, Belfast, has put it, 'To try and guarantee what we eat is actually what we think it is has become an enormous challenge'.

The range of infectious agents that cause illness through food is broadly similar worldwide, but the distribution and impact differ greatly between regions and countries. *Salmonella* species are probably the most common overall, but in low-income countries, *Shigella*, cholera and parasites are more common causes. The various groups of *E. coli* organisms also form a major element of food-borne illness, but they are described in the section on diarrhoeal disease, as they are also strongly associated with conditions of poor sanitation.

In the United Kingdom, the Food Standards Agency commissions regular research into various aspects of food-borne illness from leading academic groups. One key area for such research is to assess the burden of disease and identify the infectious agents involved. This cannot be simply derived from notification data because much illness associated with contaminated food goes unreported (few people seek help from health services), many of the pathogens involved are not identified and it is not easy to attribute symptoms of abdominal pain, vomiting and diarrhoea to particular foods consumed rather than due to person-to-person spread. This is why research is so valuable: information can be drawn from multiple sources, new data can be collected and advanced statistical modelling techniques can be used to make estimates.

The estimated number of food-borne illnesses acquired in the United Kingdom from known pathogens is 500,000 per annum. The true figure is likely to be much higher. Some 13 organisms are involved (Tables 3.8 and 3.9), of which the most common is *Campylobacter* (280,000) cases, followed by *Clostridium perfringens*, *norovirus* and nontyphoidal *Salmonella* species. Although less common overall, *Salmonella* and *E. coli* O157 are much more common causes of hospital admissions because of food-borne illness than *Campylobacter*, which is generally a milder illness, although still very unpleasant.

The estimated cost of food-borne illness is high, at around £2 billion to the UK economy (comprising costs to the NHS, loss of earnings and a factor for pain and suffering).

Food-borne illness rose throughout the 1990s, but after 2000, with the work of the Food Standards Agency, it fell substantially. Rates began to flatten out by 2007. Periods of increasing notifications may reflect a greater tendency for

Table 3.8 Main organisms causing food-borne illness in the United Kingdom

Bacteria	• *Campylobacter jejuni/coli*
	• *Clostridium perfringes* (enterotoxin)
	• *Clostridium difficile* cytotoxin
	• *Escherichia coli* O157
	• *Listeria* spp. (*monocytogenes*)
	• *Salmonella* spp.
	• *Shigella* spp.
	• *Yersinia* spp.
Protozoa	• *Cryptosporidium parvum*
	• *Giardia intestinalis*
	• *Cyclospora*
Viruses	• Rotavirus
	• Adenovirus

Source: Society for General Microbiology. *Food-Borne Pathogens*. Available from: https://www.microbiologysociety.org/uploads/assets/uploaded/19f1759f-cf6a-4c8d-99e810f33058f790.pdf [accessed 4 May 2017].

Table 3.9 Top four bacterial causes of food-borne illness in the United Kingdom

Bacteria	Proportion of food-borne illness caused in the UK (%)	Foods most likely to be contaminated
Campylobacter	30	Poultry, red meat, unpasteurized milk, untreated water
Salmonella	13	Meat, poultry, salads, eggs, raw egg products
E. coli O157	2–3	Meat, raw milk, salads
Listeria monocytogenes	2–3	Soft cheeses, pâté, chilled ready-to-eat products

Source: Society for General Microbiology. *Food-Borne Pathogens*. Available from: https://www.microbiologysociety.org/uploads/assets/uploaded/19f1759f-cf6a-4c8d-99e810f33058f790.pdf [accessed 4 May 2017].

the public to seek help when they have symptoms related to food poisoning, or more decisions by medical practitioners to investigate and report cases that present to them. In addition, major changes have occurred in people's eating habits. With more women working outside the home, and the development of a more leisure-orientated society, there is a greater tendency for people not to cook at home.

There are some 2200 *Salmonella* serotypes that can cause human illness. In the United Kingdom, the reported occurrence of *Salmonella* food-borne infections increased sharply in the 1980s but began to fall from 2000 onwards, stabilizing around 2005. One of the principal *Salmonella* organisms associated with illness in Britain is *Salmonella enteritidis*. Illnesses due to this one organism showed a very large increase in Britain in the mid-1980s. Illnesses caused by *Salmonella* organisms in food vary in severity but can be fatal, particularly in the elderly or the very young. Foodstuffs commonly implicated in outbreaks of *Salmonella* infection include undercooked poultry, eggs (particularly dishes prepared with raw eggs), milk and milk products.

Enteric fever is caused by either *Salmonella enterica* serovar Typhi (typhoid fever) or *Salmonella enterica* serovar Paratyphi types A, B and C (paratyphoid fever). These are identical in microscopic appearance and only distinguished by different reactions in laboratory tests. The diseases occur throughout the world, but endemic typhoid and paratyphoid have been virtually eliminated from north-western Europe, North America and Australasia. Usually, the organism is found in faeces, but it can occur in urine. A permanent residence of infection is the gallbladder, and in extremely persistent carrier states where antibiotic therapy has failed, surgical intervention to remove it may be considered. The mode of transmission of infection par excellence is by food and drink that have been contaminated by faeces of a case or carrier. Particularly implicated are those substances on which the organism can multiply: pastries, meat, milk, milk products, ice cream and raw fruit and vegetables. Contaminated water supplies have also been responsible for typhoid outbreaks.

Yersinia enterocolitica is a small Gram-negative bacillus that is found among wild and farm animals (particularly pigs), in water and sewage. It produces an illness with abdominal pain, diarrhoea and fever, most commonly in children. The clinical picture can closely mimic acute appendicitis or mesenteric adenitis. Erythema nodosum can be a complication in up to one-third of adults. The most common routes of transmission are contaminated milk or water or various foodstuffs. Another species of *Yersinia*, *Yersinia pestis*, whose reservoir is rodents, causes plague. Although a scourge of the past, it no longer occurs in Britain. It is still found in some parts of the world.

Listeriosis made headline news in Britain during the late 1980s when it was one of a number of food hygiene issues that aroused public concern and which led to urgent government action. The causative organism is a Gram-positive bacillus, *Listeria monocytogenes*, which is widely distributed in nature. The organism can grow at temperatures as low as those maintained in refrigerators, which is unusual for a microorganism. It is usually transmitted to people via foodstuffs such as some mould-ripened soft cheese, pâté, cold meats and cook–chill recipe dishes. It is mainly a danger to people whose immune system is impaired or to unborn and newborn babies, pregnant women and the very old. It is an important cause of neonatal septicaemia and meningitis and can spread from mother to fetus, either in utero or through direct contact with the mother's infected genital tract. Listeria infection in pregnant women can also cause abortion.

Protozoan parasitic organisms can cause illness if they are ingested with food or water. *Toxoplasma gondii* is a protozoan parasite found in the tissues of many animals, as well in people. Only in the cat is there a stage of development in the intestine. Hence, the cat excretes *T. gondii* as oocysts, which, when ingested by other animals, cause the disease. It may also result from the ingestion of contaminated uncooked meat.

Toxoplasmosis is found in all parts of the world, in both animals and people.

The primary infection rarely causes symptoms that are severe enough to be reported. However, infections in pregnancy can cause fetal damage and resulting congenital malformations. It is not known how often people become infested by these oocysts. It is thought that they acquire the infection directly either by ingesting oocysts from soil (e.g. during gardening) or by eating raw or insufficiently cooked pork, mutton or beef that contains the parasite. Transplacental infection occurs in humans when the pregnant mother acquires a primary infection. The fetus can be affected at any stage of pregnancy but is most at risk during the first trimester, when infection can lead to fetal death. Congenital infection may also give rise to chorioretinitis, cerebral calcification and hydrocephalus in up to 60% of survivors. These severe consequences have led to a call for a national screening programme to combat this disease. The most important means of preventing toxoplasmosis are the thorough cooking of meat, fruit and vegetables and advising pregnant women to avoid handling cat litter, especially with bare hands.

E. coli is a bacillus frequently found in the intestine of humans and animals. The organisms are classified into broad groups; each has many serotypes. Most strains of *E. coli* are harmless, but some can cause severe disease. The various strains are detailed earlier in this chapter, in the section on diarrhoeal disease.

Some of the bacteria responsible for food-borne illness have their main impact through the production of *toxins*. For example, toxin produced by the organism *Clostridium botulinum* is the cause of an uncommon but potentially fatal illness called *botulism*. The toxin affects the nervous system. Classically, the illness is associated with the toxin accumulating in anaerobic conditions (e.g. during home bottling or canning of vegetables), but it also occurs with smoked or preserved meats and fish and a range of other foodstuffs (honey in one outbreak in the United States, and duck pâté and hazelnut yoghurt in a UK outbreak). *Bacillus cereus* produces spores and occurs widely in nature (in soil and dust). It causes two main illnesses, both self-limiting to a day or so. The *diarrhoeal-type B. cereus* illness usually shows between 8 and 16 hours after exposure and gives rise to severe abdominal pain and profuse diarrhoea. It is due to an enterotoxin that the organism releases into the bowel. It is associated with foods such as cornflour, sauces, soups and meat dishes that have been insufficiently heated. The second main presentation, the *emetic type*, starts with vomiting one to six hours after ingestion of the incriminated foodstuff. Diarrhoea is much less common with this presentation. It is typically associated with reheated rice.

S. aureus causes a range of common infections, including superficial skin infections and wound infections after surgery. It also produces food-borne illness through a toxin (e.g. when a food handler with an infected finger contaminates a foodstuff). Ingestion typically results in sudden onset (usually within one to six hours) of abdominal pain, vomiting and diarrhoea. Foods commonly incriminated include those left at room temperature for the organism to multiply, such as cakes, trifles, sandwiches and cold meats. Outbreaks are frequent in the summer, when salad lunches and cold buffets are served outdoors, such as at fetes, weddings and sporting events.

C. perfringens produces spores that are widely distributed in nature (in soil and the gut of animals). It produces an illness with sudden onset of abdominal pain, nausea and diarrhoea (not usually vomiting or fever) between 8 and 24 hours after ingestion of the infected foodstuff, typically inadequately cooked or reheated poultry or meat dishes. The spores change into the vegetative form – which multiplies during slow cooling, storage at ambient temperature and inadequate reheating. The organism then produces a toxin when in the intestine. The illness usually lasts about 24 hours and is very seldom fatal (except occasionally in the elderly).

Other toxins that are present or accumulate in food come from nonbacterial sources. There are many that can cause illness, sometimes very serious.

The *prevention and control* of food-borne illness is a complex process involving a wide range of measures. In many countries, they are part of an overall framework to ensure food safety, since not all food-related hazards are communicable diseases. A whole raft of food hygiene measures, regulatory and other, is needed to prevent and control food-borne illness. In poorer countries, where such measures are not in place, or are incompletely applied, people too often become unwell from the food that they eat. Dealing with the risk of food-borne infection means taking concerted, coordinated action from farm to fork, in other words, action at all points in the food chain, from the rearing of food animals to the process of food production, storage, distribution, sale and preparation for eating (commercially and in the home). This requires the cooperation of producers, the food and catering industries, several government

departments and nongovernmental bodies, healthcare services and local government.

In England, the need to tackle the prevention of food-borne disease across the whole food chain, from producer to consumer, was a major reason for the establishment of an independent Food Standards Agency in 1999. This followed concerns about the weakness of the regulatory system during the bovine spongiform encephalopathy epidemic. The Food Standards Agency is an independent government agency with its own nonexecutive chair and board. It seeks to protect the public interest and the consumer, and to be free of undue influence of the food or farming industry.

Some control measures address specific organisms, but the majority are common to all. Good animal husbandry, careful attention to the content of animal foodstuffs, the raising of *Salmonella*-free flocks of poultry, high standards of slaughterhouse hygiene and a range of other measures are essential steps in ensuring that when food and drinks are consumed, they are free of harmful microorganisms and their toxins. The Food Standards Agency is responsible for the Meat Hygiene Service, which inspects and regulates slaughterhouses, meat-cutting plants and other facilities and premises.

It is also important to ensure that strict control measures operate during the manufacture of food. Increasingly, food in the United Kingdom is bought in processed form. Whether this is as joints of meat or poultry, canned or frozen products or more elaborate heat-and-serve recipe dishes, measures to prevent food-borne illness must be built in at all stages of the production process. This has implications for the design of food processing plants and for the building materials used in them; for the type of equipment used and how it is maintained; for heat and other treatments given to various types of food; for the type and content of packaging materials; for operating practices for, and training of, staff; and for inspection and quality control procedures. Many of the same considerations apply to storage and distribution chains, which should maintain the food in a hygienic condition in the interval between it leaving the production plant and reaching the shop or catering outlet. Food hygiene and safety are an integral part of the food industry, but the fact that there is such a large number of producers and suppliers, and the fact that even a small lapse can lead to a serious outbreak of food-borne illness, means that the task is one of constant vigilance and improvement of standards. Correct storage, handling and preparation of food in the home, in institutions (such as hospitals and schools), and in restaurants, cafes and other catering outlets are also vital.

There is a large body of legislation relating to food hygiene and safety in the United Kingdom, much of it based on European Union law. Almost all food businesses must be registered or approved, depending on the nature of their trade, and failure to do so is a breach of the law. This provides local authorities and other food enforcement bodies with information to carry out inspections and

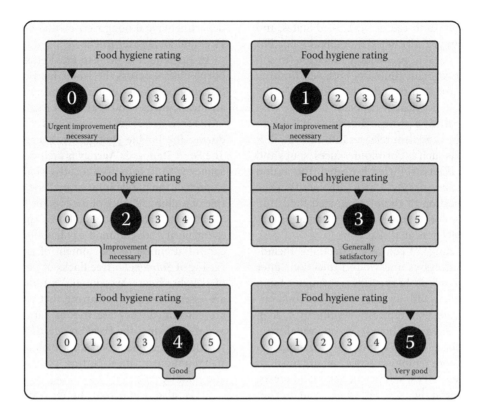

Figure 3.24 'Scores on the doors' – the UK Food Hygiene Rating system.

enforce most activities. All registered businesses are subject to unannounced inspection (Figure 3.24). With its focus on consumer protection, food legislation places obligations on food business operators to ensure the safety of food. It is an offence, punishable by fine or imprisonment, to place unsafe food on the market. The legislation also provides a range of powers to take enforcement action to ensure food business operators meet their obligations.

In the case of a large-scale food poisoning outbreak or evidence of widespread food contamination, the Food Standards Agency may issue a food alert. These provide local enforcement bodies with information or advice necessary for action to investigate problems and ensure unsafe food is not sold to the public. Where appropriate, such action is undertaken in parallel with advice issued at the local or national level to alert consumers.

Sexually transmitted infections

In the 1980s and 1990s, the whole field of sexually transmitted infections was transformed from a relatively quiet backwater of clinical and public health practice to one of major international importance by the emergence of the Human Immunodeficiency Virus (HIV). However, it would be wrong to regard the field of sexually transmitted infections, and sexual health more generally, as being defined only by this one disease, vital though it remains to prevent it, diagnose it, treat it and reduce its spread.

The World Health Organization recognizes 30 different sexually transmitted illnesses caused by infectious agents (bacteria, viruses and parasites), accounting for 1 million people worldwide being infected each day. Eight conditions are the most common: gonorrhoea, chlamydia, syphilis, trichosomoniasis, genital herpes, HIV, hepatitis B and human papillomavirus (HPV). The first four of these are responsible for about half of the burden of sexually transmitted disease. Some of the infectious agents can also be transmitted from mother to child during pregnancy or childbirth and by blood, blood products or organ and tissue transplant (e.g. HIV and hepatitis B).

The four most common infections in the United Kingdom are chlamydia (47% of diagnoses), genital warts (17%), genital herpes (7%) and gonorrhoea (7%). Assessments of the size of the problem are mainly based on data from NHS genitourinary medicine clinics. The highest incidence rates for new diagnoses of sexually transmitted infections in the United Kingdom are in young heterosexuals and men who have sex with men; in the latter group, there have been sharp rises in recent years (Figure 3.25). Among those diagnosed with syphilis or gonorrhoea, the largest proportions are among men who have sex with men: 74% and 46%, respectively.

Chlamydia infection is caused by *Chlamydia trachomatis*. It is very often symptomless, which makes transmission more likely. When symptoms occur, the most common are urethral or vaginal discharge. Its peak incidence is in men and women aged below 25 years. The most serious impact of untreated infection in women is pelvic inflammatory disease, which can cause blocked fallopian tubes and infertility or ectopic pregnancy. In men, it can progress to epididymitis

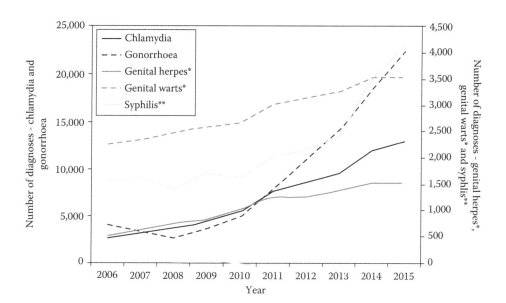

Figure 3.25 New diagnoses of sexually transmitted infections in men who have sex with men, England.

Source: Public Health England (PHE). *Infection Report: Sexually Transmitted Infections and Chlamydia Screening in England, 2015.* London: PHE, 2016.

and sometimes reactive arthritis. *Gonorrhoea* (caused by *Neisseria gonorrhea*) may be symptomless or show as urethritis with a purulent discharge. In men, untreated, the disease may progress to prostatitis or epididymitis. In women, the shorter urethra means that symptoms sometimes pass unnoticed, but ascending infection can cause pelvic inflammatory disease. In either sex, joint inflammation or meningitis can rarely occur and babies can acquire eye infections (ophthalmia neonatorum) if their mother has gonococcal infection. The disease (anorectal, pharyngeal and urethral) is much more common in men who have sex with men.

Genital herpes is caused by the herpes simplex virus (usually type 2). Type 1 herpes simplex virus, associated with cold sores, can also cause the genital form. It is a relapsing condition. The skin heals and then can break down and ulcerate long after the primary infection. Herpes is not easily treated. Antiviral drugs can sometimes be effective. The virus becomes latent in the dorsal root ganglia and can then recur at any time. *Anal and genital warts* are caused by viruses, mainly HPV. Another virus causes a warty-type infection called *molluscum contagiosum.* Anogenital warts increased during the 2000s among heterosexuals and gay men. An important association is that between certain types of HPV and the development of cervical cancer.

Although it is less common, *syphilis* (caused by *Treponema pallidum*), is a particularly serious disease if untreated. Although mainly acquired by sexual contact, it can also transmit from mother to baby via the placenta (congenital syphilis). There are three stages of the acquired disease. The primary lesion (chancre) develops as a painless ulcer on the skin or mucous membrane at the site of entry; a generalized cutaneous rash heralds secondary syphilis; the tertiary stage develops after 3–20 years and can affect bones, liver, the cardiovascular system and the central

nervous system. The patient is infectious during the primary and secondary stages of the disease and may also be intermittently infectious during latent periods.

In the United Kingdom, the prevention and control of sexually transmitted infections rests largely with the network of genitourinary medicine clinics provided around the country within the NHS. In England, local authorities are now responsible for commissioning comprehensive sexual health services for their populations, while local clinical commissioning groups and NHS England at the national level commission some specialist services.

Prompt diagnosis and investigation of people presenting is vital. Contact tracing or partner notification (as it is now more commonly called) is a key control measure requiring skill, considerable diplomacy and a workforce of specially trained nurses, health visitors or social workers.

The control measures that are required vary little between the sexually transmitted infections. Condom use – and effective promotion of this – is particularly important, certainly until partners have undergone a sexual health screen. Young adults should be encouraged to be screened for infection annually, and on change of partner. Access to sexual health services needs to be made easy, and these services need to provide rapid and confidential diagnosis, and either encourage or facilitate (depending on the diagnosis) partner notification when an infection is detected. Screening the highest-risk groups at regular intervals enhances the opportunity to diagnose infections early, especially as many can be asymptomatic. This particularly includes men who have sex with men and Black African women and men. Screening should include HIV testing, in addition to a sexually transmitted infection screen. To be fully effective, prevention programmes need to reach out beyond the clinics and other healthcare services, into the communities where those most at risk of infection reside.

A national screening programme for chlamydia (the most common sexually transmitted infection), established in the early 2000s, is aimed particularly at the under-25s. Testing kits are made widely available – not just in conventional settings, such as general practitioners and genitourinary medicine clinics, but also in young peoples' clinics, youth clubs, colleges and pharmacies. Self-testing kits can be handed in at such sites and, in some parts of the country, can be ordered online and sent back by post. Treatment is a course of antibiotics.

In the late 2000s, a vaccine was introduced for girls in secondary schools to protect against two strains of HPV that together cause three-quarters of cases of cervical cancer. The HPV vaccine has a coverage rate of 80%. The vaccine does not protect against other types of HPV, so cervical cancer and genital infection can still occur. Cervical screening and preventive measures to reduce the risk of sexually transmitted infection, particularly condom use, are both still important, even with an effective HPV vaccine.

EMERGING AND RE-EMERGING DISEASES

Plotting emerging infection occurrences on a world map (Figure 3.26) illustrates that new infections are not rare events and happen in many different places. Such infections are initially unlikely to be treatable, and no vaccine will be available to prevent and control them.

For the public health professional, or scientist, the emerging infection poses a challenge to understand the organism, its behaviour, the profile of the clinical illness it causes, the trajectory and pattern of its spread and the potential for controlling it.

There is no simple way of defining emerging diseases except that they all have some novel aspect, whether that is to do with the way that the organism transmits (e.g. developing extensive antimicrobial resistance), its geographical location (e.g. appearing for the first time in a temperate climate when it has only ever been in a subtropical area), that it has never caused human disease before (e.g. the coronavirus that produced SARS) or that it is a previously unknown organism (e.g. Nipah virus that emerged in Malaysia in 1999; its reservoir is in fruit bats and it infected people via contact with sick pigs).

Around three-quarters of the diseases that have emerged in the latter decades of the twentieth century and the first part of the twenty-first century have arisen from microorganisms crossing the species barrier from animals to people. There are many pressures (Table 3.10) that have made this more likely: changes in land use, including encroachment on forested areas; population movements; global travel; weakened public health infrastructure in areas of conflict and natural disaster; trafficking of bush meat; demand for more exotic foodstuffs and components for traditional medicines; and evolution of microorganisms themselves. Many of these influences either weaken human resistance to infection or produce conditions in which wild animals (or carcasses) come into closer contact with people and zoonotic infections are able to cross a species barrier. Or as Jim Robbins, writing in the *New York Times*, put it, 'They are a result of things people do to Nature'.

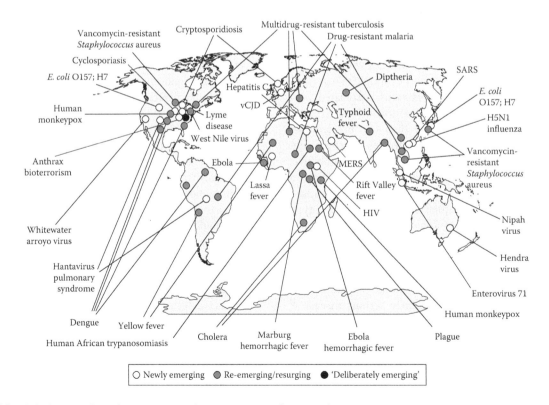

Figure 3.26 Global examples of emerging and re-emerging infectious diseases.

Source: Dr Jeremy Farrar, personal communication

Table 3.10 Factors affecting the likelihood of new infectious disease emergence

The Microbial Agent	The Human Host	The Human Environment
Genetic adaptation and change	Human susceptibility to infection	Climate and weather
Polymicrobial diseases	Human demographics and behaviour	Changing ecosystems
	International trade and travel	Economic development and land use
	Intent to harm (bioterrorism)	Technology and industry
	Occupational exposures	Poverty and social inequality
	Inappropriate use of antibiotics	Lack of public health services
		Animal populations
		War and famine
		Lack of political will

Source: Morens DM, Fauci AS. Emerging infectious diseases: threats to human health and global stability. *PLoS Pathology* 2013;9(7):e1003467.

The impact of climate change on the pattern of communicable disease has been a focus of intense study. For example, it is estimated that an increase of 2°C in average annual temperatures could alter the indigenous mosquito and tick populations in the United Kingdom. There are more than 30 species of mosquito in the United Kingdom that are generally more likely to expand their populations if warmer, wetter periods of the year extend. The possibility of dengue fever and West Nile virus becoming established would be increased; malaria is possible but much less likely. Tick-borne infections could also become more common.

Lyme disease is already endemic in the United Kingdom. It was first described in 1975 in Old Lyme, Connecticut, when several children developed acute arthritis. The causal agent in North America is *Borrelia burgdorferi*, transmitted by the bite of the Ixodes tick, which lives on wild animals (especially deer). It is not transmissible person to person. In Europe and Asia, the main organisms causing Lyme disease are *Borrelia afzelii* and *Borrelia garinii*.

Clinical manifestations are in three phases. Early symptoms may or may not include general malaise, fever and lymphadenopathy, but a key feature is the characteristic skin rash called erythema migrans. In the second phase, the infection becomes more disseminated; the rash spreads and there can be involvement of the heart and nervous system. The third phase, of late manifestations, may take years to appear, and can include arthritis as well as neurological abnormalities and heart problems. Lyme disease can be very difficult to diagnose because a tick bite can be unnoticed or forgotten and a rash ignored. So, some patients present with the symptoms of the organ or body system that has been infected. Serology is not always positive in the early phase of the disease but usually is later. Treatment is with appropriate antibiotics but often needs specialist clinical involvement. The majority of UK infections are acquired in areas such as Exmoor, the New Forest, the Lake District, the Scottish Highlands and the North Yorkshire Moors. Climate change could extend the period when ticks are active to parts of the winter and spring. There is already evidence of spread to urban areas, an adverse development that could increase with milder wetter conditions.

Once emerged, new infectious diseases can either stop transmission (this happened with SARS) or continue to transmit but at a low level (H5N1, bird flu). However, some emerged infections continue to spread and become endemic in affected areas, for example, West Nile virus. Until the end of the twentieth century, the virus was confined to tropical and subtropical areas of the world (such as Africa, Israel, India and Egypt), where it caused occasional outbreaks. Sinister signs of a major shift in the geographical occurrence of West Nile virus infection came in the summer of 1999 when a number of dead crows were found in New York City. That same year, 62 people fell ill with viral encephalitis and several died from it. Colder weather and mosquito spraying ended the outbreak in New York City that summer, but West Nile virus was established in the United States. Since this unexpected emergence beyond its traditional geographical boundaries, West Nile virus has spread extensively in North America and is now endemic in that continent. The main factors that influence the transmission of the virus are climatic conditions, population density, species of mosquitoes and the presence of susceptible birds.

Although the natural host for West Nile virus is birds, it is usually transmitted to people and some other mammals (including horses) by mosquitoes. It can also be transmitted from person to person through blood transfusion, organ transplantation, breast milk and laboratory accidents. When illness does occur, it often results in mild flu-like symptoms. Some people develop serious illness, including encephalitis, and among those who do, around 12% die. In affected areas, a number of measures are important in prevention and disease control, including advising the public to cover up at dawn and dusk (when mosquito bites are more common), using skin insect repellents and nets, draining pools of water around houses and yards, environmental control measures (mainly directed at mosquito breeding) and treatment of blood products and restrictions on blood donations.

Re-emerging infection is the term used to describe diseases that were thought to have disappeared or reduced to low levels resurging to pose a new threat to human health. Examples include syphilis in communities where men have sex with men and measles in countries where vaccine uptake levels have fallen off.

Sometimes the discovery of a new infection brings good news. Until the 1980s, gastric and duodenal ulcers were ascribed to stress, lifestyle and genetics. But in 1982, Australian microbiologists Barry Marshall and Robin Warren challenged this belief by suggesting that a particular bacterium – *Helicobacter pylori* – was in fact the major cause. The historic belief had been that bacteria could not survive for long in the acidic environment of the stomach, and so Marshall and Warren's suggestion seemed nonsensical. Over a period of many months, their evidence gradually changed the prevailing view. They managed to culture the bacterium *H. pylori* from biopsies of stomach ulcers. Famously, Barry Marshall even went so far as to drink *H. pylori* himself to demonstrate that it caused gastric irritation. In 2005, they were awarded the Nobel Prize for their discovery – and were praised for their tenacity in challenging prevailing beliefs.

It is now estimated that between one- and two-thirds of the world's population is infected with *H. pylori*. In the United Kingdom, the prevalence has declined substantially over the last decade. Although most people who are infected are unlikely ever to suffer symptoms, infection can be associated with gastritis in both children and adults. The organism is said to be responsible for approximately 80% of gastric ulcers and 90% of duodenal ulcers. It has been demonstrated that people infected with *H. pylori* are between two and six times more likely than uninfected people to develop gastric cancer and mucosal-associated lymphoid-type (MALT) lymphoma. Gastric cancer is the second most common cancer globally. Treatment of *H. pylori* infection is by means of triple therapy – two antibiotics, in combination with acid-suppressing medication. Eradication is successful in between 70% and 90% of patients, depending on the drug regimen used. The two major reasons for treatment failure are antibiotic resistance and patient noncompliance.

This introduction to emerging and re-emerging diseases has already cited examples of a range of infections that have fallen into this category. The remainder of this section tells the stories of a number of further diseases that illustrate the phenomenon of emerging and re-emerging diseases. They fit into a number of broad patterns (Table 3.11).

Ebola fever and the Viral Haemorrhagic Fevers

Some of the most dramatic emergences have been the outbreaks of haemorrhagic fevers. They produce serious, life-threatening illness and are often remembered because of television images of public health investigators clad in protective clothing, masks and breathing apparatus entering affected areas, usually in Africa. Some, such as yellow fever, have been known from early times. However, since the mid-1950s, new haemorrhagic illnesses have been recognized, many acquired from natural animal hosts. They fall into five families: *Arenaviridae* (e.g. Lassa fever),

Bunyaviridae (e.g. Rift Valley fever), *Filoviridae* (e.g. Marburg disease and Ebola fever), *Flaviviridae* (e.g. dengue fever, yellow fever, West Nile virus, Japanese encephalitis and Zika virus) and *Paramyxoviridae*.

All have a natural reservoir in an animal or arthropod species; people are never the reservoir but can be infected from it directly, intermediately through an animal that has become infected or by person-to-person spread (usually in an outbreak situation). Their geographical distribution is largely determined by the location of the habitat of the host or reservoir of the virus.

The main public health concern is that the viruses, having been transmitted from their natural host to people, are then capable of producing person-to-person transmission. This risk is greatly minimized with strict isolation of infected patients and meticulous medical and nursing procedures. Cases of this group of diseases have been very rare in Britain and imported by travellers or healthcare staff who have been in affected areas. Where person-to-person transmission occurs, diseases are infectious as long as blood and body secretions contain the virus, which can be for several weeks after clinical recovery.

Lassa fever was first isolated from an American missionary nurse in the Lassa township in Nigeria during 1969. Since then, it has also occurred in Nigeria, Sierra Leone, Liberia and elsewhere in West Africa. The reservoir for the virus is a rat, *Mastomys natalensis*. It excretes the virus in its urine. It breeds plentifully and enters dwellings in search of food. The risk for people in contact with infected fluids is quite high in affected areas.

Marburg disease is caused by a virus first described in Marburg in the Federal Republic of Germany in 1967, when 31 cases with seven deaths occurred in Germany and Yugoslavia due to direct contact with the blood, organs and tissues of a batch of African green monkeys originally trapped in Uganda. It is endemic in central and southern Africa.

Table 3.11 Key types of emerging and re-emerging communicable disease

Caused outbreaks but extinguished themselves (e.g. SARS)
Slowly and steadily increasing in parts of the world (e.g. Lyme disease)
Long established but still surging in many places (e.g. dengue fever)
Novel in character (e.g. *Helicobacter pylori*)
Can be anticipated and planned for (e.g. pandemic influenza)
Re-emerged because of broken public health infrastructure, particularly in areas of conflict or natural disaster (e.g. cholera)
Have a natural occurrence, but deliberately transmitted for malign purposes (e.g. anthrax)
Such major potential impact that are threat to global security (e.g. antimicrobial resistance, Ebola fever)

Hanta viruses produce two main haemorrhagic fever syndromes: one with renal features (mainly in China and Korea) and the other with cardiopulmonary features (mainly in North America). Both have reservoirs in different species of rodent.

Hendra virus and *Nipah virus* are members of a relatively new genus, *Henipavirus*; pulmonary symptoms characterize the former and encephalitis the latter. The natural reservoir for both appears to be fruit bats. Infection can be by direct contact with bat excreta or via infected animals: horses for Hendra virus (which has occurred only in Australia so far) and pigs for Nipah virus (which was first seen in Malaysia but has now emerged in Bangladesh and India).

Ebola virus causes a very serious illness with sudden onset of fever, general malaise and, in many people, deterioration with end-organ damage. It was first isolated in an outbreak of an unexplained and rapidly fatal illness in Zaire in 1976. Since that time, there have been more than 24 outbreaks; some have been in Zaire (now called the Democratic Republic of Congo), and other countries, such as Sudan, have also been affected. Before 2014, the largest outbreak, resulting in 425 reported cases, was in Uganda. The case fatality rate there was 53%, but in other outbreaks, it has ranged from 25% to 80%. Most of these earlier occurrences were smaller and fairly quickly brought under control.

Everything changed in March 2014, when an outbreak of Ebola fever of unprecedented scale, geographical spread and complexity hit four countries in West Africa. Never before had the disease moved out of sparsely populated areas into larger towns and cities. Three countries were most affected: Guinea, Liberia and Sierra Leone. There were also cases elsewhere, including in the populous Nigeria, where fortunately the outbreak was stopped quickly.

The conditions of the 2014 outbreak made its severity worse. First, national authorities and global health agencies recognized the onset of the outbreak late. Second, the countries mainly affected had very poor health infrastructure. People with Ebola fever need modern high-technology intensive care if they are to have a chance of survival. Such facilities did not exist. Worse still, Ebola patients also need strict isolation to avoid the disease transmitting to other patients and staff. Many past outbreaks were related to hospitals in Africa where unsatisfactory practices spread the disease. Such hospitals acted as amplifiers of the infection, with many secondary cases. In 2014, this was exactly the position in the facilities that were available. Third, the level of fear and mistrust within many communities was so high that cases were concealed from the authorities. The crucial function of surveillance, to understand the progress of the epidemic, could not then operate effectively. Health education about the disease and its mode of transmission and instruction on basic hygiene measures to reduce personal risk were slow to get off the ground at the community level in the countries. Particularly persistent was the high risk of catching the disease from handling the dead, a practice that for cultural reasons was very difficult to stop.

Ebola quickly became a global health crisis, with concern focused not just on the humanitarian element of it but also on the potential of it to spread to more countries and even become established as a pandemic if the virus were to mutate. A great deal of international donor aid, expert advice and support, rapidly erected hospital facilities and volunteer staff from charities and Western countries flooded into the affected areas. Among the dead were many local healthcare workers (it has been estimated that they were 20–30 times more likely to become infected than the general population). This degraded the affected countries' ability to mount a response even further. Foreign health workers also became infected, and some were airlifted to their own countries for specialist care, including some from the United Kingdom who were treated in the national isolation unit at the Royal Free Hospital in London.

The epidemic remained stubbornly resistant to control and continued to infect people, although gradually declining in some countries. By March 2015, a year after its onset, there had been around 25,000 reported cases of Ebola fever and 10,000 deaths. The true figure for both is certainly very much higher. Even at this point, the authorities in Sierra Leone were enforcing a three-day lockdown to restrict 2.5 million people to their homes in an attempt to limit the ongoing spread of the disease. It is difficult to imagine the trauma to the small communities struck down by Ebola, and remaining in fear of it a whole year on. Families have lost many members, children have been orphaned, livelihoods have been lost and funeral after funeral has torn apart the continuity of everyday life. The fine granularity of people's circumstances is not often visible to the rest of the world. When the media do report small occurrences, such as the temporary wooden markers on the graves of victims being eaten by termites in Nzerekore, Guinea, in February 2015, leaving the graves unidentifiable, the terrible reality of life under the tyranny of a rampant communicable disease is all too evident.

It is believed that the first case of Ebola fever in this huge outbreak was a two-year-old boy in Guinea who died of the disease after handling bat faeces. He used to play by a hollow tree that was a favourite gathering point for local children, but also a natural habitat for thousands of bats. Children caught the bats and villagers would often cook and eat them.

All past occurrences of Ebola, where a source has been identified, have involved a direct interaction between people and animals. For example, in one earlier outbreak, hunters killed, dismembered and ate a gorilla. They and others died from Ebola fever. It is estimated that a third of the world's gorilla population has been killed by Ebola virus infections. The extent of the reservoirs of Ebola virus is not fully understood. More than one animal host probably makes up the reservoir. Fruit bats are one population that is known to harbour the virus without dying from it. It is possible that wild pigs might also do so, but so far this is only a hypothesis. Infected apes and chimpanzees can certainly transmit the disease to people.

The 2014–15 Ebola crisis is a clear warning to the global community. While one of the declared priorities is to develop a vaccine – a necessary and predictable reaction – the other long-term goals must surely be to create much greater capacity and capability in responding to global public health emergencies, to move faster to strengthen healthcare systems in the poorest countries of the world and to get a better understanding of all the consequences of blurring of the boundaries between the natural world and that built by humankind, and where possible, to push back against forces that are shrinking ecosystems.

Severe Acute Respiratory Syndrome

In March 2003, the World Health Organization alerted the world to a new disease. The disease did not have a name and was given one based on the symptoms it produced – a severe respiratory illness with atypical pneumonia. The infectious agent could not be identified initially.

The first case of SARS occurred in Guangdong Province, China, in November 2002. Other cases occurred in China through the autumn of 2002 and into the first two months of 2003. Two notable incidents occurred during this early phase. First, a SARS victim hospitalized in Guangzhou, China, transmitted the virus to 50 hospital staff and 19 relatives. Second, a medical professor from Guangzhou with respiratory symptoms travelled in mid-February 2003 to attend a wedding at the Metropole Hotel, Hong Kong. He stayed only one night, but at least 16 other guests and 1 visitor were infected as a result – signifying the start of international spread. The professor was admitted to hospital and died 10 days later.

Another man who became infected at the Metropole Hotel was admitted to hospital but recovered. The importance of his condition was not recognized, and as a result, he infected 143 people, including healthcare workers. Meanwhile, a woman who had stayed at the Metropole Hotel had travelled back to her home in Toronto, Ontario. She passed the infection to four members of her family. This was to be responsible for a large outbreak in Canada.

During March 2003, outbreaks occurred in Singapore, Vietnam and Taiwan. Cases continued to occur in these and other countries, as well as in China, through April 2003.

There were further high-profile outbreaks. A housing complex in Hong Kong – Amoy Gardens – was the focus of one. A man from Guangdong Province who visited Hong Kong twice a week for kidney dialysis stayed with his brother in an Amoy Gardens apartment. He was infected with SARS, and an outbreak affected 329 residents of the housing complex; 42 of them died.

In Toronto, more than 250 people fell ill, 44 died and 10,000 people were put in quarantine. A particularly serious aspect of the outbreak was in-hospital transmission: 100 staff at the Scarborough Hospital, Ontario, caught SARS.

In total, there were more than 8000 cases of SARS worldwide, 774 deaths and reports of the disease in 37 countries before it was stopped from spreading.

The SARS epidemic caused massive upheaval, not just economically and socially but also in the scrutiny that it brought to bear on international public health systems. Within countries and areas such as Canada and Hong Kong, there were major independent reviews of the public health infrastructure, policies, governance and accountability arrangements for the prevention, investigation and control of infectious diseases. Across countries, attention focused on the gathering and exchange of surveillance and laboratory data so that the world could have early warning of such outbreaks in the future. Efforts have been made subsequently to remove barriers for reporting of data (especially a tendency in some countries towards inappropriate secrecy) and to strengthen laboratory links between countries.

The exact source of the SARS virus, a coronavirus, has not been proven, but could be yet another example of transmission from animals to people. The use of a wild, exotic animal (the civet cat) for food is a strong possibility, and in turn, this animal may have acquired the virus from a bat (as its natural reservoir). Coronaviruses cause a range of human infections, including the common cold. The strain that was responsible for SARS is another example of an infectious agent that crossed the species barrier, unexpectedly and unpredictably. The SARS story is a modern classic of an apparently new disease emerging suddenly. Important lessons that must be applied in the future have been learned from the SARS experience (Table 3.12).

Since the last case in this SARS epidemic, there has been no re-emergence of a disease that caused such alarm internationally. However, in 2012, another previously undocumented coronavirus was linked to cases of a new serious respiratory syndrome that arose in Saudi Arabia. It is called Middle East respiratory syndrome coronavirus (MERS-CoV). Since this disease emerged, by April 2015, more than 1000 confirmed cases had occurred and there had been more than 400 deaths. Most illnesses have been in Saudi Arabia, but sporadic cases have arisen in nine Middle Eastern countries, while 14 other countries have

Table 3.12 Key lessons from the experience of Severe Acute Respiratory Syndrome (SARS) in 2003

Early sharing of surveillance data between countries and with the World Health Organization
Getting virus isolates to specialist laboratories quickly is vital
'Never say never' about the possibility of animal to human transmission
Strong public health systems and clear accountability within countries is important
Travel restrictions and advisories are always controversial and need careful consideration
Early, accurate public information and regular updates are key to retaining public confidence
Global coordination of response is pivotal to success

detected imported cases in returning travellers. The average case fatality rate is reported as 39%, although it is not known whether there are asymptomatic cases; if so, the true case fatality rate is lower. Like with SARS, there has been cross-infection involving hospitalized cases transmitting the disease to other patients and healthcare workers. So far, there have been no reports of person-to-person spread in any community, nor airborne transmission; if either were to happen, this would be a sinister development likely to turn the disease into a global threat.

The source has not been conclusively determined, but people who have had close contact with asymptomatic dromedary camels appear to be at increased risk, leading to the hypothesis that camel excreta, milk or carcasses may have infected people. No reservoir has been firmly established, but some of the scientific work on the genetics of coronaviruses points to species of Middle Eastern bats.

In common with other emerging communicable disease problems of the twenty-first century – for example, SARS and Ebola fever – the Middle East Respiratory Syndrome has become increasingly political, with criticisms of the Saudi Arabian government and of global health governance in failing to control the epidemic and identify its source and routes of transmission.

Influenza

Influenza viruses are divided into three main groups: influenza A, B and C. The type A viruses cause most outbreaks and epidemics of influenza. Influenza B and C viruses infect people only. Influenza A viruses can also infect birds and other animals, such as pigs and horses. The ability of influenza A viruses to jump between species is important. It greatly helps them evolve into new strains, capable of producing large-scale outbreaks or even pandemics of influenza.

Influenza viruses are passed easily from person to person through the air when someone who is infected with the virus coughs or sneezes (droplet infection) or when someone touches a surface contaminated by the virus. Influenza viruses usually have an incubation period of between one and three days. They cause symptoms of variable severity, including headache, sore throat, cough, muscle and joint aches, running nose, weakness and fatigue.

Influenza viruses have two glycoproteins on their surface – a haemagglutinin and a neuraminidase. These are the antigens that characterize the particular strain of influenza virus. There are 16 different haemagglutinins and nine neuraminidases. These antigens produce an antibody response when someone becomes infected.

The convention is to give each influenza virus an H number and an N number to define its subtype. The numbers refer to the particular haemagglutinin and neuraminidase involved. A name is sometimes used to define the variant (which differs antigenically within subtypes). Thus, the influenza A virus that caused the pandemic in 1957 was an H2N2 subtype, and the variant was called Asian influenza.

Influenza viruses are very unstable antigenically. They are frequently transformed into new variants and, less often, into new subtypes. When a new variant arises that is antigenically different to the currently circulating subtype, antigenic drift is said to have occurred. The virus has changed its structure, but the H and N numbers stay the same. This happens periodically with influenza A viruses that cause seasonal or winter influenza. Such a virus tends to cause a larger outbreak than normal, because fewer people have immunity to it. The size of the outbreak and the severity of symptoms vary greatly, and depend on the degree of cross-infection by (or vaccination against) the previous variant, as well as environmental and other factors.

A second and more dramatic type of transformation of the protein structure of the influenza A virus is the so-called antigenic shift. This produces an entirely new subtype, meaning that the H and/or N numbers change. Then, the population has very little immunity, since the subtype is so different to strains to which people have been previously exposed (either in nature or through vaccination). As a result, the virus spreads widely and usually causes a pandemic (a worldwide epidemic).

These transformations of the influenza A virus occur in one of three ways. The most common way for antigenic drift to occur is through adaptation of the virus during the normal process of viral replication. The most common way for antigenic shift is through a process of reassortment – an exchange of genetic material between two different influenza viruses, often a human one and an animal one. A person or an animal (such as a pig) can act as a *mixing vessel* for the two viruses. Less commonly, an antigenic shift is caused by genetic adaptation of a bird (or other animal) influenza virus to become a human influenza virus. This route of transformation is thought to have created the 1918 Spanish influenza pandemic, and it generally results in a virus that causes more severe infections and more deaths than a virus resulting from reassortment.

KEY DISTINCTION: SEASONAL, AVIAN, ANIMAL AND PANDEMIC INFLUENZA

It is important to distinguish clearly between three different influenza situations. Seasonal influenza is an illness caused by influenza viruses of a subtype that has usually been around for a number of years, and to which the population has a relatively high level of immunity (because it either has had an influenza illness caused by the virus or has been vaccinated against it). When people are infected, many illnesses are mild – although some people get serious complications, and in some sections of the population (the very young, the very old and those with chronic diseases) there are deaths.

Avian influenza is an illness of birds (wild and domesticated). It transmits easily from bird to bird but can only infect people with difficulty (typically those who are in close contact with infected poultry). Avian influenza viruses are, however, candidates to reassort with human influenza viruses and so to generate an antigenic shift (a new subtype of influenza causing a pandemic). The same is so for influenza viruses that initially affect animals, such as pigs or horses.

Pandemic influenza is an illness of people caused by the emergence of a new influenza virus subtype to which the population has no (or little) natural immunity. This happens by reassortment or mutation (as discussed above). Large numbers of people become ill, and the number of deaths is substantially above the number seen in a normal flu season. Pandemic strains of influenza cause more illness and deaths among children and young adults than do seasonal strains.

PANDEMIC INFLUENZA: PAST AND FUTURE

Four past pandemics of influenza have been well documented. Three were in the twentieth century and one was towards the end of the first decade of the twenty-first century (Figure 3.27).

The first was caused by the H1N1 subtype of influenza A. It emerged in 1918 as the *Spanish influenza*. The prospect of any event similar to the Spanish influenza pandemic is much feared, because of its severity. Between 1918 and 1919, the influenza virus responsible infected an estimated 20% of the world's population and killed 40 million to 50 million people. A significant feature was that it affected young adults (20- to 40-year-olds) disproportionately.

To some extent, the severity of the Spanish influenza pandemic was accentuated because it fell in an era when levels of general population health and nutrition were much poorer than they are today, and when there was an absence of the benefits of modern medicine (such as antibiotics and intensive care units). Nevertheless, there is evidence that the virus itself was capable of producing much more serious illness than occurred in later pandemics. This was probably because it produced a much greater and earlier viral invasion of the lungs rather than the upper respiratory tract.

Studies of the influenza virus recovered from bodies frozen and preserved in the permafrost in Alaska have allowed scientists to genetically map the Spanish influenza virus. It is almost certain that it arose through mutation (genetic adaptation) from an avian influenza virus rather than through reassortment. This could explain its virulence and the high mortality it induced.

The second pandemic of influenza in the twentieth century happened in 1957–58. It was caused by the H2N2 subtype of influenza A virus and was dubbed *Asian influenza*. As expected, it caused much more widespread and serious illness than seasonal influenza, but it caused a much milder pandemic than the Spanish influenza 40 years previously. The Asian influenza pandemic began in the Far East in May 1957. The first cases in Britain were seen in June of that year, in limited outbreaks. When the schools opened in September, the number of infections surged to reach epidemic levels. There was a second wave at the beginning of 1958. During the autumn and winter of 1957–58, there were approximately 50,000 influenza-related deaths.

The third influenza pandemic of the twentieth century came a decade later, in 1968–69. It was caused by a H3N2 subtype of the influenza A virus and was called *Hong Kong influenza*. The first isolation of the new virus in Britain was in August 1968. Throughout the autumn of 1968, and into the winter and spring of 1969, there were more cases and local outbreaks, but there was no large-scale epidemic in Britain in this first year. This was in marked contrast to the situation in the United States that same year, where there was a large epidemic with high attack rates and many deaths. North America was unusual compared with other temperate parts of the world in suffering a high impact from Hong Kong influenza during the winter of 1968–69. It was the following winter of 1969–70 that the virus caused major epidemics in Britain and other European countries. This pattern of spread was very different to the Asian influenza pandemic and illustrates how unpredictably influenza viruses behave.

Given the regular cyclical occurrence of pandemics, the first twenty-first-century pandemic of influenza was regarded by experts as inevitable – its occurrence was known in advance to be a case of 'when and not whether'. By the mid-2000s, this serious threat to the public health was at the top of the agenda for national governments. This was for a number of reasons: (1) there was a realization

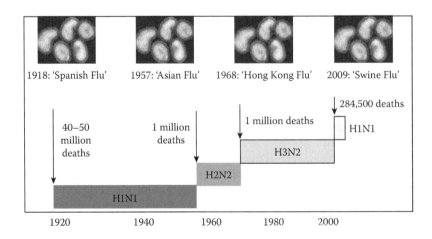

Figure 3.27 Influenza pandemics of the twentieth and twenty-first centuries.

that a pandemic had the potential to cause large numbers of deaths and major economic damage, and a desire to mitigate these effects; (2) the mobilization of international leaders to address the threat of terrorism (including bioterrorism) led to the scrutiny of other risks; and (3) there was sensitivity among politicians – in the light of SARS and Hurricane Katrina – about criticisms in the media that they lacked competence and had been complacent in responding to major emergencies. There was a great deal of international cooperation in planning for the next pandemic, led by the World Health Organization.

However good the plans may be, there is nothing that can turn back a pandemic of influenza when it emerges. To be effective, a vaccine needs to be genetically specific against the subtype and strain of the virus. These cannot be known in advance. Modern science cannot yet provide a broad-spectrum influenza vaccine that protects against all known and unknown subtypes and strains of the influenza virus. So any new subtype of influenza (i.e. antigenic shift) means that populations around the world are immediately vulnerable and remain so until a vaccine is available. When a new strain emerges, a vaccine is likely to take three to six months to produce. By this time, the pandemic will be well underway in many countries. Nevertheless, a vaccine will still be worth having in order to protect those who have not yet been affected. Unfortunately, the poorer countries of the world may not be in a position to purchase the large stocks of vaccine necessary to protect their populations.

The main countermeasure that can be prepared in advance is antiviral drugs. In many countries, including the United Kingdom, these are stockpiled in advance, for distribution when the pandemic arrives. Antiviral policy is not straightforward. First, the drugs must be given in the first 24–48 hours of symptoms developing; otherwise, they will not be effective. Second, they do not cure influenza, but simply shorten the duration of the attack and possibly its severity. Third, drug resistance can develop.

Other elements of preparedness include raising public awareness and educating people about the benefits of good hygiene (which does have an impact on slowing spread). This involves having good public messaging in place, to be deployed at different phases of the pandemic hitting a country.

Local health and social care services must have their own plans in place, which assess capacity and contingencies and are well rehearsed. Business and essential service continuity is also very important, and detailed plans need to be made to ensure this.

THE 2009 PANDEMIC

In the planning period before the first twenty-first-century influenza pandemic arrived, most attention was focused on the spread of a particular avian influenza virus (H5N1) that emerged in China in 1997, causing outbreaks of illness and death among poultry and wild birds. In May 1997, in Hong Kong, the virus was transmitted from poultry to people. A 13-year-old boy died, and a further 17 people

were affected. The Chinese authorities carried out a large-scale slaughter of poultry and the outbreak was controlled. After that, H5N1 spread widely in the wild bird population around the world. There have since been many outbreaks in different countries among domesticated birds. There have also been cases of illness and death among people. Many experts regarded this H5N1 avian influenza virus as the prime candidate to reassort with another influenza virus and cause the first influenza pandemic of the twenty-first century.

In the event, this was not what happened. When the first influenza pandemic of the twenty-first century emerged, it had no relationship to H5N1. The first cases of a new swine influenza type A (H1N1) virus were confirmed in Mexico and the United States on 23 April 2009. In Mexico, the early reports were of 149 deaths from 878 reported cases, suggesting a relatively high case fatality rate. The first two confirmed UK cases were only four days later (on 27 April 2009), in a couple who had returned to Scotland from Mexico. This shows just how quickly, in an era of international travel, a virus can move across the world. The first case in England was after only two more days; this time it was a schoolchild in Devon.

By 1 May 2009, the virus had been transmitted to affect a first person who had not travelled outside the country. The pandemic of the influenza A (H1N1) virus became established. A similar pattern of transmission was emerging in European countries and many other parts of the northern hemisphere.

It was also becoming clear that the new pandemic virus was producing milder illness than in any of the three twentieth-century influenza pandemics. However, its pattern was typical of a new subtype of influenza type A occurring through antigenic shift. It produced higher rates of illness among children and young adults than among older adults. There were many hospitalizations and deaths in these younger age groups, although fewer than in previous influenza pandemics; worldwide, 80% of deaths from this new pandemic influenza were in people aged below 65 years. This is in marked contrast to seasonal influenza, in which the majority of deaths are in older people.

The emergency response to the 2009 influenza pandemic in the United Kingdom worked well. It was led by the chief medical officers of each of the four UK countries, with policy and overall coordination by the government's emergency committee COBRA.

The plan that had been prepared and rehearsed several years previously was implemented successfully, with some modifications and new measures being introduced. The key features were high-quality surveillance data; weekly media briefings by the chief medical officer for England; extensive use of antivirals for cases and, initially, for contacts of cases; fast tracking of vaccine development; the establishment of a telephone advice line through which antivirals could be authorized (this relieved pressure on health services); regular meetings of the cross-government coordinating committee, COBRA; and regular contact with other countries through the European Commission and the World Health Organization.

The influenza A (H1N1) virus continued to cause infections and some deaths for two more winters, with its distinctive pandemic profile of attacking younger people.

PANDEMIC PREPAREDNESS

Table 3.13 shows the lessons that should be learned from the experience of the 2009 pandemic, to inform pandemic influenza preparedness for the future. The intervals between the four modern influenza pandemics were 40 years, 10 years and 40 years. There is no minimum or maximum interval – such is the unpredictability of the influenza virus. Following the 2009 pandemic, the next could come relatively quickly or not arrive for decades. Equally, the subtype of virus that will cause it cannot be predicted. It could be sparked by two prominent bird influenza viruses, H5N1 and H7N9 (still circulating worldwide), exchanging their genetic material (reassorting) with other influenza viruses. Or it could come from a source unrelated to these two viruses.

In the long term, the only sure protection from the illness, death and economic effects of an influenza pandemic is a broad-spectrum vaccine that can be given in advance. This is not currently possible but is the subject of intensive scientific research. In the meantime, governments need to ensure that up-to-date plans are in place to deal with the next influenza pandemic, whenever and wherever it may strike.

Antimicrobial resistance

In 1928, the year he was appointed professor of bacteriology, Alexander Fleming made a chance discovery that was to open up a new frontier in medicine. While he worked in his laboratory at St Mary's Hospital in London, unbeknown to him, a fungal spore floated through the window and landed in a Petri dish upon which he was growing colonies of the bacterium S. aureus. Some days later, Fleming noticed that where the mould was growing, bacteria had disappeared. This was not an experiment that Fleming had planned, but he quickly realized the need to study the phenomenon further. The mould was identified as *Penicillium notatum*.

It was over a decade later that scientists led by Dr Howard Florey developed and purified the substance in the mould

Table 3.13 Key elements of pandemic preparedness, incorporating lessons from the 2009 influenza pandemic

- A pandemic can occur at any time
- Clear, frequent public communication is crucial
- The response should aim to be precautionary, proportionate and flexible
- The response should use established systems and processes wherever possible
- Simulation exercises can help guide preparedness plans, but the reality is always different

into the drug penicillin – it could break down the walls of bacterial cells, killing them with great efficiency. The drug became available in large quantities towards the end of the Second World War and was life-saving in treating many infected battlefield injuries. The founding author of this book, Raymond 'Paddy' Donaldson, was one of penicillin's first users. As a young officer in the Royal Army Medical Corps (RAMC), during the Second World War in the Far East, he was called to see an important local dignitary. The man was semi-comatose and near death from meningitis, but an injection of the novel drug penicillin saved his life; as he rose from his bed like Lazarus, family and supporters in the room wept, fainted and cried out, 'A miracle, a miracle'.

By the mid-1950s, penicillin-resistant strains of S. aureus had become common. This did not arouse much concern, as so many new classes of antibiotics were discovered and manufactured during the 1960s, 1970s and 1980s. When an organism became resistant to penicillin, there was another antibiotic to use instead. But then the pipeline of new antibiotics began to falter. Almost 30 new antibiotics were licensed for therapeutic use between 1984 and 1988. Between 2004 and 2008, there were just three new antibiotics. Antibiotics give a lower return on investment than many other drugs, and so pharmaceutical companies lost interest in developing new ones.

In turn, the growth of antibiotic-resistant strains of bacteria has risen greatly. Many infections are now unresponsive to first-line antibiotics, and there are fears that some diseases previously curable with antibiotics will become entirely untreatable (Figure 3.28). It is not just bacterial infections that are affected in this way – those caused by viruses, bacteria, fungi, protozoa and helminthes are increasingly insensitive to medicines that used to kill them. The wider term *antimicrobial resistance* encompasses the range of infective agents and the medicines that cannot now treat them.

CAUSES OF ANTIMICROBIAL RESISTANCE

Pathogenic microorganisms develop resistance to drugs through mutations in their genetic material, or exchange of such material with similar organisms. This is essentially a process of evolution, in which the organisms with these key changes to their genetic make-up selectively survive. They multiply so rapidly that the process of evolution seems to be in fast-forward.

So why is antimicrobial resistance becoming so common? The reasons are multiple. They have to do with the widespread use of antimicrobial agents in patient care, in farming, in agriculture and in aquaculture. The World Health Organization estimates that antibiotics are used in greater quantities in food-producing animals than in medical practice. The purpose of using them in animals is to prevent disease and promote growth. This is misuse if the drugs are not given to treat individual sick animals but mass administered to many animals. Many of the same drugs are used to treat human disease, and many of the organisms that infect animals infect people as well. Antibiotics are also

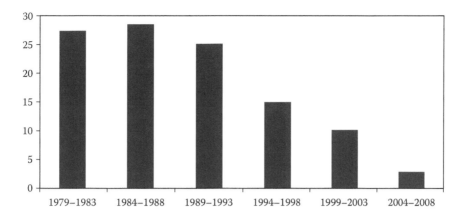

Figure 3.28 Number of new antibiotics licensed in the United Kingdom.

Source: Medicines and Healthcare products Regulatory Authority.

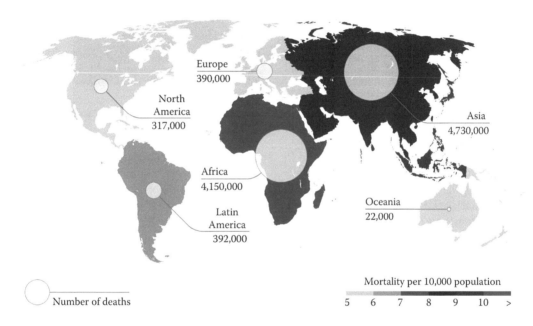

Figure 3.29 Potential annual deaths due to antimicrobial resistance by 2050.

Source: Her Majesty's Government and Wellcome Trust. *Antimicrobial Resistance: Tackling a Crisis for the Health and Wealth of Nations.* London: Her Majesty's Government, 2014.

used in fish farming and in agricultural spraying – of fruit trees, for example.

In medicine and healthcare, antibiotics are also misused in ways that promote resistance. The problems include overuse of antibiotics in situations where they are not clinically required, inappropriate use of antibiotics in an attempt to prevent infection, pressure from patients to be given an antibiotic when it is unnecessary, insufficient dosage or length of treatment and poorly educated prescribers.

THE BURDEN OF HARM

The growth of antimicrobial resistance has far-reaching consequences. Patients take longer to recover and have prolonged hospital stays. When the treatment of serious infection is slowed or even prevented, this can lead to long-term

disabilities or the need for disfiguring surgery. Healthcare systems have to bear substantial additional costs as a result of all this. There is an impact on the wider economy due to lost productivity.

The burden of disease – and risk – is not known for every individual resistant organism, but in cases where it has been assessed, it is substantial and predicted mortality in the future is substantial and global in its sweep (Figure 3.29). The Centers for Disease Control and Prevention in the United States has published a list of 18 antimicrobial threats that are placed in one of three categories: urgent, serious and concerning (Table 3.14). The lists have been drawn up for the United States, but most of the threats apply to many other high-income countries, including the United Kingdom. Many of these antimicrobial resistant infective

Table 3.14 Organisms of greatest drug-resistance threat.

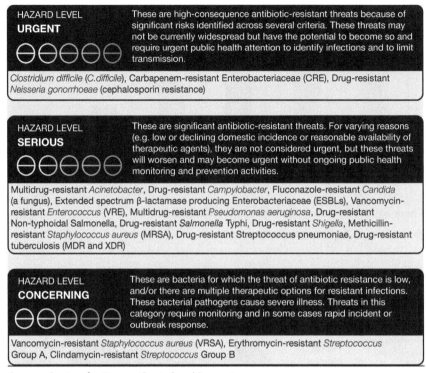

HAZARD LEVEL
URGENT

These are high-consequence antibiotic-resistant threats because of significant risks identified across several criteria. These threats may not be currently widespread but have the potential to become so and require urgent public health attention to identify infections and to limit transmission.

Clostridium difficile (*C.difficile*), Carbapenem-resistant Enterobacteriaceae (CRE), Drug-resistant *Neisseria gonorrhoeae* (cephalosporin resistance)

HAZARD LEVEL
SERIOUS

These are significant antibiotic-resistant threats. For varying reasons (e.g. low or declining domestic incidence or reasonable availability of therapeutic agents), they are not considered urgent, but these threats will worsen and may become urgent without ongoing public health monitoring and prevention activities.

Multidrug-resistant *Acinetobacter*, Drug-resistant *Campylobacter*, Fluconazole-resistant *Candida* (a fungus), Extended spectrum β-lactamase producing Enterobacteriaceae (ESBLs), Vancomycin-resistant *Enterococcus* (VRE), Multidrug-resistant *Pseudomonas aeruginosa*, Drug-resistant Non-typhoidal Salmonella, Drug-resistant *Salmonella* Typhi, Drug-resistant *Shigella*, Methicillin-resistant *Staphylococcus aureus* (MRSA), Drug-resistant Streptococcus pneumoniae, Drug-resistant tuberculosis (MDR and XDR)

HAZARD LEVEL
CONCERNING

These are bacteria for which the threat of antibiotic resistance is low, and/or there are multiple therapeutic options for resistant infections. These bacterial pathogens cause severe illness. Threats in this category require monitoring and in some cases rapid incident or outbreak response.

Vancomycin-resistant *Staphylococcus aureus* (VRSA), Erythromycin-resistant *Streptococcus* Group A, Clindamycin-resistant *Streptococcus* Group B

Source: Centers for Disease Control and Prevention

agents are found in healthcare settings, particularly hospitals, but many also circulate in communities.

The treatment of three of the most prominent communicable diseases globally – malaria, HIV and tuberculosis – has been beset by resistance. Resistance has been recorded for all classes of antimalarial drugs. Chloroquine resistance particularly has become common in many malaria zones around the world. Resistance levels to first-line HIV treatments have been as high as 20% in some countries. Tuberculosis resistance is particularly serious with MDR-TB and so-called XDR-TB emerging.

STRATEGIES TO COMBAT RESISTANCE

There is no single measure to control the growth of antimicrobial resistance. Despite past overreliance on new therapeutic options, it is still important to promote innovation in diagnostic and treatment technologies. Novel approaches – through fields like genetics, immunotherapy and vaccine science – could yet yield major breakthroughs in capacity to disable pathogenic organisms. Such innovation requires strong partnerships between the biotechnology industry, universities, scientists, governments, philanthropists and charitable foundations.

At the clinical level, a range of measures (some of which also control infection generally) can have an impact on antimicrobial resistance. Strong hand hygiene programmes reduce transmission of organisms, including resistant ones such as MRSA. Appropriate environmental cleaning and decontamination – especially in healthcare facilities – also plays an important role in reducing the risk of transmission of some resistant microorganisms (e.g. vancomycin-resistant enterococci). Screening of patients admitted to hospital, as

well as isolation of colonized or infected patients, also plays an important part. Ultimately, though, the more appropriate use of antibiotics in patient care is essential (so-called *rational use* or good *antibiotic stewardship*). Such approaches involve educating patients, the public and health professionals; ensuring high-quality medicines; improving compliance with treatment protocols; and limiting the use of drugs where resistance is growing most rapidly.

Controlling antibiotic use in animal husbandry, agriculture and aquaculture is arguably even more complex because it is closely linked to the massively important and political question of food production. Many approaches have been tried worldwide with varying degrees of success, including raising awareness, education, regulations to restrict use, alternative methods of improving animal health and more effective vaccination.

No action can be successful without a strong system of surveillance of humans, animals and the environment. It should cover antibiotic usage, tracking and profiling microorganisms, and assessing the burden of disease caused by resistant organisms.

The UK government produced an antimicrobial resistance strategy covering the period from 2013 to 2018 with seven key action areas:

1. *Improving infection prevention and control practices* in human and animal health.
2. *Optimizing prescribing practice* through implementation of antimicrobial stewardship programmes that promote rational prescribing and better use of existing and new rapid diagnostics.

3. *Improving professional education, training and public engagement* to improve clinical practice and promote wider understanding of the need for more sustainable use of antibiotics.
4. *Developing new drugs, treatments and diagnostics* through better collaboration between research councils, academia, industry and others, and by encouraging greater public–private investment in the discovery and development of a sustainable supply of effective new antimicrobials, rapid diagnostics and complementary tools for use in health, social care and veterinary systems.
5. *Better access to and use of surveillance data* in the human and animal sectors.
6. *Better identification and prioritization of research needs* to focus activity and inform our understanding of antimicrobial resistance. This may identify alternative treatments to new drugs, as well as new or improved rapid or point-of-care diagnostic tests for humans and animals.
7. *Strengthened international collaboration* working with and through a wide range of governmental and nongovernmental organizations, international regulatory bodies and others to influence opinion, galvanize support and mobilize action.

Many governments and global health bodies have produced similar strategies and action plans. However, most official reports are tentative in the action targeted at farming and agriculture. In contrast, a more robust approach is taken by nongovernmental organizations with an interest in this area of public health policy. For example, an alliance, Save Our Antibiotics, formed by three organizations (Compassion in World Farming, Sustain, and the Soil Association), has advocated for much more stringent action, using the rationale that factory-farmed animals are at high risk of infection because they are caged or penned in crowded, stressful circumstances; weaned early; and physiologically stretched to enhance productivity. As a result, animals' immune systems are often weakened, and farming uses antibiotics preventively to compensate for poor conditions where animals are likely to become sick. The alliance has called on the European Commission and member states to reduce antibiotic use in agriculture to a minimum, including setting reduction targets and closing loopholes where antibiotics can still be used as growth promoters on farm animals. They also make recommendations aimed at veterinary surgeons, farmers and pricing policy.

ORGANIZATIONS AND REGULATIONS

Several organizations share responsibility for the surveillance, prevention and control of communicable disease. Their ability to do so is necessarily underpinned by law, enabling them to take action such as closing premises that represent a threat to the public health and, in extreme circumstances, restricting the movement of individuals who present a similar threat.

Public Health England

Public Health England was created in April 2013, as a part of major structural reform of the health services in England under the *Health and Social Care Act 2012*. Public Health England has a very broad remit, with health protection being one key part. With the creation of Public Health England, almost all of what had previously been the Health Protection Agency (HPA) became part of this new organization – as its health protection directorate.

The Health Protection Agency was created in 2003. It had the following main health protection functions, which remain the same with its move into Public Health England: to advise the government on public health priorities, policies and programmes; to deliver services and support the NHS and other agencies to protect people from infections, poisons and chemical and radiation hazards; to respond to new threats to public health and provide a rapid response; and to provide important and authoritative information and advice to the public and professionals. The creation of the Health Protection Agency was an important development because for the first time, it combined functions for the surveillance, prevention and control not just of infectious diseases but also of other public health threats (such as radiation and chemical hazards).

During the first decade of the twenty-first century, the Health Protection Agency used its new capability successfully in responding to a number of public health emergencies, including the international outbreak of SARS, the poisoning of a Russian with the radioactive substance polonium-210 and contingency planning for pandemic influenza. It also played a major role in developing the mandatory surveillance system for healthcare-associated infections in England in support of the government's programme to reduce these infections.

At the front line of England's health protection service are 29 local health protection teams – each covering a population of 1 million to 3 million people. The local health protection team coordinates all activity in the area, and has three elements:

1. A round-the-clock on-call service that is informed of cases of notifiable infectious disease by doctors and laboratories
2. A surveillance function, using notifications and other clinical and laboratory data, to monitor trends in the area, report this to the regional and national level and instigate further investigation or action
3. A systems-strengthening function, which works with NHS and other services to improve the prevention of infectious disease and the ways through which infections are detected, notified and responded to

The work of health protection teams differs somewhat depending on the characteristics of the local area. In London, more time is spent on tuberculosis, for example. In coastal areas, ensuring effective port controls is an important part of the work.

Table 3.15 Infections typically dealt with by local health protection teams on call in England

Meningitis
Food poisoning, including E. coli, Salmonella
Legionnaires' disease
Measles
Rubella
Scarlet fever
Tuberculosis
Whooping cough
Diarrhoea and vomiting outbreaks, often norovirus
Scabies
Hepatitis B
Returning travellers, e.g. risk of rabies after bite, Giardia
Invasive group A streptococcal disease

A local health protection team is equipped to deal independently with most infectious disease situations in its area. Consultants in Communicable Disease Control lead each team. When there are unusual cases, outbreaks or incidents, the team can call on regional or national support. Some of the most common infections dealt with by local health protection teams on call in England are shown in Table 3.15.

Local health protection teams play a key role, but are just one part of a much larger system in which many people in a number of different agencies contribute towards the prevention and control of infectious disease.

In addition to its 29 local teams, Public Health England has a number of specialist health protection services operating at the national level. These have four main functions:

1. To conduct national-level surveillance for each infection
2. To provide specialist support to local health protection teams in their management of cases and outbreaks of particular infections – by producing written guidelines and by providing additional advice as required
3. To operate specialist laboratories, including reference laboratories
4. To manage problems best dealt with at the national level, such as preparedness for and response to seasonal influenza, people exposed to rarer imported disease (e.g. Lassa fever) and chemical incidents or radiation (which require very specialist knowledge)

There is also a regional tier within the system, which coordinates the work of local health protection teams and provides regional-level surveillance (such as for the whole of London).

Local government

Local authorities in England are empowered to take action to control notifiable diseases within their boundaries. They are required to appoint a proper officer for this function.

Some delegate this authority to their local health protection team, while others retain the function in-house. The local authority can appoint more than one proper officer and can define the limits of their responsibilities, so it does not follow that all proper officers of this function have the same powers. Scotland, Wales, Northern Ireland make their own different arrangements; for example, Scotland has retained a central health protection function.

The structure of local government varies, but the department concerned with communicable disease control is that containing environmental health services. Its function is usually led by a Chief Environmental Health Officer. Local authorities have a wide range of duties covering most aspects of environmental protection. The duties include the registration, inspection and investigation of food premises; involvement in the investigation of outbreaks of certain infectious diseases (mainly those which are food-borne); monitoring and dealing with other environmental hazards; and responding to concerns and enquiries from the public about environmental food-quality matters. Legal powers of enforcement and prosecution with respect to the control of communicable diseases rest mainly with local authorities and their proper officer.

In addition to the formal infectious disease control responsibilities, local health services and health boards have an important role in promoting health, preventing disease and securing care to meet the population's needs. Thus, surveillance of infectious diseases, the identification of particular problems and the planning of preventive measures are key roles.

Health services also have responsibilities for the treatment and care of people with illnesses caused by infectious diseases and parasites. The general practitioner, with the support of the primary care team, is the person who treats the majority of cases in the community. Only serious cases or those with complications are admitted to hospital. The fall in the incidence of serious infectious diseases over the years has led to fewer hospital beds being required for treatment. Many general hospitals are able to provide only limited isolation facilities, but specialist advice and care is provided by specialist infectious disease physicians or physicians with a special interest in infectious diseases, as necessary.

Since 2004, all NHS bodies in England have been required to appoint a Director of Infection Prevention and Control (DIPC). Each major hospital or group of hospitals has a hospital infection prevention and control committee consisting of senior professional staff and reporting to the director. The committee meets at regular intervals and keeps problems in relation to infection in the hospital under review. The day-to-day work is carried out by an infection control team comprising an infection control doctor, usually a consultant medical microbiologist on the hospital staff, and infection control nurses, often led by a nurse consultant. They are responsible for surveillance and feedback on the levels of infection (e.g. in intensive care units and other high-risk areas, as well as general wards), and they deal with outbreaks when they occur and monitor compliance with infection prevention and control procedures and protocols. Reports from the committee and the director of infection prevention and control are standard agenda items for NHS trust board meetings.

World Health Organization and Interntional Health Regulations

Communicable diseases do not respect international borders, and the explosion of air travel has allowed them to spread far more rapidly than ever before. Global surveillance and response mechanisms are therefore vital.

The World Health Organization, established in 1948, is a United Nations agency with its headquarters in Geneva, Switzerland. It is responsible for providing leadership in global health, setting norms and standards, providing technical support to countries and assessing trends in health and disease. Its remit is much wider than infectious diseases, but it does have a key role in surveillance, coordinating action and identifying new and current threats. It works closely with national governments and other international health bodies.

In the summer of 2007, a new set of *International Health Regulations* agreed on by the World Health Assembly (the governing body of the World Health Organization) came into effect. They had not been reviewed since 1969. The earlier regulations had applied mainly to three infectious diseases – cholera, plague and yellow fever. The current *International Health Regulations* are much broader and require member states of the World Health Organization to report 'any public health emergency of international concern', whether it is biological, nuclear or chemical, irrespective of origin or source. The new regulations strengthen the ability to reduce global health risks and prevent national outbreaks or incidents spreading internationally.

Each country has to designate a focal point to be accessible 24 hours a day and to notify the World Health Organization if any two of the following four criteria for assessment and notification are fulfilled:

1. Is the public health impact of the event serious?
2. Is the event unusual or unexpected?
3. Is there a significant risk of international spread?
4. Is there a significant risk of restrictions on international travel or trade?

For the most serious instances, the *International Health Regulations* allow the World Health Organization to declare a Public Health Emergency of International Concern. Such a declaration can be made in situations that are serious, unusual or unexpected; carry implications for public health beyond the affected country's national borders; and may require immediate international action.

The need for such mechanisms makes clear, as amply illustrated throughout this chapter, that communicable diseases remain a very substantial threat to public health.

CONCLUSIONS

In 2015, the G7 group of industrialized nations turned its attention to global health and set three priorities: neglected tropical diseases, pandemics and antimicrobial resistance. This stood out because the modern emphasis in global health has been on the growth of noncommunicable diseases. The G7's declaration is an important reminder that while noncommunicable diseases have been the global rising tide of the twentieth and early twenty-first centuries, communicable diseases remain the rock on which human health frequently founders.

CHAPTER 4

Non-communicable diseases

INTRODUCTION

The architects of the British National Health Service (NHS), founded in 1948, firmly believed that the need and demand for it would fall. They saw it, in the long term, as a health maintenance service. Their thinking was dominated by the experience of the nineteenth and early twentieth centuries, in which infectious diseases were what mattered for health. The worst aspects of these were steadily brought under control with a combination of improved sanitation, clean water, childhood vaccination, safer childbirth and, to a much lesser extent, modern hospital care. Policymakers and planners of the post–Second World War welfare state failed to foresee the tidal wave of so-called 'diseases of civilization' that came to dominate healthcare in the developed world in the remainder of the twentieth century. So big are the numbers of people affected by cancer, heart and respiratory disease; dementia; mental illness; and diabetes that they are the main reason for a twenty-first century healthcare debate that has centred on how to sustain the provision of care as its costs continue to mushroom.

Non-communicable diseases (sometimes called *chronic diseases*) are very different from communicable diseases. They develop over much longer periods, and often cause disabling illness long before they cause death. The seismic shift from communicable to non-communicable disease has been accompanied by two changes in how people experience ill health. First, living with disease and its consequences (poor quality of life, physical and mental incapacity and disability), rather than immediate death, is the more typical experience. Second, many people now live with more than one long-term condition simultaneously (so-called *multimorbidity*). This means that the healthcare and other health-improving measures most needed today are markedly different from a century ago, when the thrust was a do or die approach to protecting the population from the impact of communicable diseases.

The same shift in disease burden has occurred globally (Figure 4.1). The World Health Organization estimates that 80% of deaths from non-communicable diseases now occur in low- and middle-income countries. In the United Kingdom, just four diseases are responsible for more than 40% of all the premature mortality caused by non-communicable disease. These are ischaemic heart disease, lung cancer, stroke and chronic obstructive pulmonary disease (COPD).

A large part of this non-communicable disease burden can be ascribed to a small number of risk factors. A meeting of the United Nations General Assembly in 2011, taking a global perspective on non-communicable diseases, declared that four major behavioural risk factors could be modified by intervention: tobacco use, harmful drinking, unhealthy diet and low physical activity. This necessarily puts emphasis not on the individual diseases themselves, but on the underlying risk factors that contribute to them.

TRENDS IN THE UNITED KINGDOM

Two big killers cause half of all deaths in the United Kingdom today: cancer and cardiovascular disease.

The term *cardiovascular disease* encompasses separate conditions that affect the heart and blood vessels, with many pathophysiological features and risk factors in common. *Ischaemic heart disease* is the leading cause of death among this group. Its symptoms (classically angina) cause disability, and its sequelae – myocardial infarction and heart failure – cause disability and death. *Stroke* creates a premature mortality burden that is half that of ischaemic heart disease. The other cardiovascular diseases, including *peripheral vascular disease* and *aortic aneurysm*, are important but cause less premature mortality (less than 10% that of ischaemic heart disease).

Men are at greater risk of cardiovascular disease than women. It causes one in three premature male deaths, and one in five premature female deaths. Many such deaths could be prevented. This chapter describes six risk factors for non-communicable disease as a whole – smoking, physical inactivity, obesity, diet, hypertension and harmful alcohol consumption. Each is a major risk factor for cardiovascular disease, and attenuating them would reduce premature mortality substantially.

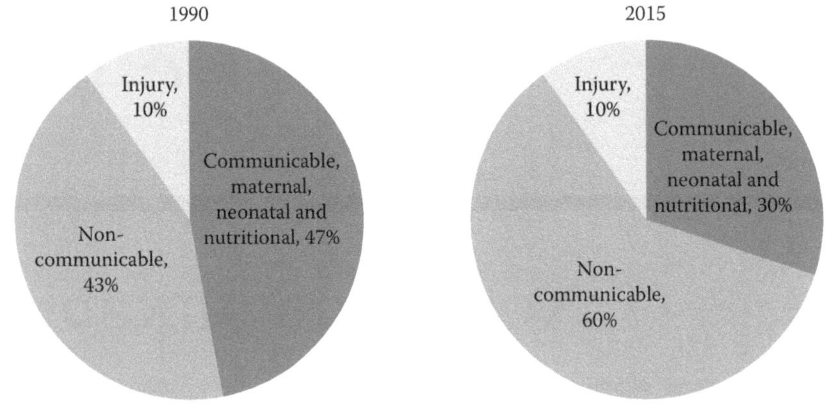

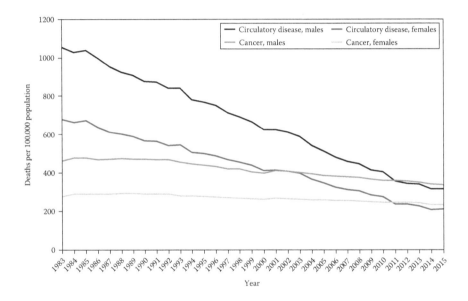

Figure 4.1 The growth of non-communicable disease as a proportion of the total global disease burden.

Source: Institute for Health Metrics and Evaluation.

Figure 4.2 Age-standardized mortality rates due to cancer and cardiovascular disease, England and Wales.

Source: Office for National Statistics.

One in three people will develop cancer during their lifetime. Around 300,000 cases of cancer are diagnosed every year in the United Kingdom. There are more than 200 types of cancer, but just four sites – lung, large bowel, breast and prostate – account for more than half. Lung, colorectal and breast cancer are also the top three cancer causes of premature mortality. Tobacco is responsible for an estimated quarter of all deaths from cancer.

The incidence of cancer increases with age. Two-thirds of cases occur in people aged 65 years and older. The incidence of cancer is going up; this is mainly an impact of population ageing. If the age structure of the population had not changed, the incidence of cancer would have been stable for the last 20 years. Increases in the age-specific incidence of some cancers – malignant melanoma and liver and oral cancers – have been offset by decreases in the incidence of others, such as stomach, bladder and lung cancers.

Over the last quarter of a century, the premature mortality caused by cardiovascular disease and cancer has greatly reduced (Figure 4.2), mainly through advances in therapy and in the organization of medical care. Reduced levels of smoking have also contributed. Ischaemic heart disease has shown the most impressive reduction. Its annual burden, measured as years of life lost, was halved over the two decades that followed 1990. This compares very favourably with most other parts of the industrialized world. UK life expectancy at birth went up by four years in the same time period (from 75.7 to 79.9 years); the reduction in death from cardiovascular disease was the major reason.

Premature deaths from cancer have also fallen over the last quarter of a century, but less so than cardiovascular disease. At the turn of the millennium, cardiovascular disease was the number one cause of death in the United Kingdom and cancer the second. The reverse is now true. When cancer displaced cardiovascular disease from the top of the mortality league table, some media reported this as if the amount of premature mortality caused by cancer had increased. This is not the case. It has decreased, but less markedly than that of cardiovascular disease. Progress in tackling cancer has not been uniform. Premature mortality from both lung and breast cancer was reduced by a quarter over the 20 years spanning the turn of the millennium. Over the same period, mortality rates for colorectal cancer fell by just 10%, particularly because delayed diagnosis remains a problem.

Overall, these changes have driven a marked overall decrease in the premature mortality that non-communicable diseases cause. In 1990, non-communicable diseases caused the premature loss of 11.3 million years of life. Over the next 20 years, this figure fell by a third – to 7.6 million years. This number continues to decrease, but non-communicable disease still causes the premature loss of more than 7 million years of life every year in the United Kingdom.

Throughout the world, just four disease processes result in more than 80% of the deaths from non-communicable disease (Figure 4.3). In addition to cardiovascular disease and cancer, these are diabetes mellitus and chronic obstructive pulmonary disease.

Diabetes mellitus causes both premature death and disability. Type 1 diabetes (formerly called *juvenile-onset diabetes*) is an autoimmune condition, whose incidence has changed little over recent years. It may be triggered by a virus in susceptible individuals. Most (around 90%) new and existing cases of diabetes are type 2. The name for this variant of the disease used to be *maturity-onset diabetes*.

This is a particular misnomer given that many cases now occur at younger ages, fuelled by the epidemic of obesity. Some 3 million adults in the United Kingdom are known to have diabetes. This number has doubled over the last 20 years. If the current trend continues, it will be 5 million in 2025. Another 1 million people may have undiagnosed diabetes. It is more common in people of South Asian and Caribbean origin.

The impact of diabetes is mainly through its micro- and macro vascular complications. They include sight loss, kidney disease, ischaemic heart disease, stroke, peripheral vascular disease and peripheral neuropathy.

Chronic obstructive pulmonary disease is largely caused by smoking, but air pollution and some industrial settings can induce it. It has decreased as the prevalence of smoking has fallen, but remains relatively common. It can cause many years of disability before death, and so its overall burden on population health is substantial.

Even though it is not a disease, injury is responsible for much death and disability globally. Its prevention, particularly in relation to accident prevention, is a traditional and important area of public health policy and practice. For these reasons, it is covered in this chapter on non-communicable diseases.

Traditionally, the burden of non-communicable disease has been considered almost entirely through these major causes of mortality. It is now increasingly realized that non-communicable disease also creates a very substantial burden of disability. While premature mortality has decreased, the disability burden has barely changed. The diseases that

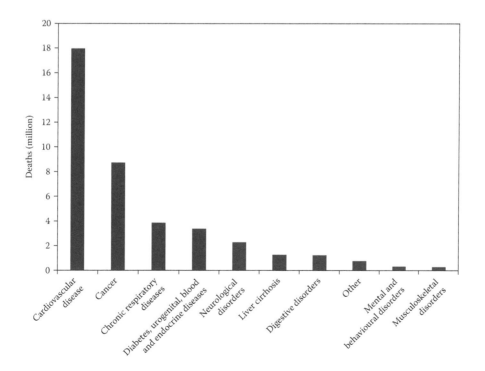

Figure 4.3 Non-communicable diseases responsible for 40 million deaths globally, 2015.

Source: Institute for Health Metrics and Evaluation.

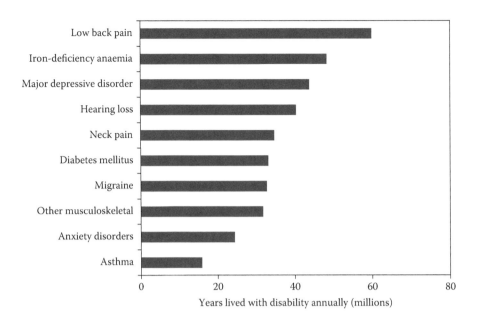

Figure 4.4 Leading causes of disability burden globally, 2015.

Source: Institute for Health Metrics and Evaluation.

cause most of this disability burden are not the same diseases that cause most of the mortality burden. The greatest disability burden comes from musculoskeletal diseases (Figure 4.4). Both in the United Kingdom and globally, low back pain is chief among these. Osteoarthritis and neck pain are other major contributors.

The world over, public health professionals tend to focus on the noncommunicable diseases that represent the greatest burden in the population. This is understandable. Doing so, though, must not cause other diseases that affect the lives of millions to be forgotten. Chronic kidney disease is an important example. This is a progressive disease, classified by stages. Early-stage disease is common, its incidence increasing with age. It causes no symptoms, but sufferers are monitored and have their blood pressure controlled if needed. End-stage disease typically comes after many years of deterioration, but can occur more rapidly. It is much rarer, but its impact severe. Sufferers need either lifelong dialysis treatment or a kidney transplant. The full range of non-communicable diseases is vast – from Parkinson's disease to epilepsy, and asthma to inflammatory bowel disease. Together, the non-communicable diseases create substantial demand on healthcare systems.

Depression, anxiety disorders and Alzheimer's disease contribute to mortality, but particularly to morbidity. In the United Kingdom, and globally, depression is responsible for the second greatest burden of morbidity after low back pain. These diseases are often considered within the umbrella of non-communicable disease. In this book, though, as is common practice, they are covered in Chapter 9, on mental health.

The non-communicable diseases are sometimes referred to as diseases of affluence, but today this is a rather outmoded term, since within the United Kingdom,

the burden of non-communicable disease falls far more heavily on the worst off. This is discussed in depth in Chapter 5.

RISK FACTORS

A small number of underlying risk factors collectively cause a substantial amount of non-communicable disease within the population. They overlap between the main non-communicable diseases. In the United Kingdom, the five risk factors that create the greatest disease burden are poor diet, smoking, high blood pressure, obesity and overweight, and alcohol and drug use (Figure 4.5). These same five are top ranking across most of the high-income countries of the world, and are now having an increasing impact in low-income countries too. The risk factors fall into three groups (Figure 4.6): *behavioural* (e.g. poor diet, smoking, physical inactivity and excess alcohol consumption), *biological* (e.g. raised serum cholesterol, genes and high blood pressure) and *environmental* (e.g. microorganisms, radiation and asbestos). Such a classification is a traditional way of dividing up risk factors of disease for descriptive study or analytical purposes. The reality is much more complex because factors within these three broad domains interact and influence each other, as well as promoting particular disease outcomes. There are also a number of social determinants of health that underpin the development of these risk factors, set out in detail in their own chapter. Age is probably the greatest risk factor of all, and is fully described in Chapter 11.

A risk factor for a disease is something that increases an individual's chances of developing that disease. For example, the major risk factors for cardiovascular disease are older age, male gender, family history (genetics), diabetes,

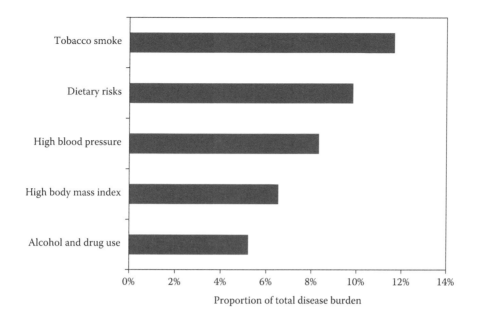

Figure 4.5 Proportion of disease burden in the United Kingdom attributable to the leading risk factors, 2015.

Source: Institute for Health Metrics and Evaluation.

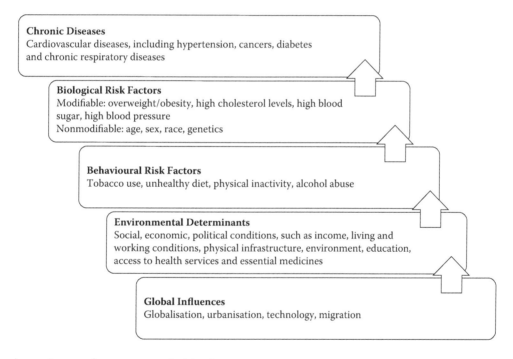

Figure 4.6 Key determinants of non-communicable disease.

Source: Pan American Health Organisation. *Regional Strategy and Plan of Action on an Integrated Approach to the Prevention and Control of Chronic Diseases.* Washington, DC: PAHO, 2006.

smoking, diet, hypertension and physical inactivity. The relationship between several of these and the risk of death from cardiovascular disease is shown in Figure 4.7. From a population health perspective, the more common these risk factors are, the more prevalent the disease will be. Age, gender and genetics are of less practical interest because they are not modifiable (although the scope of genetic intervention in the light of scientific developments is difficult to predict). Some

risk factors are disease states in their own right. For example, obesity is a risk factor for diabetes, which in turn is a risk factor for cardiovascular disease.

The risk factors described here are a big part of the story of non-communicable diseases, but not the whole story. If it were possible to eliminate each of these six risk factors from the population, this would substantially reduce the burden of non-communicable disease – but not to zero. Healthcare

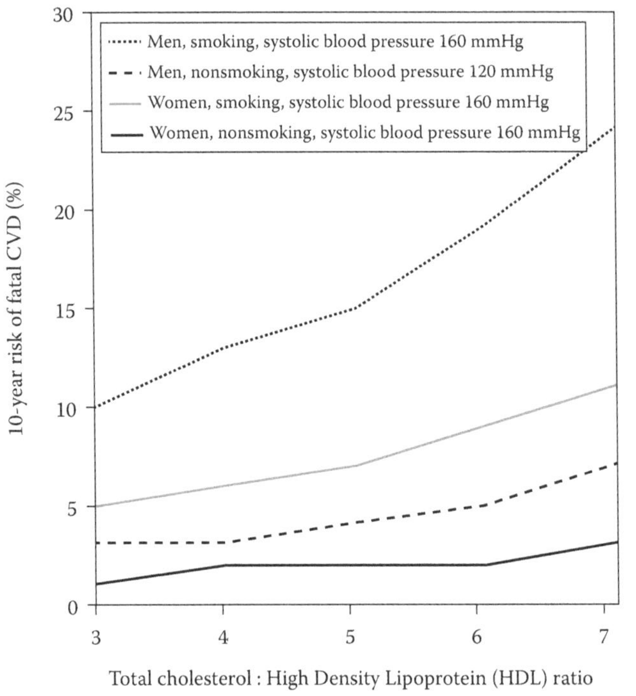

Figure 4.7 The relationship between blood cholesterol, gender, smoking, blood pressure, and 10-year risk of fatal cardiovascular disease (CVD).

Source: Graham I, Atar D, Borch-Johnsen K, et al. European Society of Cardiology (ESC) Committee for Practice Guidelines (CPG): European guidelines on cardiovascular disease prevention in clinical practice: executive summary: Fourth Joint Task Force of the European Society of Cardiology and Other Societies on Cardiovascular Disease Prevention in Clinical Practice. *European Heart Journal* 2007;28(19):2375–414. With permission.

systems able to detect and treat non-communicable diseases are therefore much needed, as described later in the chapter.

Food

In global terms, what food is produced; how it is grown, processed and distributed; and then the ways in which it is accessed and consumed have massive implications for the health of populations, the environment and economies. The design and implementation of successful, cost-effective strategies to reduce unhealthy diets and promote healthy ones would transform human health in a profound and positive way. The public health perspective takes in the problems of over nutrition, under nutrition (including deficiency diseases) and food safety. The last two are dealt with in other chapters, but here, the relevance of diet and nutrition to remaining free from, or delaying the onset of, the major non-communicable diseases is covered. The Nurses' Health Study has enrolled more than 200,000 female registered nurses in the United States. Every year, from 1980 onwards, each participant has completed a detailed questionnaire about her diet. Occurrences of death or significant disease are detected in follow-up so that, over time, patterns have begun to emerge. High intake of red meat carries a greater risk of developing breast or bowel cancer than a low intake. Those who eat more oily fish have a lower risk of

coronary heart disease and stroke. Those who eat more vegetables – particularly green leafy vegetables – have a lower risk of subsequently developing cognitive impairment. These, and other large-scale studies, have consistently shown that key features of the modern North American and northern European diets increase the risk of heart disease, obesity, diabetes and certain cancers. In particular, they involve an excess of high-energy foodstuffs and contain too much meat (particularly processed meat), the wrong balance of fats and not enough fish, nuts, fruit or vegetables. In contrast, the average diet of people in other parts of the world, for example, southern Europe (the Mediterranean diet), is more conducive to good health. The great concern is that as low-income countries become more successful economically, the forces of globalization will shape their citizens' diets and eating patterns in the former rather than the latter direction.

Discussions about the public health implications of diet often centre only on the topic of obesity. Obesity is certainly a major challenge, and nutrition contributes substantially to it. Other aspects of nutrition also have important health effects, and so it is inappropriate for obesity to dominate debate and policy action on nutrition.

Besides water, the human diet has two essential components: macronutrients and micronutrients.

MACRONUTRIENTS

Carbohydrates, fat and proteins are the three macronutrients.

Carbohydrates in the diet come from plants such as rice, grains and root vegetables and are the body's source of glucose and energy to fuel cell functions. The more complex forms of carbohydrates occur in foods like bread, pasta and rice. The simpler forms – essentially sugars – are typically in soft drinks, biscuits and sweets, and when consumed, the glucose is quickly released and absorbed into the bloodstream, causing the blood sugar level to rise sharply. By contrast, eating a plate of whole grains with their more complex chemical structures results in slower breaking down and release of glucose, with consequent more gradual rise in blood sugar concentration. Rapid rises in blood sugar level are generally bad. A high blood sugar level damages blood vessels. As the blood sugar level rises, the pancreas responds by producing insulin. This is a signal to cells to absorb sugar from the blood. If a person eats a lot of simple carbohydrates, his or her pancreas produces a good deal of insulin. Eventually, the body's cells stop responding. This insulin resistance is the basis of type 2 diabetes. In recent years, there has been particular concern about the insidious and pervasive use of fructose (a simple sugar that causes a rapid rise in blood sugar level) in foodstuffs. It is better to obtain the body's glucose requirement from more complex carbohydrates, such as whole grains. An improvement in classifying sources of carbohydrates as either simple or complex is the glycaemic index. It rates them from 0 to 100, depending on speed of blood sugar rise. Eating high glycaemic index foods increases the risk of heart disease, type 2 diabetes and obesity, while eating low-score foods helps to control type 2 diabetes and weight.

Fat in the diet comes from both animal (e.g. meat, eggs and cheese) and vegetable (e.g. nuts and pulses) sources and is of four main kinds – monounsaturated, polyunsaturated, saturated and trans. In earlier scientific studies, no account was taken of the different types of fat. Researchers simply looked at the total volume of fat consumed. Subsequent research has collected data to enable distinctions to be made and has shown that monounsaturated and polyunsaturated fats, derived from plant sources, are generally good, reducing the risk of heart disease and diabetes. The other two tend to promote the occurrence of non-communicable diseases, particularly the trans fats (created by industrial hydrogenation processes). The foods of a Mediterranean diet are high in 'good' fats – olives, fish, nuts, seeds and fish – while many UK diets are too high in 'bad' fats – red meat, butter and cheese. There is a common public misconception that a low-fat diet is a good diet. This can cause health-conscious people to reduce their intake of good fats as well as bad. Also, choosing low-fat foods as the healthy option is not always best since many contain large amounts of harmful simple carbohydrates to enhance taste in the absence of fat.

The body can make most of the fats that it requires by reconstituting other fats, but not omega-3 fatty acids. They are vital for cellular function and, eaten in sufficient quantities, reduce the risk of heart disease and stroke, and possibly some cancers. Oily fish, such as salmon and tuna, is a great source of omega-3 fatty acids. There are two major types of cholesterol in the bloodstream: low-density lipoproteins (LDLs), which carry cholesterol from the gut to the rest of the body; and high-density lipoproteins (HDLs), which carry it from the rest of the body to the gut for disposal. LDL is therefore 'bad' cholesterol, because it results in cholesterol being deposited in cells and arteries. But HDL is 'good' cholesterol, because it clears cholesterol away from cells and arteries. A person's level of LDL cholesterol is affected by dietary intake of fat and carbohydrate more than the type or amount of cholesterol consumed. This is counterintuitive and a difficult health message, but the approach on cholesterol is to follow the advice on fats and carbohydrates, choosing the good versions of each.

Dietary *protein* is the major building block of muscle, and is broken down into energy and amino acids, 20 in all, 10 of which are essential. From amino acids, many other proteins – vital for cellular processes – are built. Fish, poultry and beans are healthier sources of protein than red meat (beef, lamb and pork). This is not because of the proteins themselves (there is little difference, in health effect, between them). It is because of what comes with the protein. For example, red meat typically contains fat as well as protein, much of it saturated fat. Processed meat also often contains substantial amounts of sodium.

MICRONUTRIENTS

Vitamins and minerals are essential to life. If they are absent from the diet or present in insufficient quantities, disease can result. Vitamin D deficiency causes rickets, vitamin B12 deficiency results in pernicious anaemia, and most other vitamins, if deficient in the diet, cause an adverse health outcome.

OTHER KEY DIETARY COMPONENTS

People who eat a diet with plentiful fruit and vegetables are rewarded with lower blood pressure and a lower risk of heart disease, stroke, digestive disease, some cancers and vision loss (through cataracts and macular degeneration). Major cohort studies from the United States and Europe have compared people who eat more than five portions of fruit and vegetables a day with those who eat fewer than three. The higher-consumption groups had a 20% lower risk of both coronary heart disease and stroke than the lower-consumption group. The main health-boosting contents of fruit and vegetables seem to be fibre, vitamins and minerals.

Sodium is one of the main electrolytes within the human body. When people eat a large amount of salt, it cannot be immediately excreted by the kidneys and so remains in the bloodstream. This causes the kidneys to retain water too, in an effort to keep the sodium appropriately diluted. This increases the blood pressure. High pressure is not good for the vessels within which blood travels. So, high salt consumption, largely through its effect on blood pressure, increases the risk of coronary heart disease and stroke. In the INTERSALT Study, during the 1980s, researchers collected a urine sample from 10,000 people in 32 countries. They analysed the amount of sodium in the urine, a reflection of dietary sodium intake. It varied across countries. Populations with greater sodium intake had higher average blood pressure levels.

ACTION TO IMPROVE DIET

A goal to shift an entire population's eating patterns to higher consumption of fruit, vegetables, whole grains and fish, and to lesser consumption of animal fat, salt and trans fats is highly ambitious but necessary. There is no single intervention that can produce such change across a population. Doing so requires concerted action on many fronts.

Dietary guidelines

The UK government was one of the first in the world to establish *guideline daily amounts* to help guide consumers in making decisions about their diet. These were a statement, for men and women separately, of the amount of calories, protein, carbohydrates, sugars, fat, saturated fat, salt and fibre that represent a healthy diet. They became widely incorporated into food labels, and have gone some way towards improving dietary literacy. In 2014, guideline daily amounts were replaced with *reference intakes*, with the aim of simplifying the information. These state a single value for adults rather than separate values for men and women. The actual values are now set by European law. They come with two disclaimers – (1) that they are guidelines, not individual advice, and (2) that the values for fat, saturates, sugars and salt are maximums, not targets to aim for.

Price and taxes

A growing amount of research evidence shows that the price of foods has an impact on people's purchasing decisions. A government could use taxes to alter food prices, and thereby shape consumption patterns. Countries including Denmark, Hungary and France have already taken such an approach. They have primarily focused on calorific foods in order to tackle obesity. These are the so-called 'fat taxes' and 'sugar taxes'. However, there is also the potential to tax foods that are unhealthy for other reasons than their calorie content. The idea of governments using taxes to change behaviour is controversial. That, more than uncertainty about effectiveness, is the reason that the strategy is not more widespread. Government taxation policy and payments already affect the price of food in areas unrelated to health (e.g. agricultural subsidies and import and export duties). The more novel and controversial suggestion has not to do with the means through which a government should interfere with food prices, but the purpose of such measures.

Food labelling

Twenty years ago, a health-conscious person browsing the supermarket aisles had to pick up each item of food, turn it over to read the back label and interpret for himself or herself the relevance of the ingredients listed. Today, the task is far easier. The nutrition information is summarized in a standard table. Reference intakes (previously guideline daily amounts) are there to see (Figure 4.8). The item's energy and macronutrient content is stated as percentage contribution to an average adult's daily requirement. Increasingly, traffic light colouring is used – highlighting high salt, sugar or fat percentages in red, and lower percentages in green. The key information is on the front of the pack, as well as the back. European law now predominantly sets out the food labelling requirements, although the traffic light system is a UK government addition. A law was introduced in the United States in 2014 requiring that calorie information be displayed in food outlets, but there is currently no similar legislation in Europe.

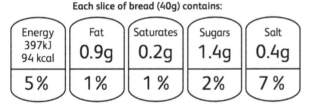

Each slice of bread (40g) contains:

Energy 397kJ 94 kcal	Fat 0.9g	Saturates 0.2g	Sugars 1.4g	Salt 0.4g
5%	1%	1%	2%	7%

of an adult's Reference Intake.
Typical values (as sold) per 100g: Energy 993kJ/235kcal

Typical values	Per 100 grams	Per slice
Energy	1588 kJ	397 kJ
	376 kcal	94 kcal
Fat	3.6g	0.9g
Saturates	0.8g	0.2g
Carbohydrate	80.4g	20.1g
Sugars	5.6g	1.4g
Protein	12.0g	3.0g
Salt	1.2g	0.4g

Figure 4.8 Reference intake label: example.

Source: Food and Drink Federation. Food labelling: A tool to help improve the food literacy of consumers. Available from: http://www.foodlabel.org.uk/label/front-of-pack-labelling.aspx (accessed 28 May 2017). With permission.

Marketing to children

In the United Kingdom, the law now restricts advertising of foods high in fat, salt or sugar during children's television programme. Similar rules apply to radio. This does not entirely prevent advertisers from reaching children, and many go to great pains to do so. The tight rules apply to programmes made for children but not, for example, to Saturday night programmes made for families (which many children watch). Social media offers further substantial opportunities for advertisers to reach their audience. There will doubtless be further developments in the law to catch up. A similar game of cat and mouse was evident when laws on the advertising of tobacco were introduced. Children are highly susceptible to the influence of advertising. Advertising to children, including through sponsorship, establishes long-lasting habits and brand loyalties. Food marketers will continue to want to reach children, and regulating their activities will be essential to achieve much-needed improvement in children's diets.

Education

Sound, unbiased information is a key component of action to improve a population's nutritional status. Providing nutrition advice is not straightforward. Government and public health agencies' usual approach is to provide a list of tips or a visual representation of the optimal balance of foods within the diet. Short and memorable tips can work well. In many countries, the aim of increasing intake of fresh fruit and vegetables is built around the five-a-day healthy eating message (encouraging everyone to eat at least five portions of fruit or vegetables per day).

Food in schools

Schools have a particular responsibility to introduce nutrition and health issues in the health education curriculum. In England, nutrition is part of the national curriculum in primary school and the early years of secondary school. The intention is that by the age of 13 years, children can prepare food, follow recipes, know the major elements of nutrition information that are available to consumers and understand what constitutes a healthy balanced diet.

It is vital to avoid children being taught one thing in the classroom and seeing something quite different in the canteen. Nutritional requirements in schools have improved somewhat in recent years. Schools must provide at least two portions of fruit and vegetables with every meal, and meat or fish that meets quality standards. They are also not allowed to sell fizzy drinks, crisps, chocolate or sweets in school meals or in vending machines. Budget limitations prevent most schools from serving culinary masterpieces, but it is essential that children be encouraged to develop positive attitudes towards eating for health, and become used to healthy food from an early age.

Improving processed food content

When most food was cooked at home from raw ingredients, people could see what they were eating. Over the last few decades of the twentieth century, processed food became increasingly popular – first as ingredients for recipes (such as jars of sauce) and then as entire meals (helped by the advent of the microwave oven). Exactly when scientific understanding of nutrition and its importance was starting to blossom, control over food content shifted away from the individual and family into the hands of the food industry.

Manufacturers and purveyors of processed food, including pre-prepared ingredients and meals, have two considerations in mind – to cater to taste so that the food will sell and to minimize production costs. This has resulted in food that is higher in calories, saturated fat, salt and sugar than is optimal for health. In the United Kingdom, a concerted effort has been made over the last 20 years to reduce the amount of salt in processed foods, for the sake of improving health. In the first decade of the twenty first century, the average daily salt intake in Britain was reduced by 1 g. This is a sizeable change – enough to prevent 6000 fatalities from heart attack or stroke every year. It was achieved through collaboration between the food industry, government, nutrition experts and consumer bodies.

There is increasing controversy about how governments should engage with the food industry. Some say that the achievement in reducing salt intake demonstrates the value of a collaborative approach without heavy regulation. This is currently most governments' preferred approach. For example, an Access to Nutrition Index is used to rank food and drink manufacturers on performance against the problems of obesity and under nutrition. The idea is that rankings like this, made publicly available, put pressure on manufacturers to justify their policies and practices. In the United Kingdom, the Public Health Responsibility Deal provides a mechanism for food producers and retailers to pledge improvements. But none of the pledges have yet been significant, in comparison with the problems that they need to deal with.

Many public health professionals now view this style of approach as an inadequate response to the unrelenting march of obesity. Many call for governments to take a harder line with industry – to regulate marketing, nutrition content and labelling. The food industry has substantial power. It is dominated by multinational companies that are small in number but enormous in size. In the United States, more than half of all food sold comes from just 10 companies. They have great influence over what people eat worldwide. Whether through a gentle collaborative approach or by governments taking a substantially harder line, engagement with the food industry is vital.

Availability of fruit and vegetables

Availability of healthy food is another concern. Some programmes have tackled this directly   such as the School Fruit Scheme, which provides daily fruit or crunchy vegetables to the youngest group of primary school children. As with many other lifestyle-related issues, the greatest challenges are with the most deprived social groups within the population. The issue of poverty, the extent to which a limited household budget is spent on food (particularly for its younger members) and the presence of 'food deserts' in many disadvantaged communities are major concerns when considering the public health problems of some parts of the population in Britain. For children in particular, what their parents can afford and choose to give them to eat is an important part of their early dietary experience. The differential adoption of healthy eating among better-off groups in the population has the potential to further increase health inequalities in the future (Figure 4.9). Among the wealthier, there has been substantial growth in demand for organic produce, and the development of home delivery box schemes is evidence of a growing desire among many people to improve the quality of the food that they eat.

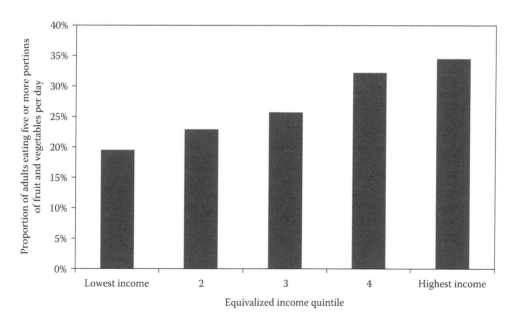

Figure 4.9 Fruit and vegetable intake by income level.

Source: Health Survey for England, 2011.

Limiting accessibility of fast food

Recent years have seen a sustained increase in the proportion of people's dietary intake that comes from food eaten outside of the home. Particular concern has focused on fast food outlets, which tend to provide food that is high in fat and salt, and low in fruit, fibre and vegetables. Such outlets are far more concentrated in deprived areas.

Local authorities have the power to exert some control over the location of such outlets, because new outlets require planning permission from them. A small number of local authorities have used this power to prevent the opening of new fast food outlets within, say, 400 m of schools and colleges. The idea is that this discourages school children from making unhealthy choices at lunchtime and on their way home from school. But despite several years of discussion, this idea has not yet been widely implemented across the country.

It is not only public health professionals talking about the need to shift the population's diet. A diet that contains less meat, more fruit and vegetables and less processed food is not just a healthier one but also a more sustainable one for a planet with a growing population and finite resources.

Smoking and tobacco control

Smoking is still a principal cause of premature death and preventable illness globally. Tobacco smoking is responsible for an estimated 100 million deaths across the world every year. In the United Kingdom, it kills 100,000 people every year. One of every two continuing smokers will die prematurely as a result of smoking. On average, smokers die 10 years younger than nonsmokers. It is also responsible for half a million hospital admissions every year, and costs the NHS an estimated £3 billion. In the United Kingdom, people in routine and manual socio-economic groupings are much more likely to smoke than those in professional and managerial groupings (yet another example of health inequalities). Many more men than women used to smoke, but the gap has narrowed considerably during the twenty-first century.

Cigarette smoke contains some 4000 chemicals. Those in its vapour include carbon monoxide, ammonia, nitrogen oxides and hydrogen cyanide. There are more than 3000 chemicals in cigarette smoke particles, including tars and the more than 50 known carcinogens. Nicotine is present in both the vapour and particulate phases of cigarette smoking. Nicotine addiction is the main reason that smokers keep smoking. Carbon monoxide, nitrogen oxides and other chemical constituents of the smoke are dangerous to cardiovascular health because they reduce oxygen transport in the blood, increase the stickiness of platelets (they are then more likely to clot) and adversely affect serum lipids. Smoking is associated with increased risk of developing or dying from a wide range of diseases, including heart disease, stroke, respiratory disease and six major cancers. Women who are smokers have more low-birthweight babies and more thromboembolic disease (particularly if taking the oral contraceptive pill). There are risks to nonsmokers through passive smoking (inhalation of the components of cigarette smoke in the environment). There is an increased risk of upper respiratory disease in children living in a household where the adults smoke. The direct costs of treating smoking-related illness and the wider cost to society are huge, estimated as £15 billion in the United Kingdom.

In the first 30 years of the twentieth century, advertising, sponsorship and celebrity endorsement were heavily used to promote smoking (Figure 4.10). Cigarette manufacturers

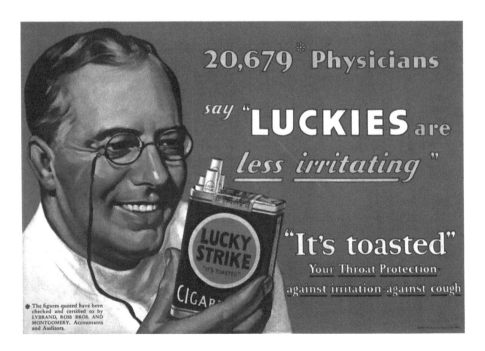

Figure 4.10 An advertisement for cigarettes featuring strong endorsement from the medical profession, 1930.

Source: Stanford University. *Stanford Research into the Impact of Tobacco Advertising.* Available from: http://tobacco.stanford.edu/tobacco_main [accessed 4 May 2017].

deliberately targeted young men at first, and later young women. By 1910, 100 billion cigarettes were being smoked annually. During the First World War, cigarette smoking was marketed at serving soldiers and sailors. Free cigarettes were sent to the front line. The increase in cigarette smoking was unprecedented.

By 1950, the world was smoking more than 1600 billion cigarettes every year. By the end of the century, this figure had risen to 5500 billion. The increase reflected growth in both the number of smokers and the number of cigarettes being smoked by each of them.

The health impact of this explosion of cigarette smoking on health is unmistakable in hindsight, although it took half a century to establish causation beyond doubt. Lung cancer was a rarity before 1900. Only about 140 deaths were ever reported worldwide. Within 30 years, however, it had become the second most common cancer among European men. A similar pattern was seen with coronary heart disease. This was first diagnosed in a living patient in 1910, having first been described in postmortem studies in 1876. It rapidly became the most common cause of premature death in men.

Despite these changes, the role of smoking was hardly recognized at first. Although Isaac Adler in the United States suggested a connection with lung cancer in 1912, the first serious studies of smoking and disease causation were carried out in the 1930s by German researchers. By 1939, Müller was able to conclude that 'the extraordinary rise in tobacco use' was 'the single most important cause of the rising incidence of lung cancer'. These early findings tend to be left out of accounts of tobacco and health because of their association with the Nazi era. Research elsewhere was delayed, sometimes as a direct result of tobacco industry lobbying. As a result, general recognition of the health consequences of smoking was not achieved for another 20 years. Two landmark studies were published in 1950 – one from the United States by Wynder and Graham and one from Britain by Doll and Hill. Both strongly suggested that smoking causes lung cancer. Follow-up studies, particularly a cohort study of British doctors by Doll and Hill, established this beyond reasonable doubt. Further research soon implicated smoking in coronary heart disease, and other diseases were inexorably added to the list.

The policy response to this new research, during the 1950s and early 1960s, was slow. In part, this can be attributed to the malign influence of the tobacco industry on the British government, well described in the book *The Nation's Doctor*. When the minister of health, Iain MacLeod, reluctantly held a press conference in February 1954, his thrust was to downplay the implications of the research while smoking four large cigarettes, lighting each from the embers of the last. The Royal College of Physicians of London produced a landmark report, *Smoking and Health*, in 1962 that put great pressure on the government to take strong action. Public awareness and attitudes started to change as smoking began the long journey towards social unacceptability, a journey that is still far from complete today. The role of independent

bodies like the Royal College of Physicians, Action on Smoking and Health (ASH), the Medical Research Council and cancer charities has been essential in keeping tobacco control policy in the United Kingdom at the forefront of government thinking.

In the United States, the law allows companies to be sued by, or on behalf of, a large group of people. A series of these collective lawsuits (known as class actions) have been brought against tobacco companies. The lawsuits started in the 1950s, spurred on by the first scientific evidence linking smoking with lung cancer. For decades, the tobacco companies succeeded in fighting most of them off. They sought to discredit the scientific evidence, and to argue that smokers take the risk. In the 1990s, the tide turned against them. In 1998, 46 states collectively heard a case that accused tobacco companies of producing a product that caused ill health and created substantial healthcare costs. The tobacco companies lost this case. The settlement totalled some $200 billion, and also restricted tobacco companies' ability to advertise their products.

A year later, the U.S. Department of Justice filed a case accusing the country's largest tobacco companies of racketeering – specifically, of conspiring to mislead the public about the health problems associated with smoking for more than half a century. The tobacco companies lost. The ruling forced them to make further changes to their advertisements, to include clear statements about the harms of smoking. It even ruled that their adverts should incorporate a statement that tobacco companies 'deliberately deceived the American public' – on this final point, a very lengthy appeals process is still ongoing.

When the New Labour government came to power in 1997, there was a big surge forward in action on smoking in the United Kingdom, with the publication of the first ever White Paper on tobacco control. The initiative was somewhat marred when the government appeared to cave in to pressure from Formula 1 motor racing bosses to delay requiring them to stop tobacco company sponsorship in line with the new policy framework. Nevertheless, the first decade of the twenty-first century was the most active in the history of tobacco policy-making in the United Kingdom.

The strategy that has been adopted in the United Kingdom has seven main strands:

1. *Stopping promotion of tobacco*: A comprehensive ban on advertising of tobacco products covers all media (printed, visual and audio) and the Internet; sports and event sponsorship; point-of-sale restrictions on how tobacco can be displayed in shops, supermarkets and other retail outlets; and brand extension to non-tobacco goods.
2. *Making tobacco less affordable*: Taxation has been consistently used to keep the price of tobacco at a sufficiently high level to discourage people from buying cigarettes and other tobacco products. However, this has stimulated a strong illicit trade in tobacco with profiteering from importing tobacco illegally and selling it

tax-free. Tackling this illicit trade is an important part of the overall tobacco control strategy.

3. *Effective regulation of tobacco products*: Regulations dictate the warnings that must be displayed on tobacco packs. Initially, written warnings such as 'Smoking kills' were required, and then pictures were also added. Subsequently, there has been a drive in some parts of the world (notably Australia) to introduce laws to make plain tobacco packaging mandatory. Similar legislation was introduced in the United Kingdom in May 2017. The law dictates that people under the age of 18 years cannot buy tobacco. The content of tobacco products is also regulated to some extent. While establishing the regulations is important, enforcement of them is equally vital if they are to be effective.

4. *Helping smokers to quit*: Nicotine is highly addictive. Nicotine replacement products can help people stop smoking. So too do support and counselling services and some medications. The United Kingdom has invested heavily in a network of smoking cessation services provided through the NHS. They mainly function on a group basis. They have played an important part in reducing the prevalence of smoking in the United Kingdom in recent years. They can also provide nicotine replacement therapy or drugs. A comprehensive smoking cessation service also involves providing self-help materials to individuals, and information in print or online. In addition, quit lines are available to provide advice and support to people by phone. To achieve the greatest population benefits, each individual should have a range of options and be able to readily access those that suit them best.

5. *Reducing exposure to second-hand smoke*: Since 2007, smoking in most buildings used by the public, including pubs, bars and restaurants, has been illegal. Thirty years ago, even offices and aeroplanes were perfectly acceptable places for people to smoke. Passive smoking was a substantial cause of ill health. Bans on smoking in cars are in place in some U.S. states, including California, as well as in some parts of Canada and Australia. In England, it is illegal to smoke in cars if they are carrying children as passengers. Similar legislation is underway, or in place, in other parts of the United Kingdom. Legislation to tackle second-hand smoke exposure means that people spend a smaller proportion of their daily lives in areas where smoking is allowed. This makes smoking more inconvenient and difficult, and less socially acceptable. The smoke-free legislation has been welcomed not just by non-smokers, but also by smokers. This is not surprising when one considers that two-thirds of smokers report that they would like to give up, and this legislation helps them to do so.

6. *Effective communication*: Having restricted tobacco companies' ability to communicate with the public, the UK government established its own communications strategy. Delivered through the various media, government-backed messages of this kind have been broadcast for decades. Their sophistication has increased markedly. At first, they were simple public information campaigns, seeking primarily to communicate information. Now they use advanced social marketing techniques to understand key audiences more deeply, and so target messages to them. The social marketing strategy has had four main aims: to motivate smokers to think about quitting smoking, to provide information helping people to make their quit attempts successful, to discourage young people from taking up smoking and to establish smoking as something that is *not* the norm. Tobacco companies themselves have helped to spread these messages, forced to do so by legislation. Cigarette and other tobacco packets provide warnings on the risks associated with smoking. Before advertisement and sponsorship was banned outright, there was a period when these were accompanied by similar warnings. Every advert was a public health message creating the platform for massive policy change.

7. *Information and research*: High-quality data to track smoking behaviour, public attitudes, tobacco sales figures and quit rates are just some of the data necessary to manage a tobacco control programme and continuously improve it.

This multipronged approach has enabled important synergies. For example, preventing tobacco advertising or increasing the price of cigarettes influences individual behaviour directly, but also helps establish new social norms that make it easier to gain acceptance of a policy of smoke-free public places. In turn, their creation makes people want to quit smoking, and they are more likely to do so successfully because smoking cessation services are readily available. In addition to delivering the components of a tobacco control strategy to a consistently high standard, it is essential to innovate. Keeping up the drive and commitment to get smoking prevalence even lower fosters the creativity to design new initiatives, whether eye-catching new adverts or substantive interventions such as extending smoke-free public places.

The World Health Organization has led the global fight against tobacco-related illness and death, creating the *Framework Convention on Tobacco Control*. This legally binding international treaty contains provisions aimed at reducing the supply of, and demand for, tobacco, as well as a range of other measures. The convention came into force in 2005 following its adoption by the World Health Assembly in 2003. As countries ratified it, they were legally bound by its provisions. Its profound, and far-reaching, nature make it a landmark development in tobacco control and international public health more generally. However, achieving full compliance with the measures in the treaty remains a major challenge.

Faced with tough public health programmes in Europe and North America, backed by legislation, tobacco companies have closed in on the poorer countries of the world. They have been able to use decades of sales and marketing

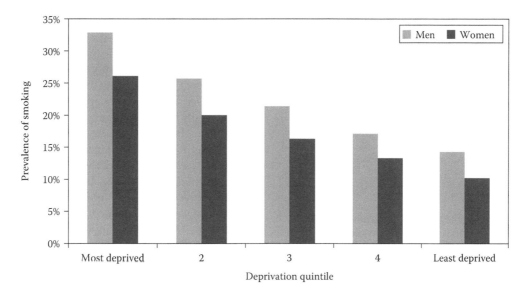

Figure 4.11 Smoking prevalence in the United Kingdom by deprivation.

Source: Office for National Statistics.

experience built up in high-income countries. The opportunities for them are major, as growing economies provide citizens with more spending power. For example, more than half of men in China now smoke, and this is a source of massive profits for tobacco companies.

In countries of the world, like the United Kingdom, where the prevalence of tobacco smoking has fallen considerably, there is important discussion to be had about what the endpoint should be. It is important to understand prevalence within subgroups of the population (Figure 4.11). The idea of aiming for a tobacco-free future is increasingly popular. The state of Tasmania, Australia, for example, is considering banning cigarette sales to anybody born after the year 2000, by effectively increasing the legal sale age by a year, every year from 2018. The aim would be that those born in 2000 would be the tobacco-free generation, and that this would continue for subsequent generations. While the attraction is clear, some feel that imposing a complete purchase ban on adults in unacceptably prohibitive. The proponents can certainly expect fierce opposition from the tobacco industry.

Complicating the situation, e-cigarettes have become increasingly popular in recent years. An e-cigarette is a battery-operated device that looks like a cigarette and releases a dose of nicotine in vapour form when the user inhales on it. Their advent has created a division of views in the public health community. On the one hand, e-cigarettes provide nicotine unaccompanied by the more harmful chemicals of tobacco-based cigarettes, and so are better for the individual user than smoking is. Much like nicotine-containing patches, they can play a part in quit attempts. On the other hand, the fact that they look like cigarettes makes some nervous that their increasing popularity could reverse the trend of smoking becoming more socially unacceptable, or could mean that e-cigarette users, particularly young people, move on to smoking cigarettes later in a gateway effect. Such worries

have led New York City to include e-cigarettes in its ban on smoking in public places. The same move is being debated elsewhere. In England, e-cigarettes are now regulated by the Medicines and Healthcare products Regulatory Agency (MHRA) and cannot be sold to under-18s.

Physical inactivity

Since the Industrial Revolution, technological innovation has reduced the need for physical activity to carry out work and domestic tasks and to move around. Labour-saving devices in the home, motorized transport and the automation of agriculture and industry have all played their part. Today, physical activity is often associated with exercise sessions – time at the gym or playing sport. But the underlying problem – the reason why gyms are needed– is that the relationship between people and their environments has changed. Many experts see the gym as a superficial solution to a deeper problem, and advocate major changes in the built environment and in social norms, so that physical activity is an integral component of all aspects of modern life.

The strong relationship between physical activity and health is well established. In an early, landmark study in 1966, Professor Jerry Morris compared the mortality from heart disease between London bus drivers and London bus conductors. The key difference between the two groups was that as bus drivers sat still at the wheel all day, their conductor colleagues were constantly on their feet selling and checking tickets, up and down the stairs and around the bus. Morris showed that heart disease mortality was significantly lower among bus conductors than bus drivers (Table 4.1). One in 10 bus drivers aged 50–59 years died of heart disease, compared with 1 in 20 bus conductors of the same age.

Table 4.1 Mortality from heart disease among London busmen

Age (years)	Drivers (rate per 100 men in five years)	Conductors (rate per 100 men in five years)
40–49	7.6	1.6
50–59	9.8	5.1
60–69	7.9	7.4

Source: Morris JN, Kagan A, Pattison DC, Gardner MJ, Raffle PA. Incidence and prediction of ischaemic heart-disease in London busmen. Lancet 1966;288(7463):553–9.

Table 4.2 Proportion of population of England who are inactive as measured against government guidelines

Women	45%
Men	33%
Girls	84%
Boys	79%

Source: Health Survey for England, 2012.

In many modern societies, physical inactivity is common and creates a major disease burden (Table 4.2). It causes an estimated 6% of the global burden of coronary heart disease, 10% of both breast and colon cancer and 7% of type 2 diabetes. In sum, it is responsible for 9% of premature mortality globally – 5 million deaths every year. There is strong evidence connecting physical inactivity with depression, coronary heart disease, colorectal cancer, breast cancer, type 2 diabetes, osteoarthritis, osteoporosis and low back pain. The positive effects of regular physical exercise include reduction in the symptoms of depression and anxiety, and improvements in self-esteem.

The World Health Organization recommends that adults should have at least 30 minutes of moderate-intensity physical activity on at least five days every week, or 20 minutes of vigorous-intensity physical activity on at least three days every week. A statistic called the *metabolic equivalent minute* (MET) quantifies the energy used in different physical activity patterns. One MET is the energy used when a person sits quietly. Vigorous activity uses approximately eight times as much, and therefore achieves eight METs. Moderate activity achieves four METs. For the more technically inclined, the World Health Organization recommends that any pattern of physical activity is appropriate providing it achieves 600 METs per week (which is equivalent to 30 minutes of moderate-intensity activity on five days). Until recently, the UK government guidelines recommended activity of at least moderate intensity for at least 30 minutes on at least five days per week. These guidelines have now been updated to recommend two and a half hours of moderate-intensity physical activity (such as cycling or fast walking) per week, or one and a quarter hours of vigorous-intensity activity (such as running), or an equivalent combination. This aligns with the greater flexibility of the World Health Organization's formulation – how the activity is spread through the week, and its intensity. The UK government also recommends that children aged 5–18 years are physically active for at least an hour a day.

International studies suggest that one-third of adults worldwide do not achieve these recommended levels of physical activity. The prevalence of physical inactivity varies markedly by world region – from 17% in Southeast Asia to 43% in the Americas. Levels of physical inactivity in the United Kingdom are among the highest in the world. Physical activity – particularly vigorous physical activity – declines markedly with age. In England, it halves between the 16–34 years' age group and the 65–74 years' group.

Physical activity data predominantly rely on self-reporting. This can mean overestimation. The Health Survey for England has compared self-reports with data collected by accelerometry. While 39% of men and 29% of women aged 16 years and over reported that they met the government's recommendations for physical activity, the accelerometer study found that just 6% of men and 4% of women actually achieved these levels.

Physical activity is more than sport and formal exercise. Individuals' activity is substantially determined by their job (sedentary or active) and by their means of transport (active, such as cycling and walking, or motorized). The level of a person's physical activity is related to his or her age, sex, genetics, health status, motivation and self-efficacy. It is also related to wider influences, such as peer and family attitudes, societal norms and the physical and work environments. Programmes to increase physical activity in the population must go beyond encouraging individuals to become more active and also address access to spaces and facilities, opportunities and barriers, particularly for those in disadvantaged communities.

For many people, the motivation to become more physically active is tough to generate. This is the challenge that public health practitioners face, as activity-sparing technologies continue to proliferate. Physical inactivity is a prime example of a population health problem that demands a multisectoral solution. The physical environment is vitally important. There need to be accessible safe green spaces, and safe paths and cycle lanes. The physical environment also extends indoors – the design of buildings encourages, or discourages, people to take the stairs instead of the lift, for example. Leisure facilities can be subsidized. Simple measures can make the healthier choices easier, for example, a grant-assisted cycle purchase scheme. Schools play a crucial part – from physical and classroom-based education to after-school sports. Schools and employers can both take steps that encourage and enable people to commute using active rather than motorized transport – such as providing cycle storage and changing facilities and, in the case of schools, organizing safe local walking options.

Mass media campaigns play a part in providing information, and in communicating the benefits of physical activity (and harms of inactivity) using social marketing techniques. Health professionals and others can opportunistically provide brief advice or exercise on referral. Some people also benefit from wearing a pedometer or a smart wristband that monitors their level of activity and gives feedback through a computer or smartphone. This technology is growing and being heavily used. Its impact as a feedback to the inactive could be substantial, but is as yet unchartered territory.

Alcohol use

The relationship of societies and their citizens with alcohol varies widely around the world and has also differed at points in history. In some places, heavy consumption of alcohol is a deeply ingrained social phenomenon. In others, religious observance means that few people drink it at all. Hogarth's *Gin Lane* marked the despair of the 'gin crazed' poor of eighteenth-century England (Figure 4.12). The Hollywood movie escapades of Al Capone symbolize a different page in a history book in which a government's attempt to solve its country's problems with alcohol by prohibiting it ended in spectacular failure. The pattern of drinking, and the age groups that drink most, also varies. For example, there is major concern about the phenomenon of binge drinking in some northern European countries like the United Kingdom, while this has been much less common in southern Europe, where people tend to drink mainly with meals. A Scottish teenager may feel that the purpose of drinking is to get drunk, while this will seem a bizarre notion to an Italian teenager, who, while used to a glass of wine at family mealtimes, would spend an evening with friends chatting in a coffee shop in preference to a drink-fuelled tour of bars and clubs. However, it has been argued that these differences are narrowing as the forces of globalization and social networking drive youth cultures to converge. The policy response to the problems caused by overuse of alcohol has often been weak and confused, perhaps reflecting the wariness at targeting a product that in moderation can be life enhancing and engender social cohesion. The impact of robust policies on tobacco control compared with the weaker approach on alcohol is clear: there has been a sharp decline in cigarette smoking, while alcohol consumption increased markedly in the 1990s and early 2000s then subsequently fell (Figure 4.13).

The harm that excess alcohol consumption causes is clear, confirmed by research evidence, and wide ranging. It affects individual health (increasing the risk of liver disease, cardiovascular disease, diabetes, cancers of the breast and gastrointestinal tract and mental illness) and one's ability

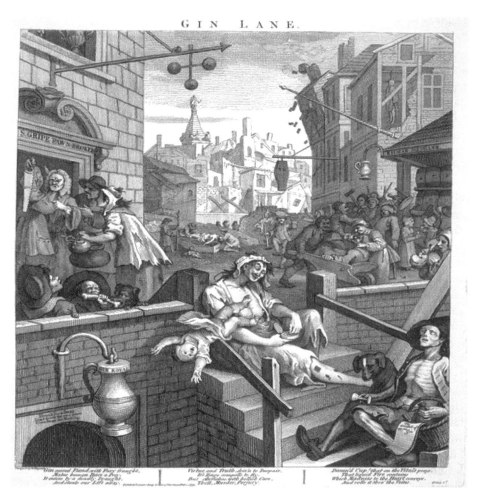

Figure 4.12 Hogarth's Gin Lane.

Source: British Museum.

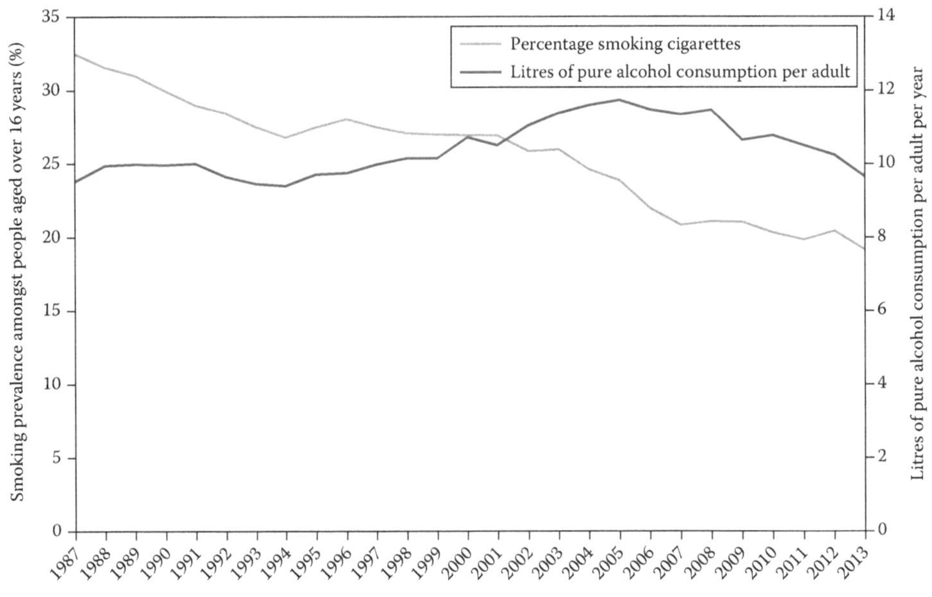

Figure 4.13 Changes in smoking and alcohol consumption in the United Kingdom.

Source: Her Majesty's Revenue and Customs (alcohol); NHS Digital (smoking).

to function socially and economically. In ballpark health terms, the World Health Organization estimates that alcohol is responsible for 2.5 million deaths globally per year. Consumed excessively and by enough people, alcohol also causes extensive social harm through accidents and violence, unwanted pregnancies, crime, antisocial behaviour and worklessness. Half of all assaults in England and Wales are related to alcohol. In Scotland, half of people reported suffering some kind of problem or disturbance due to someone else's drinking during a year.

Three main spheres of behaviour have been described: intoxication, excessive use and dependence. Excessive use is measured against official guidelines for maximum recommended consumption. Dependence is a medical diagnosis based on evidence that an individual is addicted to alcohol. Consumed in very small quantities, alcohol seems to have some health benefits for individuals, reducing the risk of cardiovascular disease in particular. The more we learn, the smaller the beneficial dose – if any – seems to be. There is no safe level for cancer risks, and as consumption rises beyond a low level, the benefit is quickly replaced by harm. Drinking among the very young is of particular concern – not just because the physical and psychological damage of drinking at a very early age is likely to be greater than among mature adults.

There is also an enormous variation between communities in the death rates associated with alcohol. Death rates are up to threefold higher for women and fivefold higher for men in the most deprived areas of the United Kingdom compared with the least deprived.

The United Kingdom is unusual in placing emphasis on drinking at sensible or responsible levels as the basis of its public campaigning on alcohol. This adopts the principle of self-monitoring, using units of alcohol to assess consumption

and to keep to safe or sensible limits. In the United Kingdom, a unit is 10 ml or 8 g of pure alcohol. Some sources of confusion for drinkers are the differing sizes of glasses in pubs and restaurants and the increasing strength of wines and beers on sale.

There has always been recognition of the dangers of long-term high alcohol consumption and of the immediate consequences of impaired performance in areas such as driving, but more recently, attention has been focused on *binge drinking*. This term describes the consumption of a substantial amount of alcohol over a short period of time, such as an evening. Guidelines now recommend that neither men nor women should drink more than 14 units of alcohol per week, and that it is best to spread drinking evenly across the week and to have some drink-free days.

National policy and governmental-level action can take one of two main perspectives: the population health approach, aiming to reduce overall consumption, or the harm reduction approach, targeting the medical and social harms caused by alcohol misuse rather than alcohol as a product. The following are strands of a comprehensive policy.

EDUCATION AND INFORMATION

From school onwards, every opportunity should be taken to ensure that people are appropriately informed about alcohol and its potential harms. The concept of units is a particularly important part of this, in the United Kingdom and many other countries. It is intended to help people be aware of how much alcohol they are drinking, and to be able to relate a range of drinks to a guideline about what level of alcohol consumption is harmful. In the United Kingdom, law mandates display of alcohol content in percentage terms. Most bottled and canned alcoholic drinks also display their unit content and the government recommendations on unit intake. The provision of information has been a key part of the alcohol industry's 'responsibility deal' with government. Although information is important, the evidence that it changes alcohol consumption is somewhat weak, compared with the impact that price and access have on consumption. The rules on alcohol labelling are actually less stringent than those on food labelling. The law requires neither full content nor calorie information.

PRICING

There is a close, observable relationship between the price of alcohol relative to disposable incomes, alcohol consumption and alcohol-related harm indicated by deaths from chronic liver disease. Put simply, if people have more disposable income or there is a fall in the price of alcohol in real terms, it is likely that consumption of alcohol will rise (Figure 4.14) and there will be a corresponding increase in the harm produced by it. Alcohol is not expensive to produce, and the price of alcohol is largely determined by the amount of tax the government decides to put on it.

If price is to be used as a harm reduction measure, it makes sense to consider the price per unit of alcohol. This is because the degree of harm is determined by the amount of actual alcohol consumed, not by the overall volume of the beverage or its type. Despite the application of taxes (whose amount generally depends on volume and type of beverage, rather than directly on its alcohol content), some drinks are available that contain a substantial amount of alcohol at a low price. In other words, they have a low cost per unit of alcohol. The establishment of a minimum price per unit of alcohol is therefore a logical idea. This is a more intelligent, targeted approach than simply increasing taxes across the board. People who consume a harmful amount of alcohol tend to choose drinks priced at a lower cost per unit than those who consume alcohol in moderation. A minimum price per unit policy would therefore affect harmful drinkers more than moderate drinkers.

There is strong evidence to support the idea that introducing a minimum price per unit would reduce consumption among heavy consumers. The measure has been implemented in Canada. In one province, a 10% increase in the minimum unit price reduced consumption of beer by 10%, spirits by 6% and wine by 5%. This may not sound like much, but its effect is magnified because this reduction is concentrated among the heaviest consumers. Across the country as a whole, this 10% increase in minimum unit price resulted in directly attributable alcohol-related mortality falling by a third.

In the United Kingdom, the policy idea is a matter of ongoing debate and commentary. High-quality economic modelling studies and international evidence support the idea. When, in 2013, the Coalition Government dropped proposals to legislate for a minimum price per unit, significant controversy centred on suggestions that alcohol manufacturers and retailers had strongly influenced that decision.

REGULATION OF SALES AND ACCESS

Access to alcohol is a crucial determinant of consumption. Premises must be licensed to serve alcohol, and the license state whether the alcohol sold may be consumed on the premises, off the premises or both. Licenses are granted by the local authority. Traditionally, pubs were required by law to stop serving alcohol at 11:00 p.m., although many bars and clubs were licensed to serve into the early hours of the morning. In the early twenty-first century, the UK government introduced so-called '24-hour drinking laws' intended

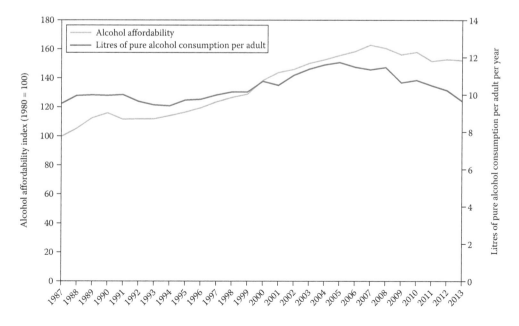

Figure 4.14 Alcohol affordability and consumption over time, United Kingdom.

Source: Her Majesty's Revenue and Customs (consumption); NHS Digital (affordability).

to relax the 11:00 p.m. finish time. Part of the idea was that this might help change social norms, creating more of a café culture in which alcohol can be consumed in a relaxed way throughout the day and night, rather than a culture in which there is a rush to 'drink up' at the end of the night. The evidence suggests that this did not work.

One of the conditions of all alcohol licenses is that alcohol must not be served to people under the age of 18 years (except that those aged 16 years and above may consume alcohol with food in some premises, with adult supervision) or to adults known to be buying on behalf of those aged under 18 years.

Another important aspect of access is that alcohol should not, by law, be sold to people who are already intoxicated. In some countries, such as New Zealand, this is stringently enforced. In the United Kingdom, this license condition is regularly flaunted. In a recent study, 80% of bars tested in a sting operation sold alcohol to those appearing extremely drunk. In 20% of cases, they actually tried to upsell them from the requested single measure to a double. In a typical year, less than a dozen people are prosecuted for selling to drunks. This is not good. Intoxicated people are highly vulnerable and may hurt themselves, hurt others and be hurt or even sexually assaulted by others. It should be a matter of greater concern that this law, in place to protect them, is basically not being implemented.

MARKETING

Extensive advertising restrictions have played a key part in the success of tobacco control, but have not been replicated (yet) for alcohol in the United Kingdom or in many other countries. Alcohol brands continue to be advertised widely, and to sponsor sporting and other high-profile events. Some elements of alcohol marketing have been the subject of pledges made by the alcohol industry – such as not using advertising sites within 100 m of schools, a sponsorship code that aims to promote responsible drinking and publicizing the Drinkaware campaign within advertisements.

BLOOD ALCOHOL LIMITS FOR DRIVERS

A familiar, long-standing and noncontroversial element of alcohol harm reduction strategies is to impose a legal blood alcohol level limit for drivers. Such a law is in place in almost every country. The variation is in what that limit is, how widespread detection efforts are and how fierce are the penalties imposed when the law is broken. The United Kingdom now has one of the highest blood alcohol legal drinking levels in Europe. A growing body of opinion would have it reduced from the current 80 mg/100 ml to 50 mg/100 ml, which it already is in Scotland.

INDIVIDUAL TREATMENT SERVICES

In addition to the enormous burden placed on health services by the short- and long-term effects of alcohol, there is also an important role for health services and other organizations in the identification of alcohol problems and intervention to resolve them. This is a particularly important role for primary care services, where an approach based on the brief interventions model is possible. One major review of the cost-effectiveness of alcohol treatment concluded that investment in evidence-based alcohol treatments could save £5 for each £1 spent. Help for people who have become dependent on alcohol, or who are suffering serious effects because of excessive use, can include treatment services (inpatient, residential, outpatient and day care) that can provide detoxification programmes, family therapy and other specific treatment and support services. Few local services are based on health service initiatives alone. The most successful are those in which the emphasis is on close collaboration between health, local authority and voluntary organizations skilled in these areas of service.

Obesity and overweight

In 1980, only 7% of adults in the United Kingdom were obese. Over the next third of a century, this number skyrocketed, quadrupling to 28%. The prevalence of obesity increases with age, at least until the age of 65 years. At starting school, 1 in 10 children are obese. Six years later, as they move on from primary school, this rises to one in five.

Projections suggest that by 2050, more than half of adults will be obese. If this proves correct, obesity will, in the space of just 70 years, have gone from being a problem affecting just 1 in 14 adults to being the norm. Being above healthy weight (although not to the extent of obesity) already is the norm. Two-thirds of men and more than half of women in the United Kingdom are currently overweight.

Obesity is a major epidemic in many countries of the world (Figure 4.15). Globally, an estimated 1.9 billion people (40% of the population) are overweight and 640 million (13%) are obese. The prevalence of obesity varies from 1%–2% in Ethiopia to 60%–70% in Samoa and Tonga.

Being obese reduces an individual's life expectancy by three years on average. Severe obesity reduces it by eight years. This is because it increases the risk of diabetes fivefold, heart disease more than twofold and colon cancer threefold. Obesity is also a major risk factor for the most common disabling conditions in the United Kingdom– back pain, osteoarthritis and mental health disorders. In total, obesity costs the NHS £5 billion per year and is responsible for 16 million sick days. Healthcare costs for obese individuals are 30% greater than for those of healthy weight.

The most common measure of overweight and obesity is the body mass index (BMI). This is calculated by dividing a person's weight in kilograms by the square of his or her height in metres. The BMI is used to define *obesity* and *overweight* and then to assess the status of the population. Other measures, such as body fat, show a more direct correlation with risk, but are less easily measured on a population basis. The World Health Organization defines overweight as a BMI equal to or over 25 and obesity as a BMI equal to or over 30.

Obese people have tended to be viewed negatively by society: as gluttons who are lazy and lack self-control.

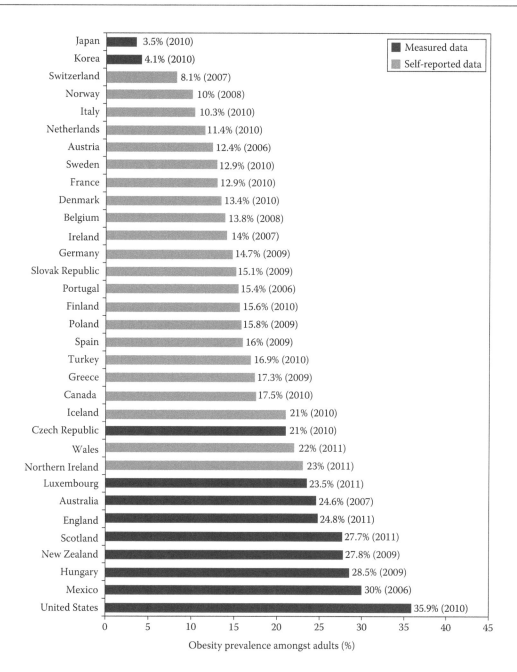

Figure 4.15 Adult obesity prevalence in selected countries.

Source: National Obesity Observatory, using data from Organisation for Economic Co-operation & Development.

Now that obesity is so common, that stigma no longer fits easily with public perceptions. More importantly, attributing the explosive phenomenon of population obesity to tens of millions of weak individuals is simplistic. It also provides little idea what can be done to tackle it. There is a clear generational dimension, with the strongest predictor of childhood obesity being parental obesity. This results from social, biological and environmental factors. Basic interventions such as good maternal nutrition, breastfeeding and healthy weaning have all been linked to healthy weight later in life.

The immediate reason why people become obese is a simple one – their calorie intake exceeds their energy expenditure, and so they accumulate body mass. The reason why

obesity is spreading throughout the population can also be simply stated – average energy intake is increasing and average energy expenditure decreasing. The first part of this equation has already been covered in this chapter's discussion of diet, and the second part under physical activity. Each of these two topics is far from simple – and the deeper reasons behind the growing tide of obesity are yet more complex still.

A huge worldwide research endeavour continues to try to elucidate the biological mechanisms that cause an individual to become obese. Thus, research covers neurosciences – examining how hunger and satiety are controlled and regulated by the brain; genetics – seeking to identify the genes that are associated with overweight and obesity (more than 30 genes have been discovered that facilitate weight gain); and biological – describing pathways through which body fat is laid down. Such work is important and will ultimately provide greater scientific understanding of the molecular basis of obesity. This may benefit the treatment of obese individuals. It may yield novel pharmaceutical agents that are effective in blocking weight gain. Along with the diet and slimming industries and bariatric and cosmetic surgery, pharmaceuticals are hugely lucrative. However, this is unlikely to provide solutions at the population level. As Thomas Farley, a New York City health commissioner put it, 'We will reverse this epidemic not with a better microscope but with a better macroscope – not through genetics or physiology but through sociology and economics'.

The UK government commissioned a special foresight project on obesity that produced an expert scientific review in the late 2000s called *Tackling Obesities: Future Choices*. It powerfully showed the many factors, 108 in all, in the human environment that are causing obesity to become widespread (Figure 4.16). There is a complex web of links between them, and this is the real point in considering the causes of obesity in a population; it is wrong to think of a simple list of factors and misleading to believe that a few targeted interventions will work. The environment is obesity creating, or *obesogenic*. This perspective challenges the old idea that obesity is predominantly about individual choice. In an obesogenic environment, it is inevitable that a population will have a preponderance of overweight and obesity. Of course, there is an important element of individual choice in whether a person becomes obese, but faced with the strength of forces encouraging them to eat more and move less, it is very difficult to assert that choice.

The factors involved in the obesogenic world can be seen as clusters with many complex and subtle interactions:

- *Food production*: Food producers face commercial pressure to grow their business and make a profit. They therefore aim to increase the efficiency of food production, by both minimizing the cost of ingredients and maximizing the volumes of food produced. Globally, the food production system is producing processed, affordable food in unprecedented volumes.
- *Food consumption*: Many foods today are energy dense and served in larger portions than in the past. Food is abundant and exists in greater variety than ever before. Constantly exposed to food, and influenced by its marketing, people take advantage of its easy accessibility to eat more and often. They are driven to energy-dense foods by their ubiquity and cheapness. Convenience is highly valued in today's world. People have less time to cook and fewer have the skills to do so. More consume fast food. In too many places, for too many people, food has become fuel. Traditional nutritional values like the pleasure of eating, a family atmosphere at mealtimes and the highly knowledgeable school dinner lady have been cast to the four winds.

- *Physical activity environment*: The amount of physical activity an individual does depends considerably on his or her environment. Dangers (real or perceived) in the environment reduce people's physical activity, as do labour-saving devices in the home. The availability of playing fields and safe green spaces, the establishment of cycle lanes and places to park bikes and the extent to which people have access to opportunities for physical activity (such as sports classes and clubs) do not begin to match what is required for a truly active population. Indeed, the whole urban and architectural landscape of modern Britain is a major contributor to the obesogenic environment.
- *Individual activity*: The amount of activity that an individual does is in part determined by how much activity his or her parents did, and therefore the behaviours that he or she learned in early childhood. Across society, there has been a major shift from sport participation to sport viewing. Children's experience of sport is increasingly through virtual reality games, rather than in fields, gardens and streets.
- *Physiology*: Many factors to do with an individual's biology impact on his or her energy intake and expenditure, such as genes that regulate how fat is metabolized and how individuals perceive fullness after eating. The truth is that it is much easier for humans to gain weight than to lose it.
- *Individual psychology*: Low self-esteem and high stress both impede people's ability to consciously control their energy intake, and can make them more ambivalent about the fact that they are gaining weight. In part, this lack of self-control can derive from early childhood experiences, as is explored in Chapter 5. For many, food plays an important psychological role as a reward, compensator or stress buster.
- *Social psychology*: Collective societal beliefs about food and weight are shaped considerably by the media and through education. These collective beliefs have an impact on other areas, particularly individual psychology and food consumption patterns.

The physical, social and economic environment has changed remarkably over recent decades, and with it, the increasing prevalence of obesity. Taking a holistic and environmental view of the genesis of obesity does not mean that focusing on the role of individuals has no value. Not everybody who is exposed to the obesogenic environment becomes obese, and it is important to look at why this is so. Evidence-based individual behavioural change programmes can have some impact. Individuals with morbid obesity have traditionally been treated in clinical services, but increasingly those who have less pronounced obesity are opting for bariatric (weight-loss) surgery to insert a gastric band or remove or bypass part of their stomach. Some are doing this in early middle age after little attempt at modifying their diet and physical activity patterns. Research shows sustained weight loss and reduction in diabetes after such operations,

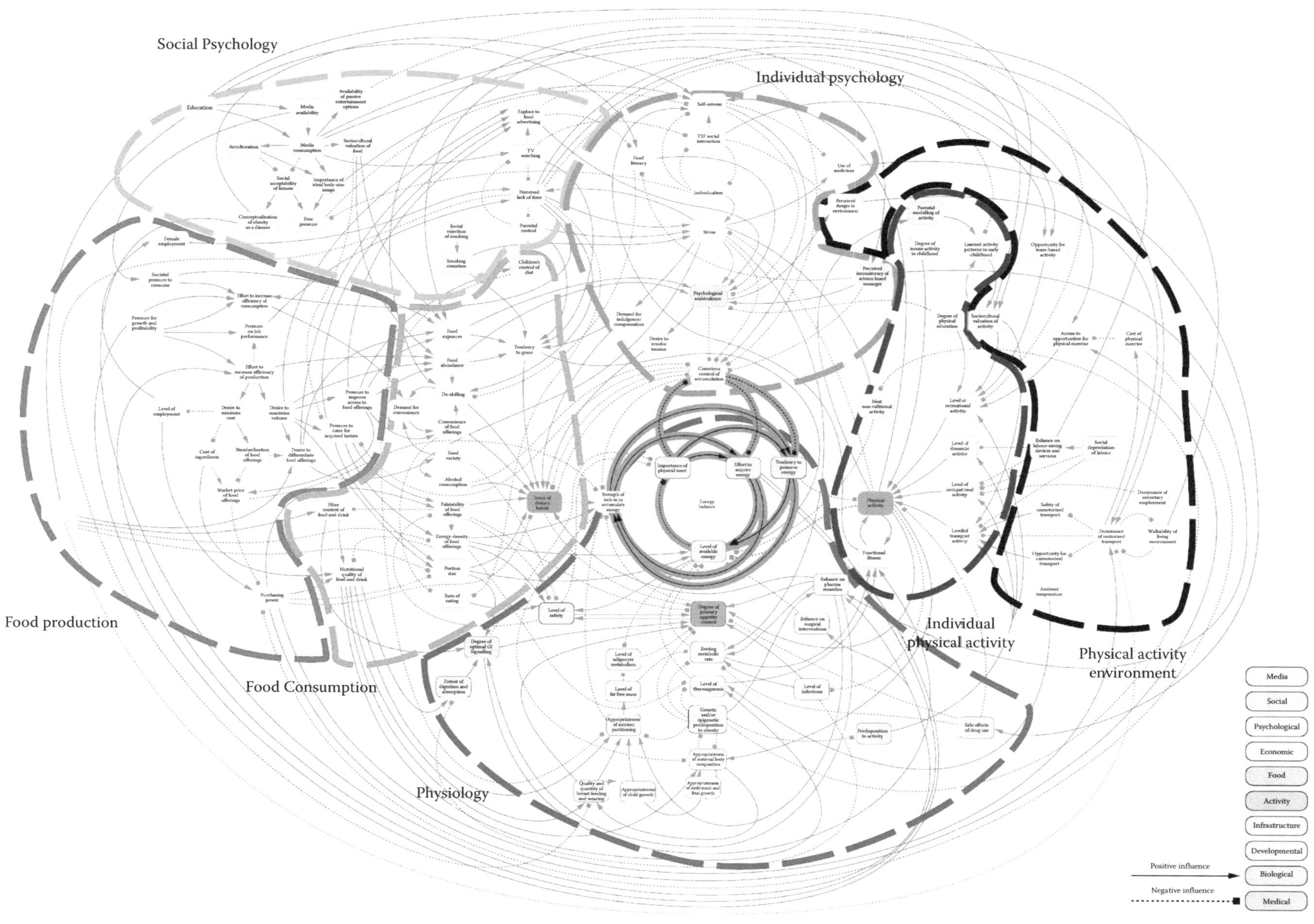

Figure 4.16 The obesity systems map.

Source: UK Government Foresight Programme. *Tackling Obesities: Future Choices.* 2nd edition. London: Government Office for Science, 2007.

but long-term studies are needed to properly establish the risks and benefits.

Mounting a policy response sufficient to make any dent in the growing tide of obesity is a daunting challenge. To date, policy discussion has largely focused on the issue's two major components – diet and physical activity. The major policy thrusts for each of these have been discussed separately within this chapter. Two things are crucial. First, there is no hope of tackling obesity without operating at the environmental level – getting to grips with the physical, economic, political and social factors that are driving the epidemic and offer some levers with which to affect it. Second, the scale of the challenge demands bold action in response – population and politics will be essential ingredients if the obesogenic environment is to be fundamentally deconstructed.

High blood pressure

As blood circulates, it exerts physical pressure on the walls of the vessels through which it travels. If this pressure is too high, it damages those vessels over time. High blood pressure therefore causes cardiovascular disease – most commonly, stroke and ischaemic heart disease. All else being equal, a person with high blood pressure is three times more likely to have a stroke or heart attack than somebody with normal blood pressure.

There is a continuous relationship between blood pressure and these adverse outcomes – as it increases, so does the risk. Historically, it was usual in medical practice to think of blood pressure as binary – of someone either having high blood pressure or not. In the United Kingdom, for many years a person was said to be hypertensive if his or her blood pressure was greater than 140/90. There was an inherent problem with this approach to hypertension. The cut-off point was rather arbitrary. A person with a blood pressure of 139/89 was deemed normal, and a person with a blood pressure of 141/91 deemed hypertensive and in need of treatment. In reality, the person deemed hypertensive had a risk of cardiovascular disease barely distinguishable from that of the person deemed normal. Similarly, the person deemed normal had a substantially greater risk of cardiovascular disease than somebody else normal whose blood pressure was, say, 125/75.

In today's medical practice, this approach is becoming more nuanced. The diagnosis of whether a patient has hypertension in need of treatment now takes into account a number of the patient's other risk factors, not just his or her blood pressure. A highly effective means of reducing an individual's blood pressure is to prescribe blood pressure–lowering medications. Prescribed widely within the population, these medications substantially reduce the incidence of stroke and heart disease, and mortality, in the population as a whole. Many such drugs (antihypertensives) are available. The introduction of antihypertensive medication has been one of the major causes of improved life expectancy over the last 40 years in the United Kingdom and many other high-income countries.

The fact that these medications exist is not sufficient, on its own, to control hypertension within a population.

Doing so also requires a healthcare system that is highly effective at detecting and treating hypertension. Detection is a challenge because hypertension is almost always asymptomatic. In the United Kingdom, as in many other affluent countries in recent years, a great deal of emphasis has been placed on case finding of hypertension in primary care – that is, checking people's blood pressure both opportunistically (when they are seeing a general practitioner or other healthcare professional, whatever the reason) and systematically (as part of a programme of health checks in which people of higher-risk age are invited to participate). Once detected, the hypertension must then be treated. This may not happen if the healthcare system fails to adequately follow up an abnormal blood pressure reading, if the patient does not attend follow-up appointments or if the patient is prescribed medication but does not take it. The last of these is a common problem, not helped by medication usually having to be taken for life despite the patient feeling no symptoms. Finally, the treatment must be sufficient to reduce the blood pressure – ideally back down to the normal level. In more than half of cases, this requires taking two or more drugs.

Until quite recently, data followed a so-called *rule of halves* in the detection, treatment and control of blood pressure within the population. Of all those in the population with hypertension, just half knew that they had high blood pressure. Of those who were aware of it, just half were treated. And of those treated, in just half was the treatment sufficient to control the hypertension. The net effect of the rule of halves was dismal – just one-eighth of those with hypertension had it controlled.

Progress has been made, consigning the rule of halves to the history books in many high-income countries. But substantial room for improvement remains, which explains why hypertension continues to be one of the top six factors creating non-communicable disease burden within the population. In England, 70% of those who have hypertension are now aware of it. Of those aware, 80% are treated. And of those treated, two-thirds are controlled (Figure 4.17). Each of these figures is better than the rule of halves, but the net effect is still that just over one-third of those with hypertension now have it controlled.

The detection and treatment of hypertension in individuals is not the only way to tackle the burden of hypertension within the population. People are more likely to develop hypertension the greater above normal their weight is, the more salt that is in their diet, and the less exercise they do. A population-level approach tackles each of these issues on a large scale and reduces the number of people who become hypertensive. It has the additional positive effect of lowering blood pressure even among those who would be said to have a normal blood pressure, decreasing their risk of ill health.

The two approaches to tackling blood pressure within a population – giving medication to those with the highest blood pressures and taking measures to reduce the blood pressure of all – are classic examples of high-risk and population strategies of disease prevention, concepts that are discussed later.

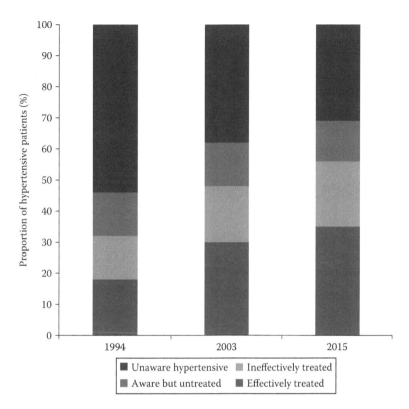

Figure 4.17 Improvement in the management of hypertension in England.

Source: NHS Digital.

UNINTENTIONAL INJURY

The terminology applied to this area of health has changed over the years, with the word *accident* being replaced by *injury* and a distinction being drawn between unintentional and intentional injuries. The term 'accident' has been used to imply an event that happens purely by chance. This is reflected in the phrase 'accidents do happen', but injuries do not occur at random. Some groups of the population – for example, children, older people or those in particular occupational groups – are at much greater risk than others.

Age is a strong determinant of unintentional injury. First, it influences exposure to particular hazards. Second, it relates to skills, competence and attitudes in particular activities. The young child and the older person, for different reasons, are at greater risk as pedestrians than others in the population. Young children are still developing physically, mentally and socially and are poor judges of dangers such as speed or distance; in addition, their attention wanders easily. An older person may have limited mobility and failing hearing or eyesight. Third, age may influence ability to withstand physical trauma and the severity of the resulting injury.

As a public health problem, injuries have been the subject of detailed study internationally, including ways to classify them. An agent that produces an injury can be considered one of five forms of energy: mechanical, chemical, thermal, electrical or various forms of radiation (e.g. ultraviolet rays or X-rays). The sudden and harmful transfer of these types of energy to a person causes the injury (Figure 4.18). For instance, a teenager might get on a friend's motorcycle without any lessons or instruction and crash into a parked car, breaking his leg (mechanical energy); a toddler might open and drink from a bottle of turpentine that her mother is using for decorating and be poisoned (chemical energy); an elderly woman might drop a smouldering cigarette into her lap after she has fallen asleep in her chair and sustain a deep burn on her thigh (thermal energy); a middle-aged man might cut through a cable on his lawnmower and receive an electric shock (electrical energy); the pale-skinned holidaymaker from Britain, with little previous exposure to the sun, might sunbathe on a Greek island beach and be seriously sunburned (solar radiation). The size of the transfer of energy, its duration, its distribution and the body's ability to resist it are all factors that determine the type and severity of the resulting injury. The energy source has produced the injury through a transmitting agent or vector. In the five examples, the agents were the motorcycle, the turpentine, the smouldering cigarette, the electrical cable and the sun's rays.

An individual's susceptibility to injury is important in determining the outcome. Everyone, every day, is in contact with many forms of energy. If the energy source is under control, it is not usually harmful. However, when it exceeds the ability of its user to control it, an injury can happen. The balance between an energy source and the person

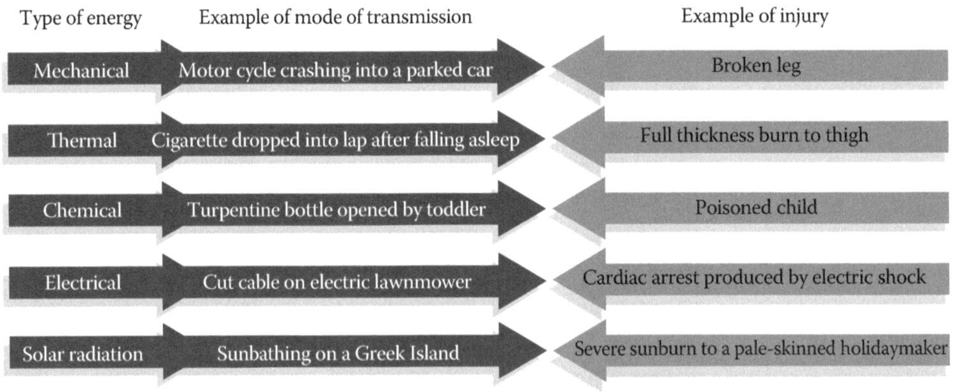

Figure 4.18 A concept of unintentional injury based upon the exchange of one of five forms of energy with the human body.

Source: Haddon W. The changing approach to the epidemiology, prevention, and amelioration of trauma: the transition to approaches etiologically rather than descriptively based. *American Journal of Public Health* 1968; 58(8): 1431–8.

controlling it is therefore a crucial one. The balance can be tipped in favour of the energy source when it suddenly becomes stronger or more difficult to control. For example, a car skidding on an icy road risks causing the driver or the passengers injury as the mechanical energy source becomes uncontrolled. The balance can also be altered if the person controlling the energy source lacks sufficient skill, the necessary physical attributes or the relevant experience to exert full control over it. An elderly woman with arthritic hands who picks up a heavy frying pan full of hot oil risks a scald injury due to her reduced capacity to exert full control over a source of thermal energy. A young, physically able person would not have such difficulty.

This description of injuries as interchanges of energy between their source and a man, woman or child is not just an interesting theoretical idea. It has proved to be an excellent basis for planning comprehensive action to reduce the consequences of such impacts. Many past approaches to prevent injuries were based on the concept of injuries arising from acts of carelessness or stupidity, so that solutions were those based on people taking much greater personal responsibility for their actions. Education, particularly of young children, regarding individual behaviour and safety still remains an important component of injury control strategies. Yet, additionally, today's thinking places greater emphasis on safer products and planning and construction of the built environment, drawing on methods of research, innovation and design from within fields such as science, engineering and psychology. This stems from recognition that if a major proportion of car crashes, for example, cannot be prevented by educating people to drive more carefully, structural modifications to reduce and distribute impact forces might at least minimize injuries and enhance the chances of survival.

This approach has been developed to identify three critical stages to an injury: pre-event, event and postevent. The factors that determine what will occur and what its impact will be are influenced by the interplay between a diversity of elements at each of these stages. This concept has been developed into a matrix that can help in understanding the causes of unintentional injuries and, even more importantly, can assist in designing prevention and control measures.

These ideas are illustrated in a matrix applied to a car crash (Figure 4.19). The pre-event stage (in this example, precrash) involves all the influences that determine whether the collision will occur in the first place, including the human factors (e.g. how good the driver's eyesight is, how experienced and skilled the driver is and whether he or she has been drinking alcohol). Other important precrash factors will include the functioning state of the vehicle, as well as aspects of the physical and sociocultural environment (e.g. tyre pressure and tread, effectiveness of brakes, provision of zebra crossings and adequacy of road surfaces).

As the collision takes place, its seriousness and the severity of injuries sustained by those people involved through the transfer of mechanical injury to their bodies will also be determined by the same groups of influences: human (e.g. whether a seat belt is worn), vehicular (e.g. how crash resistant the car body shell is), physical environment (e.g. whether crash barriers are present alongside the road) and sociocultural environment (e.g. attitudes to seat belt wearing).

Postcrash, a range of factors will determine whether those injured survive the crash and, if they do, how well they recover or are free of long-term disability. It is here that vital issues such as rapid response by the trauma services come into play.

This emphasizes that a comprehensive strategy to reduce the toll of injury, disability and premature death arising from car crashes should not just involve measures directed at drivers themselves. It should also include targets for improved vehicle construction and design so that, as far as possible, drivers and passengers are packaged to withstand the mechanical energy released if the car should crash. Similarly, roads that permit clear visibility and have well-constructed surfaces, good signposts, clear lane markings and adequate crash barriers are also factors that, if targeted in an injury prevention programme, would contribute to the saving of lives and prevention of serious injuries.

Injury is a major global health problem that affects all countries and results from a wide range of causes.

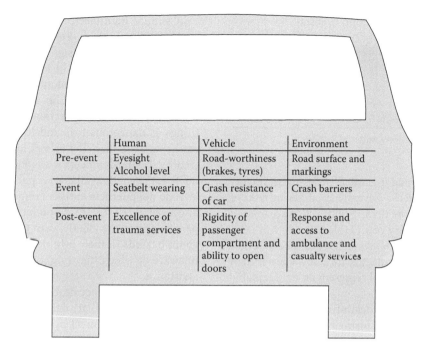

Figure 4.19 The accident prevention matrix applied to road accidents.

Source: Adapted from Haddon W. Advances in the epidemiology of injuries as a basis for public health policy. *Public Health Reports* 1980; 95: 411–21.

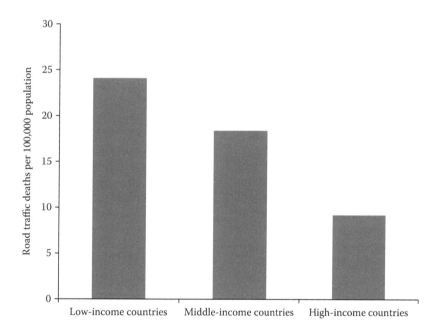

Figure 4.20 Incidence rate of road traffic deaths, in high-, middle-, and low-income countries.

Source: World Health Organization (WHO). *Global Status Report on Road Safety 2015.* Geneva: WHO, 2015. With permission.

Injury results in the loss of an estimated 5 million lives annually. Road traffic injuries account for 1.2 million deaths annually worldwide, while 50 million suffer nonfatal injury. Almost 80% of the world's road traffic deaths occur in low- and middle-income countries, even though these countries only account for half of vehicle usage (Figure 4.20). In England and Wales, each year, just over half a million deaths are attributed to 'accidents, poisoning and violence'. Injuries account for approximately 13% of years of life lost under the age of 65 years, and are a particularly important cause of preventable death and incapacity in the younger age groups. There are also substantial numbers of nonfatal injuries each year, leading to considerable health service expenditure. Causes of injuries include road traffic collisions, falls, poisoning, drowning and fires. They occur in the home, on the roads, in a variety of outdoor locations and in the workplace.

Table 4.3 Injuries and deaths among cyclists, United Kingdom, 2014

	Adults	Children
Killed	107	6
Seriously injured	3090	273
Slightly injured	15,684	1726

Source: Royal Society for the Prevention of Accidents.

Particular categories of road users (e.g. pedestrians, motor-cyclists, pedal cyclists and car drivers) have differing risks of dying or being injured. More than 19,000 cyclists are injured in the United Kingdom every year (Table 4.3).

Injury as a cause of death in Britain has declined in recent decades. Motor vehicle traffic deaths are at lower levels than in many other countries but still represent an unacceptably large public health problem.

The risk of serious injury or death from motorcycling is 100 times greater than the safest form of travel by road (bus) and 25 times greater than driving a car. At the same time, car advertising reflects an increasing concern about safety features. Rigid passenger compartments and front and rear crumple zones are almost standard, while seat belts fitted in both the front and back of new cars are now a legal require-ment in Britain. Furthermore, even more sophisticated safety features are becoming widespread, such as antilock brakes, collapsible steering columns and inflatable driver crash airbags. However, despite improvements to car design, travelling in motor vehicles still accounts for a substantial number of deaths each year. The largest proportion of these deaths occurs to those between 15 and 24 years of age and is probably connected to young people's relative lack of driv-ing experience and also to the element of risk-taking.

Road traffic collisions cause about a quarter of all deaths of children under the age of 15 years. While the rate of death and serious injuries on the road is lower in Britain than in most other European countries, the rate of pedestrian deaths among children is comparatively high. Indeed, pedestrian road collisions are the single most commont cause of injury-related death in children, accounting for 40% of all injury-related deaths in the 5- to 14-year age group and more than 20% of injury-related deaths in the younger and less mobile children from one to four years of age.

While the numbers of transport-related deaths are greatest among young males aged between 15 and 24 years, the age-specific rate of mortality is slightly greater in males aged 85 years and older. The increased frailty of elderly people and their reduced ability to recover from serious injury means that they are more vulnerable in the case of a collision. Legislative measures in Britain have included the mandatory wearing of crash helmets by motorcyclists, compulsory wearing of front and rear seat belts by driv-ers and passengers in cars and making driving a car while using a mobile telephone an offence. These measures have sometimes been controversial at their inception, since they have been said to reduce individual liberty.

A similar multifaceted approach is required to prevent non-transport injuries. For example, in domestic injuries, improvements in the design of buildings and products can reduce the risk of injury. In some areas, this may be backed up by legislation or by voluntary codes of practice agreed with manufacturers. Public awareness of these hazards has helped to encourage action to prevent the sale of such things as dangerous toys and to introduce the childproof medicine container. The role of local authorities and their trading standards officers is an important element in ensur-ing that the goods available for purchase by people at a local level do not put them at risk of injury. Local authorities have also been at the forefront of offering home check schemes, particularly to the elderly, with the goal of advising people about hazards in their own homes of which they might be unaware or which they might be unable to rectify without assistance.

Strategies to reduce deaths and injuries in the workplace rely on a strong legislative framework. Appropriate training is an important element in workplace safety. Unlike health education aimed at the general public to prevent injuries in the home or on the roads, education of the person at work can be a mandatory component of training programmes in which knowledge and skills are formally assessed. As such, it has the potential to be more effective than popu-lation health education programmes. Factory design, oper-ating procedures and adequate maintenance of machinery are also important measures in preventing injuries in the workplace. Special measures are required for occupations or processes where there are particular hazards. The most suc-cessful programmes are undoubtedly those where an orga-nization's management demonstrates a strong commitment to occupational health and safety.

The transfer-of-energy idea has been used to provide a comprehensive injury prevention framework. In it, there are 10 types of strategy for intervening to control the release or impact of energy (Table 4.4). This approach allows all options to be carefully thought through prior to designing the particular programme.

PREVENTION, DETECTION AND SLOWING DISEASE PROGRESSION

Reducing the risk of non-communicable disease and premature death from it, and slowing its progression through good clinical management are the roles of preven-tion. Traditionally, prevention has been classified into three types:

1. *Primary prevention*: This approach seeks to actually prevent the onset of a disease. The ultimate goal is to alter some factor in the environment, to bring about a change in the status of the host or to change behaviour so that disease is prevented from developing. Many of the triumphs of public health in the past, relating to the infectious diseases, were brought about through primary prevention.

Table 4.4 Accidents as energy forces: countermeasures to prevent injury

Countermeasure	Accident type	Example
1. Prevent the creation of a form of energy in the first place	Poisoning caused by a chemical agent	Stop production of the agent
2. Reduce the amount of energy marshalled	Hot water scald	Limit temperatures in hot water systems
3. Prevent the release of the energy	Mauling by wild animals	Caging tigers
4. Modify the rate of release of energy from its source	Fire started by electric kettle boiling dry	Shut-off valve on the kettle
5. Separate in space and time the energy source from the individual who might be harmed	Burn from hot fat in frying pan	Keep toddlers out of the kitchen when cooking
6. Interpose a barrier between the energy source and the susceptible individual	Child poisoned by tablets	Child-proof medicine container
7 Modify the basic structure of the hazard	Strangulation of baby in cot sides	Narrow space between bars in cots
8. Strengthen the resistance of the susceptible individual	Head injury in child cyclist	Widespread use of cycle helmet
9. Counter the damage done by the energy source	Lacerating wound due to broken glass	Apply first aid to stop further loss of blood
10. Stabilise and rehabilitate the person damaged by the energy	Multiple injuries in car crash	Rapid transfer to major accident and emergency department and provision of care

Source: Adapted from Haddon W. On the escape of tigers: an ecologic note. *American Journal of Public Health and the Nations Health* 1970;60(12):2229–34.

2. *Secondary prevention*: This level of prevention aims to halt the progression of a disease once it is established. The crux, here, is early diagnosis followed by prompt, effective treatment. Secondary prevention aimed at apparently healthy, asymptomatic members of a population is a special case with a set of criteria for deciding whether it should be introduced. This aspect of secondary prevention is usually called screening and is discussed in the next section.

3. *Tertiary prevention*: This level is concerned with high-quality clinical care of people with an established disease, to minimize further progression to disabilities and complications. Preventive activity at this stage also aims at improving the quality of life, even if the disease course itself cannot be altered.

Many different approaches are available in primary prevention of non-communicable diseases within a population. These range from social marketing to taxation, from urban redesign to psychotherapy and from medication to education. Two common threads run through the different risk factors: (1) the powerful impact that price, availability and marketing have on behaviour and (2) the unfortunate fact that public health interests are often at odds with commercial interests. Action is needed throughout the life course. As Chapter 5, on the social determinants of health, describes, interventions in early life are particularly important.

High-risk and population approaches to primary prevention

Preventive interventions and programmes focus either on individuals or on whole populations and subgroups within them. Individual-level action is often focused on those at greatest risk of developing disease, and termed *high-risk* strategies. For example, those with high blood pressure are identified and their blood pressure brought under control with medication, so reducing their risk of heart attack and stroke. Smokers are offered counselling and medication to help them stop; those with severe obesity are offered surgery.

The high-risk strategy is a good and effective one, but it has a problem – it is not only those with high blood pressure or extreme obesity who are at high risk of strokes and heart attacks. Many people who are mildly overweight or have even normal blood pressure also have heart attacks and strokes. In fact, people with normal blood pressure have more strokes than people with hypertension do. This phenomenon may sound counterintuitive, but occurs because there are many more people with normal blood pressure in the population than there are people with hypertension. For each individual with normal blood pressure, the risk of having a stroke is lower, but it is not zero. This is known as the *prevention paradox* – that a large number of people at low risk may give rise to more cases of disease than a small number at high risk.

The prevention paradox exposes the shortcoming of the high-risk strategy – that it ignores the majority of the population and, in so doing, does nothing to prevent the majority of strokes. The answer lies in adopting a population strategy approach. As described earlier, there is a continuous relationship between blood pressure and stroke; the concept of hypertension is in one sense an artificial one. If a person's average blood pressure can be lowered by 2 mmHg – from 138/92 to 136/90, say – his or her risk of having a stroke decreases. The risk reduction for this individual is very small. But if the blood pressure of everybody in the population could be lowered by 2 mmHg, the risk among the population as a whole would be substantial. It has been calculated that such a change would reduce the incidence of stroke by 15%. In other words, by reducing each individual's risk by a very small amount, the risk for the population as a whole can be reduced by a substantial amount.

The population strategy and high-risk strategy are depicted in Figure 4.21. The high-risk strategy targets the upper tail of the population. The population strategy reduces everybody's blood pressure, shifting the curve to the left. The high-risk strategy takes the traditional medical approach of thinking about an individual. The population strategy requires focus on the whole population. One option would be to give the entire population antihypertensive medication. This has the problem that medication costs money and has side effects. Both the side effects and cost are acceptable when the medication results in a substantial reduction in an individual's risk, as it does when given to high-risk individuals. But they become far less acceptable when given to people who can expect to gain far less individual benefit from the medication.

Some characterize the high-risk and population strategies as alternatives. Both play an important role.

Population-level approaches suffer from a different set of problems than individual-level approaches. They are often controversial, particularly when they involve taxes or legislation. When governments employ such measures, they risk criticism for creating a Nanny State. Such measures can be highly effective. In the United Kingdom, the most notable success has been in tobacco control. A shift in social norms has been accompanied by successive layers of legislative action, and the prevalence of cigarette smoking has fallen. Legislation that is controversial at the time can seem benign in retrospect. Changing the law to enforce seat belt wearing was held back for too many years. It had to be introduced in stages, yet few would turn the clock back now. The same could be said of the more recent legislation on smoke-free public places, although there are still pro-smoker groups who talk about repeals. Today, the heated debates are about introducing a minimum price per unit of alcohol and taxing unhealthy foods.

Both individual-level and population-level approaches to prevention have a further barrier in common. Prevention receives only a fraction of the funding that is allocated to the treatment of diseases that have already developed. This does not adequately reflect the potential of preventive interventions. There is a psychological and political reason for this. There is a deep emotional appeal to the idea of saving lives. But when most people think of saving lives, they imagine individual people. They think of heroics – of high-technology hospital services that rescue people from the brink of death. They think about immediate results. When politicians are making decisions about how to allocate financial resources, they have a natural human bias towards treatment services and away from preventive services. This reflects not just their own preference, but also that of the electorate. The problem for prevention is that it can be shown statistically to

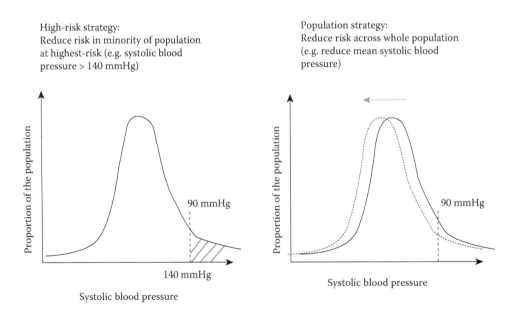

Figure 4.21 The high-risk and the population strategies of prevention.

save thousands of people's lives, but we will never know which people they were. Moreover, the benefit may take decades to realize. Saving lives visibly, as a hospital does, has far more intuitive appeal to it than saving lives invisibly, as prevention programmes do.

A small group of American researchers, led by Deborah Small, professor of marketing at the Wharton School, University of Pennsylvania, conducted a clever psychological experiment that illustrates the human tendency to favour *identifiable victims* – individuals with whom we can feel an emotional connection rather than statistics, with which we cannot. This is true even when those statistics represent many times more human lives. The study separated participants into two groups. Each individual was given $5 and asked whether they wished to donate it to a charity. In a leaflet, Group A was told about one girl. The appeal began, 'Any money that you donate will go to Rokia, a seven year old girl who lives in Mali, Africa. Rokia is desperately poor and faces a threat of severe hunger, even starvation'. Group B, by contrast, was told about a nationwide problem: 'Food shortages in Malawi are affecting more than three million children'. Those in Group A gave more than twice as much money as those in Group B. Small and her colleagues explained: 'People pay greater attention and have stronger emotional reactions to vivid rather than pallid information'.

The identifiable victim effect becomes even stronger when money starts to run short. If a hospital is short of funding and not able to provide a high-quality service, this quickly hits the headlines. The public sees identifiable victims, and wise politicians try to step in to solve the problem as quickly as they can. If a preventive health programme is short of funding, nobody sees the victims. This is a great challenge that public health professionals face. Charged with improving the health of the population to the greatest extent possible, the profession needs to find ways to overcome the identifiable victim effect.

Screening: Detecting disease in its presymptomatic phase

In its widest sense, the term *screening* implies the scrutiny of people in order to detect the presence of disease, disability or some other attribute that is under study. It has been defined as:

The systematic application of a test or inquiry to identify individuals at sufficient risk of a specific disorder to warrant further investigation or direct preventive action, amongst persons who have not sought medical attention on account of the symptoms of that disorder.

The metaphor of a sieve is often used to bring this definition to life (Figure 4.22).

With chronic degenerative disorders, often first seen in their later stages, this may seem to be a logical extension of clinical practice. This argument, coupled with the fact that many population surveys showed a high frequency of previously unrecognized abnormalities, led in the early 1960s to the advocacy of presymptomatic screening for different diseases on a large scale. This proved to be a flawed approach. As the concept of screening was explored in greater depth, it became clear that just because technology allows a disease to be identified before symptoms develop, this does not mean that apparently healthy people in the general population should all be tested.

There is a crucial distinction between systematic screening, in which members of a geographically defined population are indeed called by invitation to be offered screening (e.g. a cervical cancer test), and opportunistic *case finding*, in which people attending a health facility – such as a general practitioner's surgery or a clinic – for one purpose may be offered a screening test (e.g. a blood pressure measurement).

A number of criteria, first drawn up by Wilson and Jungner for the World Health Organization in 1968, were

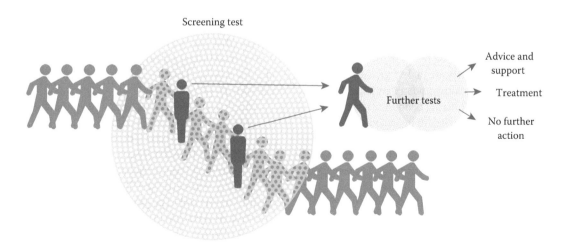

Screening test

Further tests

Advice and support

Treatment

No further action

Figure 4.22 A screening test acts like a sieve, selecting people who need further investigation.

Source: Public Health England (PHE). NHS population screening explained. Available from: https://www.gov.uk/guidance/nhs-population-screening-explained [accessed 7 July 2017].

used to help governments and health organizations to decide whether to screen:

- *Is the disease an important health problem?* Before channelling resources on a large scale, the problem must be deemed to be a serious one. Nevertheless, importance is a relative concept. Some health problems may be important because they are very common. Others, although rare, may have serious consequences for the individual or society as a whole.
- *Is there a recognizable latent or early symptomatic stage?* In order to detect a disease in its early stages, there must be a reasonable time period during its natural history when symptoms are not manifesting themselves.
- *Are facilities for diagnosis and treatment available?* If a screening programme were to reveal large numbers of patients with a particular disease, facilities to provide the necessary follow-up investigation and treatment would have to be available.
- *Has the cost of the programme been considered in the context of other demands for resources?* At no time in the foreseeable future are there likely to be unlimited resources that would permit every proposal to be followed through. Proposed expenditure on any one health option must therefore be weighed against other proposals.
- *Is there an agreed policy on whom to treat as patients?* This brings in the question of borderline cases. In any population, disease exists in a spectrum of severity. At the less severe end of the spectrum, there is a problem of differentiating people with the disease from normal people. Strict criteria must therefore be laid down about what constitutes the particular disease, before screening is carried out.
- *Does treatment confer benefit?* This is perhaps the most important consideration of all, and it raises fundamental ethical principles. The presymptomatic screening of people for the presence of disease differs from normal medical practice. In the usual situation, patients make contact with a doctor because they have recognized that they are ill and in need of medical care. The doctor attempts to formulate a diagnosis and give the best treatment available to the patient, based on the doctor's experience and current medical knowledge. In the screening situation, the 'patients' have not recognized that they are ill. In fact, they probably believe themselves to be healthy, and not patients at all. The screening programme, in offering people the opportunity to be screened, implies that a health benefit will result - that early treatment of the disease (if present) is linked with favourable outcome. The reality is that only in a few diseases is there any convincing evidence that striving for early diagnosis on a total population basis, and hence early treatment, affects the outcome for the patient. Thus, it is essential, before embarking on a screening programme for a particular disease, to review all the evidence and decide whether early diagnosis and treatment will truly benefit the person being screened, or whether, on the other hand, the outcome is no different for a person detected through screening than for someone who is treated at such time as

the condition manifests itself clinically. The phenomenon by which a screening test simply makes evident at an earlier stage a disease without actually affecting its course (but apparently leads to longer survival because of the earlier detection) is known as *lead-time bias*.

The Wilson and Jungner criteria have subsequently been developed further, and a new list of criteria is shown in Table 4.5.

RUNNING A SCREENING PROGRAMME

Identifying, inviting and informing

The first stage in a screening programme is the identification of the population to be offered screening. Decisions about the age at which screening should start or stop have huge resource consequences. Having agreed on the population, individuals have to be identified, bearing in mind that those most in need may be most difficult to identify (e.g. because they are homeless). Members of the public also need to be clearly informed not only about the possible benefits of screening but also about the risks and limitations.

Choosing the screening test

Having decided to embark on a programme to screen for the presence of a particular disease in a population, the next issue centres on which test to choose for the purpose. Usually those proposing to carry out the screening will have a particular method in mind for detecting the disease, whether it is a blood test, a urine test, an examination or a questionnaire. When making the choice, however, a number of general criteria should be borne in mind. The test should be economic and one that can be carried out rapidly by trained nonmedical personnel. It should be acceptable to the majority of people, and this usually rules out very painful or time-consuming procedures. The test should be reliable; in other words, the same result would be expected if repeated by a different observer altogether or by the same observer on a number of occasions. Finally, and most importantly, the validity of the test must be known. By validity is meant the test's ability to measure or discover what the investigator wants to know. How good is the test at discriminating between people who have the disease and people who are healthy? Validity is usually expressed through sensitivity and specificity.

Applying a screening test to a population may divide people into four possible groups (Figure 4.23). First, there are people who have the disease and give a positive result on screening (*true positives*); second, there are people who are healthy, or nondiseased, and give a negative result on screening (*true negatives*). If a screening test were ideal, these would be the only categories of people who exist. No test is perfect. So, two further categories are possible: people who, despite having the disease, are classified as healthy by the screening test (*false negatives*) and healthy people who are classified by the screening test as diseased (*false positives*).

The concepts of *sensitivity* and *specificity* take account of these problems (Figure 4.24). The sensitivity of the test is

Table 4.5 Criteria for appraising the viability, effectiveness and appropriateness of a screening programme

The test

There should be a simple, safe, precise and validated screening test.

The distribution of test values in the target population should be known and a suitable cut-off level defined and agreed.

The test, from sample collection to delivery of results, should be acceptable to the target population.

There should be an agreed policy on the further diagnostic investigation of individuals with a positive test result and on the choices available to those individuals.

If the test is for a particular mutation or set of genetic variants the method for their selection and the means through which these will be kept under review in the programme should be clearly set out.

The intervention

There should be an effective intervention for patients identified through screening, with evidence that intervention at a pre-symptomatic phase leads to better outcomes for the screened individual compared with usual care. Evidence relating to wider benefits of screening, for example those relating to family members, should be taken into account where available. However, where there is no prospect of benefit for the individual screened then the screening programme should not be further considered.

There should be agreed evidence based policies covering which individuals should be offered interventions and the appropriate intervention to be offered.

The screening programme

There should be evidence from high quality randomized controlled trials that the screening programme is effective in reducing mortality or morbidity. Where screening is aimed solely at providing information to allow the person being screened to make an "informed choice" (such as Down's syndrome or cystic fibrosis carrier screening), there must be evidence from high quality trials that the test accurately measures risk. The information that is provided about the test and its outcome must be of value and readily understood by the individual being screened.

There should be evidence that the complete screening programme (test, diagnostic procedures, treatment/ intervention) is clinically, socially and ethically acceptable to health professionals and the public.

The benefit gained by individuals from the screening programme should outweigh any harms for example from overdiagnosis, overtreatment, false positives, false reassurance, uncertain findings and complications.

The opportunity cost of the screening programme (including testing, diagnosis and treatment, administration, training and quality assurance) should be economically balanced in relation to expenditure on medical care as a whole (value for money). Assessment against these criteria should have regard to evidence from cost benefit and/or cost effectiveness analyses and have regard to the effective use of available resource.

Implementation criteria

Clinical management of the condition and patient outcomes should be optimized in all healthcare providers prior to participation in a screening programme.

All other options for managing the condition should have been considered (such as improving treatment or providing other services), to ensure that no more cost effective intervention could be introduced or current interventions increased within the resources available.

There should be a plan for managing and monitoring the screening programme and an agreed set of quality assurance standards.

Adequate staffing and facilities for testing, diagnosis, treatment and programme management should be available prior to the commencement of the screening programme.

Evidence-based information, explaining the purpose and potential consequences of screening, investigation and preventative intervention or treatment, should be made available to potential participants to assist them in making an informed choice.

Public pressure for widening the eligibility criteria for reducing the screening interval, and for increasing the sensitivity of the testing process, should be anticipated. Decisions about these parameters should be scientifically justifiable to the public.

Source: National Screening Committee, Public Health England.

a measure of its ability to detect the disease when present. A highly sensitive test would have no (or very few) missed cases (false negatives). The specificity of the test is a measure of its ability to identify healthy people as nondiseased. A test of high specificity would have no (or few) people wrongly labelled as diseased (false positives). It is seldom possible to have a test that is 100% sensitive and 100% specific. Usually, a compromise level must be agreed on. Figure 4.25 shows (diagrammatically) different levels of sensitivity and specificity.

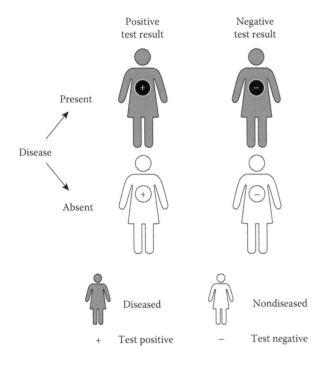

Figure 4.23 Possible outcomes of a screening test.

A level of 60% sensitivity or specificity would be unlikely to be acceptable. A level of 90% might possibly be, depending on the disease in question, but a higher level than this would usually be sought. In making a decision on what levels of sensitivity and specificity will be accepted, the practical implications of the choice must be realized. A sensitivity below 100% means that some people with the disease will be missed, and the consequences of this depend on the particular disease concerned. A specificity below 100% means that some healthy people will be told that they might have the disease, with the ensuing anxiety that might result from this. It is important to stress that screening tests cannot be regarded as diagnostic, and those people with positive results must undergo further examination and investigation to establish a definitive diagnosis.

A further measure of a screening test is its *positive predictive value*. This estimates the probability, given a positive test result, of the individual in question actually having the condition. This is sometimes confused with sensitivity, but sensitivity is the probability, given that an individual has the condition, that he or she will have a positive test result. Positive predictive value depends on both the sensitivity and specificity of the test, as well as the prevalence of the underlying condition. The higher the sensitivity, specificity and prevalence, the higher will be the positive predictive value.

Great benefit would result to the patient, to the standard of medical practice and to the health service if more was understood about many of the diagnostic tests and examinations in common use today. For example, if we are told that an analysis of chemicals in a person's exhaled breath can identify oesophageal cancer, we might not accept that at face value without asking, 'How good is the breath test at diagnosing oesophageal cancer?' 'How does it compare with other diagnostic techniques?' 'How many cases of

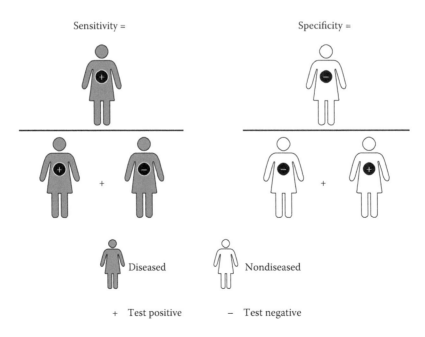

Figure 4.24 Results of a screening test showing sensitivity and specificity.

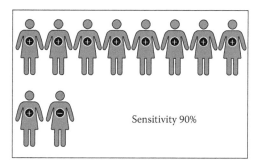
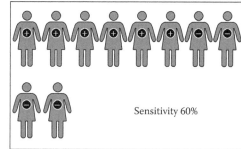
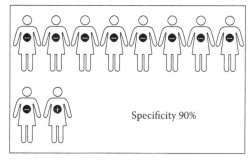
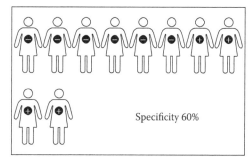

Figure 4.25 Differing levels of sensitivity and specificity.

oesophageal cancer do I fail to identify if I only investigate them by doing a breath test?' The question of the validity of a screening test, as expressed in sensitivity, specificity and positive predictive value, thus has great relevance in clinical medicine. Knowledge of these principles is of value beyond the arena of population screening.

Diagnostic phase of a screening programme

The screening test by itself usually identifies a subset of the population that requires more detailed investigation. Some screening programmes (e.g. screening programmes to reduce the risk of stroke by lowering blood pressure) proceed straight from the screening test to the intervention, such as advice on lifestyle and drug treatment. However, most screening programmes have a further diagnostic stage (e.g. colposcopy and cervical cone biopsy in the cervical screening programme).

Treatment phase of a screening programme

Once a diagnosis is made, there are two options. One is to refer the person for usual care. The second is to offer treatment within a service particularly aligned with the screening programme. Many screening programmes have taken this extra step to ensure that the quality of treatment service offered meets accepted standards for two reasons. First, it is felt that if individuals are invited to come for screening, there is a greater responsibility on the health service to ensure that treatment is of high quality. Second, the introduction of a screening programme based on systems thinking allows those who pay for or manage healthcare to involve clinicians providing treatment in a review of the service they offer, and this provides a stimulus for more explicit measurement of quality, and therefore the introduction of steps to improve it.

Evaluation and quality assurance

It is obviously essential for screening programmes to be evaluated, but many screening programmes have made the jump from evaluation to quality assurance. Evaluation implies measurement to ensure that performance improves continuously against explicit standards, and that those standards are themselves reviewed regularly to set higher challenges for the screening programme when performance improves to a level at which the previously set standard becomes inadequately challenging. Quality assurance must permeate all aspects of the programme.

Many screening programmes in health services around the world have been introduced in the past before there was a proper understanding of the basis upon which they should be evaluated. Policy on population screening is concerned with not just whether to introduce new programmes, but also the attitude that should be taken towards existing programmes (Table 4.6). This is a difficult area because stopping a programme would be portrayed by sections of the media as withdrawal of a service and may produce adverse public reaction. Moreover, in countries that do not have national health systems, it is less easy to regulate the offering of screening tests to healthy populations by private sector providers.

Many of the criteria to be taken into account when evaluating the case for a population screening programme have been described in the foregoing sections of this chapter, but the main areas that must be addressed are set out in Table 4.7.

SCREENING PROGRAMMES IN THE NHS

Calls for the introduction of new population screening programmes have become increasingly common as technological advances have produced relatively cheap, noninvasive diagnostic tests that provide early markers of the presence of disease.

It is often difficult to win the public argument that early diagnosis of illness is generally good but seeking to establish population screening to detect asymptomatic disease is sometimes bad. There is no better example of this than prostate cancer. It is a common cause of illness and death in older men, and there is a blood test to detect it. However, the complications of treatment – particularly impotence and urinary incontinence – are greatly feared. There has been a great deal of lobbying of the British government, and others around the world, to introduce routine screening for prostate cancer. Such campaigns often have considerable celebrity backing, often from high-profile individuals who have themselves had the disease. Their case often seems very compelling: 'If I had been diagnosed early, I would have been able to survive longer'. Some prostate cancers are very aggressive, invading and spreading rapidly, but most are slow growing and remain in the prostate gland. These slow-growing cancers, particularly in older men, are unlikely to cause health problems, and there is a risk of overtreating them. A metaphor is helpful in considering these two types of prostate cancer. They have been dubbed 'tigers' and 'pussycats' to describe their different propensities to grow and spread. When prostate cancer is detected very early, and it is still unclear whether the tumour is a tiger or a pussycat, men are faced with a

difficult decision. Their cancer may never trouble them. Treatment may not prolong their life but may cause harm, such as impotence or incontinence. Studies suggest that as many as one in three men treated for prostate cancer may have serious complications. On the other hand, they may have a tumour that will turn out to be a tiger and progress rapidly and threaten their life.

Within the United Kingdom, the need to have an orderly and scientific approach to calls to introduce population screening was addressed by the establishment in 1996 of the National Screening Committee (NSC). The committee advises the government on the case for implementing new screening programmes and modifying or withdrawing existing ones. After reviewing the scientific evidence and consulting experts, the committee makes one of five recommendations about the proposed programme:

1. Systematic population screening recommended
2. Systematic population screening not recommended
3. Systematic population screening not recommended but clinical practice guidelines covered by National Institute for Health and Care Excellence (NICE) should be followed
4. Systematic population screening not recommended but committee risk management guidance should be followed
5. Pilot of screening recommended

The National Screening Committee keeps the case for screening in a wide variety of conditions under regular review. The number of conditions where it has been considered but not recommended far outweighs those conditions where a screening programme has been put in place (Table 4.8).

Returning to the example of the case for population screening for prostate cancer, the UK National Screening Committee rationale not recommending universal screening of men for prostate cancer was because

- The test is not effective enough and does not identify a large proportion of men who in fact have prostate cancer.

Table 4.6 Broad public health policy options when taking an evidence-based decision about a population screening programme

- The proposed programme should not be introduced.
- The proposed programme should be introduced, provided that the skills and resources are available to ensure adequate quality standards.
- The programme that is currently being offered to the population should be stopped.
- The policy for a programme currently being offered to the population should continue (with modification as appropriate).

Source: Department of Health (DH). *First Report of the National Screening Committee*. London: DH, 1998.

Table 4.7 Evaluation of a proposed screening programme: summary of aspects to consider

Aspect	In particular
Research evidence	Of benefits and risks
Priorities and other strategies	Importance of the health problem, whether other control strategies (e.g. primary prevention, treatment) are more appropriate
Properties of the test	Validity (false positives, false negatives), positive predictive value, convenience, safety, acceptability
Clinical consequences	Effectiveness, acceptability, cost, side effects of diagnosis and treatment following screening positive
Resources	Costs of testing, organization of the programme, diagnosis and treatment of the cases of disease detected
Quality assurance	System needed to monitor, assure and improve quality if programme established
Ethical and moral	Confidentiality of data

- A positive test will lead in most cases to a biopsy, which seldom gives a definitive answer and leads to anxiety and further investigations.
- Research indicated that for every 100,000 men at age 50 years offered screening, 748 would end up being treated. The men accepting screening would have their lives extended on average by a day – while 274 men would be made impotent, 25 would be made incontinent and 17 would have rectal problems as a result of the treatment.

NHS HEALTH CHECKS

In 2009, the NHS introduced a policy that each 40- to 74-year-old with no previous diagnosis of vascular disease should be invited for an examination every five years to see whether they have an undetected major non-communicable disease or any of the main risk factors. It is a universal risk assessment and risk management programme. The aim is to reduce mortality, prevent or delay the onset of disease and improve health for a range of conditions: diabetes, heart disease, dementia, cancer, stroke and kidney disease. Key risk factors assessed include smoking, hypertension, obesity, physical inactivity, alcohol, poor diet and high cholesterol.

This NHS Health Check programme has aroused controversy among public health professionals. At first sight, it seems to be a form of case finding. However, the target population is not actively seeking healthcare. In many ways, the

programme is a type of population screening and should fall squarely within the framework for deciding whether it is justifiable. It does not fulfil all of the World Health Organization criteria for initiating a population screening programme. Moreover, critics of it point to the research evidence from other countries that appears to show little benefit. The alternative view is that the programmes in other countries are dissimilar in important ways, that NHS Health Check is new and different and that it is too early to assess its full impact.

CONCLUSIONS

Non-communicable diseases are the major causes of premature death and poor health throughout the modern world. A comprehensive approach to non-communicable disease control has many strands encompassing surveillance, research, prevention, diagnosis and treatment.

Just two disease processes – cardiovascular disease and cancer – create more than half of the non-communicable disease burden. The most substantial contribution to this burden comes from a relatively small number of modifiable risk factors. There is very significant potential to improve the population's health by tackling them. In the United Kingdom, the evidence is that just 5% of people are physically active to the extent that is optimal for health; nearly two-thirds of those with high blood pressure are not appropriately diagnosed, treated and controlled, despite the ready availability of medication to do so; and more than half of the adult population is overweight, making this the norm. This simultaneously demonstrates the potential rewards of getting to grips with these issues, and the difficulties inherent in doing so. Tackling them requires a range of approaches, at both the individual level and the population level. Many population-level approaches attract controversy and create difficult decisions for governments about what level of intervention is appropriate. Tough though this political territory may be, any country serious about better population health must traverse it. Over the coming years, as some countries show commitment to the public health agenda and others do not, attention will increasingly be focused on societal norms, values and expectations about health, disease and quality of life. Meaningful change can only occur if political and public will come together.

Table 4.8 National systematic population screening programmes in the United Kingdom

Recommended by National Screening Committee (NSC) and operational	Examples of those considered by NSC and not recommended
Breast cancer	Autism
Bowel cancer	Atrial fibrillation
Cervical cancer	Kidney disease
Diabetic retinopathy	Osteoporosis
Abdominal aortic aneurysm	Prostate cancer
Wide range of antenatal and newborn examinations and tests	

Source: Public Health England.

CHAPTER 5

Social determinants of health

INTRODUCTION

An individual's health is substantially influenced by his or her social situation. The chance of developing any given disease is affected by income, occupation, neighbourhood, upbringing and a multitude of other factors. In sum, they have a significant impact on how many years he or she can expect to live. These factors are collectively termed the social determinants of health. They vary markedly between countries, but also between people living in the same country and even the same town. They result in substantial variation in health, often referred to as health inequalities. Differences in income, power and wealth are key elements in determining the scale of health inequalities in a country.

The modern perspective on health inequalities in the United Kingdom came to public and political prominence in the 1980s through the report of a government-appointed working group generally known after its chairman, Sir Douglas Black, as the *Black Report*. The group was established in 1977. By the time the report was complete, there was a new government, headed by Margaret Thatcher. It did not endorse the group's recommendations. The government deliberately published the report on a Bank Holiday weekend and made it available in only limited numbers. This only served to make it a *cause célébre* ever after.

The Black Report demonstrated that health had improved overall since the welfare state was introduced, but that there were widespread inequalities in the distribution of ill health and death. At the time, the main measure of social position in official statistics was social class, based on occupation. The Black Report showed a gradient of mortality down the social classes, such that the mortality rate for men in the lowest social class was twice that of men in the highest social class, and that this gap was increasing. Black and his colleagues found that this gradient of mortality by social class was consistent across age and gender groups, and for a very wide range of specific causes of death. The same pattern was found for illness, as well as for deaths. The Black Report stands as a striking testimony to the degree and consistency of inequalities in health.

The persistence of three- or fourfold variations in health and mortality between groups in society has remained a consistent finding, despite improvements in the overall health of the population evident through the twentieth century and into the twenty-first (Figure 5.1).

In recent years, discourse about the social determinants of health has emphasized two important dimensions. First, Sir Michael Marmot (a leading thinker and researcher in this area, based in the United Kingdom) in particular has emphasized that people exist along a *social gradient*, and that tackling the social determinants of health cannot simply focus on those who are the most deprived but must also aim to elevate those in the middle of the gradient towards its top end. This is a relatively subtle point, but challenges the traditional primary focus only on the poor. Second, the World Health Organization's Commission on the Social Determinants of Health (also chaired by Sir Michael Marmot) highlights the need to focus not just on social determinants, such as income and education, that affect individuals directly but also on the determinants of those determinants – ultimately, the distribution of power, money and resources at the global level.

Health inequalities are something that many public health practitioners feel very strongly about. Their existence – and magnitude – is often seen as a matter of social injustice. Since the publication of the Black Report some 40 years ago, life expectancy and health have improved substantially in the United Kingdom, as elsewhere. But the gap between the most deprived and the least deprived remains as marked as ever.

SOCIAL POSITION AND DEPRIVATION

In the United Kingdom, during the twentieth century, the measure used to explore the relationship between health and social factors was *social class*. Since 1851, British government statisticians had explored population data using occupation and industry to characterize the population. The breakthrough came when the government constructed an official measure of social class based purely on occupation. It was first introduced in 1913 by the registrar general but had been developed in 1911 by a medical statistician in the registrar general's office, THC Stevenson. He grouped occupations into a hierarchy of five social classes (from

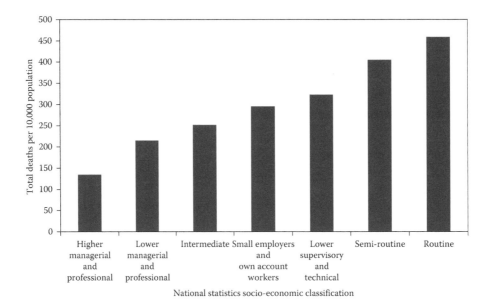

Figure 5.1 Age-standardized mortality rates for men aged 25–64 years, England and Wales, 2008–2010.

Source: Office for National Statistics.

professional to unskilled manual). Down the years, analyses of indicators of health, such as the standardized mortality ratio, demonstrated a consistent gradient of decreasing level of health from social class I to social class V. There were very few exceptions in which particular diseases or causes of death were commoner in the upper social classes. Official statistics record occupation in the census and on death certificates, and parental occupation on birth and marriage certificates. Statisticians therefore have much routine data already at their disposal. Occupation is a very convenient measure of social status, but it does have drawbacks; for example, about a third of the lives of modern Britons fall after the state retirement age, when it is much less straightforward to define them by their occupation.

The registrar general's classification of social class was in use for nearly a century, together with another official measure (introduced later) called socio-economic status. Both classifications were replaced in 2001, after extensive expert review and statistical testing, by the National Statistics Socio-economic Classification (NS-SEC). This is also based on occupation, but the characterization of occupation is much more rigorous and derived from employment relations and conditions of employment (e.g. economic security, prospects for advancement and location in systems of authority). This creates 40 basic categories that can be aggregated into 14 operational categories and 9, 7, 5 and 3 classes. The most commonly used is the nine classes (Table 5.1). Much of the data on social determinants of health and health inequalities use the NS-SEC. Older research papers, official reports and textbooks contain data presented using the earlier registrar general's classifications that were in use between 1913 and 2001.

Outside the field of official statistics, a very diverse approach has been taken to characterizing an individual in social terms; indeed, different academic disciplines vary greatly in their approach. The index most widely used is socio-economic status (usually comprising occupation, education and income). Academic critiques have pointed out that this concept confuses two elements: a person's position within the social structure and the prestige accorded to them. Much of this has to do with the purpose of the classification. The primary purpose may be explanatory (this is particularly important in fields such as social science and psychology), observational (e.g. to explore differences and trends in health statistics) and practical (to respond to need or plan services). The key step is to carefully define terms when constructing or using any measure. When Goldthorpe, a leading social scientist in this field, was asked, 'How many classes are there in contemporary British society?' he responded, 'As many as it proves empirically useful to distinguish for the analytical purposes in hand'.

Other well-respected classifications have broadened out from occupation. For example, the Cambridge Social Interaction and Stratification (CAMSIS) Scale emphasizes the similarity of lifestyle in a continuous measure of social and material advantages and disadvantages. The MacArthur Foundation Research Network on Socioeconomic Status and Health developed a subjective measure of social standing. Survey respondents were asked to position themselves on two ladders: one a socio-economic ladder and the other a community ladder. In the first, the majority of individuals used material wealth, occupation and education to position themselves on the socio-economic status ladder, while a quarter mentioned spirituality or ethical values and a fifth giving to others or their level of health. The way that individuals placed themselves on the community ladder ('community' interpreted by most as neighbourhood, town or city, but by some as religious or cultural group) was very different.

Table 5.1 The National Statistics Socio-economic Classification

Analytic class	Examples of occupations	Percentage of population in 2011
1. Higher Managerial and Professional	Directors and chief executives, civil engineers, medical practitioners, architects	10
2. Lower Managerial and Professional	Teachers, quantity surveyors, public service administrative professionals, social workers, nurses, IT technicians	21
3. Intermediate	Graphic designers, medical and dental technicians, local government clerical officers	13
4. Small Employers and Own Account Workers	Shopkeepers, dispensing opticians, farmers, self-employed taxi-drivers	9
5. Lower Supervisory and Technical	Bakers and flour confectioners, plumbers, electricians employed by others, gardeners	7
6. Semi-routine	Pest-control officers, traffic wardens, scaffolders, farm workers, veterinary nurses, shelf fillers	14
7. Routine	Hairdressing employees, sewing machinists, hotel porters, road sweepers, car park attendants	11
8. Never worked and long-term unemployed		6
9. Full-time students		9

Source: Office for National Statistics.

Wealth, education and occupation were given little weight compared with being a good citizen or good neighbour, giving to others or being respected. In general, the subjective ratings of socio-economic status were as good as, if not better than, objective measures in determining health outcomes.

An alternative approach to analyses based on an individual's social profile is to examine the social circumstances in which populations live. Often, the information resulting from such analyses is displayed in maps. This has a strong historical tradition. Charles Booth (1840–1916) was a successful businessman who was deeply moved by the profound poverty of the people in his native Liverpool when he campaigned unsuccessfully in Toxteth to win the parliamentary seat. Later, based in London, he commissioned a survey, *Life and Labour of the Population of London.* As part of this, he published the *Poverty Maps of London.* Today, a range of indicators is used to describe the deprivation status of populations, largely based on variables recorded in population censuses and other routine data sources. The indicators differ according to the concept of deprivation that underlies them (e.g. encompassing wealth, income, social isolation and environment) and according to which measures are selected to reflect this concept (such as employment status, overcrowding or car ownership). There is something of a gap between the concepts of deprivation and the measures that are available to reflect them. The concepts are often quite complex (and sometimes not made explicit), and the measures are generally restricted to those collected routinely by governments. As a result, all the various indices and scores are to some degree indirect indicators rather than direct measures.

Historically, British society has been divisible into those of working, middle and upper class. These descriptors are now outdated. Many would struggle to say which class they are in, and the middle class covers a vast range of occupations, incomes and lifestyles. In 2013, the British Broadcasting Corporation (BBC) and collaborators attempted to devise a new social class structure that more accurately captures the complexities of today (Table 5.2). It describes groups in terms of their financial, social and cultural capital.

Two deprivation indicators dominated British public health research and surveillance in the late twentieth century. These were the Townsend Material Deprivation Score and the Jarman Underprivileged Area Score (both named after the researchers who first put them forward). In Scotland, the Carstairs Score is more commonly used.

The Townsend Material Deprivation Score is based on four census variables – the percentage of private households with more than one person per room, the percentage of private households with no car, the percentage of private households that are not owner occupied and the percentage of residents eligible for employment who are unemployed. These four factors were explicitly selected to reflect different aspects of material deprivation and are combined into a single overall deprivation index. This index was used in a prominent study, conducted by Peter Townsend and colleagues in 1988, at a time of great controversy about the relationship between deprivation and health. They looked at the populations of 678 local authority wards in the Northern Health Region of England, a region that included some highly disadvantaged areas. When they ranked the council

Table 5.2 Modern ideas of social class

Group	Description	Percentage of population in 2013
Elite	Most privileged group with highest financial, social and cultural capital	6
Established middle class	Largest class group – less wealthy than the elite but high social and cultural capital	25
Technical middle class	Small group – well-off but not as social, emerging cultural interests such as gaming	6
New affluent workers	Generally young with moderate income but socially and culturally active	15
Traditional working class	Oldest average age with low financial, social and cultural capital	14
Emergent service workers	Young with low income but very social and cultural	19
Precariat	Most deprived financially, socially and culturally	15

Source: Adapted from BBC Great British Class Survey.

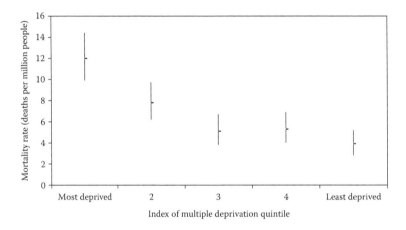

Figure 5.2 Mortality during the 2009 H1N1 influenza pandemic, by deprivation, England.

Source: Rutter PD, Mytton OT, Mak M, Donaldson LJ. Socio-economic disparities in mortality due to pandemic influenza in England. *International Journal of Public Health* 2012;57(4):745-50. With permission.

wards according to their index (based on the 1981 census), there were remarkable correlations with premature death rates, chronic ill health and low birthweight. If the health experience of the 136 wards with the best health record had applied to the 788,000 people in the worst 136 wards, there would have been significant benefits: fewer premature deaths, less sickness and disability and fewer low-birth-weight babies at high risk of complications.

The Jarman Underprivileged Area Score was not actually constructed as a measure of deprivation but as a measure of general practice workload. The variant of the Jarman Underprivileged Area Score in common use is based on eight variables, which were derived from a study of general practitioners' subjective expressions of social factors among their patients that most affected the need for primary care services and therefore their workload.

The most commonly used measure today is the Index of Multiple Deprivation (IMD). This combines 37 separate indicators of deprivation, grouped into seven domains. The separate indicators are combined to produce a total score – the higher the score, the greater the degree of deprivation. In this index, the seven domains of deprivation are income; employment; health and disability; education, skills and training; barriers to housing and services; crime; and living environment. The indicator data are routinely collected by a variety of government departments.

Analyses that use the Index of Multiple Deprivation (and similar indices in other countries) generally have two features: (1) they are based on area of residence rather than specific individuals and (2) they generally divide the population into quintiles or deciles (i.e. 5 or 10 groups). They are based on area of residence because the Index of Multiple Deprivation is not a measure that applies directly to individuals but to a population living in a particular area. An example is shown in Figure 5.2. Statistics are produced by the central government department of

Communities and Local Government every three years and provide very granular data on every local authority in England and Lower Layer Super Output Area (LSOA), of which there are 32,482.

The pattern of deprivation (Figure 5.3) generally highlights foci of deprivation in inner cities in London and the north and relatively high levels of poverty in coastal areas (e.g. Clacton and Essex). The analyses allow policymakers and planners to target resources and services to where they are most needed. Scotland, Wales and Northern Ireland each have their own Index of Multiple Deprivation. The Office for National Statistics also produces area classifications based on groupings of geographical areas that have key characteristics in common with the population concerned. These groupings seek to identify particular groups of people most likely to share certain behaviour patterns.

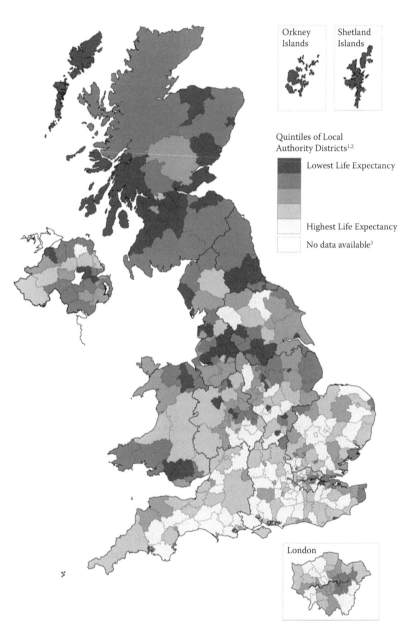

1. Local authority districts (LADs) include unitary authorities, London boroughs, metropolitan districts and non-metropolitan districts in England and Wales, council areas in Scotland and district council areas in Northern Ireland.

2. Each quintile comprises 81 LADs with the exception of the quintile with the lowest life expectancy, which has 80.

3. Life expectancy figures are not available for City of London or Isles of Scilly because of small numbers of deaths and populations.

Figure 5.3 Life expectancy by local authority district, United Kingdom.

Source: Office for National Statistics; Contains National Statistics data © Crown copyright and database right 2014; Contains Ordnance Survey data © Crown copyright and database right 2014.

MAJOR HEALTH DETERMINANTS

Although many positive and negative health outcomes can be observed among individuals, communities and populations, there are four endpoints that dominate the health landscape of nations: infant and child mortality, progressive chronic diseases, illness-related disability and premature death. Whether these occur, on what scale and to whom is down to a complex interaction between biological and genetic factors, health-related behaviour, socio-economic circumstances, and geography. These influences operate right across the life course from *in utero* to the frailty of advanced years.

In other chapters, the behaviours (smoking, lack of physical activity, calorie-dense diet and unprotected casual sexual intercourse), the risk factors (high blood pressure and elevated serum cholesterol) and the morbid states (obesity) that can cause devastating health outcomes have been described in detail. The remainder of this chapter explores the powerful underlying determinants of health and the way that they shape health inequalities.

Income

With higher income comes better health. The gradient is steep at first and flattens off as income rises. This is because receiving an extra £1000 would have a greater positive health impact for somebody on a low income than for somebody on a higher income. The relationship between income and health exists across the whole spectrum of income. The most adverse impact, of course, is for those at the bottom of the spectrum – people living in poverty.

Poverty is generally defined in one of two ways. *Absolute poverty* is an inability to meet basic needs. There is some variation in how basic needs are defined, but they are generally taken to include shelter, food, water and warmth. This implies that poverty is the same the world over. The alternative concept is one of *relative poverty*. This views those in poverty as living below a minimally acceptable standard of living, and accepts that this standard differs from one place to another. In the United States, it is common for the poorest people in society to own a car. In most sub-Saharan African countries, a person owning a car would never be considered poor.

Measuring how many people live in poverty requires a practical definition of what income level constitutes poverty. The sum of the costs to an individual (or household) of meeting their basic needs is used to create a definition of the absolute poverty level. A relative poverty level is generally defined as a fraction of the country's median income. The European Union, for example, defines those who earn less than 60% of national median income as living in poverty. By this measure, approximately one in seven people in the European Union live in poverty.

Being born into poverty increases the risk of many adverse health outcomes as an adult, including, for example, being obese. There are two primary explanations for why this is the case. The first is related to imperfect social mobility – that poor children are more likely to become poor adults and poor adults are more likely to be obese. This is the *social trajectory* model. An alternative explanation, though, holds even if children escape poverty themselves. The *sensitive period* model suggests that children whose mothers are undernourished while pregnant, and who themselves are undernourished as infants, develop a *thrifty phenotype* – that is, their regulation of energy expenditure changes to compensate. As adults, they are therefore more likely to become obese. The most sensitive period seems to be early in intrauterine development.

An individual's income level is a powerful predictor of mortality and morbidity, as has already been described. Further, the concept of *relative* poverty means that low income has an impact on an individual not just because of how low that income is in absolute terms but also because of how low it is relative to the rest of society. An increasing, although still controversial, body of evidence demonstrates that income inequality does not have an adverse impact on just the individuals at the bottom end of the spectrum, but across populations as a whole. Distribution of income within a society has been shown to correlate with life expectancy – it has actually been shown that the spread of income correlates more strongly with poor health than the average income level does. This phenomenon is increasingly relevant in today's world. Income inequality has risen over recent decades.

Three main mechanisms have been suggested to explain why income inequality can damage population health. First, it could be explained by the concave relationship between individual income and health. This is known as the *absolute income effect*. The additional health benefit for each pound of additional income is most pronounced at low-income levels and decreases at higher levels – a law of diminishing returns. The greatest health benefit would therefore be achieved if everybody's income were equal. Any distribution that is more uneven effectively removes income from those at low levels, where it is doing most to improve health, and redistributes it to those at higher levels, where it has a smaller effect on health. Researchers in New Zealand have estimated that reducing income inequality there by 10% would yield a 4% reduction in total mortality – an effect equivalent to preventing 350 road traffic accidents per year.

Second, the *relative income effect* involves social comparison and positional competition. Individuals on lower income compare themselves to the wealthier in society and feel relatively deprived, and this has a real impact on their health. The higher-income individuals, of course, compare themselves with most of society and feel a degree of satisfaction as a result. But their degree of satisfaction is less than the low-income individuals' degree of dissatisfaction, and so the net effect across the whole population is a negative one. As income inequality rises, it creates a bigger gap between an individual's income and that of others with whom they compare themselves, and so the magnitude of this effect increases.

Finally, the *contextual effect* theory proposes that a spread in income levels reduces the cohesiveness of a society, with less cohesive societies having more social isolation and, in turn, poorer health.

The evidence base is still evolving, and there is argument about the relative importance of these three effects. Whatever the mechanism, though, the implication is the same: the greater the discrepancy between the least well-off and the best-off in a society, the higher the overall levels of ill health and premature death. Overall, some leading thinkers in this field argue that the degree of variation in income levels in a society may have as much impact on health, or more, as an individual's absolute income – although this is controversial.

The Gini coefficient is a measure of inequality in income or wealth. It ranges from zero, expressing total equality, to one, maximum inequality. Worldwide, countries' Gini coefficients range from 0.25 (Sweden) to 0.65 (Seychelles) (Figure 5.4). The Gini coefficient is calculated by plotting graphically the income distribution of a country (or other area). This is then compared with the line of perfect equality. The Gini coefficient describes the difference between the actual distribution and this perfect line.

The Gini coefficient is the main measure of income inequality, but others also exist. The Robin Hood Index, for example, describes the proportion of aggregate income that would need to be redistributed from rich to poor households to attain perfect equality of incomes.

Education

Education is a significant predictor of health status (Figure 5.5). This is true both at an individual level (those who progress to higher education have better health than those who do not) and at a population level (countries that spend more per capita on education have better health). There are two explanations for the relationship between education and health. The first is that education imparts knowledge; more highly educated people are better informed about health and can make better lifestyle choices, recognize the symptoms of disease earlier and use healthcare more effectively. The second is that educational achievement generally brings higher income, less chance of unemployment and enhanced living conditions.

Another theory suggests that the relationship between education and health is not truly causative, but that it is confounded by intelligence. In other words, people of higher intelligence are more likely to both progress further through the education system and make better lifestyle choices, leading to education and health being positively correlated without one actually causing the other. On balance, the evidence weighs against this explanation. In cohort studies that have adjusted for individual educational attainment, there appears to be no relationship between intelligence and better health directly. The true relationship, it seems, is that higher intelligence leads to greater educational attainment, which in turn improves health.

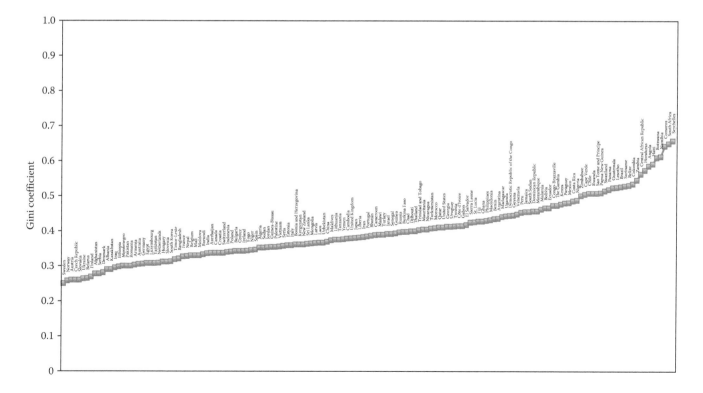

Figure 5.4 Income inequality, as measured by the Gini co-efficient, by country.

Source: World Bank. *The Growing Danger of Non-Communicable Diseases: Acting Now to Reverse the Course.* Washington DC: World Bank, 2011.

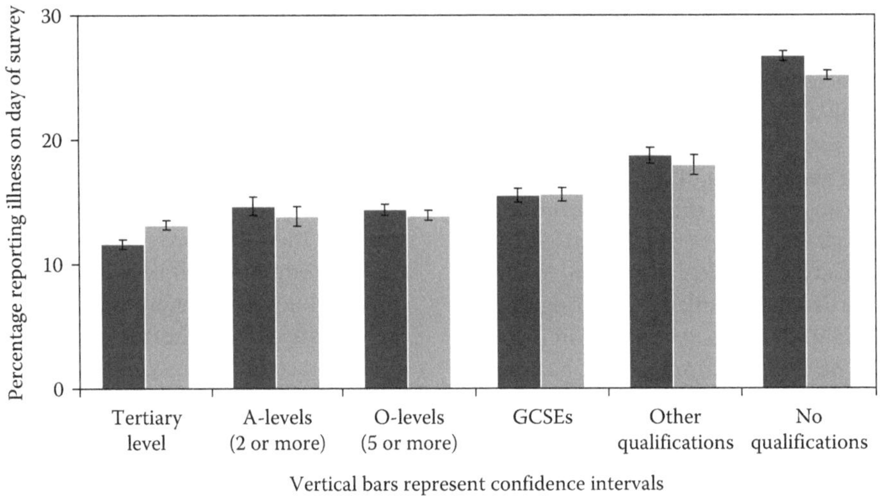

Figure 5.5 Educational attainment and health.

Source: The Marmot Review. *Fair Society, Healthy Lives.* London: The Marmot Review, 2010. With permission.

There is a good deal of evidence to support a final, perhaps less obvious, theory about the relationship between education and health – *the self-control theory*. It asserts that as well as imparting knowledge, the education system teaches people to be patient. It teaches people to defer gratification. Simply put, there may be more immediately appealing options for a child than doing their homework, but reward (good grades, parental approval and greater future potential) comes later if she can apply herself now. The skill of self-control is important to health. The immediately appealing options are to sit on the sofa, eat tasty (but calorific) food and enjoy smoking and drinking alcohol. Those with greater self-control are more able to forgo these immediate pleasures for the sake of their future health, or even just how they will feel tomorrow. The theory therefore goes that education improves health in part by improving self-control.

It seems that early experiences are particularly important in shaping an individual's self-control. The evidence suggests that preschool education, particularly if directed explicitly at teaching patience and self-control, can be effective in shaping these behaviours throughout life.

Occupation

The relationship between occupation and health is important and complex. It involves hazards in the workplace, workload, the chronic stress associated with the structure of many jobs and working conditions and the adverse effects of being out of work. For those in work, the state of being employed plays a very important part in their lives. It has many positive benefits, providing income, financial security, healthcare (in some countries), self-esteem, purpose and opportunities for leisure. For those without work, particularly those who are unemployed over the long term or young people who have not ever had a job, the negative forces of low income, apathy, hopelessness and lack of self-confidence

and self-worth are difficult to bear and can be a source of poor mental and physical health and toxic levels of stress. Although some jobs are associated with poor health, unemployment is generally far worse. When a person becomes unemployed, his or her risk of suicide increases, as does his or her cardiovascular mortality risk. Underemployment, not just full unemployment, has been similarly associated with worse mental health. At population level, this is of particular concern when economic recessions hit – they tend to create more unemployment, more underemployment and greater job insecurity, and so negatively impact on health. Data tracking the 2008 global financial crisis showed rising levels of poverty among children and adults with disabilities.

To a large extent, the general relationship between occupation and health is simply a reflection of the relationship between income and health. Those in higher professional groups earn more than those further down the hierarchy. Similarly, there is a relationship between education and occupation, but this is not the whole explanation. The early studies of Whitehall civil servants began in 1967. The first involved a cohort of nearly 20,000 male British civil servants. It demonstrated a significant relationship between occupation within the civil service and mortality. The strength of this relationship is striking when it is considered how much this cohort has in common. All lived in the same city (London), had similarly sedentary jobs, free of environmental hazards, and earned a respectable wage. Yet there was a fourfold difference in mortality between those at the top of the hierarchy and those at the bottom. Later studies started to explore the reasons for this. The key element appeared to be that job strain varied substantially between different jobs. The general public understanding of job-related stress focuses on the degree of demand associated with a job – the need to work fast, to deal with conflicting priorities and to handle an excessive amount of work. This is an element but is not the only factor that determines job strain.

Robert Karasek constructed a model of job strain illustrating this. Jobs are described along two axes – demand and control. Control reflects the opportunity to use and develop skills, and the opportunity to make one's own decisions. The demand–control model describes four different types of job conditions, produced by the interaction between the two factors demand and control. Chief executives' jobs are high demand, high control. They need to work hard, but have the opportunity to use and develop a range of skills, and to exercise a reasonable degree of control over their own environment. By contrast, the security personnel who sit at the chief executive's reception desk have low-demand, low-control jobs. There is little active work to do, but they often have no control even over when they take a break, gain few new skills and have little opportunity to enjoy making an impact on the environment around them. The traditional view of stress would see the chief executive as having the stressful job, but the demand–control model of job strain makes it clear that both jobs have some strain-inducing elements. In fact, the evidence suggests that the security person's job (in the passive quadrant of the 2 × 2 table in Figure 5.6) has a higher degree of strain than the chief executive's (in the active quadrant). The worst combination is a job with high demand and low control (a high-strain job), such as being a waitress in a busy restaurant. Probably the best combination is a job with low demand and high control (low strain), such as being a research scientist.

The mechanisms by which job strain impacts on health are almost certainly mediated through the stressor pathways described in the next section of this chapter. Other factors that create chronically stressful conditions can also have a detrimental health impact. Shift work, job insecurity, undertaking multiple jobs to make ends meet with consequent exhaustion and persistent lack of sleep, bullying and abuse in the workplace and the lack of any opportunities for career advancement all create such circumstances.

Working conditions are amenable to change through intervention by government, and through the efforts of individual employers. Paid parental (maternity and paternity leave) and sick leave is an important example – Germany, Norway, France and Sweden allow for long parental leave by law, whereas Canada, the United Kingdom and the United States allow only shorter periods. The benefit of parental leave is not solely that the mother or father can spend time with the child during the critical years of early development. It also helps parents to remain in the job market, leading to better long-term career prospects.

Understanding the elements of job strain, employers can improve the quality of work life by developing jobs accordingly. Even jobs that demand repetitive work (such as a factory line) can be redesigned to some degree, and employees can be rotated between different jobs to increase the job's demand and control. Employment policy, both at the macro, governmental level and at the micro, employer level, has an important bearing on a country's health, productivity and prosperity.

Ethnicity

There is striking evidence from many countries that ethnic minority groups have poorer health than the majority population. In the United States, for example, African Americans die earlier and suffer higher levels of chronic disease and disability than European Americans. In Australia and New Zealand, the disparity is greater still. The New Zealand Maori population lives an average of nine years less than the white population (Figure 5.7). The Aboriginal and Torres Islander populations of Australia live a staggering 20 years less than the rest of the Australian population.

In these countries and many others, there is also a strong relationship between ethnicity and socio-economic status, with those in ethnic minority groups tending to be poorer, to have fewer educational opportunities and to be unemployed or occupy lower-status jobs. Does this alone explain the life expectancy gaps? Not entirely. Data from the United States, for example, show that around two-thirds of the difference by ethnic group is explained by differences in socio-economic status, but that one-third is not.

Exactly what causes the residual difference is a matter of some controversy. Some argue that race-based differences in health may be attributable to genetic differences, but there is little convincing scientific evidence to support this. It seems clear that discrimination is at work. Discrimination involves systematic unfair treatment. It varies in form and type, depending on how it is expressed, by whom and against whom. It takes three main forms: *institutional discrimination*, which is related to policies or practices carried out by institutions; *structural discrimination*, which relates to the different ways a society

	Psychological demands	
	Low	High
Control — High	Fulfillment without undue pressure (low strain)	Pressurized but potentially fulfilling (active)
Control — Low	Unpressurized but not always fulfilling (passive)	Overloaded without compensating fulfillment (high strain)

Figure 5.6 Model of job control.

Source: Karasek RA. Job demands, job decision latitude, and mental strain: implications for job redesign. *Administrative Science Quarterly* 1979;24:285–308.

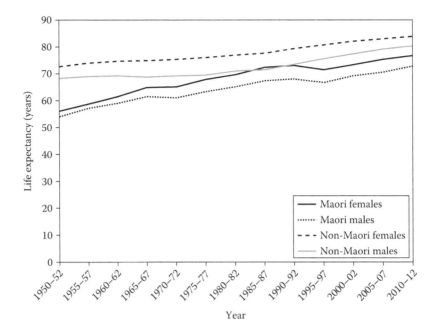

Figure 5.7 Life expectancy in New Zealand by age and ethnic group: Persistence of health inequalities.

Source: Statistics New Zealand.

promotes discrimination; and *interpersonal discrimination*, which relates to the perception of discriminatory interactions between individuals. It can have an impact on the healthcare that people receive, where they live and where they work. Discrimination can also provoke a stress response and give rise to maladaptive coping strategies, of the kind described in the biological pathways section of this chapter. In addition, some researchers have described that negative societal stereotypes can be so powerful that those to whom they refer start to themselves believe them, even to the extent that their own performance becomes adjusted to correspond to the stereotype.

In the United Kingdom, the national census has added much more precision to the definition of ethnicity as respondents are asked to choose a group that they feel fits them best. As a result, detailed data are available to enable the responses to questions on long-standing illness to be explored against ethnicity. Overall, these show considerable variation between ethnic groups. Although some ethnic groups have poorer health than their white British counterparts, this is not the case for all groups. The relative impact on health, and the contribution to health inequalities of factors such as fleeing from areas of conflict, being in an asylum centre, racism, discrimination and biological and genetic susceptibility are not well understood and difficult to deduce from official statistics. Undoubtedly, they have a bearing on the health status of these groups relative to the overall population in the United Kingdom.

Neighbourhood

Where people live makes a major difference to their health. Neighbourhoods can promote or damage health depending on their physical features, such as the quality of water and air; availability of health-promoting environments at home, work and play, such as safe, open spaces to exercise and good-quality housing; availability of services that support people in their daily lives, such as transportation, schools and public amenities; sociocultural features, including community integration; and reputation – people's perception of the area in which they live. Neighbourhoods can be assessed for their impact on health across three dimensions: the physical elements, the man-made structures and the social attributes (Table 5.3).

The quality of housing makes a significant difference to health. Rented accommodation tends to be poorer than owned accommodation – more often damp, noisy, vandalized and affected by crime, and less often having outdoor space. Research evidence has repeatedly shown that residents in poor neighbourhoods are not only personally poor, but that their neighbourhoods also tend to lack the supportive social and physical environments required for good health.

In many towns, cities and countries, there are separate geographic concentrations of wealthy and poor people. Affluent people are increasingly living and interacting with affluent people while poor people live and interact with other poor people. Poor people move to low-income neighbourhoods because of the availability of cheap and affordable housing, and people of minority ethnic groups prefer to move to neighbourhoods where lots of other people of the same group live. In general, wealthy people have more choice about where to live than poorer people do. The residents of richer neighbourhoods tend to have better health than the residents of poorer neighbourhoods. This is both because of the people (their other health determinants, such as income and education)

Table 5.3 Neighbourhood health effects

Neighbourhood feature	Hazard	Health effect
Biological/chemical environment		
• Air	• Air and water pollution	• Respiratory diseases
• Water	• Noise	• Hearing loss
• Soil	• Waste	• Sleep deprivation
	• Lead paint	• Developmental delays
	• Other environmental hazards	• Impaired cognition
Built environment		
• Housing	• Housing-related environmental toxins	• Asthma
• Transportation	• Allergens	• Obesity
• Commercial establishments	• Inadequate access to healthy food	• Alcohol and tobacco addiction (leading to liver, lung and cardiovascular disease)
• Billboards	• Increased exposure to fast food, alcohol and tobacco products	• Hypertension (due to obesity and lack of exercise)
• Parks	• Exposure to tobacco smoke	• Compromised immune system
• Libraries	• Lack of recreation	
Social environment		
• Levels of neighbourhood stress and support	• Violence	• Anxiety
• Enforcement of common rules for public behaviour	• Crime	• Fear
• Behavioural norms	• Social isolation	• Hyper vigilance
	• Low levels of interpersonal trust	• Depression
	• Public disorder	• Stress-related behaviour (over eating, smoking, addiction)

Source: Adler NE, Stewart J (eds.). *Reaching for a Healthier Life: Facts on Socioeconomic Status and Health in the US.* Chicago: MacArthur Foundation, 2007.

and because of the environment. The former is described as a *compositional effect*, and the latter as a *contextual effect*. Understanding the balance between these effects is useful. If geographic differences seem to be mainly compositional in nature, the right research and policy response would be to focus on the population's other characteristics – such as education. If they are mainly contextual, though, researchers and policymakers would focus on the health-damaging and health-promoting features of the neighbourhood environments themselves.

Contextual effects are not transient. Research has convincingly linked birthplace with health in later life. The presence of both compositional and contextual effects makes it far from straightforward to research the links between neighbourhood and health – but it is clear that these links are substantial.

Social capital and social support

The concept of *social capital* is an indication of the strength, resilience and mutual support in a community,

social or professional group. There are many formal definitions of social capital. The Office for National Statistics defines it as 'the pattern and intensity of the networks amongst people and the shared values that arise from those networks'. Where social capital is high, there is usually better health, greater educational attainment, more employment and less crime. Or as Michael Woolcock, a social scientist from the World Bank and Harvard University, puts it, communities with strong reserves of social capital are likely to be those that are 'housed, healthy, hired and happy'.

Nan Lin of Duke University has constructed a *position generator* that measures social capital as the ability of an individual to access powerful social connections. Individuals are asked to nominate members of their acquaintance network who hold valued social positions. An individual with high social capital is connected to people who have high-status or high-prestige occupations, or who can offer instrumental resources such as access to employment or money. In another *resource generator* approach, the respondents are asked directly about what resources they are able to access through people they know – in the form of information, influence or instrumental assistance.

The Organisation for Economic Cooperation and Development (OECD) describes three kinds of social capital:

1. *Bonds*: Links to people based on a sense of common identity ('people like us') – such as family, close friends and people who share culture or ethnicity
2. *Bridges*: Links that stretch beyond a shared sense of identity, for example, to distant friends, colleagues and associates
3. *Linkages*: Links to people or groups further up or lower down the social ladder

A further distinction is made between *bonding* and *bridging* social capital. Bonding social capital refers to trusting and cooperative relations within groups whose members share similar characteristics. Bridging social capital describes relations between individuals who are dissimilar in terms of their social identity and power. The distinction is important because in many disadvantaged communities, there can be plenty of bonding social capital, with members constantly helping each other, but they remain trapped in poverty unless they can access bridging social capital.

Whether describing individuals or groups, a distinction can be made between *cognitive* and *structural* social capital. Cognitive social capital refers to people's perceptions of the level of interpersonal trust, and norms of reciprocity within the group. Structural social capital refers to the externally observable behaviours and actions of people within the network, such as patterns of civic engagement. Trust is a particularly important aspect of social capital, with both cognitive and structural aspects. High levels of trust positively affect individuals' well-being and also make it easier for them to accept and give practical and financial help. Research in the United Kingdom has shown that lower interpersonal trust is associated with a greater likelihood of reporting poor general health, malaise and dissatisfaction with life.

The social support that people provide to one another helps health in a number of different ways. *Emotional support* given by close friends and relatives helps people's self-esteem and self-worth. *Instrumental support* is more practical, involving help with money or work. *Appraisal support* is help in making decisions. *Informational support* is the provision of advice. Social support therefore has *behavioural* health benefits – helping people to live more healthily because they make better decisions, are supported practically and so forth – and *cognitive* benefits from feeling supported, both at the time of receiving the support and from knowing that support is available when needed.

Some public health interventions aim directly at building social support – enabling individuals to participate in their community and build resilience through stronger social support networks. These can help to build individuals' self-confidence and well-being.

Social mobility

A major contributor to the persistence of health inequalities in a country is the extent of *intergenerational mobility*: the difference between the socio-economic status of parents and their children when they become adults. It has been repeatedly shown that there is intergenerational transmission of poverty, and of the health effects of poverty. Babies born to deprived parents are more likely to become deprived adults themselves than if they had been born to better-off parents. The degree of *social mobility* within a society determines how strongly this holds.

Looking at educational attainment, economic success and employment of adults compared with their parents allows intergenerational mobility to be contrasted between countries. The Organisation for Economic Cooperation and Development has done this and shown that:

- Parental or socio-economic background influences offspring's educational, earnings and wage outcomes across nearly all countries studied.
- Mobility in earnings across pairs of fathers and sons is particularly low in France, Italy, the United Kingdom and the United States, and higher in the Nordic countries, Australia and Canada (Figure 5.8).
- In Europe, there is a wage premium in growing up in a better-educated family and a penalty for being in a less educated family.
- The influence of parental socio-economic status on students' achievement in secondary education is particularly strong in Belgium, France and the United States, and weaker in some Nordic countries, as well as in Canada and Korea.
- Inequalities in secondary education are likely to translate into inequalities in tertiary education and subsequent wage inequality.
- At the other end of the spectrum, there is also generational persistence for below upper secondary education. This is relatively strong in certain southern European countries, Ireland and Luxembourg, and lower in France, some Nordic countries and the United Kingdom.
- Education policies play a key role in explaining observed differences in intergenerational social mobility across countries.

Towards the end of the second decade of the twenty-first century, there has been growing concern that social mobility in the United Kingdom has been slowing and the gap between the haves and the have-nots has been widening. The Commission on Social Mobility and Child Poverty has pointed out that the country remains elitist, with the majority of judges, military officers, key parliamentarians and senior civil servants having been privately educated (Figure 5.9).

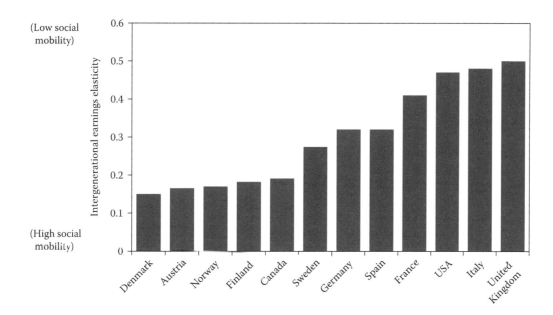

Figure 5.8 Persistence of economic advantage between generations, by country.

Source: Adapted from: d'Addio, AC, *Intergenerational Transmission of Disadvantage: Mobility or Immobility across Generations? A Review of the Evidence for OECD Countries.* Paris: Organisation for Economic Co-operation and Development, 2007.

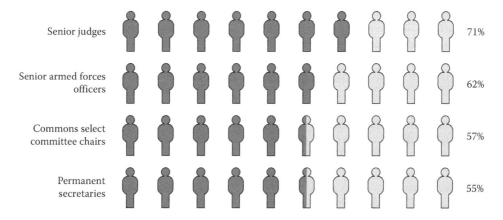

Figure 5.9 Proportion of Britain's high-ranking professionals educated at independent school.

Source: Social Mobility and Child Poverty Commission, 2014.

BIOLOGICAL PATHWAYS

Over the years, most academic study of health inequalities has focused on the associations between different characteristics of people's socio-economic circumstances and their health outcomes. Until recently, little thought was given to trying to establish the biological pathways that might mediate the social influences on health. Indeed, the disciplines of public health and the social sciences, on the one hand, and biological and clinical science, on the other, were two different worlds that perceived little relevance of each other's work to their own. This situation has been transformed by the introduction of the techniques of molecular biology and genetics. This has brought an exciting new dimension to understanding social determinants of health.

David Barker (1938–2013) put forward a theory of the developmental origins of adult disease. He maintained that nutrition in intrauterine and postneonatal life was a key determinant of later development of coronary heart disease, stroke and diabetes. This *fetal programming hypothesis*, more frequently called the *Barker hypothesis*, has become a highly influential concept in the field of social determinants of health and health inequalities, given the poor nutritional status of mothers in poorer and deprived communities. David Barker, who was based in Southampton University, England, once expressed his idea in a powerful metaphor of the car:

Across the world there is now general agreement that human beings are like motor cars. They break down either because they are being driven on rough roads or because they were badly made in the first place. Rolls-Royce cars do not break down no matter where they are being driven. How do we build stronger people? By improving the nutrition of babies in the womb. The greatest gift we could give the next generation is to improve the nutrition and growth of girls and young women.

Another major area of study relates to the concept of stress. Traditionally, stress has been understood and dealt with from the viewpoint of its clinical or behavioural consequences. The pressured company executive, the student preparing for a major examination and the athlete before an important race may all feel stressed or may appear to others as being stressed. Mostly, though, they will be responding naturally through the body's reaction to these situations. External or internal stimuli can produce a stress response that leads to the release of hormones and neurotransmitters, principally cortisol and catecholamines, that enable the body to adapt. This is part of the core process to prepare for 'flight or fight'. This acute response is both positive and necessary to deal with a challenge or threat. It is an ancient evolutionary adaptation, to enable us to run away quickly if in danger. While it is beneficial in the short term, in the long term repeated stressful stimuli, or the failure of the body's systems to regulate them effectively, can mean damage to cells, tissues and the immune system. In effect, the human body is releasing powerful hormones designed to protect and survive, but using them for psychosocial reasons. It is this *chronic stress* or *toxic stress* that is closely linked to both the social determinants of health and adverse health outcomes, such as premature death and chronic disease. Stanford neuroscientist Robert Sapolsky pointed out that only primates and human beings do this: 'We evolved to be smart enough to make ourselves sick'.

This explanation of the relationship between stress, health and disease is more fundamental than the everyday idea of stress. Two terms are frequently used in this context: allostasis and allostatic load. *Allostasis* is the set of body regulatory processes for maintaining homeostasis when there is exposure to stressors. When the stressors are repeated, allostasis cannot maintain complete control and damage starts to occur. The accumulation of this damage to cells and organs is referred to as *allostatic load*. It is sometimes referred to as 'wear and tear', although this rather trivializes the seriousness of the adverse effects. Thus, an allostatic load can build up through overexposure to stress hormones or to failure of the body to switch them off. Studies have shown that some people are very resilient and, in response to repeated exposure to stressors, can bring them quickly under control. They are in the minority.

A wide range of factors can act as stressors, but many of them are associated with social and economic deprivation. The mediation of stressors in infancy and childhood is vitally important to the future of a child. Nurturing, attachment and support are extremely beneficial, while distance, neglect, abuse and the absence of love start to build an allostatic load even at this early stage of life.

Another major finding from molecular biology has been that chronic stress reduces the length of telomeres. The telomere is the DNA–protein complex cap, protecting the end of each chromosome. Shorter telomeres are a feature of ageing and diseases associated with ageing. Studies have found them to be shorter in children living in deprived circumstances and among adults in conditions of chronic stress, such as long-term carers for people with dementia.

POLICY AND ACTION

Governments are the principal architects of a country's social environment. They determine education, taxation, employment, housing, urban planning and healthcare policy. For better or worse, these substantially shape the social determinants of health. Improving the social determinants of health is therefore a major task for government, as well as local communities and their governance mechanisms.

Not all governments accept this responsibility or hold it central to their mission. For most, employment, education, taxation and welfare are important areas of policy, but few government policymakers see, or pursue, them through the lens of improving health and reducing inequalities.

The Nordic countries have a strong record of putting social determinants front and centre. Sweden has 18 national public health objectives, of which the first five are strong solidarity and social community, strong social environments that support the individual, secure and equal conditions during childhood and adolescence, a high level of employment and a good work environment. Setting such objectives is only the start – but it is a vital step, missing in many countries.

In the United Kingdom, a series of prominent reports have made a strong case for tackling health inequalities by improving the social determinants of health. Each report has powerfully demonstrated the enormous scale of inequality as a call to action, and has coupled this with a series of recommendations to government, based on the available evidence.

For many years, the 1980 Black Report was the reference point for many who believed that health inequalities should be taken more seriously, both in the United Kingdom and elsewhere. Nearly 30 years after the Black Report, Tony Blair's incoming New Labour government commissioned Sir Donald Acheson, a former chief medical officer, to head an enquiry into health inequalities and produce a report to guide policy. His committee explored a wide range of determinants of health, and made recommendations to the government as a whole, not just the Department of Health. The three main areas of recommendations were that (1) all government policies should be evaluated for their impact on health inequalities and, wherever possible, should reduce such inequalities; (2) high priority should be given to policies aimed at improving health and reducing health inequalities in women of childbearing age, expectant mothers and young children; and (3) priority should be given to policies that reduce income inequalities and improve the living standards of poor households.

In the field of the social determinants of health, Professor Michael Marmot is today's giant. He chaired the World Health Organization's Commission on the Social Determinants of Health, which published its report in August 2008. Shortly afterwards, the UK government asked him to lead a similar review in England. Published in 2010, this review was called *Fair Society, Healthy Lives*, and is generally referred to as the *Marmot Review*.

The Marmot Review rehearses the grave inequalities in health that exist between the most deprived and the least deprived. It estimates that between 1.3 million and 2.5 million potential years of life are lost every year in England, through premature death associated with social disadvantage.

Marmot and colleagues synthesized the available evidence to recommend how the government could effectively tackle the social determinants of health. The review made recommendations in six policy areas, which tie closely to the social determinants of health explored in this chapter. These were (1) give every child the best start in life; (2) enable all children, young people and adults to maximize their capabilities and have control over their lives; (3) create fair employment and good work for all; (4) ensure a healthy standard of living for all; (5) create and develop healthy and sustainable places and communities; and (6) strengthen the role and impact of ill health prevention.

Of these six, the early years ('give every child the best start in life') is accorded highest priority, because of the potential to achieve lifelong changes most effectively and efficiently early in life. The other five areas apply throughout the life course, though, because focusing only on the early years would miss opportunities for effective intervention later in life and would seem unfair to adults for whom social disadvantage is already established.

Many of the Marmot Review recommendations are to do with how resources are allocated by government. Instead of allocating resources equally across the population, the review advocates allocating greater resources to those in greater need. This is a practical expression of the principle of equity. Marmot emphasizes that there are not two groups – the deprived and the privileged – but that there is a *social gradient* along which health improves with socio-economic status. Action cannot solely be focused on the most deprived, but must be on flattening the social gradient in health by improving the lot of everybody along it, in proportion to their need – a principle termed *proportionate universalism*.

Given that finite resources are available, spending on reducing health inequalities takes money away from activity that may more efficiently improve the overall health of the population. There is a trade-off between a *health maximization* approach and an *egalitarian* approach.

The National Institute for Health and Care Excellence (NICE) produces evidence-based guidance for local authorities on tackling health inequalities. At the global level, the Commission on the Social Determinants of Health aims to improve the social determinants of health that are visible in the conditions of daily living. These are similar to the recommendations of the England Marmot Review, but clearly apply to a broad range of countries. The five priorities are (1) to enhance equity from the start of life by removing barriers to education, particularly for girls; (2) to build living environments that promote health; (3) to create fair employment and decent work; (4) to establish social security systems everywhere; and (5) to establish universal healthcare, particularly primary healthcare.

The Commission on the Social Determinants of Health also highlights a range of social determinants that are not as immediately visible as education, work and healthcare, yet have a profound effect on health inequalities. These are to do with how power, money and resources are distributed globally, nationally and locally. The Commission calls upon the world to tackle the inequitable distribution of these vital resources. It makes a series of bold, far-reaching recommendations on areas from improving gender equity, to enhancing the use of donor funding, to improving global governance as a whole.

As with other reports in this field, the Commission on the Social Determinants of Health does not only present a list of policy recommendations. It also tries to build a case for change and to create a vision that will inspire people to make that change. It highlights that girls born in some countries today can expect to live for 45 years, while in other countries they can expect vastly more – 80 years. It presents this as a fundamental social injustice, and its plan aims to close this gap within the space of a generation.

CONCLUSIONS

In the late 1990s, the New Labour government, in an early White Paper on public health, constructed a metaphor that has since been used over and over again. It equated a journey on the London Underground to the expectation of life of populations living in the districts at each stop. A journey on the Jubilee Line of eight stops between Westminster and Canning Town resulted in a fall of one year in average life expectation at birth as each successive station is reached (Figure 5.10). It was powerful, shocking and conveyed the challenge of health inequalities in a way that resonated far beyond professional public health circles.

To understand the social determinants of health is to understand something quite profound, and quite different to how most people think of health. To many, ill health is seen solely through its proximate causes – smoking, poor diet and lack of physical activity– and its potential for treatment and cure. Understanding the social determinants of health involves a journey far upstream to the causes of illness, disability and premature death.

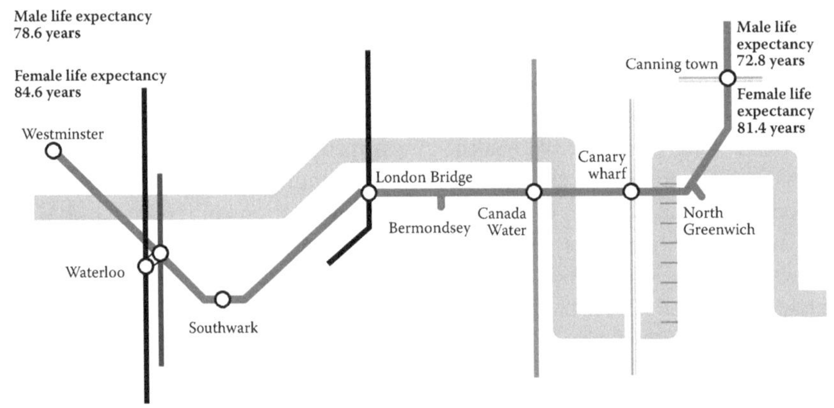

Figure 5.10 Travelling east on the Jubilee line.

Source: London Health Observatory (LHO). *Mapping Health Inequalities Across London.* London: LHO, 2001. Updated with 2000–2006 life expectancy data from Office for National Statistics.

The traveller coming out of the Jubilee Line stations to the east of Westminster and walking through the streets to find an explanation for his or her poorer health will not find the answers or the solutions in the higher prevalence of smoking, the greater numbers of people who are overweight or obese or the level of alcohol consumption. These behaviours will be more common than in the affluent areas of London, and they do have to be addressed, but they are driven by deeper social and economic ills: poverty, worklessness, a lack of opportunity, the absence of safe green spaces, the unavailability of cheap yet fresh nutritious food and a cycle of deprivation that stifles social mobility from one generation to the next. These forces and more generate the unhealthy behaviours that damage health. Even worse, they also have a direct effect, not mediated through specific risk factors; the cells, tissues and organs of the body are damaged by the effects of long-term, toxic stress that activates

biological pathways. This way of thinking would be powerfully different in itself but takes on further impetus when it becomes apparent that social conditions vary enormously, that they have a major impact, and therefore that there are stark inequalities in health. The two discourses – on social determinants and health inequalities – are different from one another, because the former would still be valid without the latter, but in practice are tightly intertwined.

Michael Marmot said that 'this link between social conditions and health is not a footnote to the "real" concerns with health – healthcare and unhealthy behaviours – it should become the main focus'. His reports, and those of Black, Acheson and others, have built the case for putting social determinants front stage. The field, by its nature, is highly political. At its core lie the same factors as lie at the heart of politics – the distribution of money, power and resources.

CHAPTER 6

Health systems

INTRODUCTION

Around the world, the health systems of most high- and middle-income countries are big, complex and expensive. In many low-income settings, the facilities, staff and resources are completely inadequate to meet the needs of the populations. Despite the stark differences in levels of infrastructure and capacity, any country's health system has special significance to its citizens. It is more than its staff, its money and its work – health systems are living products of society, reflecting beliefs, ideologies and historical events. Every one has been shaped by the population it serves, by periods of war and peace, by economic boom and bust, by the rise and fall of political theories, by the geographical landscape, by fluctuating demands and expectations, by changing laws and societal structures, by new technology – in short, by the ever-changing world. Health systems share many common aims, but there are many ways to achieve them – shaped by their societies, their histories and available funds. This makes the study of health systems complex, but also offers fertile ground for countries to learn from each other.

The World Health Organization defines health systems as 'the sum total of all the organizations, institutions and resources whose primary purpose is to improve health'. Health systems incorporate the elements that everybody sees (doctors, nurses, hospitals and ambulances), but also many vital functions that are not visible to the general public. Doctors cannot deliver high-quality care without regulation and licencing of the drugs that they prescribe. Patients cannot trust doctors unless excellent medical education is in place. Patients' experience of care depends on what services are available, where they are located and how long they have to wait to access them. All this requires planning and management, activities that are often scathingly depicted by the media as an unnecessary diversion of funds from the front line of care, yet are a vital element of a successful health service.

The values of a society fundamentally shape the interactions that occur within a health system. A patient's consultation with a doctor is underpinned by the values of equity, confidentiality, trust, respect, integrity, selflessness and safety. Health professionals uphold these values, but every part of the wider health system must also promote them; they should be reinforced by all the technical functions that determine how healthcare is delivered, from funding mechanisms, to service infrastructure, to medical training and education, to medical technology licencing, to monitoring systems, and many more.

In most countries, national governments take at least some responsibility for providing a health system. Such governments are said to have *stewardship* of the health system, and use *governance* systems to steer towards their goals. Stewardship is a political process that involves balancing competing interests from within and outside the health system. There is a constant flow of new ideas, initiatives, standards and expectations of the health system. High-income countries tend to have a multitude of agencies that do not directly deliver front-line services, but instead play discrete and important roles in the governance and regulation of the health system. Their collective role differs between countries, particularly depending on how the country's health system is (or health systems are) financed. Governments managing a state-owned health system play a very different role from those simply regulating, and shaping the market for, private healthcare providers.

Ultimately, the provision of healthcare that is comprehensive in scope, centred on the needs of patients and families, humane, safe and of high quality is a mark of a civilized society. Progress in medicine, science, technology and organizational development has delivered much in the last hundred years, but modern times continue to pose formidable challenges for those dedicated to providing the very best healthcare that the twenty-first century can offer.

IDEAL OF UNIVERSAL HEALTH COVERAGE

The World Health Organization defines universal health coverage as 'ensuring that all people have access to needed promotive, preventive, curative and rehabilitative health services of sufficient quality to be effective, while also ensuring that the use of these services does not expose the user to financial hardship'. While many high-income countries

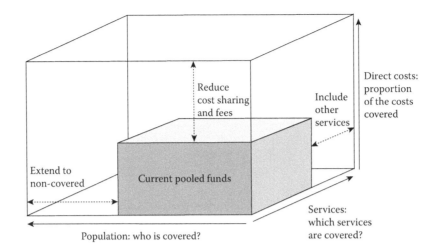

Figure 6.1 The three dimensions of achieving universal health coverage.

Source: World Health Organization. *Health Financing for Universal Coverage, Universal Coverage – Dimensions.* Available from: www.who.int/health_ financing/strategy/dimensions/en/ [accessed 13 September 2016]. With permission.

already offer their citizens access to a comprehensive range of health services without significant out-of-pocket cost, this is not the case for the majority of countries globally. Many health system goals – access, financial protection and equity – are far from being realized. Too many individuals forgo health services or pay substantial amounts to receive care.

The World Health Organization, the World Bank and many other international agencies and foundations have pledged to assist countries to reach universal health coverage. Many countries face high hurdles – political, financial and cultural – and the road to achieving universal health coverage will be a long one. The World Health Organization has posed three main questions for governments approaching the task of establishing universal health coverage (Figure 6.1):

• Which members of the population should be covered?
• What range of services are people entitled to?
• What is the extent of protection against individuals having to bear the costs themselves?

Early thinking on the goal of universal health coverage concentrated on how to reach the twin goals of coverage and financial risk protection. Latterly, much more attention is being given to the nature of the coverage: how comprehensive is the provision of services, and how good are the services that are being provided?

Countries come to the task of achieving universal health coverage from very different starting points. The United States spends more than any country on healthcare, yet large numbers of its citizens are not insured (more than 40 million in the mid-1990s). President Obama's Affordable Care Act ameliorated this but was thrown into doubt by the election of President Trump. The challenge of achieving universal coverage in that country is not only about money

and system redesign but also about overcoming political resistance and vested interests. In western Europe, coverage is pretty much universal, mainly through social insurance schemes; in the United Kingdom, the universal coverage is taxpayer funded. In all these countries, and others around the world whose citizens are currently well covered by affordable care, the challenge is to sustain universal coverage in the face of burgeoning demand and an adverse fiscal environment. The task is also to improve the quality and safety of care and make it more patient centred. In some middle-income countries, coverage is in place for part of the population but not for others (e.g. those living in rural areas). In other such countries, the system may be misaligned, with a dominance of hospital provision and no adequate primary care sector. Such countries face the challenge to even out the patchiness of provision and rebalance it. For example, in Brazil, the 1988 constitution had enshrined universal and egalitarian access to healthcare as a right of the citizen and an obligation of the State. Yet, access to care remained fragmented and too heavily based in hospitals. The government of Brazil implemented a Family Health Strategy that strengthened the primary care base of the healthcare system, expanded coverage to the poorest communities and improved some health outcomes. The programme continues. Thailand is another middle-income country that has successfully introduced universal health coverage from a situation at the beginning of the 2000s when 30% of the population was uninsured (Figure 6.2).

Many countries are still struggling to overcome the substantial barriers – financial and political – that limit access to basic healthcare services. Meanwhile, countries that have made major progress in offering all citizens access to basic healthcare services are grappling with a range of further issues. These include ensuring the appropriate range and quality of services, enhancing respect for patients' dignity and values and constantly balancing these aims with

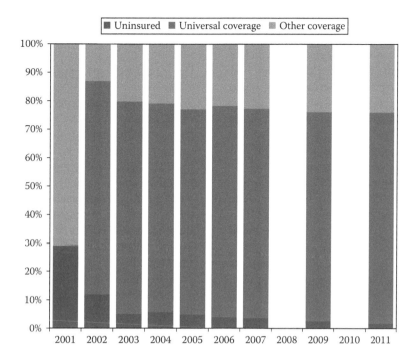

Figure 6.2 Introduction of universal health coverage in Thailand.

Source: Government of Thailand. *2012 Health and Welfare Survey.* Bangkok: Government of Thailand, 2013. With permission.

competing demands and financial constraints. Universal health coverage is simple as a concept, but the practicalities and complexities of implementation are huge. Policymakers, politicians and society as a whole all have roles to play in navigating the pathway to universal health coverage.

HEALTH SYSTEM AIMS

The Institute for Healthcare Improvement in the United States has set out an approach to delivering better health system performance. It is based on pursuing three goals simultaneously – the so-called *triple aim*. The three goals are improving the patient experience of care (including quality and satisfaction), improving the health of populations and reducing the per capita cost of healthcare.

This is a helpful view of the purpose of a healthcare system. It was driven very much by the need to find answers to the seemingly intractable question of how to control the high level of spending on healthcare in the United States (hence the third aim, expressed as reducing per capita costs).

Here, six aims of a healthcare system are set out. They broaden the perspective that must be taken if such an approach is to be relevant in all parts of the world.

Health

Most people living in a country will view the main aim of their health system as to provide care when they are ill. This is an entirely reasonable view, and indeed, most health systems are primarily health*care* systems – their major focus is on providing diagnosis, treatment and care. Most also

declare their commitment to improving the population's health and reducing preventable disease. However, the reality is mostly different: healthcare services, especially hospitals, take up the greatest share of the time of leaders and policymakers, and certainly get the lion's share of available resources. Yet, the demand for healthcare, the money spent on it and its affordability and sustainability into the future depend greatly on the numbers of people with preventable diseases that are currently not being prevented. A healthcare system cannot simply be a passive receptacle for the sick people who flow in to use its facilities and expertise. It must look upstream. Aside from specific interventions like lowering hypertension, or finding and controlling diabetes, this means reaching into the wider determinants of health, and taking a broad view of what constitutes a healthy life.

Health systems that have this necessary focus on health, as well as healthcare, have a complex job. They need to promote the multitude of factors that contribute to a healthy life, prevent the wide range of conditions that have a negative impact on health and deal with the major burden of diseases that afflict the modern world. It is much easier to adopt the wider aim of improving population health when the financial incentives support it. In many healthcare systems, the funding flows are such that hospitals and other providers of care are rewarded for treating more patients, not for stopping them from becoming patients in the first place.

Quality and safety

In the last two decades of the twentieth century and into the twenty-first, there was a growing emphasis on the nature of the care provided, not just the numbers of patients seen and treated. Most well-functioning health systems now state that they aim to deliver care through the most efficient, effective and safest means possible. There has been increasing emphasis on evaluating health services and health gained (or lost) from interventions. Health economists have led the way in demonstrating the cost-effectiveness of interventions taking into account long-term outcomes, quality of life, safety and complications alongside the initial costs. This has led to large organizations – such as the National Institute for Health and Care Excellence (NICE) in the National Health Service (NHS), described in detail later – being charged with recommending healthcare interventions that are the best option for patients, the health system and society as a whole.

A greater understanding has emerged of the range of factors that can pose a threat to the quality and safety of care:

- *Weak infrastructure*: The range, appropriateness and distribution of facilities, equipment and staff are inadequate to provide fair, suitable and timely access to required care.
- *Poor coordination*: There is poor organization or interaction between the components of care necessary to meet the needs of a patient, or group of patients, resulting in ineffective outcomes and inconvenience to patients and their families.
- *Low resilience*: The defences in place, and the design of processes of care, are insufficient to reliably protect against harm, such as that resulting from errors or from faulty and misused equipment.
- *Poor leadership and adverse culture*: The organization or service providing care does not have clear goals and a philosophy of care that is embedded in the values of the organization and visible in every operational activity.
- *Competence, attitudes and behaviour*: The practitioners and care providers working within the service lack the appropriate skills to deal with the patients that they encounter, or they are unprofessional in their outlook and actions, or they do not respect other team members or work effectively with them.
- *Suboptimal service performance*: The way that the service is designed, organized and delivered means that it does not deliver processes of care to a consistently high standard, so that over time it chronically underperforms, often in a way that is not noticed until comparative performance is looked at.
- *Slow adoption of evidence-based practice*: The service does not conform to international best practice in particular areas of care or overall.

Creating and maintaining a safe, high-quality healthcare system means addressing all these potential threats, as well as creating an environment in which quality improvement flourishes. This requires strong and clear leadership and engagement of doctors, nurses and other health professionals who are at the front line of care. The subject of quality and safety of healthcare is dealt with in more depth in Chapter 7.

People-centred care

People vary in their expectations of health services. What works for one may not be appropriate for others. Health systems are increasingly trying to provide care that is people centred and respects individuals, communities and their choices. There is still a great need to strengthen this aspect of health systems globally. Many health systems fail to meet basic standards, such as dignity and respect, when individuals receive care. A responsive health system encompasses these ideas, is flexible and can react quickly and positively to the expectations of users. It treats them with dignity, involves patients in decisions about their care, communicates clearly and upholds confidentiality.

The best services in the world today also give major priority to involving patients and families across the whole range of their activities, from board-level policymaking, to design of care processes, to quality improvement efforts, to evaluation of services, to working on reducing risk to patients as part of patient safety programmes.

There are many potential themes for family engagement in health and social care, for example, shaping and designing services, measuring the quality of care, setting standards for consultation, sharing decision-making, strengthening self-care of chronic diseases, preventing harm and giving feedback on practitioner performance. Few services do all of these, some only scratch the surface of genuine involvement and others do a few well.

Public expectations of healthcare have changed markedly. Patients are far less likely to be passive recipients of care than they were in decades gone by. Many are informed about their health and take a very active interest in the service they expect to receive. It has always been the case that patients know themselves, their bodies and their behaviours better than any health professional. By engaging individual patients and tailoring health services to them, care is most likely to be successful in achieving the desired outcomes, which may well be different even for two patients of a similar clinical profile. People-centred care is primarily about doing what is right for individuals, but because it can lead to greater patient engagement and greater efficiency of care, there is benefit for the health system as a whole too. The term *people centred* is usually preferred to the sometimes used *person centred* to better reflect the community, population-based approach to both organizing services (e.g. population stratification of risk) and improving public health.

Entitlements and protection

The health system of almost every country or region will serve a diverse group of people – in different geographical areas, in various socio-economic and cultural groups; of different genders, ages, religions and ethnicities, and of a range of cultural heritages. All these factors, and more,

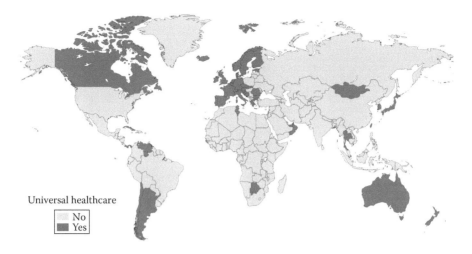

Figure 6.3 Countries with universal health coverage.

Source: McKee M, Balabanova D, Basu S, Ricciardi W, Stuckler D. Universal health coverage: a quest for all countries but under threat in some. *Value in Health* 2013;16(1):S39-45. With permission.

contribute to each person's health status and to the way in which he or she interacts with the health system.

Health systems should not just provide services but also aim to do so fairly. Ideally, no citizen who needs healthcare should be disadvantaged in receiving it by barriers related to where he or she lives, his or her social standing or his or her ethnic group. *Equity* is a very important moral principle that should underpin the design and operating system of a good health service. It is not an easy aim to achieve. Studies of healthcare access and use in different parts of the world have consistently shown evidence of serious inequalities (Figure 6.3). In the United Kingdom, equity was one of the founding principles of the NHS and has remained a fundamental tenet ever since. There has been little evidence of major or sustained reduced access to NHS treatment for those of lower socio-economic status (the main source of inequity in many health systems). However, inequity is present in the NHS, particularly geographically, as different populations get differential rates of treatment for the same condition, the so-called *postcode lottery* (Figure 6.4). Much of this has to do with funding levels of local NHS planning and commissioning bodies, the way local priorities are set or the quality of management in ensuring that services are equitable.

The dominant concern in many healthcare systems, particularly in low- and middle-income countries, is whether the poorest people are able to get the quality of care that they need as a right and an entitlement. If this is to be the case, then the next questions are how comprehensive will the offer of free care be, how will eligibility be determined, and who will pay for it? These questions are key to the provision of universal health coverage – a major goal for many low- and middle-income countries. In many countries, particularly the poorer ones, individuals can only get access to healthcare if they pay out of pocket. They can incur costs at every stage. Even in health systems that are purportedly free at the point of use, informal payments or even bribes to health professionals may be necessary to secure access. In many lower-income

countries, patients or their families can be faced with insurmountable problems in paying for treatments. The cost of cancer chemotherapy and major surgery can easily run to tens of thousands of dollars. If the health system does not cover the cost, patients and their families can face a choice between no treatment and financial ruin. There can be wider implications of such systems. For example, when China went to a largely free-market model of healthcare, its citizens, fearful of financial ruin if illness befell the family, hoarded their savings. The wider economy was affected, as people did not spend their disposable income. China established a State Council Medical Reform team in 2006 and has made progress in introducing a basic medical and healthcare package for its population while ensuring equality of access and affordability.

The United Kingdom does not put its citizens at financial risk since the NHS is largely free at the point of use. There are some costs – medicines, travel, over-the-counter treatments and perhaps lost earnings from visiting healthcare services – but these are minor. Most people in the United Kingdom cannot envisage a health system in which they had the ever-present worry about the cost of falling ill. There is an important psychological benefit to knowing that you, or your family, will be taken care of in the event of illness, without losing all your financial assets. This peace of mind – not just the healthcare itself – is an important health benefit of health systems that provide comprehensive care.

An important aim of any health system, then, is to protect the people who need it from having to face substantial payments of this kind. The financing and risk-sharing arrangements of health systems are as important as the services and treatments that they make available.

There are two broad scenarios against which to test the adequacy of financial risk protection: (1) whether a catastrophic illness or injury means that the patient or family paying out of pocket is overwhelmed by the cost of the care required, (2) whether the person's condition means that the regular out-of-pocket costs of care force the patient or family to become

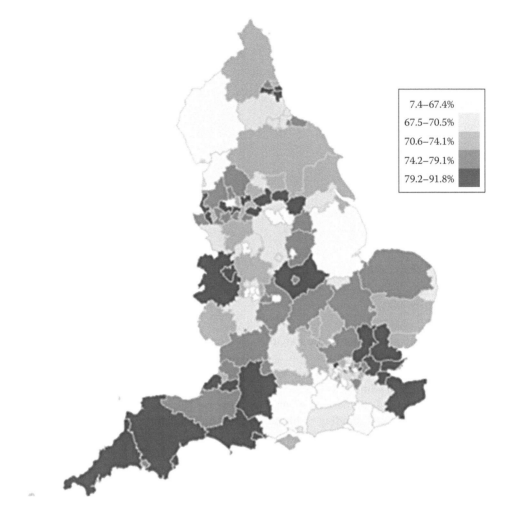

	7.4–67.4%
	67.5–70.5%
	70.6–74.1%
	74.2–79.1%
	79.2–91.8%

Figure 6.4 Percentage of the diabetic population receiving screening for diabetic retinopathy.

Source: NHS Right Care. *NHS Atlas of Variation in Healthcare.* London: NHS Right Care, 2011. With permission.

so impoverished that they slip below the poverty line. A key aim of any modern health system must be to provide its citizens, particularly the poorest, socially disadvantaged, severely incapacitated and disabled, with protection in both potential scenarios. This is at the heart of universal coverage.

Resilience

Health services tend to go about their everyday business with a good understanding of the problems that will arise: additional winter emergency admissions to hospital; the development of new drugs that could be beneficial to many patients, but are very expensive; and major failures of plant or equipment. All are examples of challenging occurrences that nevertheless can usually be dealt with in a well-managed and adequately resourced service.

Every local, regional and national health service also needs surge capacity to respond to emergencies and crises. The real difficulties arise when something happens that threatens the ability of an individual hospital or a healthcare system overall to cope. In the past, this has occurred with major outbreaks, or epidemics, involving novel or complex infectious

agents. The emergence of the severe acute respiratory syndrome (SARS) in Hong Kong, and later in Canada, caused widespread public fear and uncertainty as the virus spread among hospital patients and staff, causing deaths. The 2014 outbreaks of Ebola fever in West Africa rapidly overwhelmed health systems that were already very weak, and generated fear and mistrust of the authorities, leading some communities to hide family members who were ill. Both SARS and Ebola created worldwide concern, huge media coverage, large-scale mobilization of external aid and resources and numerous global meetings of politicians and experts. This did not prevent the health organizations in the affected areas from being in a prolonged state of crisis that damaged their ability not just to deal with those struck down with these life-threatening illnesses but also to provide care for the many other health needs in their populations. The speed of regaining control of such situations, recovering and rebuilding is much easier in a high-income country like Canada that has a well-resourced health system than in a poor country like Sierra Leone that had little even before the crisis hit.

The resilience of health organizations is not just tested by acute, unexpected events but also by circumstances that produce sustained pressure over a longer period of time. This has been the case in many parts of sub-Saharan Africa that are affected by HIV and AIDS, and have very poor healthcare infrastructure. The sheer numbers of people requiring treatment in some places have been so great that services are constantly overwhelmed and in crisis.

Economic recession can have a major impact on health systems. The collapse of the Soviet Union in the early 1990s led to economic turmoil in many countries, whose health systems were insufficiently resilient. Mortality rose – particularly from alcohol, tobacco and chronic disease–related deaths – leading to a decreasing life expectancy in former Soviet Union countries in the mid-1990s. The global recession that started in 2008 also had profound effects on health systems as public finances for health were squeezed. In many European countries, user charges were introduced for some individuals or services, investment in health services was reduced and there was significant restructuring of services.

Beyond economic shocks, events such as natural disasters and conflict pose big threats to health systems. The sheer number of injured and ill individuals following an earthquake or tsunami, for example, can quickly overwhelm services – at times when health professionals may also be missing, health infrastructure damaged and supply routes interrupted. After the acute shock, re-establishing routine care is a priority.

There are no easy answers to these challenges, but preparing for health system shocks and disasters is now an essential role for policymakers, health leaders and system managers. Making organizations and healthcare systems resilient involves many steps, including establishing sufficient resources and governance structures, ensuring flexibility and adaptability and training staff to cope.

Sustainability

Well-functioning health systems take a strong interest in both efficiency and effectiveness. Efficiency refers to the outputs that are obtained for the inputs, where the inputs are primarily considered in financial terms. The term efficiency often has negative connotations, especially when perceived as a euphemism for cost-cutting. But, the underlying principle of efficiency is key to ensuring the health system is achieving the best impact it can with the resources available.

Rightly, governments, healthcare providers and insurance companies put pressure on health systems to ensure that money is well spent. There is significant focus on ensuring that the right services are being delivered for the right cost. The methods of improving efficiency are often contentious – jobs may be lost and services reorganized – and it is up to policymakers, health professionals, managers and the populations served by health systems to agree on the best ways to make their services efficient. Efficiency is not a static concept, because the population's needs and the treatments and other technologies available are changing over time. The effectiveness of services, medicines and technologies refers to how well these interventions achieve their desired outcomes.

All healthcare systems are struggling with inexorably rising need and demand from the populations that they serve. The pressures come from population ageing, which generates rising numbers of people with frailty and multimorbidity; explosive increases in the numbers of people suffering from chronic diseases and their complications; rapid advances in technology and therapeutics; higher public expectations of what healthcare can do for them; and increases in pay and prices. Health systems will become unsustainable unless solutions can be found to reduce the impact of these pressures, since it will be unacceptable to simply increase the proportion of a nation's budget spent on health. The United Kingdom spends approximately 9.1% of its gross domestic product on health; this is close to the average for Organisation for Economic Cooperation and Development (OECD) countries. The proportion spent by countries around the world

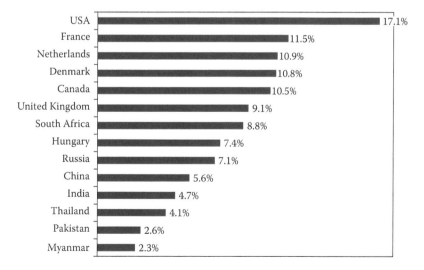

Figure 6.5 Total spending on healthcare as a percentage of Gross Domestic Product, 2014.

Source: World Health Organization.

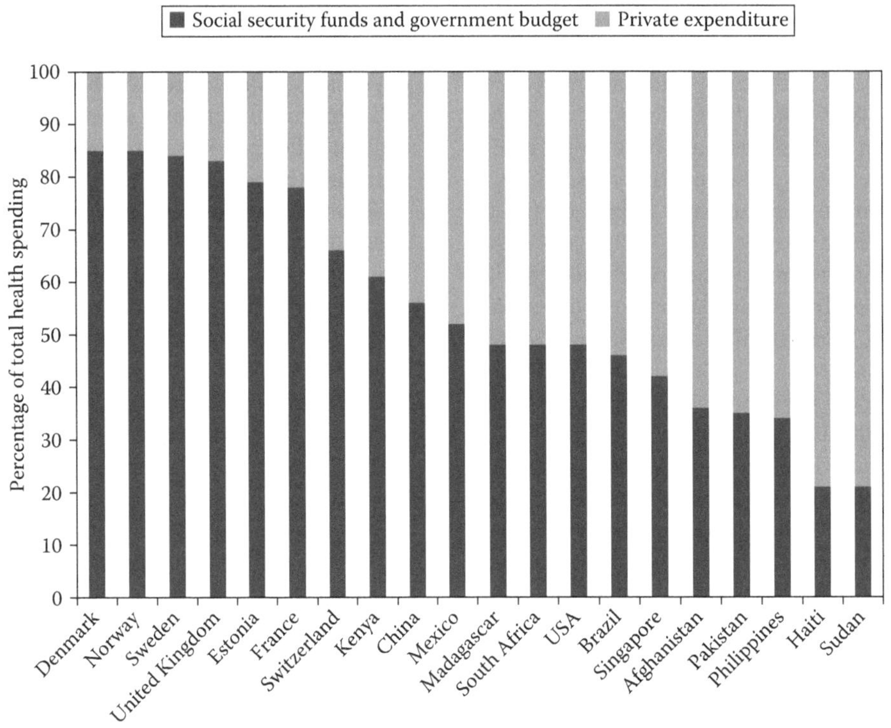

Figure 6.6 Sources of healthcare funding by country, 2014.

Source: World Health Organization.

varies greatly (Figure 6.5), as do the relative amounts from the public and private sectors (Figure 6.6). The highest proportion of health spending relative to gross domestic product is in the United States (17.1%), and among the lowest at 1.5% is Timor Leste.

A vital aim for leaders of a health system, therefore, is to make it sustainable over the long term. This will mean more effective cost containment, new care delivery models for chronic disease, more effective health promotion and disease prevention, greater self-care, a focus on effective and evidence-based services and finding new sources of funding. These are actions that have proved very difficult to formulate and implement in the past.

HEALTH SYSTEM MODELS

Health systems can be generally categorized into three broad groups based on how they are organized, operated and financed. The three groups – the social and other insurance models, the tax-funded model and the direct payment model – are based on core founding philosophies that developed over the last 150 years – workplace insurance, central funding from general taxation and market economics. Notably, much of the distinction between health system models centres on financial flows. Nonetheless, whilst offering insights into the foundations of modern health systems, these groupings are a simplification of reality. Many countries have mixed arrangements that have elements of all three models.

Tax-funded

In 1918, following the Russian Revolution, Nikolai Semashko (1874–1949) became the Commissar of Health of Soviet Russia. As part of his socialist reforms, he introduced government-run healthcare. State government took full responsibility for health services, owning the entire infrastructure, providing medicines and technologies and employing health professionals. Healthcare was provided free of charge, financed from central government funds. This was the first state-controlled health system.

Thirty years later, following the upheaval of the Second World War, the UK government created the NHS. Sir William Beveridge made the first recommendations about how the system should function, and so the Beveridge model of the NHS is named after him. Most of the assets of the NHS are owned by the state, and the majority of hospital staff is on the state payroll. Most general practitioners are independent contractors. The creation of a national health service in the United Kingdom was followed by similar tax-funded, publicly provided health systems in some other countries. Over time, most of the systems established on the Beveridge and Semashko models have changed to incorporate some form of competition, insurance and market-based economics. Since the fall of communism, completely state-controlled and state-provided healthcare is rare. For example, in the United Kingdom a proportion of state-funded care is provided in the private and independent sector.

Social and other insurance

In 1881, Otto von Bismarck (1815–1898), the Chancellor of Germany, laid the foundations for the first social security system and the formal health system in Germany. At the time, there was substantial political pressure to develop new forms of social protection for the working population. As a result, health insurance was extended across the working population. These policies represented the first steps towards a comprehensive insurance model for health coverage and laid the foundations for expansion of these policies to other populations and countries in the early twentieth century. The Bismarck model for health systems has formed the basis of health systems funded through social insurance – an entitlement to health services that is linked to employment. Contributions by employer and employee (by payroll deductions) build up resources that are held in sickness (insurance) funds that determine how they are spent. Sickness funds pay providers – most often private – to deliver healthcare.

The social insurance model has evolved substantially since the nineteenth century, and modern forms are in place in many European countries. This evolution has mainly centred on expanding health insurance to those outside formal employment, thereby promoting equity. The unemployed, those working informally, the disabled, children and the elderly previously received limited insurance coverage in many places. Now, sickness or local insurance funds often receive funding from governments to cover these vulnerable populations. Alternatively, separate insurance funds may be established covering these population groups specifically, to provide at least a minimum package of healthcare.

Many countries have either undertaken reform of traditional social insurance sickness funds or established completely new health system financing arrangements based on health insurance (as has been done in many countries emerging from the Soviet Union in the 1990s). These forms – often called *national health insurance* or *single-payer systems* – are consolidations of multiple sickness funds to a national organization. Under this model, citizens pay a compulsory insurance premium to the government itself or a government-sponsored organization in charge of collecting funds for financing health services. Many countries operate a national insurance agency or fund, preferring this to multiple sickness funds because of its economies of scale and ability to provide a more uniform service nationally. Although a national insurance model works on the principles of entitlement, insurance coverage and contracting mechanisms for health service provision, large elements of a tax-funded system are present. There is the largest degree of risk pooling (see below) possible and, as a large national entity, health insurance agencies have strong bargaining power with service providers and drug companies. Also, the insurance premiums effectively are a form of tax – as they are often collected directly from income – with the government providing funding for vulnerable and exempt groups. Service providers can be public or private, or both.

There are numerous variations on the social and national insurance models. Countries vary largely in the number of insurance funds, the exemption and inclusion criteria, the packages of service covered, the costs individuals must contribute for services and the arrangements for vulnerable populations. Insurance-based health systems are generally attractive to people and governments, and are widespread globally.

Direct payment

In many countries, the state plays very little role in the funding and provision of healthcare, and there may not be any organized system of social insurance either. In these circumstances, the availability and provision of care is mainly market driven. This is typically the case in many low-income countries, where government finances or capacity limits health system delivery. Wealthy people either take out private insurance coverage or pay directly when they or their family are ill. Poor people get no care, pay out of pocket for as much as they can afford or receive some care from charities or aid organizations. The large inequities created by market-based systems provide a strong drive to introduce universal health coverage worldwide.

HEALTH SYSTEM FINANCING

Financing lies at the heart of health systems and clearly characterizes the main models described above. The way in which money flows into and through the system varies markedly between health systems of different types and has a significant impact on the goals that the system is trying (or is able) to achieve. Importantly, financing has also to do with how individuals are protected (or not, in some systems) from financial risk, particularly from substantial, catastrophic health expenditures. The flow of money between different parts of a health system creates incentives (and disincentives) for individuals and health organizations to behave in particular ways and so is vital to the way it functions.

Health system financing has three elements: how the funds are generated and collected, how these funds are pooled and how service providers are funded and reimbursed. These three strands are interconnected, although distinguished separately here.

Raising revenue

Raising sufficient financial resources is essential to meeting health system goals. Funds can be collected in three main ways – through general taxation, by insurance schemes or via direct (out-of-pocket) payments to providers. In addition, some lower-income countries receive a large proportion of their health system funds from foreign aid or philanthropic foundations. Spending on healthcare – and the proportion funded by public expenditure – varies greatly between countries.

In the United Kingdom, NHS finances are allocated from the government budget, which comes from a range of taxes and duties (mainly income tax, corporation tax, value-added tax, business rates, national insurance contributions and council tax). There is no allocated revenue-raising mechanism that specifically funds the health system – it all comes from the general government budget (Figure 6.7). The devolved administrations of the United Kingdom also receive allocations from the central government budget for their health services. In addition to general taxation, the NHS raises relatively small amounts of income through prescription fees, providing services to private patients and dental fees and charges. These represent out-of-pocket expenditures for patients, although there are exemptions for low-income and vulnerable groups.

As well as the publicly funded health system in the United Kingdom, there is a strong independent and private health sector. This provides services – such as cosmetic surgery – not available in the NHS; it treats patients who wish to pay for private care or have taken out their own insurance, and it gives care to wealthy patients from abroad who travel to use UK qualified specialists. Increasingly, commissioners of NHS care use some private and independent sector providers to deliver it (at no cost to the patient).

Sweden, Portugal, Norway, Italy, Spain, Denmark and New Zealand have systems that are mainly funded by taxes. These can be collected at either the national level, like in the United Kingdom, or the local level, such as through local councils in Denmark. Revenue raised in these tax-funded systems is generally not earmarked for healthcare spending – the local or national government decides what portion of it should be spent on healthcare. Central to tax-funded systems is the idea of *universalism* – that all citizens are covered, whatever their contributions.

Insurance-based systems usually involve compulsory contributions that are collected from income. Unlike a tax, these funds are most often directly for healthcare funding. The norm is for both employees and employers to contribute. Some countries operate a single social or national insurance scheme (Australia, Estonia, France and Belgium), while others (such as Austria) operate different schemes in different geographical areas. Social and national insurance schemes are not generally based on individual risk, so contributions do not depend on age, weight, gender or lifestyle factors. Even though social insurance–based health systems are predominantly funded by specific contributions from employees and employers, the state often makes a contribution from tax revenues to supplement the finances and to cover populations such as the young, old and disabled, and others outside formal employment. The degree of universalism within systems funded through insurance contributions therefore depends on government regulation and input.

Private insurance schemes operate in all countries – often alongside social insurance or tax-funded schemes. The extent to which private insurance is used varies enormously, though. The United States, for example, relies heavily on private insurers. In Germany, although most of the population is covered by the public insurance scheme, around 15% of people opt for private insurance. In the Netherlands, curative and primary care services are funded by mandatory private health insurance plans, while long-term social care for the elderly and terminally ill is funded through social

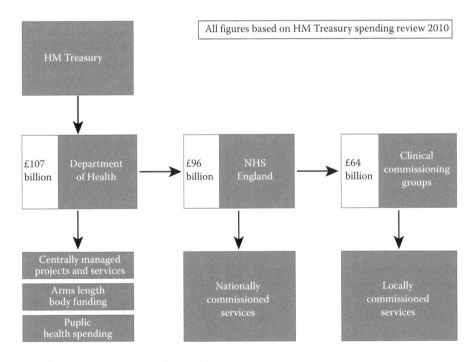

Figure 6.7 Funding flows in the English National Health Service.

Source: National Health Service (NHS). *Understanding the New NHS*. London: NHS, 2014. With permission.

insurance funds. Private health insurance plans involve individuals paying their own premiums, which are usually weighted based on their age and occupation, and in some cases pre-existing medical conditions and lifestyle factors. Individuals may pay the entire premium themselves, or employers may make a contribution.

Most low-income countries have weak arrangements for health system financing. They have neither comprehensive tax-funded nor social insurance models. Both the funding and provision of care tend to be fragmented between public, insurance and out-of-pocket funded elements. Out-of-pocket expenses take the form of direct payment (user fees) for services, cost sharing and informal payments. User fees can be encountered for all aspects of care – consultations, tests, medicines, surgery, therapies, inpatient care and so forth. Cost sharing involves individuals making a contribution towards funding their care but not bearing the full cost, but this still involves financial outlay for individuals. Informal payments (bribes, gratuities and gifts) are common in systems that have limited funding, little accountability and a culture that tolerates or expects such practice. In countries such as Chad, Guinea, Nigeria, Cambodia and Sudan, out-of-pocket payments represent more than 60% of total healthcare expenditure. The burden of such payments is concentrated in the poorest and most vulnerable populations (those on low incomes or outside formal employment), so the principle of equity is often violated in such systems.

Fund pooling

Fund pooling spreads risk across a population. This is important because many conditions can be very expensive to treat. Cancer treatments and complex surgery can cost tens of thousands of dollars. Drug costs can be high, particularly for rare conditions. If such costs were borne by the individuals unfortunate enough to suffer them, they could be impoverishing. If they are spread across a whole population, the costs, although still substantial, are manageable. The design of the fund-pooling process is important to the health system goals of equity and financial risk protection. Systems funded by insurance or general taxation are more equitable than systems in which patients pay out of pocket, because the healthcare received is separated from ability to pay.

The degree of risk pooling in a population depends on political and societal norms. In countries such as the United Kingdom, Sweden and Denmark, the whole population is covered under a national health system. The degree of risk pooling is high, and the risk is widely shared. In countries with multiple private insurance companies, coverage can be less equitable because some parts of the population are excluded from coverage. Some insurers may select healthier, and therefore cheaper, people to insure, charging unhealthier individuals more or excluding them from the insurance fund. In these situations, the unhealthiest (and often the poorest) parts of the population can struggle to find affordable coverage. To improve equity in these situations needs government legislation – such as the *Affordable Care Act* in the United States.

Distributing funds and reimbursing service providers

In many countries – although not all – there is a separation within the health system between organizations that purchase care on behalf of populations and those that provide it – known as a *purchaser–provider split*. In countries, such as the United Kingdom, with state-funded and largely state-provided healthcare, this is somewhat artificial, since the purchaser organizations and most of the provider organizations are state owned. It aims, primarily, to introduce competition between providers of services, with the goal of improving efficiency and quality. This competition is enhanced by the trend towards paying for some NHS patients to be treated by private sector providers. It also aims to make some organizations specifically responsible for studying the needs of the population and purchasing (otherwise known as commissioning) services to match.

In insurance-funded systems, the purchaser–provider split tends to be much clearer and more meaningful. In Germany, for example, the regional sickness funds (health insurance companies) negotiate contracts with healthcare providers. In France, like many other countries with a national insurance system, the national health insurance agency reimburses health service costs. The insurance organizations, and sometimes the employers that are paying the premiums for their workforce, exert considerable leverage over the provision of care in areas such as value for money, quality of care and models of service delivery. For example, The Leapfrog Group in the United States is a national coalition of employers that are healthcare purchasers. A small group of companies came together at the beginning of the twenty-first century in recognition that the industry was paying billions of dollars for employees' healthcare with no information on quality, value for money or comparative provider performance. Other companies joined as they decided to 'leap' forward to remedy this situation. Today, The Leapfrog Group is a sophisticated and important contributor to improvements to the quality, safety and efficiency of the U.S. health system.

Health systems pay for services using a variety of different funding mechanisms that have evolved. These are important because they have a substantial impact on how people and organizations within the healthcare system behave. Today's funding mechanisms continue to be developed, in the quest for an approach that best matches the health system's goals.

The main models of paying for healthcare are:

- *Global budgets* (also called *block contracts* or *budget transfers*): This is the most basic way of paying healthcare providers, and is used far less today than it was historically. A global budget allocates a set amount of funding to a provider (such as a hospital), with which all costs should be met. Global budgets can help to cap healthcare expenditure, but providers may compromise services or quality so as not to exceed their allocation. Global budgets also provide little financial incentive for providers to improve the quality of their care or the effectiveness of their services, since they get the funding anyway.

- *Fee-for-service* (FFS): The direct cost of the service is passed on to the purchaser (the patient, insurer or government). While this is a simple method for financing care, it leads to spiralling costs, as providers have an incentive to provide the most costly treatments and even unnecessary treatments. This is the dominant method for paying doctors in the United States and other private healthcare-based systems. Fee-for-service also tends to make providers focus more on the quantity of procedures and consultations than on their quality.

- *Diagnostic-related group (DRG)–based payments:* This is a more complex approach. The provider receives a set amount of money for each patient seen, based on a prior estimate of the costs of caring for a patient of that kind with a condition of that kind. Instead of having a separate price for every individual condition, conditions that cost similar amounts are grouped into a single price. Adjustments to the basic price paid can be varied if, for example, there is a complication in surgery. This method has become more common in hospitals as purchasers aim to reduce costs. This is the main way in which hospitals are funded in the United Kingdom, where the term *Healthcare Resource Groups* (HRGs) is used.

- *Capitation*: A set fee is paid to providers to cover each patient registered with them, regardless of how much healthcare that patient actually uses (which may be none). This is a common approach in primary care worldwide, in which general practitioners or family physicians are paid to provide services for patients registered with them. Capitation payments are often adjusted based on social and demographic factors of the local population, such as age, sex and deprivation.

- *Pay-for-performance* (P4P): In this approach, part of the payment for a service depends on the quality that the service achieves. Measures of quality are stipulated in advance. This has become particularly prominent as a component of primary care payments. It is used in the NHS through the Quality and Outcomes Framework (QOF) for general practitioners, and many countries have adopted similar methods. It is also being increasingly used in the purchase of hospital services.

In recent years, there has been a general transition to more complex funding models. Increasing attention is given to how local demographics affect the health needs of a population, and therefore the funding that they require. These trends have been driven by a need for greater cost-effectiveness in health service provision and to better meet the needs of patients and populations. In general, poorer and older populations require more care (and more expensive care), as do certain population subgroups, such as the disabled and unemployed. The term *case mix* is used to refer to the health needs of the population, the severity of the conditions encountered and the complexity of treating them.

STRUCTURE AND FUNCTIONING OF THE NATIONAL HEALTH SERVICE

The United Kingdom's NHS is vast. More than 600,000 people use it every day. It employs more than 1.2 million people. Globally, only the U.S. Department of Defense, the Chinese People's Liberation Army, Walmart and McDonald's have more staff. Its annual budget exceeds £100 billion. The NHS is an important part of the fabric of UK society. It is loved by the majority of the public and loathed by some commentators, who see it as an anachronism riddled with the flaws of an old-style nationalized industry. Journalists devote millions of column inches to it every year, and no politician would underestimate its importance. The NHS came into being as the United Kingdom emerged, scarred but victorious, from the Second World War. It represented a promise to the country's citizens that their healthcare would be free at the point of use, and provided according to their need, not their ability to pay.

Faced with a large and complex health system, government ministers may feel that they have far from perfect control. They do have levers that can be used to lead health systems in the desired direction. These include:

- Developing and implementing health policy
- Designing frameworks and strategies for the health system
- Overseeing the health system's functioning
- Creating partnerships and collaborations with groups and organizations outside the health system – including other government departments and civil society
- Regulating, through laws and administrative rules, many aspects of the health system, enacting appropriate penalties if they are broken
- Introducing and enforcing accountability mechanisms to hold service providers and others in the health system responsible for their actions
- Controlling the rules for the flow of money and payment systems

Used well, all these approaches can contribute substantially to the achievement of a health system's goals.

Founding principles

In the summer of 1941, the British government appointed Sir William (later Lord) Beveridge (1879–1963) to chair a committee of senior civil servants to undertake a survey of existing national schemes of social insurance and allied services and to make recommendations. The Beveridge Report, published a relatively short time later in December 1942, contained a series of sweeping proposals and recommendations that laid the foundation for the modern welfare state. He built his case around felling the five giants that were holding Britain back from prosperity: Want, Disease, Ignorance, Squalor and Idleness. The White Paper, *A National Health Service*, which was published in February 1944, ambitiously moved beyond the initial brief for a national hospital service and provided instead a plan for a comprehensive national health service.

The medical profession was initially reluctant to participate in Beveridge's plan, which required work within a state-managed system and restriction on their capacity to determine their own incomes. A Labour government was elected in 1945 and appointed Aneurin Bevan Minister of Health. This created new difficulties and resulted in a breakdown of negotiations with the British Medical Association (BMA). Bevan exploited existing divisions in the medical profession between generally wealthy consultants and comparatively poorly paid general practitioners to achieve their eventual agreement to work within the NHS.

Beveridge's original report and the 1944 White Paper formed the basis for five main acts:

1. *The Family Allowances Act 1945* provided for cash allowances to the second and subsequent child.
2. *The National Insurance Act 1946* established a comprehensive contributory national insurance scheme.
3. *The National Insurance (Industrial Injuries) Act 1946* made provision for insurance against accidents and injuries and some specified diseases due to a person's employment.
4. *The National Assistance Act 1948* finally replaced the Poor Law, placing on local authorities the responsibility for the elderly, the handicapped and the homeless and setting up a scheme for financial assistance on a national basis for those in need.
5. *The National Health Service Act 1946* created a comprehensive health service available to all citizens.

With the commencement of the NHS on 5 July 1948, the Minister of Health became statutorily responsible for providing a comprehensive health service for the population of England and Wales. All hospital property, whether it had been in the voluntary or municipal sector, came under the control of the Minister, including all but a small number of privately owned hospitals. Thus, the Government inherited a wide array of buildings and accommodation with varying origins, traditions and functions, and with differing levels of upkeep, which were spread unevenly throughout the country. However, the administrative merging of these made it possible to plan a hospital service for a locality, to begin to rationalize its distribution and to make arrangements for the training of medical, nursing and technical staff.

England was originally divided into regions with regional hospital boards. The Minister of Health appointed their chairmen and members. These regional boards appointed hospital management committees to be responsible for the day-to-day running of individual hospitals or groups of hospitals. Teaching hospitals had separate arrangements, being administered by boards of governors appointed by the Minister and responsible directly to him rather than being administered through the regional hospital boards.

Early developments

The NHS brought general medical, general dental, ophthalmic and pharmaceutical services under a national contract through local executive councils. Thus, with the advent of the NHS primary medical care was also provided free and as a right for all who wished to request it. However, Bevan's vision for a completely free NHS did not last long. The original estimated cost of the NHS was £176 million (for 1948–49). The actual cost was £225 million, grossly in excess of the tight postwar budget. As a remedial measure, charges for dental work and optical services were introduced in 1951 in conjunction with a stricter financial regime. This led to Bevan's resignation as Minister of Health. The Conservative Government introduced prescription charges in 1952. However, by 1960 it was clear that the NHS required substantial investment, and expenditure was once again allowed to rise, enabling a major hospital building programme to be started in 1962.

Health centres were a major focus for primary care for the local authorities at the time, but they were very slow to gain acceptance with general practitioners. As early as 1920, the Dawson Report had recommended that local authorities provide, equip and maintain health centres where groups of doctors and other healthcare staff could work together. One of the most widely praised was the Finsbury Health Centre in London, which was constructed to an award-winning design in 1938. Yet by 1966, only 28 purpose-built group practice premises, housing about 200 general practitioners, had been established.

The first experiments with local authority nursing staff attached to practices occurred in the late 1950s and early 1960s. General practice at this time was experiencing problems. There was a common perception that general practitioners were failed hospital doctors. General practitioners' income was wholly dependent on the number of patients registered with them, and they received no assistance from the government towards the provision of adequate premises or supporting staff. In consequence, morale among general practitioners was low. Many UK graduates emigrated to North America.

In 1966, as a result of the *Charter for the Family Doctor Service*, a new contract for general practitioners introduced major change. A three-part payment system of basic practice allowances, capitation fees and item-of-service payments was supplemented by group practice allowances and incentives for doctors to work in underdoctored areas. Partial reimbursement of the salary costs of practice clerical and nursing staff was instituted, and funds were made available for the building or upgrading of premises. These steps encouraged a trend towards group practices, the employment of ancillary staff, the imaginative development of premises and an expansion in the range of services offered to patients. Attachment of district nurses and health visitors developed steadily, and practices progressively sought to accommodate these staff in their premises. These positive developments were accompanied by the expansion of vocational training for general practitioners, which became mandatory in 1982, and the establishment of academic departments of general practice in the medical schools.

Aside from therapeutic services that were based in hospitals or general practice, the NHS laid down a range of other services concerned with the health of the population that were delivered mainly by major local authorities (counties and county boroughs). This was the only part of the new service that had specific responsibility for the prevention of disease. However, little detail was specified, giving considerable scope for innovation by individual local authorities. The authorities discharged their functions through health committees whose chief officer was the medical officer of health.

In addition to the general responsibility for developing a preventive function, local authorities were charged with providing a range of supportive services. These included a wide variety of community services (such as health visitors, home nurses, domiciliary midwives and home helps) to provide care, support and advice to people in their own homes; a responsibility for the control of infectious diseases, including through vaccination; the care of expectant mothers, infants and young children; the provision of an ambulance service; and the provision of health centres.

Following the heyday of public health in the inter-war period, the formation of the NHS made for an awkward and relatively unfocused development of the public health profession. Many authorities adopted new duties without fully considering their strategic public health function. Public health doctors attempted to reinvent their discipline as *community medicine* in the late 1960s with limited success. Medical officers of health were replaced with community physicians, but they found it increasingly difficult to balance their commitments to epidemiology and NHS resource management.

The first reorganization: 1974

Between 1948 and 1974, the health service was organized in a so-called tripartite fashion, whose three components were:

1. *The hospital service* (administered by regional hospital boards and a network of hospital management committees at a local level) and teaching hospitals (administered by boards of governors)
2. *The family practitioner services* (with contracts held by executive councils)
3. *The local authority health services* (which operated within the sphere of local government administration to provide public health services in the form of infectious disease and environmental hazard control, preventive services and community-based services)

The first major administrative reorganization of the NHS took place in 1974. Its aim was to provide a better, more sensitive and more coordinated public service. Before 1974, it had never been the responsibility, nor had it been within the jurisdiction, of any single named authority to provide a comprehensive health service for the population of a given area. As a result, it had not been easy to balance needs and priorities rationally and to plan and provide an integrated service within the resources available. From 1974, local authority health services were brought within the NHS, along with hospital services. The service was organized geographically into 14 regional health authorities, and within them were area health authorities.

In introducing proposals for a National Health Service in 1944, the government emphasized:

> The real need is to bring the country's full resources to bear upon reducing ill health and promoting good health in all its citizens; and, there is a danger of over-organisation, of letting the machine designed to ensure a better service itself stifle the chances of getting one.

The governments that followed did not heed these wise words. The changes in 1974 were the first of as many as 19 reorganizations of the NHS that would take place over the next 30 years. They changed the number and functions of administrative tiers, the way that funding flowed through the system, the balance between central and local policy-making and planning and many other detailed aspects of policy relating to clinical services.

Introduction of general management: Griffiths

Prime Minister Margaret Thatcher commissioned an NHS manpower enquiry in 1983. Its author manoeuvred it to become the National Health Service Management Inquiry, so creating space for one of the most important moments in the history of the service. The most noticeable consequence of the *Griffiths Report* was the introduction for the first time of general managers at various levels within the health service, but the enquiry exposed the lack of clear accountability, leadership and management expertise within the NHS at the time. Sir Roy Griffiths, a director and deputy chairman of J Sainsbury PLC, supermarket chain, criticized the consensus style of administration in the NHS; it gave each member of a team of equal partners (administrator, nurse, doctor and treasurer) a right of veto over decisions. Griffiths recommended a national board and chief executive officer for the NHS, and that a single general manager should be appointed to each health authority, accountable to the board and responsible for general managers at the operational level.

In this way, for the first time since 1948, there was (in theory) a clear line of accountability, with a single nominated individual at each point. In practice, there were considerable tensions, particularly between the new general managers and the professionals providing services, and the 1980s were marked by a series of clashes over financial targets and service responsiveness.

Griffiths advocated that the NHS adopt the principles and practice of modern management, and the influence of his recommendations is still being felt today. His report is best remembered for saying, 'If Florence Nightingale were carrying her lamp through the corridors of the NHS today, she would almost certainly be looking for the people in charge'.

Less well known but equally telling was another remark that he made at the time (referring to the prime minister): 'It took a grocer to teach a grocer's daughter the difference between price and cost'.

Creation of an internal market: The Thatcher reforms

The next significant shift in thinking about the structure and functioning of the NHS came as the end product of a review undertaken by the Thatcher Conservative government. This followed unwelcome publicity in the winter of 1987 that had focused on two perceived shortcomings:

1. Incidents of hospitals closing beds, deferring or redirecting admissions or sending doctors on extended leave to limit workload in order to stay within budget, despite continued real increases in health service funding.
2. The existence of perverse incentives, whereby extra workload in the most efficient, effective and sought-after hospitals was not matched by extra funding, and these hospitals were the first to have to limit their services.

The proposals ended the conflicting roles of the then district health authorities, in which operational responsibility for healthcare provision (in local hospitals) within their geographical boundaries was coupled with serving the needs of the resident population. The proposals also ended the system of funding, which was seen as offering no incentive to hospitals to treat more patients, to improve quality or to provide a wider range of services.

The 1990 reforms introduced a number of new features to the way in which the NHS functioned. Their principal thrust was to separate responsibility for purchasing healthcare from its provision. District health authorities and general practice fundholders became service purchasers, funded according to the health needs of their population. Fundholding general practices could use their budgets to purchase some hospital and community services, to cover prescribing costs and to employ practice staff. By the middle of the 1990s, some 15% of the population was served by fundholding general practitioners.

Under the *internal market* arrangements, hospitals and other provider organizations were free to concentrate on

improving the effectiveness and efficiency of healthcare in order to win service contracts, the means of agreeing on service delivery between purchasers and providers. NHS trusts were created as a new and more autonomous kind of provider of NHS services. These were described in the *Working for Patients* White Paper (and for some time afterwards in the media) as *self-governing hospitals*, which reflected the philosophy of the time: to free hospitals from bureaucratic interference by management tiers above them. They had their own trust boards directly accountable to the Secretary of State for Health and significant freedom in the way they could employ staff and invest in capital infrastructure. Trusts were dependent on contracts with purchasers for most of their income, keeping services provided in line with the requirements of the populations they served.

Despite all the reassurances that were given, many health service staff and sections of the public in Britain seemed to hold to the view that these reforms concealed a hidden agenda to privatize the NHS. In addition, where problems did occur – as they do from time to time in any health service – the media and the public were quick to attribute them to the organizational changes introduced in 1990. Moreover, the managerialism that swept into many public services in the late 1980s and early 1990s was also unpopular. The idea of salaries that were more competitive with the private sector and of employee benefits (such as company cars) was anathema to those for whom the NHS was a cherished institution sustained by the taxpayer. Money not used very directly for patient care was readily portrayed as money squandered.

Looking back on this important period in the history of the NHS, it is difficult to assess fully the benefits of the changes. It must be remembered that, at the start of the decade, many other countries were also experimenting with healthcare system reform. The changes in Britain to separate purchasing from provision of service were in keeping with an international philosophy towards the public sector. Undoubtedly, the discipline of being explicit about the cost and quality of health services was long overdue. However, the central concept of an internal market – bringing the perceived benefits of competition to a publicly funded system – increased bureaucracy and set up significant transaction costs. The introduction of a purchaser–provider split had been originally intended to create a competitive internal market to drive up quality and so increase value for money. However, the scope for genuine competition in the NHS has always been very limited. The term *commissioning* subsequently superseded *purchasing*. Commissioning involves a wider set of functions – assessing need and planning services accordingly, and the use of financial incentives to intentionally drive the system's development relating to the type of services provided, their quality and their efficiency. Despite their unpopularity, the key philosophy of the 1990 reforms has endured. No subsequent government has dismantled the NHS architecture to merge the purchasing and provision of care under one organizational structure; they remain on two sides of a fence.

New Labour's modernization programme

The Labour government that first came to power in Britain in the summer of 1997 initially ended the experiment with competition within an internal market. Therefore, new policies and legislation were introduced in the late 1990s. The internal market was declared dismantled. In reality, its core remained. The separation of planning (or commissioning) and provision of care was retained, as was the devolution of management responsibility for running local healthcare organizations. However, a new emphasis was placed on collaboration and partnerships, rather than competition.

The main elements of the modernization programme were:

- Clear national standards
- Devolution of responsibility for delivery of services to the local level
- Local planning mechanisms to draw together all relevant parties to establish how to meet health needs and how to improve health in the population served
- Grouping general practitioners and other health professionals in primary care organizations to deliver primary and community health services and to commission hospital services for the local community
- Greater emphasis on improving the health of communities through public health programmes, addressing national and local targets to reduce mortality, increasing healthy years of life and narrowing health inequalities
- Improved local partnership working (especially between health and local authorities) to create a whole-system approach to planning and delivering care, particularly for groups with multiple needs, such as older people
- A duty of quality placed on all local health organizations and implemented through clinical governance programmes
- A stronger framework of accountability for performance of local services, to be monitored, managed and independently inspected

To strengthen the modernization programme, the government published a 10-year *NHS Plan* in 2000. This followed a commitment by the then prime minister, Tony Blair, to invest more in the NHS (to European Union average funding levels) and to address public concerns resulting from a small number of high-profile service failures and from prolonged waiting times for treatment. This plan reaffirmed the commitment to the principles of a national health service free at the point of need. Emphasis was put on encouraging local solutions and redesigning existing services to meet the needs and convenience of patients. At the same time, the government published its *Neighbourhood Renewal Strategy,* which required primary care and public health practitioners to play a leading role in addressing health inequalities and regeneration with local authorities and other agencies through local strategic partnerships.

The *NHS Plan* provided a clear national vision of the need for rapid improvement in the health service. Linked to additional investment was a range of centrally set targets, including increases in the number of doctors and nurses, building up additional technology for diagnosis and treatment, and further reductions in access times for patients.

The pledge to increase the level of the United Kingdom's spending on health to the European Union member state average (about 9% of gross domestic product) was linked to the goals of the *NHS Plan.* The extra investment actually came after an independent report by the former banker, the late Sir Derek Wanless, which argued the need for it and also emphasized the importance of reform not just in the delivery system but also in preventing more ill health, conceptualizing this as a *fully engaged scenario.* Wanless later produced a second report, specifically on public health.

The *NHS Plan* was initially widely welcomed by health service staff, professional bodies and external commentators, as it recognized long-standing funding shortages and the way in which the infrastructure of the NHS had fallen behind that of many other developed countries.

The approach was successful at first. For example, long waits in accident and emergency departments were largely abolished, waiting times for cancer care rapidly fell and waiting times for planned operations in many parts of the country became very much shorter. These changes came at the expense of criticism of the way that the service operated. Too many top-down targets were seen as stultifying and oppressive to local discretion in meeting healthcare needs and in pursuing innovation. At the same time, the government remained concerned that the pace of change and improvement was too slow and was not meeting public expectation, especially given the extra public funding that had accompanied implementation of the ambitious *NHS Plan.*

From 2002 onwards, a series of structural changes and incentives were introduced to speed up change, improve services and secure greater value for money. The five key components of this reform programme were:

1. *Choice*: Guaranteeing patients needing planned operations a choice of provider.
2. *Payment by results*: A system of fixed national tariffs for treatments to ensure that money followed patients and to encourage efficiency and competition based on quality of service, not price.
3. *Independent sector treatment centres*: Central procurement of facilities for surgery and diagnostic services to add capacity, as well as to put competitive pressure on traditional NHS services.
4. *NHS Foundation Trusts*: A new, more autonomous form of NHS provider with a membership and board of governors, still part of the NHS but with more freedoms, expected to move farther and faster to achieve levels of excellence.
5. *Commissioning*: Strengthening the role of Primary Care Trusts (PCTs) and general practitioners to shape and improve services.

Towards the end of the first decade of the twenty-first century, the NHS stood part way through a period of tumultuous change. The incoming Labour government of 1997 had initially abandoned the previous Conservative government's unpopular internal market design for the health service, only to readopt it, modify it and develop it further in a quest to create a health system that could meet the needs of patients in an efficient and effective manner while still relying largely on the tax-funded approach that has been the hallmark of the British system since the NHS was created in 1948.

Centrally imposed targets, major structural reorganization, greater investment and performance management drove an initial phase of change. Processes and incentives to encourage reform, improvement and higher-quality services gradually replaced this. The intention was to create more local decision-making, greater diversity in provision, greater choice and personalization of services for patients, stronger emphasis on treatment in primary and community settings and more focus on population health and prevention of disease and illness.

In the summer of 2008, the government published the report of a review of the NHS carried out by the practicing surgeon and health minister Lord Darzi of Denham. This sought to move the NHS from a focus on *quantity* of care to *quality* of care. More important even than the specific proposals was the emphasis on making quality the organizing principle of the NHS at every level and placing clinicians at the heart of the necessary change.

Looking back on this period of unprecedented reform, it achieved many improvements and set a clear direction for a more modern style of NHS. However, major change in any public service inevitably meets resistance and easily becomes politicized. Implementation of the New Labour reforms stalled during the government's last few years in office, and the opportunity to further develop a system that was beginning to deliver sustained improvement was missed.

Coalition government and the Lansley reforms

The 2010 general election led to a coalition government formed by the Conservatives and the Liberal Democrats. Andrew Lansley MP, the long-standing opposition spokesman for health, was appointed Secretary of State for Health in the new government. Reforms to the NHS were introduced very early in the government's life, many reflecting the personal vision of Mr Lansley. Despite previous statements by senior members of the government that there would be no more top-down reorganizations of the NHS, a mere 60 days after coming to power, the government published a White Paper, *Equity and Excellence: Liberating the NHS*, that set out plans for a reorganization so big that 'it could be seen from space', according to the then chief executive officer of the NHS. Ironically, given the extraordinary turmoil the proposed reforms created, most of them had been extensively aired in Mr Lansley's speeches and documents during his long years as shadow health secretary.

The main proposals were:

- Establishing a national commissioning board, independent from the Department of Health
- Abolishing strategic health authorities and primary care trusts
- Moving responsibility for public health to local authorities
- Devolving responsibility for commissioning healthcare to groups of general practitioners
- Creating an outcomes framework through which to hold the NHS Commissioning Board to account
- Setting up an economic regulator to set prices and promote competition

The White Paper provoked huge controversy and hostile reaction, some from those who did not see the point of major, disruptive change as the country's most important public service was facing a period of fiscal austerity, and the rest from those who were deeply unsettled by what they perceived as an ideological purpose behind the reforms. It is now acknowledged that the political handling and communication of the new policies was very poor; indeed, one key figure observed that 'the ideological cart has been put before the political horse'.

The government responded to the row by pausing the legislation (an unprecedented move) and setting up a committee, the Future Forum, to look at the proposals, and enable it to 'pause, listen and reflect'. This Future Forum toned down the proposals to do with competition and recommended the establishment of additional clinical advisory mechanisms within the proposed new local commissioning arrangements. However, even taking on board the modifications that came from the forum, the resulting Bill that entered the parliamentary process was a monster; it contained 309 clauses and was dense and very difficult to follow; as a result, few people read it in its entirety, even many of those who publicly opposed it. The health minister who shepherded it through the House of Lords, Earl Howe, explained why the Bill was so complex:

> The Bill is long and complex because for the first time in statute it seeks to define the functions and duties of every element in the chain of accountability within a reformed healthcare system, and to join up those functions and duties into a coherent whole. Whereas in the past it has been possible for a government to change the NHS simply by direction, in the future it will be impossible to do so without recourse to Parliament.

A key element of the bill, that many saw as having the sinister purpose of opening the door to privatization of the NHS, was the element dealing with the role and accountability of the Secretary of State for Health. Existing legislation required him or her to 'provide' services; the proposed new legislation envisaged a role standing back from day-to-day involvement, with a duty to 'promote autonomy' among organizations within the NHS. This was the focus of much opposition to the Bill and campaigning for it to be dropped.

The Bill was subject to 1000 proposed amendments, many of which were accepted in their original or modified form, making it even more complex as it progressed through Parliament. However, the eventual Act of Parliament contained much of what had been originally proposed and had attracted such hostility. Most of the NHS budget was devolved to groups of general practitioners, the majority of whom had no experience of commissioning, planning or management. The headquarters of the NHS was outsourced to an arm's-length body, the system was to be regulated by two other arm's-length bodies, non-NHS providers would be encouraged to enter the market and the Secretary of State's role would be more hands off.

Aneurin Bevan, the health minister who introduced the NHS in 1948, memorably claimed that 'the sound of a dropped bedpan in Tredegar will reverberate around the Palace of Westminster'. No longer would a health secretary call up this metaphorical image in support of his omnipotence and omniscience. Henceforth, he or she would stand back from the day-to-day running of the NHS – in theory, at least.

NHS management

The structure of the NHS is highly complex (Figure 6.8). The description in the sections that follow is of the NHS as it is after implementing the *Health and Social Care Act 2012* that was described in the previous section. This material can never be completely up to date because the system is constantly being modified and developed. The main description is of the NHS in England. The devolved administrations of Scotland, Wales and Northern Ireland are discussed separately. Their organizational structures and operational mechanisms vary significantly, but the underlying population needs are the same and there are strong common themes in the way that the health service responds.

NATIONAL ROLES AND ACCOUNTABILITIES

Five key bodies govern and regulate how the NHS operates in England: the central government Department of Health (sets policy and objectives and allocates resources), NHS England (the national commissioning board), the National Institute for Health and Care Excellence (sets standards), the Care Quality Commission (CQC) (the regulator of quality and safety) and NHS Improvement (supports NHS

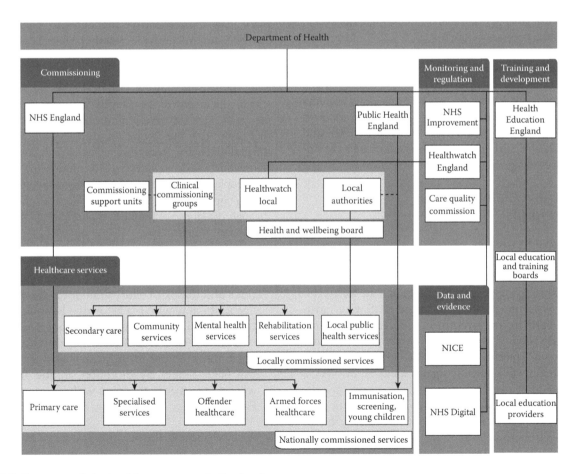

Figure 6.8 Structure of the healthcare system in England.

Source: Adapted from National Health Service (NHS). *Understanding the New NHS*. London: NHS, 2014. With permission.

providers in delivering efficiency and better quality and investigates patient safety incidents).

In England, the Secretary of State for Health is accountable for 'promoting' a comprehensive health service and 'securing' the provision of services. This is a step back from the accountability for 'providing' a health service (that was enshrined in legislation from 1948 onwards) and reflects the redefinition of powers in the *Health and Social Care Act 2012*. The Secretary of State is a Member of Parliament appointed to his or her ministerial role by the prime minister and supported in his or her role by other health ministers (currently five in number). The Secretary of State leads the Department of Health, which is run day-to-day by a Permanent Secretary (a senior civil servant).

The *Department of Health* is responsible for strategic leadership of the health and social care system. Since 2012, the Department of Health is no longer responsible for management and day-to-day running of the health system.

The Department of Health has the following stated responsibilities:

- Lead across health and care through national policies and legislation, providing the long-term vision to meet current and future challenges, putting health and care at the heart of government and being a global leader in health and care policy
- Support the integrity of the system by providing funding, ensuring the delivery and continuity of services and accounting to Parliament to represent the best interests of the patient, public and taxpayer
- Champion innovation and improvement by supporting research and technology; promoting honesty, openness and transparency; and instilling a culture that values compassion, dignity and the highest quality of care

Ultimately, responsibility for all health system goals rests with the Department of Health. Achieving these goals involves strategic leadership of the health and social care systems, which is exercised principally through the production of health policy. Producing appropriate health policy for any health system is a complicated process. In England, the Secretary of State for Health determines policy for the NHS, as well as on health matters more generally, although increasingly, NHS England is taking on more of this role. Civil servants; professional, scientific and technical staff; and health service managers all work in the Department of Health, developing policies and guidelines for the health and social care systems. In addition, special and external advisers and expert committees all advise on health policy. A parliamentary Select Committee on Health also scrutinizes and comments on the work of NHS England and addresses other contemporary themes in health and healthcare.

COMMISSIONING

NHS England is the main strategic centre for healthcare services in England. It performs a headquarters function and funds local clinical commissioning groups (CCGs) to commission services. It directly commissions certain specialist services itself, as well as commissioning primary care services; increasingly, this is either in partnership with clinical commissioning groups or by delegating fully to the latter. NHS England has taken over many responsibilities that historically belonged to the Department of Health.

Clinical commissioning groups replaced primary care trusts, but did not take on all their responsibilities. The public health responsibilities of primary care trusts were transferred to local authorities, and the commissioning of most primary care moved to NHS England. They have, though, assumed responsibility for commissioning most healthcare services for their local population. All general practices belong to a clinical commissioning group. The groups work with patients and health and social care partners (such as local hospitals, authorities and community groups) to ensure that services meet local needs. Their boards are made up of general practitioners from the local area and at least one registered nurse and one secondary care specialist doctor.

National funds are allocated between clinical commissioning groups using a formula that aims to give an equal level of services for people with equal need, and to tackle health inequalities. It builds on a formula that was used to determine primary care trust (the predecessor of clinical commissioning group) funding prior to 2013. The allocation is based on the number of people resident in the group's area, adjusted by three factors:

1. *Age*: Areas with more elderly or very young people receive a larger allocation.
2. *Need*: Areas with higher levels of particular diseases and deprived populations receive a larger allocation.
3. *Higher cost of provision*: Areas with higher costs (particularly labour costs), predominantly London and the southeast, receive a larger allocation to reflect this.

This *weighted capitation formula* gives each clinical commissioning group a target allocation. Its application produces a wide range in allocations between different clinical commissioning groups (Figure 6.9).

NHS England oversees the actions and spending plans of clinical commissioning groups from national level, and supports them in their role of securing high-quality services. The groups commission most services on behalf of patients, including emergency care, community care, planned hospital care, mental health and learning disability services in their local areas. In England, £96 billion of the £107 billion allocated to the Department of Health is passed to NHS England, as the national commissioning body. The remainder goes to local government authorities for public health, and to the administrative costs of the Department of Health and its arm's-length bodies. Of this £96 billion, £64 billion is passed to local clinical commissioning groups. The other £32 billion is spent on primary care services, public health services, services that require specialized commissioning and NHS England's administration.

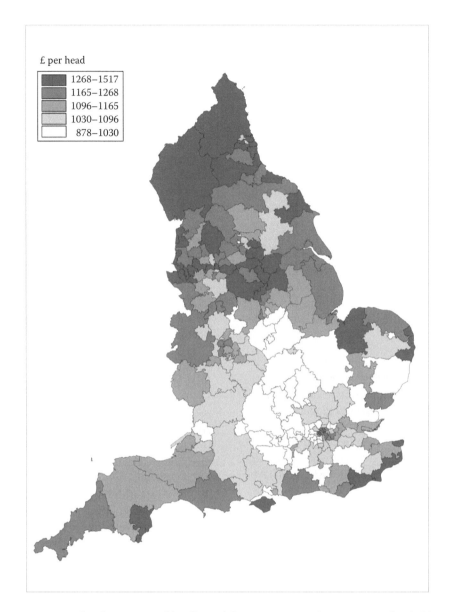

£ per head

■	1268–1517
▨	1165–1268
▨	1096–1165
▨	1030–1096
□	878–1030

Figure 6.9 Variation in per-capita funding received by Clinical Commissioning Groups in England, 2014–15.

Source: NHS England.

As part of the commissioning arrangements, a national tariff is set for hospital services; it is based on Healthcare Resource Groups. Hospital tariffs have evolved since the system was originally established in the mid-2000s. The services covered under them have expanded, there have been changes in the tariff to reflect local prices and variations, and certain services – such as rehabilitation – have been unbundled to encourage care outside acute hospital settings. The national tariff is currently set for hospitals after consultation with clinical commissioning groups and NHS England. Clinical commissioning groups then use this national tariff, and determine which providers they wish to use and what volumes they require. They also have some freedom to agree on price variations locally.

NHS England commissions primary care services from general practitioners. It uses three main contractual mechanisms:

1. *General Medical Services (GMS)*: General medical practitioners operate under a national contract, although there is some local flexibility.
2. *Personal Medical Services (PMS)*: A locally negotiated alternative to the General Medical Services contract that allows greater flexibility on what services are provided and at what price.
3. *Alternative Provider Medical Services (APMS)*: Allows competent providers from any sector (public, commercial or not-for-profit) to provide primary care services, introducing an element of competition.

General practitioners who are paid under the General Medical Services contract receive payment in a number of strands: a global sum linked to list size and workload, payment for meeting quality indicators or targets (the Quality and Outcomes Framework), payment for extra services provided and administrative payments. The majority of general practices operate under either the General Medical Services or Personal Medical Services contract.

The *Quality and Outcomes Framework* is an important part of primary care funding in England. It is a set of indicators used to create incentives to achieve higher standards of care. General practices are allocated points when indicators are met. The overall points score is used to calculate the amount of extra funds paid to each practice. Practices are not required to take part, but most do. This pay-for-performance mechanism has two elements: clinical and public health. The clinical indicators cover a range of conditions. The number of true outcome measures is quite small, with many measuring processes of care (e.g. number of people who have had a blood pressure measurement in the last five years). The Quality and Outcomes Framework is the largest pay-for-performance system in the world (about £1 billion is spent on it). Evaluations of its impact have shown only small gains in quality; this is probably because of the predominance of process indicators, the high attainment of the indicators and that there is no incentive to go beyond the target level.

New organizations have been formed to support and advise NHS England and clinical commissioning groups in the commissioning process. *Clinical Senates* provide clinical advice and support, particularly based on knowledge of the configuration of services in the wider geographical area and in complex commissioning matters. Patients and members of the public are also involved. They provide independent, strategic advice and guidance. *Strategic Clinical Networks* are advisory groups of clinical experts covering a particular disease group (such as cancer, stroke or diabetes), patient group or professional group and offer advice to clinical commissioning groups and NHS England. Their particular focus is on helping to improve care pathways. Both clinical senates and strategic clinical networks provide advice and guidance, but their involvement is not mandatory, nor can their input force clinical commissioning groups to act in a particular way.

In addition to its strategic leadership of the health system, NHS England plays an important role in directly commissioning services. The services commissioned by NHS England are specialized services, primary care services, offender healthcare and services for members of the armed forces. NHS England applies specific criteria to determine whether it will take on commissioning of a specialist service (as opposed to devolving it). In general terms, it does so when local commissioning would be inefficient. The four criteria are the number of individuals who require provision of service, the cost of providing the service or facility, the number of organizations able to provide the service or facility and the financial implications for clinical commissioning groups if they were required to commission the service or facility themselves. The specialist services that NHS England commissions are for rare conditions, and for those that need specialized teams working together. They include services for specific mental health problems, neonatal services and services for rare conditions such as uncommon cancers, burns care, medical genetics, specialized services for children and cardiac surgery. Together, they account for approximately 10% of the NHS budget.

Although Public Health England (PHE) has taken over many of the public health responsibilities in England (through funding public health services in local authorities), NHS England directly commissions some public health services, including national immunization programmes, national screening programmes, public health services for offenders in custody and sexual assault referral centres.

STANDARD SETTING: NATIONAL INSTITUTE FOR HEALTH AND CARE EXCELLENCE

The National Institute for Health and Care Excellence provides national guidance and advice to improve health and social care services, to improve the outcomes for people using these services. This is done by:

- Producing evidence-based guidance and advice for health, public health and social care practitioners
- Developing quality standards and performance metrics for those providing and commissioning health, public health and social care services
- Providing a range of informational services for commissioners, practitioners and managers across the spectrum of health and social care

NICE guidelines represent NHS England's recommendations for evidence-based care. Although NICE is accountable to the Department of Health, it operates independently and makes recommendations based on expert committees. The topics that it addresses are many and varied – across different types of health conditions, medicines, social services and broader community interventions. There are also technology appraisals, looking at the effectiveness of health devices, interventions, procedures and diagnostics. These are intended to help the NHS adopt the most clinically effective and cost-effective technologies.

NICE also has an important role in setting quality standards for health services. It devises metrics and parameters for measuring and driving improvements in quality. The Quality and Outcomes Framework for general practitioner services is set by NICE and updated annually. NICE's role is to independently and transparently produce a menu of measurement indicators that can be negotiated on by NHS employers (for NHS England) and the General

Practitioners Committee (on behalf of the British Medical Association). NICE assesses what Quality and Outcomes Framework indicators are both clinically effective and cost-effective to use and ensures that the indicators adequately reflect its own recommendations and guidelines about effective clinical care.

The newer Clinical Commissioning Group Outcomes Indicator Set (CCGOIS) is produced by NICE and used for assessing the quality of care and health outcomes achieved by clinical commissioning groups. This includes a range of indicators – such as hospital admissions for particular conditions and premature deaths from certain causes. Patient-reported outcomes and experiences of care are included. The indicator set is intended to provide comparative information for patients and health services about clinical commissioning groups.

REGULATION

The *Care Quality Commission* was established in 2009, from the merger of several bodies, as the main agency for inspecting and regulating health and social care service providers in England. It sets national standards of quality and safety and registers services that meet these standards. It has a programme of regular inspections of hospitals, care homes, general practices, dentists and home care services to make sure they continue to meet national standards. The Care Quality Commission reports on the quality of care of services, publishing this information online. This includes performance ratings.

The Care Quality Commission plays an important role in safeguarding and protecting the rights of vulnerable people, including those whose rights are restricted under the *Mental Health Act*. For service providers that are failing to meet the standards, the commission takes action based on the impact of noncompliance with standards. Where people are not at immediate risk of harm, the commission will report on how the provider is failing to meet standards, how they can achieve compliance and actions that they must undertake in a given time frame. There may be warning notices for further noncompliance. In the event of serious transgressions, the commission can issue penalty notices, remove or suspend registration (and ability to provide services) and initiate criminal law proceedings, civil law enforcement or prosecution.

NHS Improvement is the second main regulator for health services in England, although how regulatory its functions turn out to be depends on how it evolves following its creation in late 2015. It was formed from the merger of Monitor (an organization established in 2004 to be responsible for monitoring and regulating NHS Foundation Trusts in England) and the NHS Trust Development Authority (an organization set up to help NHS trusts prepare for foundation status). Monitor assessed NHS trusts that were seeking to become Foundation Trusts (and thus financially autonomous). This involved evaluating the financial management, board capability, governance and performance of these Trusts. Monitor had power to take actions if a Foundation Trust was failing to provide good-quality care. In addition to the regulatory aspects of NHS services, Monitor also set prices for NHS-funded services, tackled anticompetitive practices that were against the interests of patients, helped commissioners ensure essential local services continued if providers got into serious difficulty and enabled better integration of care so services were less fragmented and easier to access. The broad functions of NHS Improvement encompass helping providers of NHS services to become more efficient and deliver at a higher level of quality. There is also a special unit to investigate serious patient safety incidents.

The *Medicines and Healthcare Regulatory Agency* is responsible for ensuring that medicines and medical devices work and meet an acceptable standard of safety. It is also responsible for blood and blood components for transfusion, and therapeutic products derived from tissue engineering. Its main mechanism for protecting the public's health is through regulation. It also works to improve health by encouraging and facilitating the development of new and existing products.

Experts and committees advise the agency in its task of assessing all new medicines to ensure that they meet the necessary standards, and there are ongoing systems of inspection, testing and safety monitoring. Increasingly, new medicines are being licenced via a centralized European procedure operated by the European Medicines Agency (EMA), with which the agency works closely. The *Medicines Act 1968* provides the legal basis, in the United Kingdom, for control and monitoring of medicines, but European Union medicines legislation takes precedence over domestic legislation in many circumstances.

Medical devices have different legislation, and a different approach, to that for medicines. There is no UK medical devices act that is comparable to the *Medicines Act 1968*. Instead, there are a series of European Commission device directives. These require medical device manufacturers to ensure that their products are safe and fit for use. It is not clear how this will apply after Brexit.

A nonexecutive agency board, whose members bring wide external experience, oversees strategic direction and governance. The decisions taken by the agency's own staff (medical, scientific, technical and managerial) in their day-to-day work are supported by reference to advisory committees of independent experts and lay members – in particular the Commission on Human Medicines and the Committee on the Safety of Devices. Using the available scientific and practical evidence, these play a crucial role in providing advice on whether medicines and devices work and are acceptably safe. Legally, the agency's powers are vested in the Secretary of State for Health.

The agency carries out regular inspections of medicine and medical device manufacturers and suppliers, distribution and storage facilities, clinical trials, testing laboratories and blood establishments. Around 3000 samples of marketed medicines are carried out each year at manufacturers' premises, wholesalers and pharmacies. It has a particularly important role in the process of detecting untoward reactions from drugs, and adverse incidents involving medical devices. For medicines, the mechanism for doing this is the yellow card scheme that receives reports from health professionals, patients, carers and parents on suspected adverse reactions to medicines. These reports are evaluated and form part of the wider process of pharmacovigilance by which the risk or benefit of medicines is continually monitored in population use.

For medical devices, the Adverse Incident Reporting System collects reports from users on design faults, poor instructions or maintenance and incorrect use of devices. Risk assessments are carried out and further investigations undertaken with the manufacturer. Based on information gained from reports and investigations, the agency issues medical device alerts within the United Kingdom, and shares information on a range of safety issues with other authorities in Europe and elsewhere around the world. Additional safety guidance of a more general nature is published in device bulletins.

Following new regulatory requirements, the Serious Adverse Blood Reactions and Events (SABRE) system was implemented to capture individual incident reports submitted by transfusion and blood service staff. Annual summary reports are collated across the European Union. Blood establishments are subject to inspection, as are blood banks where indicated by the audit of annual compliance reports. The agency increasingly uses risk assessment methodology to maximize public health gain while minimizing regulatory burden.

The *Human Fertilisation and Embryology Authority* (HFEA) is the United Kingdom's independent regulator of treatment using eggs and sperm, and of treatment and research involving human embryos. It sets standards for, and issues licences to, centres involved in human fertilization and embryology. It also provides information for the public – in particular for people seeking treatment, donors and donor-conceived people. It plays a major role in determining the policy framework for fertility issues.

The *Human Tissue Authority* (HTA) is a watchdog that licences organizations that store and use human tissue for purposes such as research, patient treatment, postmortem examination, teaching and public exhibitions. It regulates the removal, storage, use and disposal of human bodies, organs and tissues. This includes approval for organ and bone marrow donations from living people. Its regulatory authority of these issues is conferred in the *Human Tissue Act* of 2004.

OTHER NATIONAL-LEVEL SPECIALIST FUNCTIONS

The *General Medical Council* (GMC) is the independent regulator of all doctors in the United Kingdom. It sets clinical standards and ensures doctors are qualified to work in the NHS. It does this through monitoring education and training for doctors, and ensuring doctors

are revalidated every five years. It can take action to stop a doctor working if he or she is practicing in an unsafe manner. Similar to the GMC, the *Nursing and Midwifery Council* (NMC) oversees professionals standards for nurses and midwives in the UK through training and education, and investigating those not reaching its standards. Additionally, the *General Dental Council* (GDC), the *General Optical Council* (GOC) and the *General Pharmaceutical Council* (GPhC) are in charge of regulating health professionals working in dental, optical and pharmaceutical services. The *Health and Care Professionals Council* (HCPC) regulates a wide range of allied health professionals, including technicians, therapists, scientists and dieticians.

Operating nationally and locally, *Healthwatch* is an organization designed to represent the public's view on health and social care services. View and opinions are gathered and used to inform the commissioning of services.

NHS Digital is the national provider of information, data and information technology systems for commissioners, analysts and clinicians in health and social care. Its main roles are:

- Collecting, analysing and presenting national health and social care data
- Setting up and managing national IT systems for transferring, collecting and analysing information
- Publishing a code of practice on how the personal confidential information of patients should be handled and managed by health and care staff and organizations
- Building up a database to measure the quality of health and care services
- Improving efficiency in the health system by ensuring that only essential data are collected, and that the system avoids collecting the same information twice
- Helping health and care organizations improve the quality of the data they collect and, by setting standards and guidelines, helping them to assess how well they are doing
- Creating a register of all the information collected, and publishing that information in a range of different formats so that it will be useful to as many people as possible while safeguarding the personal confidential data of individuals

Special health authorities are arm's-length agencies that are somewhat independent from ministers. They were established in 1977, although their number and functions have changed several times since. The number of special health authorities was reduced in April 2013, with a consolidation of their functions. There are now three special health authorities:

1. *NHS Blood and Transplant* safeguards the blood and transplant organ supply to hospitals across the United Kingdom by collecting, testing, processing, storing and delivering blood, plasma and tissues.

2. *NHS Business Services Authority* carries out a wide range of functions that support the NHS administratively, including making pension arrangements for NHS staff, administering the European Health Insurance Card (EHIC) scheme, managing the outsourced NHS supply chain, reimbursing pharmacists and dentists, providing the NHS *Dictionary of Medicines and Devices*, being responsibility for the NHS *Drug Tariff* for England and Wales, managing NHS student and social work bursaries and the NHS injury benefit scheme, and administering health-related services across the United Kingdom, including a low-income scheme, medical and maternity exemption schemes, tax credit NHS exemption cards (in the United Kingdom) and prescription prepayment certificates.
3. *NHS Litigation Authority* provides indemnity cover for legal claims against the NHS and assists the NHS with risk management.

Health Education England and the *Health Research Authority* were Special Health Authorities until 2015, when they became non-departmental public bodies. The former provides leadership for the education and training of the health and public health workforce. The latter protects and promotes the interests of patients, participants and the public in health research, and also undertakes ethical reviews of health services in the United Kingdom.

PUBLIC HEALTH ENGLAND AND LOCAL PUBLIC HEALTH SERVICES

The creation of Public Health England was another feature of the *Health and Social Care Act 2012*. It brought together multiple agencies (including the Health Protection Agency, the National Treatment Agency for Substance Misuse and Public Health Observatories) and additional functions that were previously carried out by the NHS, the Department of Health and several arm's-length bodies.

Public Health England's main aims are to protect health and address inequalities and to promote the health and well-being of the nation. It provides national leadership and expert services to support locally led public health initiatives and to respond to health protection emergencies. Its specific aims are:

- Making the public healthier by encouraging discussions, advising government and supporting action by local government, the NHS and other people and organizations
- Supporting the public so they can protect and improve their own health
- Protecting the nation's health through the national health protection service, and preparing for public health emergencies
- Sharing information and expertise with local authorities, industry and the NHS, to help them make improvements in the public's health

- Researching, collecting and analysing data to improve understanding of health
- Reporting on improvements in the public's health
- Helping local authorities and the NHS to develop the public health system and its specialist workforce

It has a chief executive who is accountable to the Department of Health and has an unfettered right of access to the Secretary of State and the lead minister for public health, to raise any concerns and respond personally to any issues that the ministers wish to raise. The chief executive is supported by an advisory board comprised of nonexecutive members appointed by the Secretary of State for Health. Directors coordinate day-to-day operations. Beyond administrative directors (including finance, human resources and strategy), others lead on health protection, health and well-being, knowledge and a national infection service. The health protection directorate is responsible for health protection services, establishing and maintaining best practice and providing professional advice to government, local authorities, the NHS and the devolved administrations. The directorate is responsible for Public Health England's emergency preparedness, resilience and response capabilities. Within the health protection directorate is the Centre for Radiation, Chemicals and Environmental Hazards, which provides expert advice on these specialist areas to national government and local areas as needed. The National Infection Service has responsibility for infectious disease surveillance and control, acts as the national focal point for coordinating infectious disease responses and discharges many of the United Kingdom's international infectious disease obligations. It leads the national health protection service, including the immunization programme, infectious disease public health and pandemic flu preparedness and response.

The health and well-being directorate is responsible for health improvement and healthcare public health, as well as supporting local authorities and the NHS. It does this by working with, and supporting, local authorities in delivering public health services, leading national health improvement social marketing campaigns and promoting innovation in public health delivery. It is also developing Public Health England's capability in emerging fields, including health economics and behavioural economics. The directorate also has a role in sharing lessons across the public health system, assures the quality of screening programmes and provides public health advice to support NHS England in commissioning specialized services.

The knowledge directorate is responsible for Public Health England's evidence and intelligence service, which includes research, statistics and 'know-how'. This knowledge should inform and support public health practice, and hence drive improvements in the public's health. The directorate promotes an evidence-based approach to public health practice across the system. It works with local government, the NHS and the voluntary and community sectors to provide high-quality, relevant information and intelligence. The directorate works closely with the NHS Information Centre, NICE and the Office for National Statistics (ONS).

Finally, the operations directorate is responsible for ensuring delivery of consistent high-quality services throughout Public Health England. The services include the regional centres of Public Health England, and the health and safety and microbiology services. Public Health England has four regions – north of England, Midlands and east of England, south of England and London. The regional centres are responsible for emergency planning, resilience and response strategy, and continuing the main actions of Public Health England (including professional support to the public health system, ensuring consistency of services and supporting accountability of the system) across their region. Each region has several local centres, numbering nine in total. These provide local health protection, health improvement, drugs and alcohol misuse and public health-care service. They develop and maintain key relationships with local authorities, local resilience forums, the NHS and other partners to support and influence the delivery of public health services. They provide a single point of access to the full range of Public Health England's specialist skills and knowledge.

Until 2013, public health was very clearly part of the NHS at the local level. Every primary care trust (the predecessor of clinical commissioning groups) had a director of public health, with wide-ranging public health responsibilities. The 2013 enactment of the 2012 *Health and Social Care Act* changed this, transferring the directors of public health and most of their responsibilities from the NHS to local authorities. While Public Health England provides national leadership, local authorities are responsible for local public health services. In delivering these responsibilities, they should work closely with regional teams of NHS England, NHS Trusts, Foundation Trusts, clinical commissioning groups and civil society.

The role of public health at the local level is to ensure that attention and action are focused on improving the health of local communities and reducing health inequalities. Tackling deep-seated problems like drug and alcohol misuse, teenage pregnancy and high levels of premature mortality from cancer and heart disease can only be effective through multi-agency action. It is essential also to engage local communities themselves in such programmes. Public health directors in local authorities can play a pivotal role in leading, influencing and mobilizing expertise to create effective multi-agency public health programmes, particularly in the most disadvantaged communities. They also have some responsibility for ensuring that those preventive services that are provided in primary care by general practitioners, health visitors and other professional staff are delivered effectively. Thus, they ensure, for example, that immunization uptake levels are high, that cervical cancer screening coverage is good, that people with hypertension are identified and their blood pressure is controlled and that smoking cessation clinics are working well.

PROVISION OF PRIMARY CARE

Primary care is the first level of contact of individuals, the family and community with a health system. It aims to bring healthcare as close as possible to where people live and work. At its best, it should be about prevention as well as treatment; about ongoing relationships between patient and provider, not discrete care episodes; and about patient empowerment. Primary care serves four key functions:

1. Acting as the *first point of contact* into the health system
2. Composed of care that is provided *longitudinally* (or with *continuity*) during the person's life through personal relationships between professionals and patients
3. Providing a *comprehensive* package of health services that addresses all health needs – not just clinical needs – through prevention, promotion and education, in addition to medical services in primary care and referral to higher levels of care
4. Acting to *coordinate* care throughout the rest of the health system and related sectors through integrated networks

While the United Kingdom benefits from a strong primary care system, citizens in other countries often directly access specialist services, resulting in inefficiencies and increased costs. Health systems with strong orientation to primary care are associated with better and more equitable health outcomes and higher user satisfaction. Health system costs can be reduced and health outcomes improved through focus on prevention.

For many in the United Kingdom, primary care is embodied by their general practitioner, through whom they can access the whole of the health system. In reality, primary care is all services except hospital care and is provided by a huge range of organizations and professionals. This includes pharmacists, community and practice nurses, dentists, opticians and therapists, in addition to services such as NHS 111 and walk-in centres.

General practitioners provide services for a wide range of health conditions. They run clinics, provide health education, offer advice on smoking and diet, give vaccinations and carry out simple surgical operations. They play an important role in managing health conditions and medications over time. They work closely with allied health professionals and organizations – such as midwives, therapists and social services. They act as gatekeepers to the rest of the health system and refer patients to secondary care services as needed. Practice nurses work as part of general practitioners' surgeries to provide important complementary services, including taking blood, performing diagnostic tests, managing minor wounds, giving vaccinations and providing family planning and sexual health advice. District nurses provide skilled nursing care for patients at home and in the community. They are also often based in general practices or community health services. They play a vital role in keeping hospital admissions and readmissions to a minimum and ensuring that patients can return to their own homes as soon as possible after hospitalization. They assess the needs of patients and families and monitor their care. Many of their patients are the elderly, those recently discharged from hospitals, the terminally ill and those with physical disabilities. Health visitors often operate out of general practitioners' surgeries. They are nurses who are trained to visit families with babies and very young children, and older people. They provide advice and parenting supporting, and physical and developmental checks, in addition to having a safeguarding role for vulnerable children.

NHS 111 is a nonemergency medical helpline that was established in 2014. It replaced NHS Direct. A team of trained advisers supported by nurses and paramedics staff it. It responds to public enquiries on a variety of health matters, including nonemergency healthcare and information about health conditions. It provides advice on how to act on symptoms and signs, and directs patients to appropriate services, including accident and emergency, out-of-hours doctors, walk-in centres, community nurses, emergency dentists and 24-hour pharmacies. The service provides professional advice 24 hours a day, 365 days a year. *NHS Choices* (www.nhs.uk) is a health information service on the Internet. It provides a range of information about finding and using NHS healthcare, healthy lifestyle advice (such as smoking, drinking and exercise), news on health topics and information on conditions, medicines and treatments. NHS Choices includes more than 20,000 regularly updated articles and more than 50 directories to find, choose and compare health services. The website draws together knowledge and expertise from organizations including NHS Evidence, the Health and Social Care Information Centre and the Care Quality Commission. The site offers videos, interactive tools and listings to compare services. NHS Choices aims to be a world-leading, multichannel service that will act as a 'front door' for everyone to engage with the NHS and social care. *Walk-in centres* were established in the mid-2000s to provide greater access for people with minor illnesses or injuries without the need for them to make general practitioner appointments. They are particularly convenient for people whose workplace is not near their home. NHS walk-in centres are usually managed by a nurse and are available to everyone. Most centres are open 365 days a year and outside office hours. There are about 100 such centres around the country.

SECONDARY AND TERTIARY CARE

Secondary care involves services of other specialized health professionals. Traditionally, this specialist care has been delivered in hospitals (to both inpatients and outpatients). Increasingly, though, it is being delivered in the community where some services, such as psychiatry and physiotherapy, have been located for some time.

Secondary care is needed for both acute medical conditions (those that occur in a short period of time, such as most injuries and infections) and chronic conditions (which persist for a long period). It also encompasses both elective care (i.e. planned in advance) and emergency care. The

specialisms provided in hospitals include (to name a few) cardiology, dermatology, haematology, liver surgery, ophthalmology, radiology, rheumatology, trauma and orthopaedic surgery and urology. Some hospitals are selective over the specialities they provide (e.g. cancer, cardiovascular and orthopaedic services), while some provide most or all of the range of specialist services.

For highly specialist and rare conditions, tertiary hospitals – located in urban centres such as London, Manchester and Birmingham – provide services for a wide geographical region. These services include organ transplantation, burns care, rare cancer treatments, neurosurgery and high-risk pregnancy and neonatal care. The most specialized of these services are specially commissioned through NHS England.

In England, NHS Foundations Trusts and NHS trusts operate hospitals. In 2017, there were 226 trusts providing hospital and other specialist care, including 10 ambulance trusts. Of these, 145 are foundation trusts. The remainder are NHS trusts. Originally, the purpose of the trust concept was to establish considerable managerial freedom for hospitals, community units and other providers of care or services (e.g. ambulance services) while retaining them under the overall organizational umbrella of the NHS. Each NHS trust is headed by a chief executive and a board of nonexecutive and executive directors. NHS trusts have a responsibility to maintain a balance of services for patients (depending on the type of trust) and to ensure that major investment decisions, such as new buildings and equipment or employing new specialist doctors, are consistent with local priorities.

The foundation trust concept has existed since 2003. NHS trusts that perform to a high standard can apply for foundation status. NHS Foundation Trusts are independent public benefit organizations but remain part of the NHS, subject to its standards and inspection regimes. Historically, they were not accountable to the Secretary of State for Health through the strategic health authorities, and are now not accountable through clinical commissioning groups or NHS England. Although they are not directly accountable, their services are regulated. Local people, patients, carers and staff are eligible to become members of an NHS Foundation Trust; the members elect a board of governors, who are responsible for appointing the chair and nonexecutives to the board of directors and for informing and influencing how the organization is run. NHS Foundation Trusts have additional freedoms beyond those of other NHS organizations. They are not subject to direction by the Secretary of State for Health, can borrow and invest subject to approval by the regulator and have greater operational freedom in meeting national standards.

EMERGENCY CARE

Primary care services, with referral to secondary care as needed, can deal with the majority of health problems. But some conditions require very urgent treatment, because of their severity and time-sensitive nature. Symptoms that should prompt people to seek emergency care include severe bleeding, chest pain, difficulty breathing and loss of consciousness.

In the United Kingdom, ambulance services attend emergencies at home and at the scene of accidents, stabilize the patient and transport him or her to a hospital. This service is offered through the emergency 999 number. Ambulances are no longer scoop-and-run services that simply rush people to hospital. Their trained paramedics are able to provide an increasing level of initial treatment, and in some instances assess that the patient does not need to go to hospital.

Hospitals across the United Kingdom have emergency departments, receiving patients brought in by ambulance and those who attend by themselves. In 2016, there were more than 23 million attendances at emergency departments in England.

INDEPENDENT AND PRIVATE HOSPITALS

The majority of hospitals and other service providers in the United Kingdom are operated by NHS organizations, but some services are provided by hospitals managed by the independent sector (either for-profit or not-for-profit organizations). Clinical commissioning groups may purchase services from independent sector providers. Some people also purchase private healthcare services themselves, paying either directly or through medical insurance plans.

INTEGRATED CARE

There has been a major drive in the NHS – and health systems internationally – to improve integration of care. The term *integrated care* is used frequently inside and outside the health system, but many struggle to grasp what it truly means. By addressing the fragmentation of different health services and support systems, and forming cohesive care pathways for patients, services can become more integrated. This fragmentation is commonly between primary, community and specialist services and wider systems, including education, social care and housing services. Overall, integration

is about refocusing health services to become person centred and coordinated. It involves patients being informed and in control of their care. There is continuation of, and communication between, different healthcare services.

While the drive for integration in healthcare services has existed in many forms – previously called coordinated care, care management or multidisciplinary care – in England, the Department of Health and NHS have put in place measures to promote integration. Commissioners of local services are expected to promote integrated services as much as possible where there is benefit to patients and potential improvement in health inequalities. New ways of encouraging integration are being promoted, such as capitation payment for providers covering community, primary and social care. Flexibility in guidelines and regulations allows integrated services to develop at the local level. Integrated care *pioneers and vanguards* – organizations that have successfully introduced integrated care services – are being showcased for other commissioners to learn from. In general, the trend to increase health service integration has been left up to local commissioners and service providers, with national organizations providing guidance and encouragement. This is in an attempt to promote integrated services that are tailored to local needs and situations, although the extent to which this is happening and how successful they are remains to be seen.

Integrated care is necessary for modern health systems. As health systems aim to address financial burdens from rising multimorbidities and chronic conditions, a whole-person focus and efficient health services are essential.

HEALTH WORKFORCE

The health workforce is the foundation of any health system and, for many, symbolizes what NHS and other health systems are. The workforce in any health system is huge – the NHS employs more than 1 million people (Figure 6.10). In general terms, and either directly or indirectly, NHS staff are there to ensure that the patients or users of health services receive the help that they need, and to promote, maintain

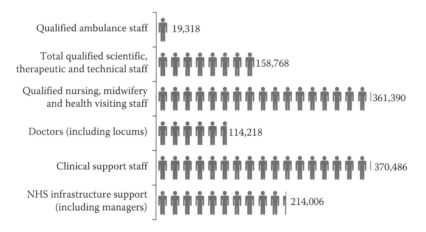

Figure 6.10 The 1.2 million employees of the National Health Service.

Source: NHS Digital.

or improve their health. The health services employ a wide range of professional staff. Doctors, nurses, physiotherapists, clinical psychologists and occupational therapists are examples, but the list is ever increasing. In addition, there are many groups of staff that perform specialist technical jobs – medical physicists and information technologists, for example. In addition to front-line clinical staff, there are health system managers and administrators responsible for functions such as finance and personnel. There are allied and auxiliary staff that support the efficient and effective running of the service by providing a key support infrastructure – for example, drivers, porters, catering staff, ward clerks, records officers, medical secretaries, engineers, laboratory technicians and public relations officers.

The beginning of the twenty-first century saw a much greater awareness on the part of the NHS of the need to identify and address the workforce implications of its policies, and the need for developing staff to be equipped for the new health policies that were being put in place. For example, the traditional role of nurses has been greatly extended into areas such as prescribing, clinical assessment of patients and providing health promotion services. These areas would in the past have been the sole province of doctors, but today nurses have a much greater degree of autonomy. Other professions have extended their roles similarly, while all healthcare professionals, including doctors, have had to further develop their skills in areas such as health promotion, information technology, evidence-based practice and counselling patients.

As the foundation of the health system, human resources are the system's most valuable asset. There is clearly a need to manage this resource well, because issues can lead to devastating problems. First, there is a need for the health professionals to 'be up to the job'. Professional qualification and training needs to be high quality, appropriate to the skill sets required and continually updated. There need to be enough professionals in the health system to meet demands, with the right mix of specialists and professions. There needs to be appropriate management of health professionals. Distribution of the workforce across the health system needs to be well managed and the right tools and resources in place to support services. Staff need to be appropriately motivated to encourage high-quality care, to reduce workers leaving the health system, and for front-line staff to actively improve the care that they deliver.

Around the world, there are major shortages in the professional healthcare workforce (Figure 6.11). There are severe shortages throughout some countries. In others, there are severe distributional inequities, with staff predominantly located in urban and wealthier areas. Problematically, health professionals are not located where they are most needed. First, there are capacity issues with training new doctors, nurses and allied health professionals – especially in resource-constrained settings. Second, much of the existing workforce is inappropriately skilled for their current roles in the health system. Historical training schemes have not equipped doctors and nurses for twenty-first-century roles, with little continuous professional training in recent decades. Third, many doctors and health professionals are leaving low- and middle-income countries to work in high-income countries where remuneration and opportunities are greater. This 'brain drain' is a substantial challenge for the countries that they leave.

Social care

The social care sector is an important complementary system to the health system. The care provided by social services has a direct impact on the health of individuals. In the United Kingdom, social services are the responsibility of local authorities. Older people, people with physical disabilities, those with mental health problems, people who misuse substances and people with learning disabilities are the main recipients of long-term care in the

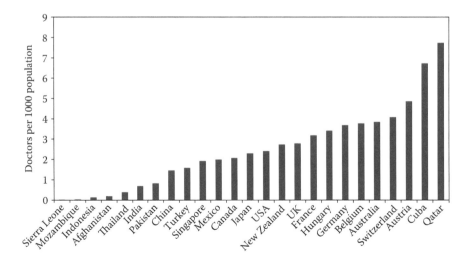

Figure 6.11 Doctor density by country, 2013.

Source: World Health Organization (WHO). *Global Health Workforce Statistics*. Geneva: WHO. With permission.

United Kingdom. This takes the form of residential care – in nursing or residential care homes – and community care – such as day centres, home help or respite care. The *Care Act* of 2014 now underpins the legal responsibilities for social care in the United Kingdom.

There is a substantial degree of overlap between the people who need social care services and those who need healthcare services. The fact that the two are run independent of one another can result in poor communication and coordination between the services. In Northern Ireland, but not in the other countries of the United Kingdom, health and social care are integrated – health and social care trusts provide both. Some parts of England are starting to experiment with pooled health and social care budgets, including through local devolution of these budgets in Manchester.

UK DEVOLVED ADMINISTRATIONS

The Devolution Acts for Scotland, Wales and Northern Ireland devolved most health and social care responsibilities. The organization of these functions differs quite markedly between the four countries, but the fundamental values are unaltered. They aim to stay true to the original ideals of the NHS while modernizing. There are common themes to the direction of travel underway in all parts of the United Kingdom, including developing primary care and ensuring that evidence transfers more rapidly into practice. The interpretation of new evidence may be different, for example, between the Scottish Intercollegiate Guidelines Network (SIGN) in Scotland and NICE in England and Wales, but such differences of interpretation tend to be variations on a theme, not different tunes.

Devolution means that there are four centres of political decision-making in the United Kingdom. The full implications of devolution are still emerging. However, even where different policy priorities may pose a challenge, they also provide an opportunity to learn and broaden the evidence base and experience of what works.

Devolution means the delegation, from Westminster to either Scotland or Northern Ireland, of powers to pass primary legislation in devolved subject areas. The Scottish Parliament and the Northern Ireland Assembly can make primary legislation on any matters not reserved for the UK Parliament. The *Government of Wales Act 2006* enables the National Assembly for Wales to ask the UK Parliament for legislative competence, and responses are made. In practice, most health and social care matters now rest with Welsh ministers.

Certain population protection functions are more effectively conducted on a United Kingdom–wide basis, and so are not devolved and remain as powers reserved to Westminster. In health, these include functions controlling and regulating medicines, medical devices, the registered health professions, abortion, human genetics, surrogacy, xenotransplantation and the prices charged for medicinal products and medical supplies.

MEASURING HEALTH SYSTEM PERFORMANCE

Health systems, as vast and complicated entities, are constantly undergoing change as policymakers, clinicians and patients attempt to steer them towards better fulfilment of their health system goals. Understanding their performance is a complex science. Technologies, medicines, management structures, payment systems, working arrangements and clinical approaches come and go frequently. Health services are being reshuffled and adapting to changes in politics, management and the populations they serve. Most problematically, expectations about what a health system is and what it should provide are always in flux.

Despite this, considerable effort goes into measuring health system performance. First and foremost, this is to inform stakeholders – that is, anyone with an interest in how the health system performs – on all aspects of the health system. This ranges from the efficiency of services, to the quality of care delivered, to health outcomes gained and patient expectations matched. All areas of the health system are up for scrutiny and evaluation. This includes the health systems goals – health, quality and safety, financial risk protection and responsiveness – but also the functioning aspects (e.g. financing and governance) and outputs (services) delivered.

There are important concepts to consider in health system evaluation and utilizing data from information systems. Often simplistic measures are used, and give only superficial understanding. Life expectancy and mortality rates give broad understanding of health outcomes in a country, but give little further insight. What is the distribution between populations and locations? Readmission rates indicate some aspects of quality of care at different hospitals, but underlying differences in the types of patients and severity of diseases encountered must be taken into account. Furthermore, means and averages only provide aspects of performance when ranges – the top and bottom performers – may in fact be more relevant. Often, data are lacking to truly understand health system performance, and so many indicators only allude to true system performance.

Underpinning thorough and useful evaluations are health information systems. The availability of appropriate, timely, accurate and in-depth data is essential for any health system. Information systems relate to every aspect of the health system and vary from patient records to financial flows to recording of hospital outbreaks to patient opinions. Many are essential in providing relevant data and information for those understanding the functioning of the health system. Many countries invest considerable resources ensuring data are collected accurately, stored confidentially and disseminated widely and promptly. There is a large amount of effort put into ensuring the capabilities of organizations to evaluate these data effectively and inform decision-making processes across the health system. The principles of evidence-based care, safety, quality and equity rely fundamentally on in-depth understanding of the health system's functioning. In countries where resources are constrained and investment and capacity in health information systems are limited, all areas of the health system suffer, further hampering health system development. Nonetheless, there is still a great need to constantly strengthen and improve health information systems globally.

CONCLUSIONS

There is no starker reminder of what an unequal world we live in than surveying countries' health systems. Paul Farmer, the Harvard University–based physician, anthropologist and global health pioneer, has said of his time in rural Haiti,

> I convinced myself, at first, that the differences in outcome must have been due to worse injuries, greater impact, more blood loss. But with time and broader experience, I was tempted to record the cause of death as: "weak health system for poor people," "fell through a gaping hole in the safety net," or "too poor to survive catastrophic illness."

Many low- and middle-income countries still have weak health systems with fragmented service provision, current or recent political instability and poor regulation over the wider social determinants of health. Expanding coverage to the poorest populations and generating finances for health systems are problems that are being tackled through combinations of private providers, health insurance systems and tax-funded care or contributions. This is in tandem with major drives to improve governance for health, service quality and provision and retention of professionals. There is still a need for focus on health promotion activities, including vaccination, taxation on unhealthy behaviours and hazards, education and incentives for health-improving activities. Health systems that are susceptible to shocks – large-scale emergence of communicable disease; natural disasters; economic, political or environmental threats – must aim to improve resilience through strong governance frameworks, improving capacity for policy formation, securing health funds, appropriate risk pooling methods and creating flexible service delivery structures.

Health systems are in constant flux as new ideas gain prominence, the health and demographic landscape of the population changes and goals and priorities shift. A great deal of effort is made to improve health systems on an ongoing basis, although a substantial proportion of major change also happens in response to major failures or scandals. Globally, there is a pressing need to strengthen health systems to meet the health needs of populations now and in the future, to reduce the occurrence of major failings in care and to equip systems with the flexibility to adapt to unexpected events.

Even in countries with stronger health systems, there are substantial challenges. Political will and major reorientation of services will be essential to forming health systems that are fit for the future.

Healthcare today is able to offer vastly more benefit to people than was ever the case in the past. New drugs are constantly becoming available. New technologies have revolutionized the treatment of many conditions. One reason why healthcare is costing ever more is that there is so much more that is worth spending money on. But with this comes tough decisions about how much to fund and through what means, and a need to make care highly efficient. The additional problem with non-communicable diseases is that many people have several of them. This phenomenon of multimorbidity does not simply mean that there are more instances of disease to treat. It means that the health system has to deal with people whose ill health is more complex because of interactions between their different diseases. Coordination between the different services – which are traditionally organized by organ system – is not straightforward and often not done well. How health systems adjust to this shift towards complex, expensive and long-term interventions is imperative for their sustainability.

Around the world, citizen views of health and healthcare are changing. The days of doctor knows best are fast disappearing. Patients are no longer passive, deferential recipients of care. The Internet has changed the understanding of health and disease. Hundreds of millions can, and do, Google their symptoms, research their medication, look for new experimental therapies and review feedback from other patients on their doctors and treatments. Patients are becoming consumers. There are increasing expectations, consumer rights and demands for information. The rise of legal cases against health professionals and providers – often in privately dominated health systems, but also in the NHS – is changing the relationship between the doctor and patient. Patients as consumers expect health services to embrace new technologies – whether they be telephone consultations, access to medical notes or an app to manage chronic health conditions. Health systems have to reorientate themselves to a consumer focus, and are being judged by the standards individuals expect of other services.

For any individual healthcare organization, such as a hospital, there are enormous consequences of the rapid growth in demand and changes in user expectations. They are under pressure to balance three imperatives: managing within a financial budget, meeting the needs of patients who present as emergencies and maintaining high standards of care for all patients – in particular, keeping response times short. These can be in conflict with one another. For example, a surge of emergency admissions during winter months due to respiratory illnesses can mean planned admissions being cancelled.

In the United Kingdom, the NHS remains a beacon of universal health coverage with maximum financial protection for those who use it. When viewed internationally, it is generally acknowledged as a relatively efficient system of delivering good health outcomes to the population. However, it is very different to the NHS in its first 50 years of existence. Today's NHS is much less centralist, less planned, more pluralistic in its provision, more consumer focused and more formally regulated. It has the serious weakness, shared by the systems of many richer countries, of not being able to ensure a consistently high-quality, safe, patient-centred standard of care during every encounter. This is why it must continue to adapt, learn and improve and create a sustainable system in the face of ever-increasing demand for more care.

CHAPTER 7

Quality and safety of healthcare

INTRODUCTION

Healthcare is complex – more so than even 20 years ago, when many of today's tests and treatments simply did not exist. Healthcare today involves more specialists than ever before, looking after patients with more conditions, on more medications, receiving their care in more locations. Healthcare offers incredible benefits, but delivering it is difficult.

In today's consumer-orientated society, one of the cornerstones of supplying goods and services is their quality. In turn, one of the principal stimuli in a market economy for improving quality and raising standards is competition among suppliers and providers to produce a better product or service as economically as possible – and to produce one that meets the expressed needs or wishes of the purchaser. Healthcare cannot be a pure consumer market, because it must always protect the needs of the most vulnerable.

In the first half of the twentieth century, in the healthcare systems of western Europe and North America, there was no formal and comprehensive approach to quality assurance and improvement. Much faith was placed in the idea that if standards of professional training and practice were high, they would ensure that the practitioner delivering the service would do so at uniformly high quality. Over time, it became obvious that the complexity of defining and measuring quality in the healthcare field is much greater than in other sectors. This was an impediment to developing formal quality frameworks for healthcare provision. Also, awareness of concepts of quality, ways to measure it and methods for improvement remained low among those responsible for organizing, funding and delivering services to patients. Even worse, the passion for quality and the belief that it should be at the core of any healthcare system rested largely with academics and enthusiasts rather than policymakers, planners and institutional managers. The latter placed more importance on meeting financial and productivity targets than on ensuring that outcomes of clinical care and patients' experience improved year on year.

All this began to change in the later years of the twentieth century and into the twenty-first century. There were four main reasons.

First, a number of quality problems were consistently revealed in studies of the healthcare systems of the richer countries of the world. They appeared intractable, and the solution to them was not primarily money. Prominent among these endemic quality problems was major variation between hospitals and geographical areas in outcomes of care that could not be explained by social, demographic or clinical differences between patient populations. Also, there was widespread evidence of slow translation, in mainstream practice, of the benefits of research into more effective therapies. Most telling were the many examples of care where the experiences of patients and their families were not of the standard that should be expected.

Second, there were instances of highly publicized failures in healthcare provision that shocked the citizens of the countries in which they happened and reverberated beyond their borders. These included high levels of postoperative mortality among children treated by the heart surgery service at the Bristol Royal Infirmary in England, with the subsequent enquiry finding a club culture that put professional interests ahead of the safety of patients; the deaths of patients in the care of a surgeon at Bundaberg Hospital in Queensland, Australia, with the enquiries finding widespread failings in the organization and leadership of the health authorities, as well as major concerns about the doctor himself; and the unnecessary removal of the uteri of many women during caesarean section at Our Lady of Lourdes Hospital in Drogheda, Ireland, with no one challenging this unacceptable practice. While the precise circumstances of each of these service failures differed, there were common features. Although problems often came to light through a serious incident or complaint, subsequent investigation showed that concerns had existed over a much longer period of time but had not been acted on. The culture of such hospitals was often dysfunctional, with cliques and factions creating divisions between different groups of staff and between management and clinicians. When confronted with serious problems in a service, managers and senior doctors were sometimes unsure what to do about them or how to resolve the difficulties.

Third, there was a growing recognition that error was much more common than had previously been recognized, that it too often led to serious harm and death, that incidents such as operating on the wrong side of the body recurred often in very similar circumstances in different parts of the world and that healthcare compared badly with other high-risk industries (such as aviation) in preventing accidents and reducing harm.

Fourth, the struggle to contain the inexorable rise in resources expended on healthcare drove policymakers to seek quality-based solutions transferable from the experience of industry that would reduce costs and increase value.

Moving into the twenty-first century, the healthcare systems of the world's richer nations espoused a vision, and a core purpose, of delivering safe, high-quality, patient-centred care to everyone. Laudable though this shift in emphasis is, many commentators remain sceptical as to whether the reality consistently matches the rhetoric. Variation in outcomes of care remains rife, few avoidable major sources of harm have been eradicated and scandals in individual hospitals continue to haunt those who claim progress. In Britain as recently as 2013, the reports of public enquiries into neglect of elderly patients in Mid-Staffordshire Hospital, and the culture that enabled it to happen, make chilling reading. Moreover, the lamentably low levels of compliance by doctors with hand hygiene protocols in some hospitals rightly leave patients and the public wondering whether they can trust the system to keep them safe.

Most of the policy, research and improvement programmes for quality and safety have been carried out in the healthcare systems of high- and middle-income countries. While the same principles are applicable to healthcare everywhere, the context is very different in the poorest parts of the world. There, access to any care at all is the key consideration. Even where hospitals and other facilities are available, there may be no running water, no clean instruments, no masks or gowns, no identification bracelets for patients, no support to repair or maintain infrastructure, no effective waste disposal and no information technology. The know-how to fix a neonatal incubator can be as important as the availability of trained clinical staff.

QUALITY CONCEPTS AND PHILOSOPHIES

Approaches to quality in healthcare, and thinking about how best to improve it, have evolved over the last 50 years. Many key ideas have originated in sectors outside health, for example, the industrial production line, the world of successful customer-focused businesses or the fields of leadership, organizational culture and team building. Others are firmly rooted in clinical traditions. Each approach has its own underpinning philosophy, its own advocates and its own story of achievement. It is striking how many of the ways of defining and improving quality are attributed to prominent individuals or entities that have conceived and championed them.

Some quality philosophies, their practical tools and their models for achieving beneficial change are transient: flavours of the year (if not the month). New ones are invented and existing ones are seen as dull and dated and become unfashionable. It is tempting to think that if an agreed international framework for defining, measuring, assuring and improving quality had been devised and universally adopted, the world's healthcare systems would perform more consistently and be more transparent and accountable.

There are many formal definitions of quality in healthcare. Most place emphasis on the goal of attaining the best outcomes for patients according to evidence-based best practice (Table 7.1). Over the years, there has also been extensive discussion of what should constitute the so-called dimensions of quality. Lists of these differ, but most include *effectiveness*, *efficiency*, *access*, *equity*, *safety* and *patient-centredness*. Such aspects work particularly well in painting a picture of healthcare at the system level.

In this section, the main schools of thought in quality are set out.

Donabedian triad

One of the most important classifications of quality in healthcare was propounded by Avedis Donabedian (1919–2000). He identified three dimensions: structure, process and outcome.

The first of Donabedian's dimensions of quality of healthcare relates to factors such as the amount and nature of facilities and staff available. This is the *structural* dimension of quality. For example, one determinant of whether a local health service is good or bad is how many hospital beds or senior doctors there are per thousand population. Such structural aspects of quality can be used to compare health services within a country or between countries. Differences can trigger discussions about the adequacy of healthcare facilities available to different populations. They can also stimulate change or improvement. Structural measures alone are not enough to judge the quality of a service. It by no means follows, for example, that one service with a higher number of surgeons per head of population than a neighbouring service will yield better results for hernia repair operations (low in-hospital complication rates and low long-term recurrence rates). Thus, while structural

Table 7.1 An established definition of quality.

The degree to which health care services for individuals and populations increase the likelihood of desired outcomes and are consistent with current professional knowledge

Source: Lohr K. Committee to Design a Strategy for Quality Review and Assurance. In: *Medicare: a Strategy for Quality Assurance. Volume 1.* Washington, DC: National Academy Press, 1990.

measures are important in assessing the quality of healthcare, they are best regarded as part of an overall concept that also embraces process and outcome measures.

The second attribute of quality is what is done for, and to, a patient or group of patients and how well it is done: the *process*. Assessment of the quality of care based on the process approach can be wide ranging. For example, the evaluation of a programme for control of high blood pressure (hypertension) might involve establishing how adequately the population at risk of developing hypertension had been identified, how thoroughly diagnostic criteria had been determined, how valid and accurate were the blood pressure readings that were taken, how other associated medical conditions were detected and managed, whether agreed treatment protocols were being followed, whether patients were complying with treatment regimes, how often patients were followed up and how adequate were their subsequent clinical assessments. All these process measures would throw light on the quality of services given to hypertensive patients. Assessing quality like this involves establishing agreed standards of good practice in the process of care concerned. Then, the actual service can be compared with these standards.

Although the process perspective on quality gives much greater insight than does the structural approach, it cannot be viewed in isolation from it, nor from the third attribute, outcome measurement. Indeed, there is no point in assessing the extent to which a process of care is in place unless the process is one that has a proven effect on an outcome of care.

The third, and final, attribute of quality in the Donabedian framework is the *outcome* of the healthcare provided to the patient. Does he or she survive the illness or disease occurrence? Does he or she get better? Are there any clinical complications? Is he or she satisfied with the care delivered? Outcome is the final arbiter of the quality of care provided. There are numerous possible approaches to defining outcomes of healthcare. One way of doing this is to think about the five D's: death, disease, disability, discomfort and dissatisfaction. For example, assessing the outcome of care for a man admitted to hospital for treatment of a ruptured aortic aneurysm might take account of whether he survived (death); whether the aneurysm was technically well corrected surgically (disease); whether he returned to normal physical, psychological and social functioning after discharge from hospital (disability); whether he remained free of residual pain (discomfort); and whether the interpersonal as well as the technical aspects of the nursing and medical care were pleasing to him, as well as the environment in which it was provided (dissatisfaction).

Donabedian also pointed out that healthcare has different attributes upon which judgements about quality can be made. The health professional's definition of high-quality care would probably rely heavily on technical considerations (e.g. how well the therapeutic or investigational aspects of the care were delivered). On the other hand, many patients would judge the care they receive based on the interpersonal or amenity attributes of their care (e.g. kindness, dignity, respect, explanation, information giving and standards of lighting, heating, food, toilet and washing facilities).

The Donabedian classification remains the most enduring and widely respected conceptual approach through which the quality of healthcare can be defined and assessed. The three attributes of quality are closely interrelated and dynamic. Determining the way in which health facilities (structural) are used (processes) to produce the end result of care for the patient (outcome) is the real route to improving the quality of care. All are important quality considerations, and it cannot be assumed that high quality in one attribute automatically means high quality in the others. For example, a surgeon may be excellent in the domains of communication and empathy with his patients but obtain less satisfactory surgical results than a colleague who is a masterly technical surgeon but treats his patients in an impersonal manner.

Avedis Donabedian remains one of the most revered figures in healthcare quality and was driven by a real passion for the subject throughout his career; he said, 'Quality is something more than an attribute. It is rather the moral force that must animate all who devote their lives to healthcare. Without a personal commitment to quality in our work, and prideful joy in accomplishing it, no amount of organizational artifice will suffice to safeguard it'.

Deming and the 14 principles: Total quality management

In the aftermath of the Second World War, the Japanese were renowned for producing cheap, poor-quality merchandise. American industry predominated in such areas as car manufacture and saw its goods as inherently superior to foreign goods in all respects. But then, over a relatively short time, Japan gained a major share of the North American and, indeed, world markets. The story of how it did so is instructive. It produced and exported merchandise that competed with alternatives on quality and reliability – not simply on price. American consumers began to buy Japanese cars and other goods in preference to those manufactured domestically. The dramatic turnaround in the competitiveness and market position of Japanese industry was grounded in the adoption of simple principles and methods of quality improvement.

Ironically, the man credited with transformation of postwar Japanese industry was not Japanese; he was an American who was largely unknown in his own country. W Edwards Deming (1990–1993) was welcomed and ultimately revered by industrial and political leaders in Japan. He was an engineer and statistician by training and had worked for the U.S. Census Bureau. Deming's approach was based on the idea that, by continually improving the processes of production, expensive consequences such as scrapping defective products, expenditure on warranty agreements and remanufacturing will be avoided. Concentrating on quality yields improvements in productivity, market share and profitability. This is often called total quality management (TQM) or continuous quality improvement (CQI), although today these terms are used generically, rather than exclusively to describe Deming's work.

The traditional approach to quality control in industry was based on the concept of inspection to detect defects. This has major disadvantages. First, it does not gain commitment of the whole workforce. Instead, quality is seen as the business of a separate quality department or inspector. This makes a workforce feel that they are not trusted and implies that they will only achieve a high standard when being watched or inspected. Second, when the process of manufacture is not properly designed and the raw material is inadequate, no amount of inspection will remedy the problem. This approach inspects out poor quality rather than building in good quality to the systems of management and production.

Deming urged reduced dependence on inspection and instead championed involving the whole workforce, using their knowledge and expertise of manufacturing processes to constantly improve them and eliminate defects, errors and poor products. He saw the top management of an organization and the culture it creates as crucial. The overall benefit for a company was the success of its business. Reduction in errors and defects not only increases quality, but also reduces costs (from remanufacture, replacement goods and inspection), improves profitability and, by satisfying customers, gains more market share.

Deming's philosophy was very comprehensive and, in its complete form, was set out in 14 essential principles. At its heart were several fundamental messages: (1) Quality problems were seldom the fault of staff at the front line but almost always lay in a poorly designed system that was management's responsibility to get right. (2) The workforce should be valued, respected and engaged in the business of continuous quality improvement. (3) Measurement was essential to process control and improvement. Deming learned about statistical assessment of performance (Figure 7.1) from the work of Walter Shewhart (1891–1967).

As the impact of Deming's work in Japan became clear, he was increasingly asked to transform companies in his own country. His quality philosophy had, and continues to have, a profound influence on manufacturing and service industries around the world. Some healthcare organizations have adopted it in its entirety, but more often, many of the key principles and methods (e.g. the plan, do, study, act [PDSA] cycle) have been embedded in other quality improvement approaches. Many would acknowledge Deming as the first quality guru. People took up his work with missionary zeal and flocked to his lectures when he was alive. Today, Deming's work still inspires. A society is named after him, and film clips of him speaking about his ideas are frequently viewed on the Internet, where he can be seen uttering his memorable aphorisms, such as 'no instant pudding'. True success in quality improvement is indeed a long-term endeavour. Hence, one of Deming's 14 principles is *constancy of purpose*. It is surprising how this essential philosophy is so casually disregarded in so many areas of modern healthcare.

RAND's leadership on quality: The concept of appropriateness

Another way in which quality can be viewed is the extent to which the healthcare interventions of known effectiveness are properly applied in the case of individual patients. The main concept involved here is *appropriateness*. This is one of the key areas explored over many years by the RAND Corporation and the leader of its health programmes, Robert H Brook. The appropriateness of care can be judged by whether the health benefit expected exceeds the anticipated negative aspects of that care by a sufficient amount. Of course, a number of perspectives can be taken on that idea of 'a sufficient amount'. It can be judged clinically, by the patient or from a societal viewpoint, or any combination of the three.

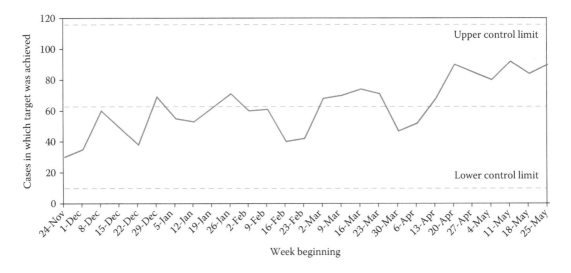

Figure 7.1 A control chart showing achievement of 90-minute 'door to balloon' time for primary angioplasty in one hospital in the treatment of myocardial infarction.

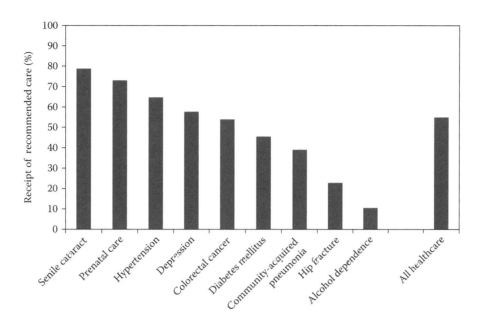

Figure 7.2 A key study showing that many Americans do not receive appropriate care.

Source: McGlynn EA, Asch SM, Adams J, et al. The quality of health care delivered to adults in the United States. *New England Journal of Medicine* 2003;348(26):2635-45.

Table 7.2 Clinical governance: A definition

Clinical governance is a framework through which NHS organisations are accountable for continuously improving the quality of their services and safeguarding high standards of care by creating an environment in which excellence in clinical care will flourish

Source: Scally G, Donaldson LJ. Clinical governance and the drive for quality improvement in the new NHS in England. *BMJ* 1998;317(7150):61-5. With permission.

Appropriateness brings in three important dimensions of quality: *overuse* (providing care where the resultant harm is greater than the benefit), *underuse* (neglecting to provide particular care when it would have produced a benefit) and *misuse*. Extensive study around the world has shown that healthcare systems regularly have patients not receiving a treatment when they would have benefited from it, while others are receiving treatments when they will not derive improved outcome from them. Beth McGlynn, a colleague of Brook, carried out a seminal study that showed that half of Americans were not receiving recommended care (Figure 7.2). The misuse of diagnostic or treatment technologies that increase risks to patients highlights the concept of patient safety, which is discussed later in the chapter.

Clinical governance: The call for clinical leadership and accountability

In the 1980s and early 1990s, issues such as achieving financial balance and meeting workload targets had started to

dominate the agendas of many organizations in United Kingdom's National Health Service (NHS). At the same time, there were troubling examples of poor standards of care where doctors had not always been prepared to challenge the unacceptable behaviour of their colleagues. The concept of *clinical governance* was formulated in the late 1990s (Table 7.2) to provide a unified approach to quality assurance and quality improvement. It addressed the twin concerns that clinical values had been submerged in a managerial agenda and that doctors had to take ownership of the safety and quality of the care that they and their teams provided.

The organizations that make up any health service will vary in their performance against quality criteria. A hypothetical quality curve shows this (Figure 7.3). Healthcare organizations at the left-hand tail of the curve will be those that have demonstrated failures in standards of care, whether detected through complaints, inspection, audit, untoward incidents or routine surveillance. The challenge here is to learn lessons that can be built into future service delivery. Similarly, looking at the innovative organizations at the right-hand tail of the distribution, good practice must be recognized, the scope for more general applicability identified and methods found to transfer it both locally and nationally. This process of learning lessons – from both exemplar and problem services – was never tackled systematically before, and it was an important part of the clinical governance programmes introduced into the NHS at the beginning of the twenty-first century. In addition to addressing these tails of the quality curve, a major movement of any curve of this kind towards improved quality requires that health organizations in the middle range become engaged (*shifting the mean*). Most organizations lie

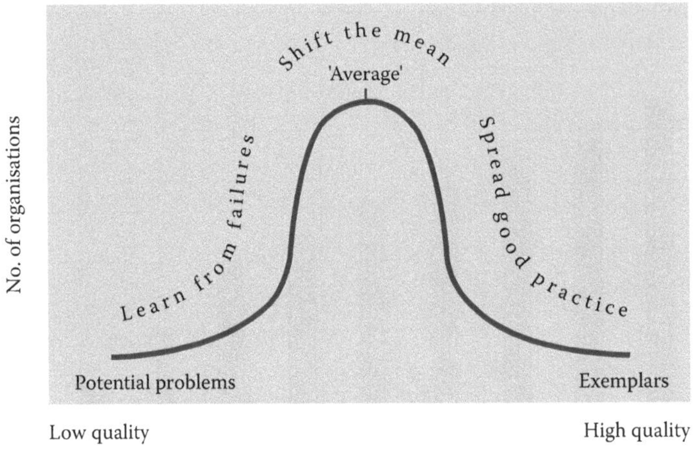

Figure 7.3 Variation in the quality of healthcare organizations and actions required in response.

Source: Scally G, Donaldson LJ. Clinical governance and the drive for quality improvement in the new NHS in England. *BMJ* 1998;317(7150):61–5. With permission.

Table 7.3 Six characteristics of high performing clinical teams

- Excellent clinical leadership
- Management goals expressed as clinical benefits
- Clinical ownership of service performance
- Day-to-day use of data and quality improvement methods
- Eagerness to compare with other services
- Patient and family involvement strong

Source: Adapted from: Donaldson LJ. *Best and Safest Care.* London: Department of Health, 2007

relatively close to the mean, so the thrust of clinical governance is to improve quality in every organization, not simply to concentrate on the best and the worst. The task is largely a developmental one – of organizations and staff. Clinical and management systems, quality improvement mechanisms and the work of teams and individuals all need to be aligned to produce a new kind of health organization.

When considering different hospitals and primary care services, the feature that distinguishes the best from the others most clearly is probably their culture. In an organization where the culture is underpinned with an understanding of clinical governance, high standards become a prevailing purpose rather than a desirable accessory. Patients measure a clinician's performance on what they understand and value. Clinicians communicate their attitude and culture in their daily behaviour when interacting with other members of their team and with patients and their families. An organization that creates a working environment that is open, participative and team based; where ideas and good practice are shared; where education and research are valued; and where blame is used exceptionally is likely to be one in which clinical governance is prospering.

Clinical governance involves the integration of many aspects of quality (including those discussed in this chapter) that had previously been dealt with in a rather fragmented way. The introduction of the clinical governance framework sought to modernize systems for quality control, incorporating established clinical standards, evidence-based practice and learning from the lessons of poor performance. Clinical governance includes all activity and information that allows an organization, and those who work within it, to assure and improve the quality of services locally. Successful clinical governance relies on proper arrangements for accountability that are seen to be effective by the public. At the heart of good clinical governance is a high-performing clinical team (Table 7.3).

When clinical governance was introduced into the NHS in the late 1990s, it sought to shatter the pre-existing medical practice paradigm that good medicine is only about treating the patient in front of you. It opened up a new vision of doctoring, a new mission of practice, that sees a broadening to also encompass a responsibility to assure and improve the quality and safety of care throughout the individual doctor's and the entire clinical team's work.

McMaster and the evidence-based medicine movement

Every day, throughout each health service in the world, hundreds of thousands of decisions are taken by doctors, nurses and other health professionals during the diagnosis and treatment of illness. No systematic approach to understanding the quality of healthcare can afford to overlook clinical decision-making.

For decades, it has been recognized that there is wide variation in such decision-making. International comparisons show, for example, that thresholds for surgical intervention in patients with broadly similar clinical problems vary greatly. Such variation also occurs between different services in the same country and even between members of the same clinical team. It has also long been acknowledged that the science and practice of medicine do not go hand in hand in the way that they should. The failure to translate the results of research into practice quickly and effectively has meant that too few patients benefit in the way that they should from medical advances. It is also one of the reasons why there is wide variation in medical practice.

During the 1990s, these observations led health leaders to look critically at how clinical practice could be made more effective. Particularly influential was the work of David Sackett (1934–2015) and his colleagues at McMaster University in Ontario, Canada. They saw the need for a revolution in medical practice rather than merely a change in emphasis. Clinical decisions in the past had relied on intuition, impression and experience. The new movement saw a future in which many more clinical decisions were based on the findings of valid research relevant to the particular patient's condition. Their first idea was to name the new concept 'scientific medicine', but this caused hostility from their colleagues at the implication that their existing practice was 'unscientific'. They settled on the term *evidence-based medicine* (Table 7.4). It rapidly gained international currency.

It is important to distinguish efficacy from effectiveness, because the two terms are often confused or misused. *Efficacy* is whether the intervention (e.g. the drug or operation) delivers a particular outcome (e.g. restoration of lost function, relief of pain or five-year survival) under ideal conditions. For example, what was the efficacy of the intervention when it was first subjected to research evaluation in a randomized controlled trial? *Effectiveness*, on the other hand, assesses how well the intervention yields the desired outcome under everyday circumstances – such as in a busy hospital service.

Evidence-based practice has been controversial in some circles. Generally, health policymakers and managers have welcomed it enthusiastically as a route to improving quality and reducing clinical variation. Within the health professions, too, it has generally been embraced – but not everywhere. Some have seen it as implying the end of clinical judgement based on experience and the dawn of cookbook medicine. This is not the aim of evidence-based practice. There is an important place for traditional skills (the art of medicine), but clinical judgements should have a strong scientific basis as well as an experiential one.

The introduction of an evidence basis to professional practice, and to healthcare more generally, is a complex task involving a number of important steps (Figure 7.4).

Table 7.4 Evidence-based medicine

A process of life-long, self-directed learning in which caring for patients creates the need for clinically important information about diagnosis, prognosis, therapy; clinicians should:
• Convert these information needs into answerable questions.
• Track down, with maximum efficiency, the best evidence with which to answer them (whether from clinical examination, the diagnostic laboratory, the published literature, or other sources).
• Critically appraise that evidence for its validity (closeness to the truth) and usefulness (clinical applicability).
• Apply the results of this appraisal in their clinical practice.
• Evaluate their own performance.

Source: Sackett DL. *Evidence-Based Medicine: How to Practise and Teach EBM.* 2nd ed. Edinburgh: Harcourt Brace, 2000.

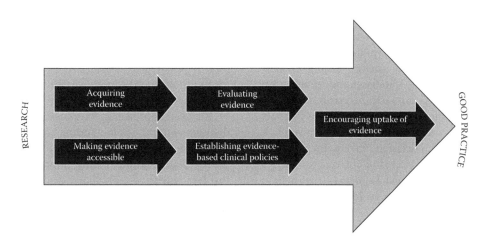

Figure 7.4 Evidence-based practice – key steps and activities.

Source: Adapted from: Donaldson LJ. *Best and Safest Care.* London: Department of Health, 2007.

Wherever there is a lack of research evidence in relation to the diagnosis or management of a particular disease, research needs to be commissioned to fill in the gaps.

Using the results of research studies to aid a clinical decision is not straightforward either. For example, a women patient aged 65 years who has suffered a number of transient ischaemic attacks may or may not benefit from an invasive carotid endarterectomy. How many studies are necessary before the correct use of the intervention is proven? How good are the studies on which current evidence is based? Does the evidence apply to all patients with transient ischaemic attacks, or were the original studies limited to selected groups of patients? These are just some of the questions that are raised when the use of information from published research studies is considered. The importance of evaluating the quality of the research evidence is now appreciated. Thus, for example, one clinical trial on the use of therapy may not have been big enough to yield a benefit in the treatment compared with the control group (if such a benefit was present). Five clinical trials may not be enough to constitute good evidence if they were all flawed in their methodological design. Part of the task of developing evidence-based practice involves ensuring that health professionals are trained in the evaluation of research evidence. Techniques and training programmes have been devised to enable health professionals to acquire so-called *critical appraisal skills*.

Different types of evidence may be available, of differing quality, depending on the state of research in the particular field. It is important to be clear what quality of evidence is being relied on to formulate a clinical policy. As the chapter on epidemiology describes, a *systematic review* is a type of secondary research that takes the findings of original (primary) research studies and carefully assesses them using a strict set of criteria. Often, this will mean pooling data from the original studies and reanalysing them, a technique called *meta-analysis*. It is important to recognize that this form of secondary research is itself open to bias if the methods are wrongly applied or if it is undertaken superficially. Just as there can be bad randomized controlled trials, there can also be bad systematic reviews and bad meta-analyses.

Clinical staff cannot be expected to undertake this evaluation themselves, from scratch, before taking clinical decisions across a busy service. Databases and information systems provide topic-based summaries of research evidence that can be made available to health professionals in short easy-to-assimilate form – summaries and advice given in a way that is of help to clinical decision makers. Increasingly, evidence is contained within electronic interfaces with the clinician – so-called *decision support systems* – that help to prompt, provide options and challenge decisions.

The Toyota Tradition: Stop the line and lean thinking

The Toyota Motor Manufacturing Company is renowned for its decades-long commitment to quality control and quality improvement. One widely cited feature of what is really a multifaceted, holistic approach to quality is Toyota's stop-the-production-line practice. Each member of staff is expected to take full responsibility for the quality of his or her work and to try never to pass on poor quality to the next stage. If something unusual happens in the manufacturing process, workers are taught that they should pull the cord. Pulling the cord stops the production line moving and sounds an alarm, bringing managers over to see what the problem is. They fix the immediate problem, and the team leader pulls the cord again to let the line continue. That way, no quality problems are passed on to the next person.

Vitally, though, the Toyota approach puts great emphasis on preventing recurrence of problems by examining the causes and taking appropriate countermeasures to correct them. Countermeasures are grouped into those involving machinery and equipment, and those involving the process flow. Toyota always seeks to find the root cause of problems. The company encourages staff to keep asking, 'Why?' Experience has been that finding the real cause will require 'Why?' to be asked at least five times before the problem is truly understood and action taken to stop it from recurring. When the pull cords were first installed, they were pulled several times in every shift. But as time went on and the underlying problems were dealt with, the line ran more smoothly and the pull cords were needed less frequently.

An equivalent approach has been implemented in some hospitals, as a means of reducing poor quality. Anybody encountering a situation of poor quality is encouraged to 'pull the cord' – usually by phoning a specific number (the cord is metaphorical rather than literal). This immediately convenes a team of people who can address both the immediate issue and its underlying causes.

The origin of *Lean*, with the help of W Edwards Deming, was also in the company philosophy of car manufacturer Toyota. The core concept is the elimination of *waste* (the Japanese term for this waste is *muda*). A car production line involves workers taking a series of steps. Many of these are valuable, contributing towards the overall goal of converting raw materials into a car. But some steps do not add value, because there is duplication or unnecessary paperwork, or because an error is made and additional work is then required to correct it. Waste occurs in a number of forms: time, money, physical resources or impaired customer experience.

The Lean approach involves assessing a process in detail, distinguishing the value-adding steps from the non-value-adding steps, and taking action to remove the latter. The practical application of this improvement model usually involves intensive workshops over three to five days, in which workers released from their normal duties map out one or more processes, identify the wasteful steps, design ways to improve the processes and then test these in practice. This is a rapid cycle process that may involve multiple iterations in changing the process and studying the result.

The original Toyota idea was communicated much more widely when business experts packaged it as

Lean thinking. This attracted great interest in the concept because business leaders saw the potential for its application to their work.

For Lean to succeed, those involved need to be willing to see their work as a process and to see utility in the concept of reducing waste. With the right attitude, organizational culture and leadership, people can see a great deal of waste in healthcare and be motivated to reduce it. Among those who do not fully understand the Lean approach and its Toyota traditions, there have been many concerns about its widespread application. There are many partial applications of Lean thinking that place the major emphasis on cost-cutting or bringing in outside management consultants to redesign processes. The true basis of Lean is a continuous quality improvement approach. It incorporates a number of different improvement models, bound together by a philosophy about processes and how best to improve them. Understanding concepts like *value, value streams* and *flow*, and how to facilitate change, is at the heart of achieving positive improvement. The full engagement of staff is essential and not something that can be sidestepped and outsourced.

Six Sigma: The Motorola and General Electric way

Six Sigma is another quality improvement method with its origins in manufacturing industry. Motorola originally developed it in the mid-1980s. General Electric, a major U.S. corporation, took it up when its charismatic chief executive Jack Welch was at the helm. This brought it to much wider attention, and subsequently many companies around the world adopted it.

Six Sigma is a statistically based idea. The approach involves measuring and reducing the variation in the performance of a process. Sigma is the Greek symbol used to denote standard deviation. The desired variation is expressed in standard deviations from the mean. A Six Sigma performance would be pretty close to perfect: 99.9999998% of results would fall within the acceptable performance limits, equating to a rate of two defects in every billion opportunities. An *opportunity* is any point in the operation of the process where and when things could go wrong. The usual tolerance level is set at less than 3.4 defects per million opportunities. If this is met, or bettered, then the system concerned will be operating at a very high level of quality. There is great variation in rates of defects between industries, with healthcare being one of the worst.

The Six Sigma approach uses a set of tools and methods, including an improvement cycle based on *define, measure, analyse, improve, control.* It is used extensively in the manufacturing industry. Its application to service industries, including healthcare, depends on the amount and quality of available information about the inputs and key processes that determine results. Six Sigma is a very data-driven approach to quality improvement and cannot really be used where appropriate data are lacking.

Clinical standards and audit

Three concepts are firmly part of the traditional ethos of clinical quality: *standards, practice guidelines* and *clinical audit.* There are many definitions, but those developed by the U.S. Agency for Healthcare Research and Quality (AHRQ) are widely used.

According to AHRQ, standards are 'authoritative statements of satisfactory levels of performance that can range from minimum, through acceptable, to excellent'. Standard setting is something for all members of a clinical team to aim for, but it should be based on the best available medical evidence and knowledge. Many professional bodies – such as, in the United Kingdom, medical royal colleges and specialist associations – produce standards for particular areas of clinical practice. In England and Wales, the National Institute for Health and Care Excellence (NICE) produces standards for the NHS and social care system. These are concise statements whose purpose is to drive measurable quality improvements in particular areas of health or care. They are derived from the best available evidence and developed independently, in collaboration with health and social care professionals, their partners and service users.

Clinical or practice guidelines are 'systematically developed statements to assist practitioner and patient decisions about appropriate healthcare for particular circumstances'. Their purpose is to promote good clinical performance. A wide range of professional and academic bodies publish such guidelines. The National Institute for Health and Care Excellence produces guidelines for the NHS.

Clinical audit is an improvement model, although not always described as such. It involves health professionals critically examining their own, and one another's, practice, so that the lessons learned from such scrutiny can be used to make improvements in professional practice. The process of effective clinical audit involves progressing around the *audit cycle* (Figure 7.5). Key components of the cycle are setting standards based on evidence, and then comparing current practice against these standards. Clinical audit can be an effective tool; it is the longest-established improvement model used by clinicians. Too commonly, clinical audit is seen as a one-off event of analysing current practice. It is only of use in improvement if this analysis results in changes being made, and these changes are further studied.

Institute for Healthcare Improvement: Collaboratives and the improvement model

The Institute for Healthcare Improvement based in Boston, and one of its founders, Donald M Berwick, has played a very important role in focusing the attention of leaders of health systems around the world on quality improvement.

Over the years, the Institute has developed a wide range of methods and programmes that have had a high impact on the design of healthcare. It is particularly known for using *improvement collaboratives.* These bring together teams,

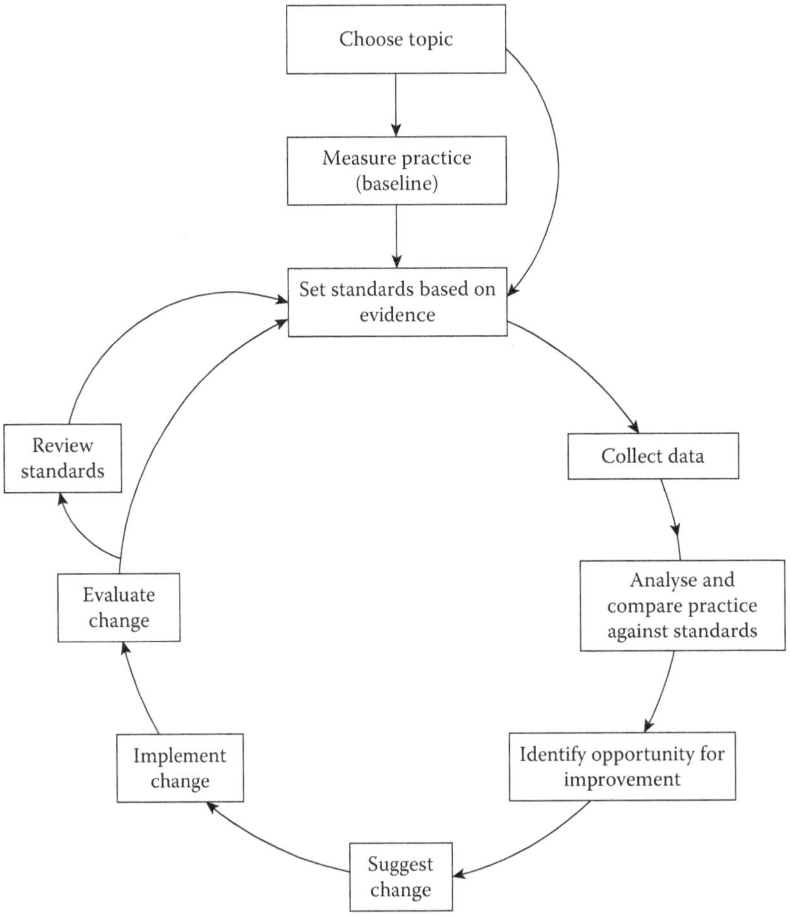

Figure 7.5 The clinical audit cycle.

typically of 25–50 people, who are working on similar projects. At a series of events timetabled over a period of several months, the teams share experiences as their projects progress, and distil best practice. Specialists in quality improvement are often present to provide advice and support. The teams could be from different wards in a hospital, from different hospitals or even from different countries.

The *model for improvement* (Figure 7.6) has become well known through the efforts of the Institute for Healthcare Improvement but was actually developed by the U.S.-based Associates in Process Improvement. Their work, in turn, draws particularly on the teachings of W Edwards Deming. The model for improvement is simple. It guides the project team through three questions: What are we trying to accomplish? How will we know that a change is an improvement? What changes can we make that will result in improvement? The idea is that these questions facilitate discussion within the team, help identify the key data that are needed and force clarity about what the problems and potential solutions are. The questions are useful in a vast range of different areas. The problem at hand might be long waits for orthopaedic operations, poor patient experience in a particular ward or variability in the prescription of appropriate antibiotics within a medical unit. All these, and many more, are amenable to improvement starting with the three questions.

The second half of the improvement model is the *'Plan, Do, Study, Act' (PDSA)* cycle. Based on answering the three questions, the team plans what they can change about their current system that might result in the desired improvement. Examples might include introducing an antibiotic protocol, or changing the anaesthetic rota to allow more orthopaedic operations to be completed in each operating session. The plan is implemented (do). Its effect is then studied, using the data measures that the team decided on when they answered the question 'How will we know that the change is an improvement?' They then act on their findings, perhaps making further amendments, and so enter a further PDSA cycle. The intention is to move rapidly around the cycle. Several iterations are often required before a process change results in the best possible improvement.

Some view such models with scepticism, because they can appear little more than common sense. This is an unfair criticism. When people try to make improvements without following a model such as this, they too often leap into the stage of changing something without working through the vital underpinning questions, and then do not follow through to understand whether the change has worked, whether it has truly created an improvement and whether further improvement is possible. The value of models such as this is that they are indeed simple – but not simplistic.

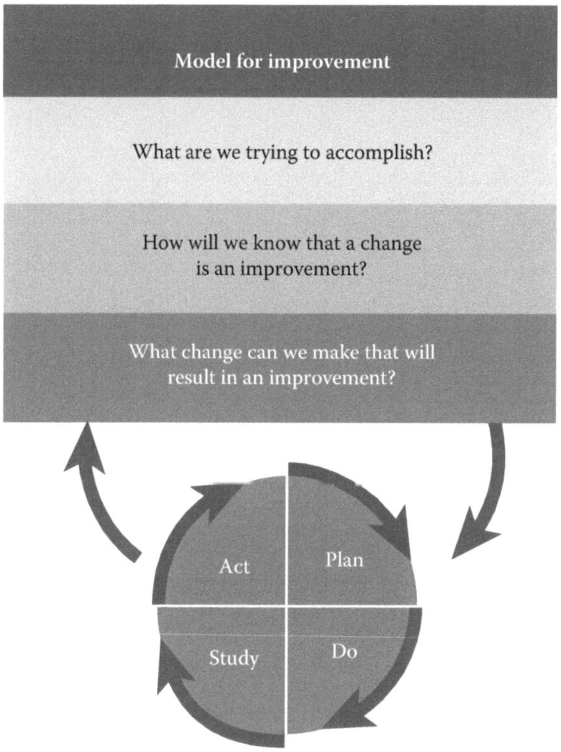

Figure 7.6 The Model for Improvement.

Source: Langley GJ, Nolan KM, Nolan TW, Norman CL, Provost LP. *The Improvement Guide. A Practical Approach to Enhancing Organizational Improvement.* San Francisco: Jossey Bass, 1996. With permission.

Don Berwick has worked extensively in the NHS in England and Scotland, facilitating change through large improvement collaboratives in fields such as primary care and cancer services.

Standardization: The world of checklists and standard operating procedures

Traditionally, medicine has not embraced the need to standardize procedures carried out in healthcare. This approach has been used in other sectors to assure the quality of products and services, as well as to reduce risk in situations where safety is paramount. In the early years of the twenty-first century, though, some developments started to challenge the status quo in healthcare.

Drawing parallels with the importance of checklists used in the airline industry, the World Health Organization devised and implemented a *safe surgery checklist*. It is a list of seven items that should be completed before a patient is given an anaesthetic, a further seven before the operation starts and five before the patient leaves the operating theatre. All are simple, such as 'Has the patient confirmed his/her identity?' and 'Does the patient have an allergy?' Without the checklist, good healthcare professionals do these things most of the time. But they do not do them all the time – with the result that some people have the wrong

operation, or are given a drug to which they are allergic. Initial research suggested that using this checklist could reduce the risk of surgery-associated death. Subsequent studies have also found reductions, although the size of the impact has varied. The checklist is now a beneficial, established part of surgical practice as long as it is used correctly. The World Health Organization went on to develop a safe childbirth checklist.

A different approach to standardization of practice has emerged with the concept of the *care bundle*. This is a small set of evidence-based interventions for a particular patient population and healthcare setting. One of the first, and best-documented, applications of a care bundle was to reduce central-line-associated bloodstream infections in intensive care patients. Professor Peter Pronovost, a critical care physician at Johns Hopkins Hospital in Baltimore, has led the work. He is also director of the Armstrong Institute for Quality and Safety and a global patient safety leader. He reduced the incidence of central-line-associated bloodstream infections by two-thirds in intensive care units across the state of Michigan (Figure 7.7), saving 1500 lives and $100 million annually. This involved no new clinical intervention – just a set of tools to help health professionals reliably apply best practice when inserting, and then maintaining, a central line. The initiative has been applied widely in other parts of the United States and elsewhere in the world, with similar impact. What has been learned from the implementation sites is that it is not enough to make staff aware of the bundle and require them to use it. Such an approach will meet with resistance and noncompliance. Cultural change, organizational development, staff engagement and team building must be introduced alongside the technical intervention of the care bundle.

Bundles, checklists and standardized operating procedures are particularly helpful in reducing inappropriate variation in the treatment given to patients. When a patient in hospital develops sepsis, very good research evidence shows what treatment he or she needs. Every medical student is taught how to treat sepsis, and the knowledge is retaught and retested in specialty exams. But when a patient becomes septic, does he or she reliably receive this treatment? No. This effect is compounded when there are several different elements to the treatment of a condition. In sepsis, for example, there are four main actions that should be taken within the first three hours. Each of these is done most of the time. But if, for example, each of the four actions is done in 80% of cases, the likelihood of all four actions being completed is just 40%. Increasing standardization – whether through a care bundle, a computerized order set or a checklist – can greatly increase successful outcomes of care, including saving lives.

PATIENT SAFETY

A careful, conscientious approach to clinical practice has always been part of the training and ethos of health professions. Similarly, reducing risks and seeking maximum benefits has been essential when introducing new medicines and

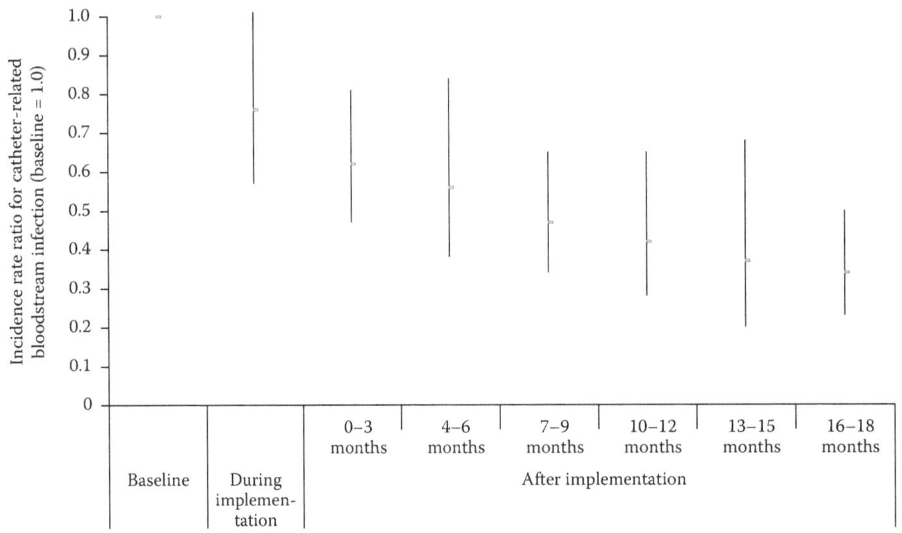

Figure 7.7 An intervention to reduce the incidence of catheter-related bloodstream infection in the intensive care unit.

Source: Pronovost PJ, Needham D, Berenholtz SM, et al. An intervention to decrease catheter related bloodstream infection in the ICU. *New England Journal of Medicine* 2006; 355: 2725–2732.

equipment into the healthcare arena. Yet, these traditions have not prevented the daily occurrence of harm to patients around the world. The question of patient safety came to the attention of the public, clinicians, health leaders and politicians as a result of two influential reports published at the beginning of the twenty-first century. The first, in the United States, was an Institute of Medicine report called *To Err Is Human*. In this report, it was estimated that as many as 98,000 deaths occurred in the United States every year as a result of medical error. The report equated this to one jumbo jet crashing every day of the year. The shock and outrage produced continues to drive action to reduce the risks of healthcare. Around the same time, the chief medical officer for England (one of the authors of this book) published *An Organisation with a Memory* in the United Kingdom. Both reports set out a direction for making healthcare safer and called for patient safety to be given priority in the provision of health services, in research and in the education and training of health professionals. Within a few years, the World Health Organization had launched a major programme on patient safety that moved action to a global level.

Burden of harm

At the outset of the patient safety movement, the term *error* or, more often, *medical error* was used to describe adverse outcomes caused by mistakes or flaws in the delivery of care. Today, the broader term *harm* is more often used to describe the diversity of things that go wrong in healthcare with consequent impact on patients. Other terminology – for example, *incident*, *adverse event*, *near miss*, *close call* and *never event* – is used when discussing patient safety, but there are no universally agreed formal definitions of these terms.

Studies of the care of hospital patients around the world have shown the occurrence of harm ranging from

3.5% to 20%, about half of it avoidable. Based on a crude average of these research studies, many people quote 1 in 10 hospital admissions as involving error in the patient's care as a ballpark figure.

There is consistency in the types of harm that occur in high-income countries. In low-income countries, the lack of infrastructure, facilities and access throw up very different sources of harm. In North America, Europe, Australasia and many parts of Asia and the Middle East, the analysis of information in incident reports and the findings of patient safety research studies show a strikingly consistent pattern. Patients in hospitals around the world die unnecessarily, and are avoidably injured or disabled, due to acquired infections, falls, missed and delayed diagnoses, poor clinical management of acute illnesses, pressure sores, mistakes in the administration of medicines or in the conduct of procedures, faulty or misused equipment, inexperienced and incompetent staff and many other factors. The amount of each type of harm varies, but the overall burden has changed little over the last decade despite the unprecedented priority that has been given to patient safety within these health systems. Little is known about the level and nature of harm in primary care, although more attention is now being given to it.

The patient safety research agenda set by the World Health Organization reflects both the big gaps in present knowledge and the differing needs, priorities and concerns between low-, middle-, and high-income countries (Table 7.5).

Importance of systems thinking

In the past, healthcare systems showed little sign that they could learn systematically from their mistakes. They did not enable the bad experience of one patient to be used to make

Table 7.5 Priorities for patient safety research

Low-income countries	Middle-income countries	High-income countries
1. Counterfeit and substandard drugs	Inadequate competencies and skills	Lack of communication and coordination (including coordination across organizations, discontinuity and handovers)
2. Inadequate competencies and skills	Lack of appropriate knowledge and transfer	Latent organizational failures
3. Maternal and newborn care	Lack of communication and coordination (including coordination across organizations, discontinuity and handovers)	Poor safety culture and blame-oriented processes
4. Healthcare-associated infections	Healthcare-associated infections	Inadequate safety indicators
5. Unsafe injection practices	Maternal and newborn care	Adverse drug events due to drugs and medication errors
6. Unsafe blood practices	Adverse events due to drugs and medication errors	Care of the frail and elderly

Source: World Health Organization (WHO). *Global Priorities for Patient Safety Research*. Geneva: WHO, 2009. With permission.

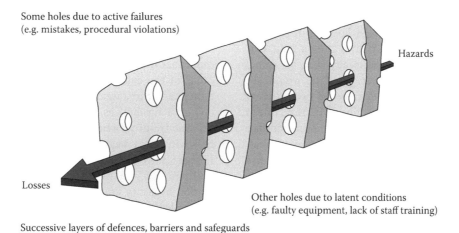

Figure 7.8 The Swiss Cheese model of accident causation.

Source: Adapted from Reason J. *Managing the Risks of Organizational Accidents*. Farnham: Ashgate Publishing, 1997.

the care of future patients safer. This is still the case in many places.

At the beginning of the twenty-first century, a new kind of thinking was introduced to healthcare. In the past, errors leading to medical accidents and harm to patients had been seen as parochial, one-off events that were unlikely to be repeated. A new view began to emerge when experts in other fields of risk and accident science began to take an interest in healthcare. Prominent among these was Professor James Reason of the University of Manchester in England. His view of accident causation compares the risks of something going wrong to the holes in the slices of a Swiss cheese, a powerful metaphor (Figure 7.8). The solid parts of the slices of cheese are the systems defences, and the holes are the vulnerabilities. Unlike the holes in real Swiss cheese, the holes in the imaginary slices of cheese – the organization's system

– are constantly opening, closing and shifting position. Danger arises when a set of holes line up. Some of the holes – the risks – are caused by unsafe actions committed by individuals. These are slips, lapses, mistakes or violations of procedures. However, many more are due to so-called *latent conditions*. These are factors in the system – such as lack of training, poor equipment and absence of procedures – that create preconditions for failure. When human error occurs in the presence of these latent conditions, a serious incident can happen. The importance of the Swiss cheese analogy is that it helps to encourage systems thinking and a preventive approach based on anticipating risks and trying to reduce them.

A *system*, whether in healthcare or any other sector, is composed of the processes, actions, interactions, interventions, ways of working, technology, relationships and human

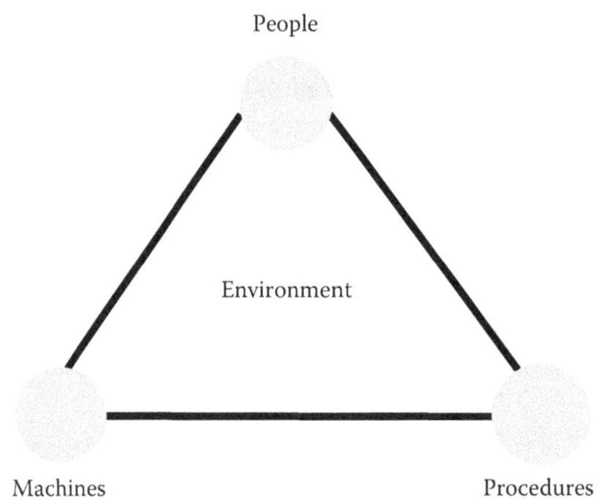

Figure 7.9 Thinking Systems: Interfaces and Interactions.

behaviours that produce results, intended and unintended. Primarily, it is an interaction between people, procedures and machines, with the crucial influence of the physical and social environment playing a key role (Figure 7.9).

This systems perspective was taken in the investigation of the tragic death of a teenager in a hospital in the East Midlands area of England in 2001. He was given a drug, vincristine sulphate, by injection intrathecally (into his spine) when it should only ever have been given intravenously. For treatment of his cancer, he in fact needed two different drugs, one to be given intravenously (vincristine) and one to be given intrathecally. The two syringes looked very similar. He was given the vincristine by the wrong route, so a treatment that was intended to play a part in saving his life was responsible for his paralysis and death. In short, a mix-up proved catastrophic for the teenage patient.

Professor Brian Toft carried out the investigation, and his report is still the best of its kind in the public domain. It reveals a classic accident with some 40 things that went wrong. He concluded, 'The evidence presented to this inquiry suggests that the adverse incident that led to Mr Jowett's death was not caused by one or even several human errors but by a far more complex amalgam of human, organisational, technical and social interactions'.

Two junior doctors committed the error when they administered the medication by the wrong route, but their error was provoked by a system riddled with weaknesses. It was *error prone*. The vulnerability of such patients to this form of harm is emphasized by around 70 similar incidents having been reported worldwide at the time (others may have gone unreported). This is a very rare but catastrophic event. But it was not a one-off, special event to be regretted and nothing else. If the same kind of harm occurs to different people in different places at different times, then there will be common factors and, potentially, a systemic cause (an *error trap*). The solution needs to address the underlying weaknesses in the system that provoked the particular error.

In the case of the vincristine administration errors, work was subsequently undertaken to devise a standard protocol for intrathecal chemotherapy; however, the ultimate need was for a design solution that made it impossible to connect an intravenous syringe to a spinal tap device. This has taken a long time to develop but is now commercially available.

So, while on the surface serious medication errors like this seem to be tragedies caused by human error, doctors making fatal mistakes, investigations almost always reveal a cause that is far from being a simple human error. The true cause of the catastrophe in the vincristine incidents was human error in a weak system: a weak safety culture, weak operational practices, weaknesses in the presence of protocols and training, weaknesses in communication and weaknesses in the packaging and design of drugs and equipment. In short, the cause is comprehensive systems weaknesses.

There is a very nasty twist in this tale. In 2007, information began to emerge from China of cases of paralysis among leukaemia patients who had been treated in hospital with the drug methotrexate. This drug is given by the intrathecal route, as part of chemotherapy regimes. It is now clear that in the manufacturing plant of a large Chinese, state-owned pharmaceutical company, methotrexate had become contaminated with traces of vincristine, which was also being manufactured at the plant. At one stage, Western media outlets were reporting that 107 patients had been harmed. It is not known whether this is the true figure, nor how many people died. The global number of cases of vincristine-related serious harm and death, which had accumulated one by one over four decades, tripled in a period of weeks. No one predicted it, and it is doubtful that anyone even thought about such an upstream element, so remote from the clinic, playing such a dramatic part in a story that seemed to be well understood. It is a true object lesson in the importance of deep understanding of systems if serious harm in healthcare is to be eliminated.

In taking on board a philosophy of systems thinking, this does not mean that the role of the individual is unimportant or that it should be ignored. Healthcare systems need well-trained, careful, competent, well-supervised staff, just as airlines need highly skilled, safety-conscious pilots.

Learning from other high-risk industries

Accidents that kill and seriously injure people happen in many service industries, particularly transport. In many such high-risk industries, major improvements in safety have stemmed from catastrophes. In aviation, for example, the Tenerife air disaster was a seminal moment in the process of change (Table 7.6). In the offshore drilling industry, the Piper Alpha accident in 1988, in which 167 oil rig workers died, stands out as an event that led to major change. In rail safety, in the United Kingdom, accidents at Clapham in 1988 (35 killed, 500 injured), Ladbroke Grove in 1999 (31 killed, 520 injured) and Hatfield in 2000 (4 killed, 30 injured) put the rail industry under sustained public and media pressure to make big improvements.

Some, but not all, of these events led to transformational change in the level of safety in the industry concerned. Lessons learned, and action taken, were global, not just limited to the country in which the accident occurred. They are characterized by rigorous, deep investigation following the accident, and establishment of the range of factors that contributed to its causation. As a result, many strands of action were initiated across all areas of risk, directed at aspects such as organizational culture and priorities, inspection and testing of equipment, competence of staff, leadership, education and training, standard operating procedures and, particularly, measures based on an understanding of human factors. In the healthcare field, it is uncommon to find events in which the quality of investigation and identification of action to reduce risk have led to industry-wide transformation of patient safety. Much can still be learned by healthcare from the experience of other high-risk industries (Table 7.7).

That is not to say that accidents no longer happen in these other high-risk industries, nor to assume that people are not harmed. The Transportation Board of Canada shows this only too well with its report on a derailment and explosion

Table 7.6 The Tenerife air disaster of 1977

The biggest loss of life in a single civil aviation crash – 583 people – took place on Sunday 27 March 1977 at Los Rodeos Airport, Tenerife. A number of aircraft had been diverted there after a bomb exploded at Gran Canaria Airport. After lengthy delays, two aircraft were preparing for take-off: KLM Flight 4805 and Pan Am Flight 1736. The airport was a small one with just one runway and the air-traffic controllers were not used to being in charge of so many planes. When Gran Canaria Airport was re-opened allowing normal service to resume, a thick fog descended over Los Rodeos Airport; it was so bad that the two planes getting ready to depart could not see each other, nor could the control tower see the planes. There was no ground radar. The Pan Am plane was directed to a turning off the take-off runway onto the parallel runway to enable it to come up behind the KLM plane and wait for it to take-off first. The Pan Am pilots could not be sure where they had stopped given the extremely poor visibility and their own unfamiliarity with the airport layout. A series of communications took place between the pilots of each plane and the control tower. The KLM pilot believed that he had been cleared for take-off but subsequent analysis showed that there were misunderstandings and miscommunications leading to KLM Flight 4805 taking off with the Pan Am plane sitting on the runway. There was also the suggestion that the co-pilot and the flight engineer did not feel able to challenge the pilot's decision to take-off because they were in awe of his seniority. Both planes tried to avert the collision but it was impossible. Everyone on the KLM flight was killed but there were some survivors on the Pan Am plane. The crash shocked the airline industry, especially as the KLM pilot was one of the most senior and respected pilots in the world. Following the investigations, the rules for communication were standardized. No longer would informal instructions like "OK" be accepted as a basis for action. Also, the whole question of the inter-relationship of the crew members was addressed leading to the approach of Crew Resource Management. Many people lost their lives in this accident but the industry-wide changes that it provoked undoubtedly made air travel safer thereafter.

Table 7.7 Examples of safety-enhancing measures used routinely in aviation that are used in healthcare only partially or not at all

Measures	Use in aviation
Checklists	Used extensively throughout the flight
Crew resource management	Training in errors and teamwork
Sterile cockpit rule	Nonessential activity not allowed at times when maximum concentration is required
Standard layouts	No variation between aircraft
The black box	Records incidents for detailed analysis
Incentivized no-fault reporting	To encourage learning

Source: Lewis GH, Vaithianathan R, Hockey PM, Hirst G, Bagian JP. Counterheroism, common knowledge, and ergonomics: concepts from aviation that could improve patient safety. *Milbank Quarterly* 2011;89(1):4-38.

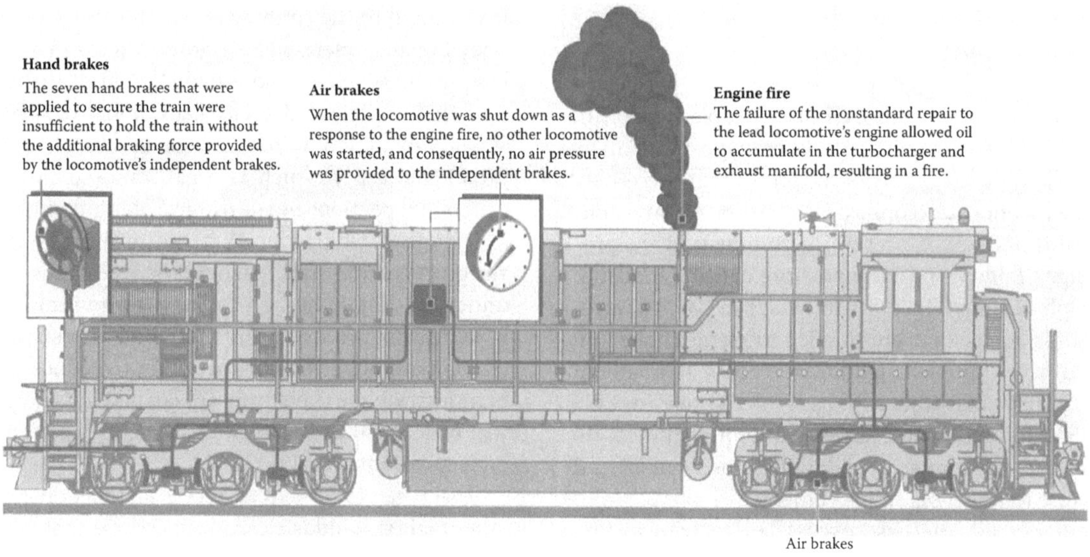

Figure 7.10 Lac-Mégantic: Anatomy of a Disaster.

Source: Toronto Globe and Mail. With permission.

of a runaway freight train in Lac-Mégantic, Quebec, on the night of 5 July 2013. The train carrying 7.7 million litres of volatile petroleum crude oil was parked up overnight on a slope, partway through a long journey across North America. Railway regulations require that handbrakes alone should be strong enough to hold a parked train, and that this must be tested before leaving the train stationary. That night, a test was indeed carried out by the engineer before he went off duty. Apparently unaware that the air brakes had also been left on, he was falsely reassured about the adequacy of the handbrakes. His test suggested that the handbrakes of seven cars were holding the train satisfactorily when, in fact, the air brakes were playing a part (Figure 7.10). The investigation of the accident subsequently showed that between 18 and 26 handbrakes would have been necessary to keep that number of engines and cars from moving.

Later in the evening, a fire broke out on the lead locomotive and the local fire brigade put it out. The firefighters used the emergency fuel cut-off switch to shut down the lead locomotive. They also moved the electrical breakers inside the locomotive cab to the off position, to eliminate a potential ignition source. They then sought advice from a track foreman, who had been dispatched to the scene by the railway company; however, he had limited experience on the relevant technical matters. The train was judged safe to leave parked up until the journey was resumed in the morning. With the engines shut down, air was no longer being pumped in air brakes. They leaked air and weakened, and the handbrakes alone were not enough to hold the 1.4 km train. It rolled down the hill, picking up speed, and derailed on a bend, at 1:15 a.m. on 6 July. As it plunged towards the town, its petroleum cargo ignited into a huge fireball. Deaths, injuries and destruction followed.

The analysis of events in Canada that night is particularly instructive. They show all the ingredients of a classic accident:

18 causes and contributory factors. While the weakness of the brakes was at the heart of the causation of the accident, there were multiple factors that came together to make it happen. The metaphorical Swiss cheese was full of holes. Weak safety training, failure to use a siding to park the train rather than the main track and inadequate oversight by the federal regulator were just some of these contributory factors. As is often the case, in major accidents, there was something buried in the system from a past action that surfaced to devastating effect. The lead locomotive, the one that caught fire, had a repair eight months before the accident that was substandard: an epoxy resin was used as a sealant (apparently to save time), but it did not stay secure, leading to critical leaks in the engine. James Reason's term *latent factors* perfectly fits this example. There is usually no single explanatory cause for a catastrophic event. Instead, there is a complex interaction between varied factors, some related to human behaviour, others to technological and sociocultural factors and still others to organizational and management weaknesses. The response to the Lac-Mégantic accident illustrates the rigorous standard of investigation that is seldom a feature of the approach to serious incidents in healthcare.

A major lesson from another high-risk industry, again the airline industry, came in the late 1970s when NASA reviewed all past air crashes and found that poor communication, weak leadership and team dysfunction were at the heart of these accidents' causation. This led to the introduction of special training programmes called *crew resource management*. The wider concept of *human factors* has developed greatly since this work in the 1980s. The International Ergonomics Society defines human factors as 'ergonomics (or human factors) is the scientific discipline concerned with the understanding of interactions among humans and other elements of a system, and the profession that applies theory, principles, data and methods to design in order to optimize human well-being and overall system performance'.

This field of scholarship grew in part from studying accidents, particularly in aviation, and recognizing that even highly skilled, conscientious pilots flying normally functioning planes still sometimes crashed. Charles Hopkins, technical director of the Human Factors Society group that investigated the Three Mile Island nuclear power plant disaster in 1979, said, 'The disregard for human factors in the control room was appalling. In some cases, the distribution of displays and controls seemed almost haphazard. It was as if someone had taken a box of dials and switches, turned his back, thrown the whole thing at the board and attached things where they landed'. In the airline industry, redesigning cockpits and instrument layout to reduce the likelihood of errors, addressing weaknesses and ambiguities in communications between members of the flight crew and establishing strict protocols for the handling of emergencies, all backed up by extensive simulation training, have greatly improved safety. The human factors approach and expertise is increasingly being used in healthcare. It should be an essential component of investigating serious adverse incidents but is not always. It can also be used proactively within a hospital or other health organization to look more fundamentally at procedures and ways of working.

Reporting, investigating and learning

There are a number of ways to identify harm in healthcare and investigate its causes. Greatest attention has been given to establishing routine systems for the reporting of incidents from the front line. Globally, incident reporting systems vary greatly in the nature of the data captured, the extent of public release of information, whether reporting is voluntary or mandatory and the depth of investigation undertaken. Most reporting systems start by defining in general terms what should be reported. Terminology varies – *adverse event, incident, error* and *untoward incident* are all in common use internationally. The epithet *serious* can be applied to any of the terms.

The largest national system in the world was established in the NHS in England and Wales as a result of the report *An Organisation with a Memory*. It is called the National Reporting and Learning System (Figure 7.11). NHS staff members are encouraged to make an incident report of any situation in which they believe that a patient's safety was compromised. In this system, a *patient safety incident* is defined as 'any unintended or unexpected incident which could have, or did, lead to harm for one or more patients receiving NHS care'.

Worldwide, the problems associated with incident reporting are remarkably consistent, whatever system design is adopted. First, underreporting is the norm, although its degree varies. This seems to depend on the prevailing culture and whether incidents are seen as an opportunity to learn or as a basis for enforcing individual accountability and apportioning blame. It also depends on staff perceptions about the difference their report will make and how easy it is for them to convey the information that they are required to. Reporting rates are much lower in primary care services than in hospitals. Second, given the volume of reports made, there are often insufficient time, resources and expertise to carry out the depth of analysis required to fully understand why the incident happened. Third, the balance of activity within reporting systems goes on collecting, storing, and analysing data at the expense of using it for successful learning. Indeed, there are relatively few examples worldwide of major and sustained reductions in error and harm resulting because of lessons learned from reporting.

The main purposes of a patient safety incident reporting system are a public accountability function, a response to

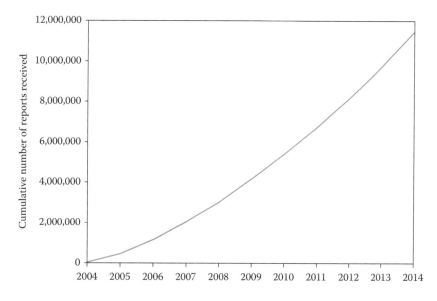

Figure 7.11 Patient safety incident reports made to the National Reporting and Learning System for England and Wales.

Source: National Reporting and Learning System (NRLS). *Annual Report 2014.* London: NRLS, 2015.

the patients and families, a communications alert route, a barometer of risk of care and, more importantly, a foundation for learning.

There are various approaches to investigation, of which *root cause analysis* is particularly widely used. This technique, borrowed from other high-risk industries, involves studying an incident's causation by repeatedly asking the question 'Why?' to get past the superficial explanation for why harm occurred (often 'human error') to understand the deep, systemic issues – the root causes – underlying this. There are many different frameworks for applying root cause analysis to an incident of harm, but most helpful is to identify the main categories that can then be used to explore detailed contributory factors. An example is shown in Figure 7.12; in this case, a *fishbone diagram* is used to facilitate the process.

Incident reporting systems are criticized because the major degree of underreporting means that the rate of harm cannot be meaningfully estimated. Indeed, an increase in the rate of reporting more often represents an improvement in the safety culture, with staff becoming more willing to report, than an actual increase in the incidence of harm.

Retrospective review of a sample of patient records is a different way to estimate the incidence of harm, and was the method used in the studies that have estimated the extent of harm in several different countries, but this depends on how much is actually recorded in the medical notes. The Institute for Healthcare Improvement has developed the *Global Trigger Tool* to assist this process. A *trigger* is an occurrence that is fairly readily seen by looking through the patient record, and which may indicate that an adverse event (which is often more difficult to spot) has occurred.

Transfer of a patient to a higher level of care is one example of a trigger – this does not always indicate that an adverse event has taken place, but it merits a closer look. Guided by the trigger tool, or another method, the reviewer records the number of adverse events and their severity. From this, an estimate can be made of the rate of harm (e.g. adverse events per thousand patient-days) and tracked over time.

There is no general agreement on what other sources of routine data will give a valid and reliable assessment of the level and types of harm occurring within healthcare. Such sources will vary according to the kinds of data collected on patients' contacts within the health system concerned, but broadly they should seek to identify and aid the prevention and mitigation of all aspects of harm.

The evidence base for solutions that reduce the risk of particular types of harm is not as strong as it could be. Those with strong confirmatory evidence are relatively few in number. As a result, staff investigating incidents, whether by root cause analysis or less rigorous means, are left to formulate their own solutions, which is often on the basis of common-sense reasoning.

Simulation and human factors training are two approaches particularly used to improve safety, but also of value in other areas of quality improvement more broadly. The concept of using simulation is borrowed from other high-risk industries, most notably the airline industry. Pilots practice emergency scenarios, such as engine failure and fire, in highly sophisticated simulators. Trainee pilots learn to fly simulators before they fly real planes. The fundamental concept of simulation is that it allows skills to be honed in a safe environment, before they are applied in a

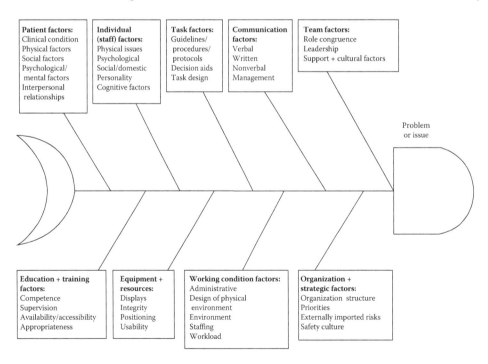

Figure 7.12 Root Cause Analysis.

Source: National Patient Safety Agency. *Root Cause Analysis Investigation.* Available from: www.nrls.npsa.nhs.uk/resources/collections/root-cause-analysis/ (accessed 28 May 2017).

real environment. It is increasingly used in healthcare – so that, for example, a new doctor's first severely unwell patient is not a real one, and a surgeon's first stitch, cut and even entire operation is not on a real patient either. Simulation allows groups of healthcare professionals to apply and hone these skills in a safe environment.

The process of improving safety involves important stages of activity, which must all be aligned if it is to be successful (Figure 7.13).

Patient safety cultures

There is widespread acknowledgement that organizational culture is very important to the consistent delivery of safe care. Most discussion of this subject centres on the dangers of the so-called *blame culture*. Setting up an expectation that doctors or nurses will not make mistakes is entirely unhelpful. The expectation exists because it is a reassuring one – that a healthcare professional who makes mistakes is an exception. Nobody wants to confront the alternative – that a person who makes

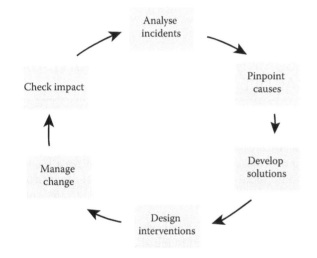

Figure 7.13 Patient safety: a cycle of improvement.

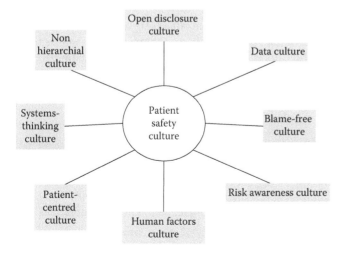

Figure 7.14 Patient safety culture has many strands.

mistakes is the rule, not the exception. They are fallible human beings working in complex systems. To err is, indeed, human.

When a loved one comes to harm, his or her family will often find the idea that nobody should be held to account a bitter pill to swallow. The natural human tendency is to look for somebody to blame. However, experience from other high-risk industries shows that an atmosphere of blame and retribution surrounding error is counterproductive. It makes individuals fearful of admitting mistakes. It creates a strong incentive for staff to keep quiet when things go wrong. Who would choose to report if they know that the full burden of blame will land on their shoulders? As a result, in a predominantly blame culture, little will be learned that could reduce risk for future patients.

Patient safety experts advocate that healthcare organizations should declare a policy of a *no-blame culture*. In such environments, when something goes wrong, the emphasis is on learning, not judgement. The concept of a no-blame culture is often misunderstood. It does not mean that no one is ever held accountable. There will always be instances in which individual professionals have truly fallen short in their responsibilities or capabilities – when there has been negligent practice, reckless behaviour or wilful disregard of advice or established procedures. So it is inappropriate to provide them with complete amnesty. Some prefer the term *just culture*. In a just culture, staff are able to report and discuss incidents knowing that the entire system, not just their personal contribution, will be subject to review, and that often the greatest fault lies with the system, not with individuals. But they also know that instances of unacceptable individual failing will also be dealt with.

Maintaining a no-blame or just culture involves walking a narrow tightrope. To one side lies a culture in which scrutiny, rather than learning, predominates. Individuals are punished, and the system does not learn. To the other side lies a culture in which the need for conscientious, competent and careful staff is not fully recognized and concern about personal failings is dismissed too readily. In many countries, the prevailing political, media and public climate is towards too readily apportioning blame. In the presence of a high-profile case of harm to a patient, it can take a great deal of courage by a hospital chief executive to reinforce the moral position of not blaming an individual when the system is the problem. The pressure to capitulate and hang an individual out to dry can be enormous.

The relevance of organizational culture to patient safety goes beyond even the important questions of blame, openness and learning. Culture means the ideas, beliefs and behaviours that are the norm for that organization and the people working within it. It is sometimes summed up as 'the way we do things around here'. To which some would add 'when no one is looking'.

The culture of a hospital or other healthcare organization is often viewed as a single entity. In reality, though, such organizations are made up of many different professionals and other groups of staff, each with their own traditions, customs and practices. In thinking about the action needed at the organizational level to promote safer care, it is often helpful to concentrate on the different strands of the culture that contribute to the whole (Figure 7.14).

For example, valuing data or being a patient-centred organization each requires passionate, committed leadership; the engagement of staff; and expert advice and facilitation, among other things. Achieving a 'data culture' in which staff want to measure and assess their service, compare it with others, make plans for improvement and have access to evidence is a formidable task, but the benefits for improving patient safety are very great.

Towards high-reliability organizations

The patient safety movement (recognition of the scale of harm, concerted action to address it and even the term *patient safety*) has developed since the beginning of the twenty-first century. There are some examples of initiatives that have substantially reduced the risk to patients, but being a recipient of healthcare remains a somewhat hazardous pursuit. The greatest successes have been in specific, controlled environments – intensive care units

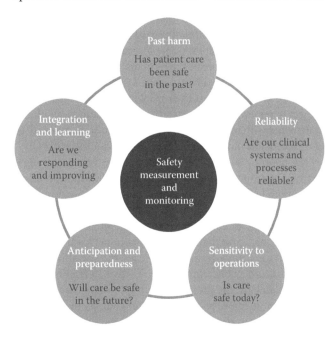

Figure 7.15 A framework for measuring and monitoring patient safety.

Source: Health Foundation. *A Framework for Measuring and Monitoring Safety: A Practical Guide.* London: Health Foundation, 2014. With permission.

and operating theatres in particular. There has been less success in reducing harm across care boundaries. Patient safety has received more attention in secondary care than in primary care, where even incident reporting systems remain little used. The transformations of care delivery that are much needed – in particular, moving more care into people's homes – are even less well understood in safety terms, and likely create new risks in a low-visibility environment. Healthcare has not yet matched the focus or record on safety that is seen in other high-risk industries.

It is for these reasons that rather than directing all activity on learning from serious incidents, some leaders in healthcare are embracing the approach (again derived from outside healthcare) of building *resilience* into their organizations. From this, the concept of the *high-reliability organization* has emerged: one that is constantly looking for risks and hazards and making changes to ensure that they do not become future sources of harm (Figure 7.15). Karl Weick and Kathleen Sutcliffe in their book *Managing the Unexpected* give many examples of this philosophy and set out the key characteristics of a high-reliability organization (Table 7.8).

ASSURING THE QUALITY OF INDIVIDUAL PRACTICE

The delivery of high-quality healthcare does not depend only on creating health organizations with the leadership, culture and systems to ensure and improve the standard of services they provide. It also requires a focus on the individual health practitioner to ensure that mechanisms are in place to assure the quality and safety of his or her practice.

The quality of individual practice is developed, maintained and improved through the provision of education and training programmes. In the United Kingdom, these aim to be career-long, with continuing professional development reinforcing and extending knowledge, skills and values.

In other high-risk industries, there are regular assessments of individuals' skills and competence, as well as their health. This is not the case in healthcare in many parts of the world. Until recently in the United Kingdom, for example, once someone was trained and in independent practice,

Table 7.8 Five principles of high reliability organizations

Principle	Amplification
An interest in failure	Consider any failure however small an opportunity to reduce risk
A reluctance to simplify	Use different information sources and encourage different points of view
A sensitivity to operations	The highest hierarchical levels must stay in contact with front-line operations
A commitment to longevity and resilience	Foster the ability to maintain or retain stability of operations after a major event
Respect for expertise	Empower experts regardless of their place in hierarchy

Source: Weick KE, Sutcliffe KM. *Managing the Unexpected: Resilient Performance in an Age of Uncertainty.* San Francisco: Wiley, 2007.

they would not be independently assessed for the rest of their career. In the same period, an airline pilot would be assessed roughly 100 times in a simulator and by independent observation. The result is that many patients around the world do not know whether their doctor is a good doctor. They have to take it all on trust. In some countries, this is changing.

In a reform of medical regulation in the United Kingdom, doctors' fitness for continuing practice is regularly assessed. The system is called *revalidation* and is overseen by the General Medical Council, with the involvement of NHS and private sector employers, the medical royal colleges and patient representative groups. It involves two separate processes: *relicensing* (confirming that a doctor's practice is in line with the General Medical Council's generic standards) and *recertification* (confirming that doctors on the specialist and general practice registers conform with standards appropriate to their specialty). Doctors have to pass these checks periodically if they are to remain on the medical register. The new system is a major revolution in medical regulation and gives the medical profession and the public more objective assurance than in the past that a doctor is up to date and practising safely and to acceptable standards.

Mechanisms are also needed to address situations in which a healthcare professional's performance is so poor as to give rise to concerns about patient safety or the effective functioning of a clinical team or service. This is not something that is dealt with comprehensively in many parts of the world. A national professional regulator, broadly equivalent to the United Kingdom's General Medical Council, usually deals with the most serious problems where such a body exists. The General Medical Council has health and fitness-to-practice procedures that are used when complaints or concerns are raised about a doctor's practice. The presence and scope of such functions varies greatly around the world. In the United Kingdom, there are nine councils, including the General Medical Council, that regulate health professions. Three of these are the Nursing and Midwifery Council, the General Optical Council and the Health Professions Council (which covers a wide range of professions allied to medicine). The Council for Healthcare Regulatory Excellence (CHRE) is an independent body (accountable to Parliament) with an oversight function for the individual health professional regulators. The council has a number of discrete statutory functions, such as promoting the interests of the public and patients, reviewing fitness-to-practice systems of individual regulators and identifying learning points. It also seeks to promote good practice and harmonize functions across the regulators.

There will always be a proportion of the workforce whose performance falls below what is required but does not, at first sight, seem serious enough to be referred to a statutory professional regulator. This is a situation for the employer to deal with, and the chief executive of a hospital (or other healthcare organization) will usually rely on the human resources department to lead on evaluating the problem and identifying the action to be taken. However, many such

organizations now have a clinical management structure. Members of professional staff in such situations may report to a clinical director. When there are more serious performance concerns, a board-level medical or nursing director may become involved, depending on the circumstances. The performance problem becomes much more serious if it is judged to compromise patient safety. Such problems can be complex and difficult to unravel. In England and Wales, a special body was set up to provide expert advice to NHS employers in the assessment and management of such cases (but only for doctors, dentists and pharmacists). The National Clinical Assessment Service (NCAS) does not take over the role of an employer, nor is it a regulator. It aims to help the employer by giving advice in resolving performance issues locally and carrying out objective assessment. Following assessment, the service will advise the referring organization on appropriate courses of action, which could include recommendations for remedial training. In serious cases, the General Medical Council will also become involved and will consider whether issues with a doctor's professional conduct, performance or health are serious enough to affect their licence to practice.

Although problems with clinical performance affect only a small proportion of the workforce, they can lead to harm to patients. It is important to recognize them early and intervene. They can be a source of great tension, especially if they occur in a small clinical team. The main categories of problem encountered in a doctor's poor performance in the NHS are shown in Table 7.9.

PATIENT AND FAMILY INVOLVEMENT

Chapter 6, on health systems, has a section describing the main themes of patient and family involvement to which a modern health service should be orientated. Specifically in relation to quality and safety, the traditional interface with patients and families is through feedback on their experience of care. There is a great deal of development work to improve the way that patient experience is captured. Increasingly, experts and others seeking to develop better, more relevant measures of the quality of healthcare are returning to the challenges of measuring the third element of Donabedian's triad – outcome – but doing so in a way that captures the patient's perspective. The International Consortium for Health Outcomes Measurement has done extensive work on this. The consortium defines outcome as 'the results people care about most when seeking treatment, including functional impairment and the ability to live normal, productive lives'. Figure 7.16 shows one domain in which a range of different outcomes has been defined in consultation with clinicians and patients. The NHS in England is experimenting with the use of *patient-reported outcome measures* (PROMs). These aim to be more patient centric than traditional clinical outcome measures in two ways. First, they measure aspects that are important to patients – such as quality of life and their sense of overall health, rather than purely narrow technical measures of treatment success. Second, as

Table 7.9 Top-level categories of concerns about NHS doctors referred to a national service because of poor performance

Top-level category	Examples
Clinical difficulties	Weak record keeping, poor diagnostic and treatment decisions, serious departure from protocols
Governance/safety issues	Poor responses to complaints, serious lapses in infection control
Behaviour other than misconduct	Poor communication with colleagues and carers, erratic or aggressive behaviour towards others
Misconduct	Fraud and financial irregularities, inappropriate sexual behaviour, bullying and harassment
Health problems including substance misuse	Cognitive, sensory or physical impairment due to alcohol or drug misuse, stress and burnout, bipolar disorder
Work environment influences	Inability to cope with workload, dysfunctional team-working, unresponsive to corporate policies
Personal circumstances not ill-health	Relationship problems, family illness and bereavement, money worries

Source: Donaldson LJ, Panesar SS, McAvoy PA, Scarrott DM. Identification of poor performance in a national medical workforce over 11 years: an observational study. *BMJ Quality and Safety* 2014;23:147-152. With permission.

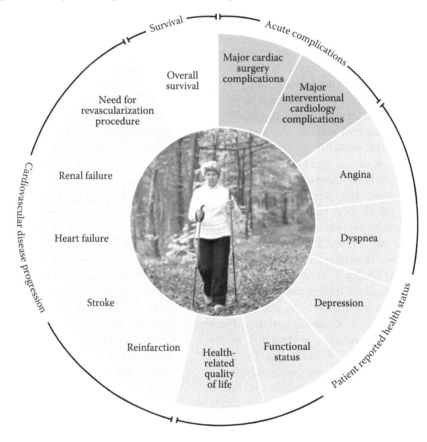

Figure 7.16 Measures of health status defined as important by patients with coronary artery disease.

Source: International Consortium for Health Outcome Measurement 2015. With permission.

the name suggests, they are reported directly by patients, through questionnaires. The NHS is dipping a toe in this promising, but complex, area by using patient-reported outcome measures just for hip and knee replacements, hernia and varicose vein operations.

The English NHS also now uses a friends and family test as an overall measure of patient satisfaction with services. Patients are asked, 'Would you recommend this service to friends and family?' Staff are also asked the same question about the service in which they work. The concept of this measure is drawn from commercial marketing practice, in which consumers are commonly asked the same question about products and services.

Patient stories can play a particularly important role in motivating healthcare professionals to change. Hearing patients' experiences of healthcare – both positive and negative – provides much greater motivation to people than abstract metrics do. However, narrative accounts of care are difficult to aggregate, and so this valuable source of information is more usually deployed in education and training sessions where they can create deep insights for staff and students into how it feels to be a patient in their system.

When patients are asked in surveys what they expect from a complaint system, they usually respond by saying an explanation, an apology and a reassurance that improvements to the service will be made based on their experience. A good complaint system has the following features: satisfactory local resolution of the majority of complaints; speedy response times; excellent communication with patients; good record keeping; apologies made in person by the senior staff involved, not on their behalf; accurate monitoring of the numbers and categories of complaint; and effective learning from the themes identified through analysis of complaints.

The NHS in England encourages patients to voice any concerns early, and directly, with front-line staff. Informal, local resolution of problems saves every concern becoming a time-consuming complaint. If patients feel unable to do this, if an attempt to do this fails or if the issue is more serious, there is a formal complaint procedure. Patients are encouraged to make a complaint to the service provider. If they feel unable to do this (perhaps because they are concerned that doing so may affect their ongoing care), they can complain to the commissioner of the service. The Patient Advice and Liaison Services (PALS) employ NHS staff who help patients to resolve concerns and, if necessary, make complaints.

An NHS constitution was introduced in 2009 setting out patients' rights, including in relation to complaints. Patients have a right to have their complaint dealt with efficiently and be properly investigated, know the outcome of any investigation into their complaint, take their complaint to the independent Parliamentary and Health Service Ombudsman if not satisfied with the way the NHS has dealt with the complaint, make a claim for judicial review if they think they have been directly affected by an unlawful act or decision of an NHS body and receive compensation if they have been harmed.

The organizations around the world that represent patients and families who have suffered harm have made a very strong case that incidents of error, harm and poor-quality care should be disclosed by the healthcare provider concerned. This can be seen as a moral responsibility, as well as a move towards greater openness. It also seeks to break down the wall of secrecy and silence that continues to surround so many adverse events, reinforced by a legal approach of defending the provider in a very robust fashion. This traditional way of handling the event can unleash a second wave of psychological and emotional trauma to add to the original damage caused to the patient. In the United Kingdom, a statutory duty of candour has been introduced to the NHS, so that proactive disclosure is mandatory.

In the most forward-looking healthcare systems, the agenda on empowering and engaging with patients and families is much broader and more ambitious. At the level of a healthcare organization, it includes a strong system of patient experience data benchmarked against comparable organizations. It also involves working with and involving patients and families in the planning and design of services and in the governance structures. Ultimately, the goal of achieving truly patient-centred care must sit within an overall strategic framework for modern healthcare (Figure 7.17).

BUILDING QUALITY AND SAFETY INTO HEALTHCARE

Strategies and practical actions to improve the quality and safety of healthcare must operate at different levels in a system. The *macrolevel* is the whole healthcare system and the social, economic and political environment in which it operates. The *mesolevel* is the organization, such as a hospital delivering care or an organization commissioning care, while the *microlevel* is the front-line clinical team.

System level

Within an existing system, quality improvement is neither easy nor straightforward. It involves changing complex systems and – harder still – making people change their behaviour, and even beliefs. *Change management* is the field of management science that studies and describes such endeavours. The vast majority of change efforts fail. A common reason for failure is that people try to change the technical elements of a system, without paying sufficient attention to the people factors. Change management gurus provide models that can be genuinely useful if properly applied – such as John Kotter's eight-step model (Table 7.10). These focus a great deal of attention on the need to communicate and lead. Change is more likely to occur if those who are being asked to change understand the problems of the current situation and the urgency to change it, and believe that there is a better alternative that they can work towards. Change is not an easy process for people, so they must feel motivation to get through it.

Those leading a health system have some key roles in the process of improving quality and safety. First, they must set overall goals for the system. The choice of goals and how they are prioritized very much depends on the context. Well-chosen and well-formulated goals for quality and safety improvement should address the major burdens of harm and the important areas where quality regularly falls below best practice. Good goals should be applicable at the system level but also relevant to quality improvement when disaggregated to the service delivery level. For example, a system level goal of 'To slow the progression of chronic disease' is relevant, powerful and potentially transformational because it creates the possibility to prolong life, improve quality of life and reduce demand for healthcare. It can also be used at the clinical front line where staff can develop their own

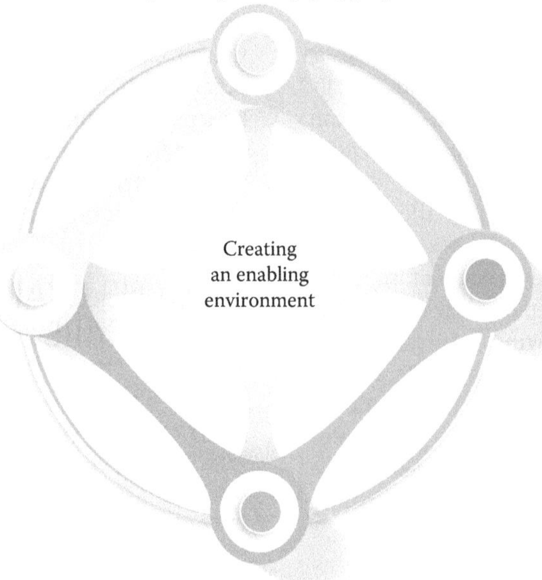

Figure 7.17 Important elements of creating people-centred and integrated health services.

Source: World Health Organization (WHO). *Global Strategy on People-Centred and Integrated Health Services: Interim Report.* Geneva: WHO, 2015. With permission.

Table 7.10 The eight-step model for leading change

1. Establish a sense of urgency
2. Form a powerful guiding coalition
3. Create a vision
4. Communicate the vision
5. Empower others to act on the vision
6. Planning for and create short-term wins
7. Consolidate improvements and produce still more change
8. Institutionalize new approaches

Source: Kotter JP. Leading change: Why transformation efforts fail. *Harvard Business Review* 1995; 73(2): 59–67.

action plans and redesign their services to address the goal as it applies at their level and for the chronic diseases that they look after. Some would also say that goals should have ability to inspire: what the management guru Jim Collins called big hairy audacious goals (BHAGs).

Second, the system level is the best place to state, communicate and promote the values of healthcare. Values are not like improvement goals. They are generally timeless. They are less often measured but can be and should be, though measurement is more difficult. They are discussed in more detail in Chapter 6.

Third, the system level is the best place to deal with configuration of healthcare services. This is an important determinant of their quality and safety, which is often in the hands of the most senior leaders, and often politicians, in any healthcare system. The concentration of specialist services is particularly important, and is a political hot

potato. In general, facilities dealing with a larger volume of cases achieve better outcomes for their patients. This applies to many cancers, heart and neurological conditions requiring surgery, severe traumatic injuries, revision of joint surgery and many rare and complex conditions generally. An example is shown in Figure 7.18. The solution to this is to concentrate expertise, specialist equipment and facilities in a smaller number of places. But, despite the beneficial outcomes, sometimes the difference between life and death, patients do not always want to travel farther and clinicians with small caseloads do not want to relinquish the special interest. Healthcare leaders have an important role to play in communicating with the public about the trade-offs between convenience of access and quality of care. Such communication is seldom well handled. As a result, there are many areas in the world where patients receive inadequate care or even have poor survival because clinical and local politics preclude major changes being made to the configuration of services, even when the current configuration is extremely suboptimal. Moving and closing down services is always controversial, the evidence is often disputed and save-our-hospital campaigns are started in towns and cities.

Fourth, the system level is also the right place to address one of the biggest challenges of quality and safety improvement: how to bring the benefits of successful change achieved in one place, or known evidence-based interventions, to everywhere: so-called *scaling up* or *spread*.

The starting point for considering this is the work of the psychologist Everett Rogers, whose book *The Diffusion of Innovation* introduces the famous adoption curve with its

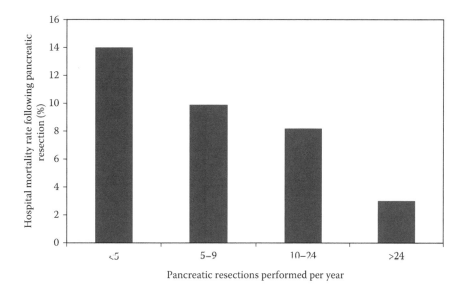

Figure 7.18 The association between case volume and mortality for pancreatic resection.

Source: van Heek NT, Kuhlmann KF, Scholten RJ, et al. Hospital volume and mortality after pancreatic resection: a systematic review and an evaluation of intervention in the Netherlands. *Annals of Surgery* 2005;242(6):781–90.

early adopters and *laggards* (Figure 7.19). Rogers gives a very extensive and detailed treatment of the subject with numerous examples from different fields. He uses the term *innovation* broadly to mean something new, for example, a change in behaviour, a new practice or take-up of a new product. He argues that the target of the change (e.g. a group of people, an organization or a society) should be seen as a social system. This must be understood if successful spread is to be achieved.

There are a number of ways that spread can be achieved, of which the improvement collaborative approach, mentioned earlier, is one. Most cited examples in healthcare are drawn from the systems of high-income countries. However, the benefits of modern quality improvement methods can be brought to bear to tackle the major challenges of low-income countries. The programme outcomes depicted in Figure 7.20 resulted from an improvement collaborative to spread a practice innovation (in this case, a care bundle) to reduce postpartum haemorrhage in the third stage of labour among mothers in Niger. This is a common cause of maternal mortality throughout Africa. Teams worked through how to implement the practice and overcome barriers such as difficulty in accessing oxytocin, women arriving at the health facility after delivery and time constraints. The improvement was brought to the care of many women with a very positive impact.

Within healthcare organizations

Healthcare organizations can also set goals to which their constituent parts contribute. For example, a hospital may set a goal of reducing mortality, to be achieved through a portfolio of different quality improvement projects. The Department of Surgery can work to improve deep vein thrombosis prophylaxis, the Department of Medicine could implement a pneumonia care bundle and all departments might improve their reliability by better observing patients and taking prompt action if a patient is deteriorating. Each of these has separate project-level goals, but each also contributes to the organization-level goal of reducing mortality. A structured approach such as this is better than simply having a collection of unrelated projects. An organization may wish to set several goals – some to do with safety, some to do with patient experience, some to do with clinical effectiveness.

In addition to providing this direction, hospital (or other healthcare organization) managers can facilitate success by investment, so that people responsible for quality improvement have the training, support and time to do it properly; selecting a small number of improvement models and tools for use within the organization, so that staff gain familiarity with them over time; ensuring that staff have access to data that are as close to real time as possible, to understand current performance and to guide improvement; and making quality improvement important, by visibly taking an active interest in it from the board level downwards, making it part of every staff member's performance appraisal, and using it in promotion decisions.

In short, the leadership of healthcare organizations can put in place and develop an organized, structured approach to quality improvement, as well as promoting an organizational culture that is centred on the needs of patients and the philosophy of continuous improvement.

On the front line

As has been described, there are important actions that managers can take across whole organizations and healthcare systems to facilitate and support front-line quality improvement. Ultimately, though, quality improvement

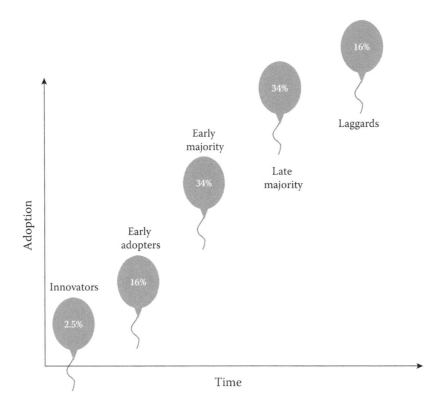

Figure 7.19 The adoption of innovations by groups sequentially (percentages of total population).

Source: Adapted from Rogers EM. *Diffusion of Innovations.* London: Simon and Schuster, 2010.

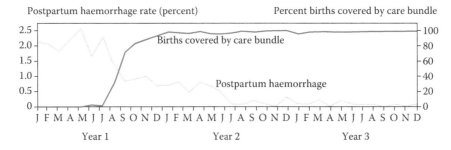

Figure 7.20 Implementation of a care bundle in labour reduces postpartum haemorrhage incidence, Niger.

Source: Massoud MR, Donohue KL, McCannon CJ. *Options for Large-scale Spread of Simple High-impact Interventions: Technical Report.* Bethesda: University Research Co, 2010.

must be a front-line pursuit. It needs to be done by those who deliver care, tackling one problem at a time, through one project after another.

Almost without exception, successful quality improvement projects use a clear improvement model – that is, they choose a particular process to follow as their guide to undertaking the project. For any given project, many such models could potentially be appropriate. The important thing is to choose one, and use it rigorously. Many of those in common use are described in the first half of this chapter, including the model for improvement, rapid process improvement weeks (part of the Lean approach), Lean and clinical audit.

As well as using a clear, well-developed model, successful projects also tend to have three further characteristics. First, they use data – to understand the situation before they make any changes, and to track progress as they proceed through the project. Second, they are done by the right team – what constitutes the 'right team' depends on the local context, but it is usually important that the relevant front-line clinicians are centrally involved, and that they are trained in quality improvement methodologies or supported by those who are. Third, they make effective changes to the system. Too often, poor quality is documented but no change is made, or the change that is made does not have the desired impact, or is not sustained.

Data and information

W Edwards Deming famously said, 'In God we trust. All others must bring data'. Too often in healthcare, management decisions are made on the basis of gut feeling and anecdote. To some extent, this also applies to clinical decisions. Good data, used to provide information and insight, are vital to quality improvement. Data can show what the current situation truly is, and they can show improvement as it happens.

One of the authors (LJD) visited a hospital in North America that has regularly ranked among the highest in performance on quality. A striking feature was the extent to which statistical data depicting performance were displayed on wall charts in clinical areas. When asked how the hospital had managed to get clinicians to embrace data so extensively, the chief of service replied, 'We have made it a scientific activity'. In other words, clinicians who had traditionally regarded quality and service performance data with disdain, and part of the dirty management world, had come to see it as essential to improving their clinical service. This transformation to what we have dubbed *clinical dataphilia* is still in the minority of health systems worldwide. Yet, it is an essential step in making quality improvement a mainstream element of clinical practice.

The amount of data available within healthcare systems has exploded over recent years, as it has in other areas of modern living. It must be converted into valid and reliable information that is of value to policymakers, healthcare system leaders, clinicians, patients and the public. This is a massive but essential step in developing a high-quality, safe health system. The range of data that specifically provide measures of quality and safety is rapidly expanding. There are choices to be made about what frameworks are chosen to provide structure to the data gathering and analysis, which particular measures are chosen and whether there

are adequate sources of data to construct them. A key decision is to be clear about what purpose the measures will be put to, especially to distinguish between data that will guide judgements on whether quality and performance are good, bad or mediocre and data that will be a trigger for quality improvement activities (Table 7.11). Overall, quality and safety data in healthcare can be collected and used for four main purposes: accountability, improvement activities, choice and assessing progress against goals. Then, there are different types of data that are relevant, for example, clinical effectiveness data, patient experience data, patient safety data, health service access data, efficiency and productivity data.

Data can be presented and displayed in many different ways. *Statistical control charts* were pioneered by Walter Shewhart (1891–1967). He advocated the use of the control chart in identifying scope for improvement of industrial processes (Figure 7.1). This method is of particular value in quality improvement. Graphs display a single measure over time. It is very rare to see a straight line – there is almost always variation. In interpreting a control chart, the key distinction is between random (*common cause*) and meaningful (*special cause*) variation. Common cause variation occurs by chance; special cause variation occurs because something is truly different. For example, 310 people may attend an emergency department one weekday, 330 the next and 321 the next, purely as a result of chance. Nobody would expect exactly the same number of patients to attend every day. But if 310 attend one weekday and 620 attend the next, this is likely special cause variation – perhaps there was a major accident on the second day, or a neighbouring hospital's emergency department was closed. Common cause variation is usually of little interest in quality improvement. Special cause variation, by contrast, is almost always of value. It represents an important change in the measure of interest. The observed improvement (or deterioration) may

Table 7.11 Characteristics of indicators used for judgement and improvement

Indicators for judgement	Indicators for improvement
Unambiguous interpretation	Variable interpretation possible
Unambiguous attribution	Ambiguity tolerable
Definitive marker of quality	Poor data quality tolerable
Good risk-adjustment	Partial risk-adjustment tolerable
Statistical reliability necessary	Statistical reliability preferred
Cross-sectional	Time trends
Used for punishment/reward	Used for learning/changing practice
For external use	Mainly for internal use
Data for public use	Data for internal use
Stand-alone	Allowance for context possible
Risk of unintended consequences	Lower risk of unintended consequences

Source: Raleigh VS, Foot C, *Getting the Measure of Quality – Opportunities and Challenges.* London: Kings Fund, 2010.

have resulted from a deliberate change that has been made to a process or system. Or it may have another explanation, worthy of investigation because it may provide a clue about how to deliberately improve performance.

The reporting and payment mechanisms within a healthcare system need to signal that quality is important, and provide an incentive to improve it. In England, Commissioning for Quality and Innovation (CQUIN) payments and Never Events are two examples of this. CQUIN payments allow commissioners to specify certain quality targets for providers to meet, and make payment contingent on achieving these. *Never Events* are serious patient safety incidents – such as wrong-site surgery – that should be entirely preventable. If one occurs in the NHS, this appears on the public records of the organization where it happened, and that organization is not reimbursed for the care related to it. However, routinely available data can have limitations if they are used for quality improvement. This is particularly so for studying postoperative complications, a key measure of the quality of surgical care. Hospital Episode Statistics, used in the NHS in the United Kingdom to record administrative and clinical data on hospital patients, appear to be very poor in accurately capturing certain major adverse surgical outcomes compared with a well-established clinical quality database.

Publicly reporting quality data is, in theory, a means of encouraging individual doctors and organizations to improve. This seemed to work well when cardiac surgery mortality data were reported, which first happened in New York shortly before the turn of the century. It is more difficult for areas of healthcare with less immediate outcomes. It is also not clear that the public gives these data much credence – perhaps the greatest value is in motivating physicians to understand and improve their own performance.

Quality improvement is not just common sense. Change efforts often fail. As with anything else in medicine and in life, there are approaches that are more likely to produce success. Studying what these approaches are is complicated. The success of any given quality improvement project depends on the intervention itself, on the skills and time commitment of those doing the work, on the leadership and culture of the organization and on all manner of contextual factors. For example, a single stubborn, determined individual can either bring a project to its knees or drive it to success, depending on whether he or she is for or against it. Any number of factors can either promote or impede success in this way. *Improvement science* applies research methods to study all this, and help understand which approaches work best.

INSPECTION AND REGULATION

Some healthcare systems around the world work in conjunction with a regulator of quality and safety so that a body, separate from those managing the system, assesses its performance. They vary greatly in the approach taken to regulation and in their power within the healthcare system.

The Joint Commission, in the United States, is one of the longest standing; it sets standards of performance, and then inspects based on those standards and accredits hospitals and other organizations that meet them.

There is a general presumption that a regulator of healthcare will be independent, open and transparent in its operation. Most regulators declare that they are, and operate on this basis. Public perceptions may differ. Trust matters, and any evidence that the regulator is colluding in concealing problems or being too cosy with the providers of care can be very damaging to its public credibility and indeed its viability. So, a regulator is expected to make judgements and criticisms without fear and favour. Certainly, it should stand well above the political process, however uncomfortable that may be for the government of the day.

A good regulator should also have the capability, capacity and procedures to react quickly if there is some serious failure in standards of care or safety. In its day-to-day surveillance function, it should also have the right, reliable data to be able to identify shortfalls in quality at an early stage. Generally, regulators try to be proportionate and risk based in their surveillance and inspection functions. This is a more controversial area. In the first decade of the twenty-first century, the powers of regulators were drawn on the basis that they should not introduce red tape that stifled innovation. In the United Kingdom, this light-touch philosophy was extended to the way that public sector regulators were set up and resourced. Then came the global banking crisis of 2007, when it was obvious that regulation in the financial sector had been too superficial. The widespread failure of standards of care in the Mid-Staffordshire NHS hospital, in England, was the subject of a major public enquiry that uncovered some failings in regulation, along with many other contributory factors. These developments led to the strengthening of health and social care regulation in England with more inspection, including unannounced inspection.

CONCLUSIONS

For most of the twentieth century, quality and safety improvement in healthcare was the sole preserve of academics and enthusiasts. During the twenty-first century, quality and safety have increasingly moved into mainstream thinking about healthcare management and delivery. In many other industries, quality and safety have for decades been absolutely central to how organizations are managed, but this cannot yet be said of healthcare.

One of the most powerful statements about healthcare quality was made by Paul Batalden, from Dartmouth University, Hanover, New Hampshire, and a long-time associate of the Institute of Health Improvement: 'Every system is perfectly designed to get the results it gets'. It is through understanding how the myriad components of a healthcare system, organization or team interact to produce the outcomes that they do that care is improved and made safer.

CHAPTER 8

Maternal and child health

INTRODUCTION

The paediatrician John Apley (1908–80), who practised in Bristol, England, was famous for his aphorisms – some original, some popularizing the quotes of others. His introductory talk to each new generation of medical students began, 'Children are not mini-adults'. This is widely repeated by many today. Children are special, and *childhood* is special. With nurturing, protection, support, guidance and understanding of responsible adults, the early years are the foundations of a healthy and fulfilling life.

The lifetime health impact of the early years is profound – even from the moment of conception. A fetus's intrauterine environment affects the risk of coronary heart disease, hypertension, diabetes, stroke and cancer, years later in adulthood. Adverse events in childhood have been linked with obesity, heart disease and mental health problems as an adult. Children's early development is a strong predictor of health and success in later life.

Giving every child the best start in life should be the highest priority for every nation. The burden of childhood disease is distributed grossly unequally around the world. Two-thirds of all infant and child mortality occurs in just 10 countries. Pregnancy and childbirth still threaten the lives of both mother and baby in too many parts of the world, with deaths in labour being not uncommon, and children's funerals a feature of everyday life. Even with these stark global inequities, there is cause for optimism. Childhood and motherhood are now substantially less hazardous than they were, with remarkable improvements in survival and health over recent decades. Worldwide, the under-five years' mortality rate was cut in half between 1990 and 2015, and the maternal mortality ratio by just under half. However, there is much still to be done.

The United Kingdom is not a leader among high-income nations in child health. Five additional children die every day in the United Kingdom compared with Sweden (the country with the lowest child mortality in Europe). UNICEF ranks the United Kingdom bottom of a league of 21 developed countries for childhood well-being.

Stillbirth rates in the United Kingdom are some of the worst in high-income countries, and there is substantial variation in healthcare provision and health outcomes across the country.

The spectrum of maternal and child health runs from fertility and family planning, through antenatal care and postnatal care, into childhood and then adolescence. Children's health depends particularly on healthcare services, their health behaviours, wider determinants of health and, for some, on child and family protection services.

MATERNAL MORTALITY

An estimated 800 women die every day from preventable pregnancy-related causes – almost all of them in low-income countries. Maternal deaths are subdivided into four broad categories (Table 8.1). The World Health Organization defines a maternal death as 'the death of a woman while pregnant or within 42 days of termination of pregnancy, from any cause related to or aggravated by the pregnancy or its management, but not from accidental or incidental causes'.

Globally, there has been a huge decline in maternal mortality over recent years, with rates dropping by almost 50% worldwide over nearly two and a half decades since 1990. In 1990, it was 385 per 100,000 live births. Twenty-five years later, it was 216 per 100,000 live births. This has been attributed to improvements in the general health of women, wider availability of simple medical technologies (such as antibiotics and blood transfusion), a reduction in the number of illegal abortions and improved obstetric and anaesthetic care.

As described in Chapter 1, reducing maternal mortality was one of the Millennium Development Goals. The aim was to reduce it by 75% in the period between 1990 and 2015. The reduction of nearly 50% achieved does not hit the target, but is remarkable nonetheless. A substantial focus of policymaking and action planning must be in Africa: 36 of the 40 countries with maternal mortality rates of 300 deaths per 100,000 live births are on that continent.

Table 8.1 Subdivisions of maternal mortality

1. **Direct maternal deaths** result from obstetric complications of pregnancy, labour and the puerperium.
2. **Indirect maternal deaths** arise from an existing disease, or one developing in pregnancy whose effects were accelerated or changed by the pregnancy.
3. **Fortuitous** (or **coincidental** in the United Kingdom) **maternal deaths** result from causes not related to or influenced by pregnancy.
4. **Late deaths** occur more than 42 days but less than one year after the end of the pregnancy, and can be direct, indirect or fortuitous.

Table 8.2 Causes of maternal death worldwide

		Number	Percentage of total
Direct causes	Abortion	193,000	8
	Embolism	78,000	3
	Haemorrhage	661,000	27
	Hypertension	343,000	14
	Sepsis	261,000	11
	Other	235,000	10
Indirect causes		672,000	28

Source: Say L, Chou D, Gemmill A, et al. Global causes of maternal death: a WHO systematic analysis. *Lancet Global Health* 2014; 2(6):e323-33.

Understanding the causes of maternal death worldwide requires expert analysis because the quality of available data on causation is so variable. Such studies (Table 8.2) show that almost three-quarters of deaths are due to direct obstetric causes and just over a quarter to indirect causes. The three leading direct causes are haemorrhage, hypertension and sepsis, while among indirect causes, the precise conditions are not well defined, although HIV-related problems are prominent in many African settings.

Addressing the direct and indirect causes of maternal illness and death opens up the opportunity to reduce mortality of mothers and newborns. Measures include expanding access to facility-based care; bringing the management of more women's antenatal care and delivery into the hands of skilled midwives, nurses or doctors; and widespread adoption of evidence-based practices (e.g. sterile blades for cutting umbilical cords, drugs for treatment or prevention of postpartum haemorrhage, immediate breastfeeding, magnesium sulphate to treat pre-eclampsia, appropriate use of antibiotics and rigorous application of hand hygiene practices). At a fundamental level, the societies most affected by poor maternal, neonatal and child health will also have to fully embrace the concepts of gender equality and education for girls.

In the United Kingdom, the maternal mortality ratio was 9 per 100,000 live births in 2015. Since the 1970s, the two leading causes of direct maternal death have been pulmonary embolism and hypertension in pregnancy.

The Confidential Enquiry into Maternal Deaths examines individual cases to produce recommendations for action. It has identified potential for improvement in a range of areas, including diagnostic errors, inappropriate treatment, a need for better communication between health professionals, greater involvement of consultants during pregnancy and labour and a need to consistently recognize and act on potential problems that arise.

In recent years, the confidential enquiries have found that about two-thirds of deaths are due to medical and mental health problems in pregnancy, and one-third due to direct complications of pregnancy, such as bleeding. Three-quarters of deaths occurred in women with known pre-existing health problems. One in eleven deaths were found to be due to influenza, despite flu vaccines being made available to pregnant women.

CHILD MORTALITY

The rates of infant mortality and of deaths of children under five years of age are important indicators of a population's overall health status (Table 8.3). They, along with maternal

Table 8.3 Key measures of mortality

Mortality measures	Description
Stillbirth rate	Number of stillbirths (deaths from the 24th week of gestation) per 1000 total births in one year
Perinatal mortality rate	Number of still births and deaths up to 6 completed days of life per 1000 total births in one year
Early neonatal mortality rate	Number of deaths from birth up to six complete days of life per 1000 total live births in one year
Late neonatal mortality rate	Number of deaths between the 7th and 27th completed days of life per 1000 total live births in one year
Neonatal mortality rate	Number of deaths in the first 27 completed days of life per 1000 total live births in one year
Post-neonatal mortality rate	Number of deaths between 28 days and the first year of life per 1000 total live births in one year
Infant mortality rate	Number of deaths in infants aged less than one year per 1000 total live births in one year

mortality and life expectancy, are widely used in making global comparisons of health.

Like maternal mortality, childhood mortality has also fallen greatly over recent years, as a result of improved public health and health services, economic development, better health technologies, better nutrition, safer housing and smaller families. Like maternal mortality, the under-five mortality was the subject of a Millennium Development Goal – to achieve a two-thirds reduction between 1990 and 2015. A reduction of nearly 50% was achieved – from 91 deaths per 1000 live births in 1990 to 43 deaths per 1000 live births 25 years later. The infant mortality rate fell similarly (Figure 8.1).

Despite the improvements, approximately 6.3 million children aged under five years still die worldwide in a year – 74% within their first year of life. Most deaths in under-five-year-olds occur in sub-Saharan Africa and Southeast Asia. Only around 2% occur in Europe. As ever, such inequality is also seen within countries, not just between them. Child mortality rates are generally higher in rural areas, for poorer families and for less educated families.

A child's risk of dying is highest immediately after birth, and decreases over the subsequent days, months and years. Worldwide, the main causes of death in the first month (the neonatal period) are prematurity, infection and birth-related complications such as asphyxia. The main causes of death for infants and children aged 28 days to 4 years are infection (including pneumonia, HIV, measles and malaria), diarrhoea, congenital anomalies and other non-communicable diseases (Figure 8.2). About 45% of all child deaths are linked to malnutrition. Many of these causes are preventable and treatable.

Birth registration is a legal requirement in the United Kingdom. Every birth must be registered within 42 days in England and 21 days in Scotland. The information is collected by the local registrar of births, marriages and deaths and passed to the Office for National Statistics in England and Wales. In parallel to birth registration is the system of birth notification, which involves the midwife, doctor or other birth attendant informing authorities about the birth within 36 hours. The two systems have different purposes. Registration legally records the birth, parentage and name, and provides a birth certificate. Notification alerts health services to the birth so that the necessary care and support can be provided. If a baby dies, that death must also be registered within five days. Systems for birth and death registration vary in their accuracy and comprehensiveness internationally, which can impair comparisons between countries. Recording of infant mortality is very complete in the United Kingdom, but is not so good in some lower-income countries.

A stillbirth is legally defined as 'a child which has issued forth from its mother after the 24th week of pregnancy and which did not at any time after, having been completely expelled from its mother, breathe or show any other signs of life'. Risk factors for stillbirth include maternal smoking, obesity, age over 35 years, alcohol consumption, first pregnancy, illicit drug use, diabetes and hypertension. Infection and placental pathology account for the majority of stillbirths, but about a third remain unexplained. Stillbirths must be registered within three months. In addition to the information recorded for a live birth, data are obtained from the medical certificate of stillbirth on cause of death, gestational age and postmortem findings.

In the United Kingdom, improvements in nutrition, education, environmental conditions and medical care have brought about a substantial reduction in childhood mortality over the last century. In the 1930s, most childhood deaths in western Europe were caused by infectious disease, including pneumonia, tuberculosis, diphtheria, measles and whooping cough. As described in Chapter 3,

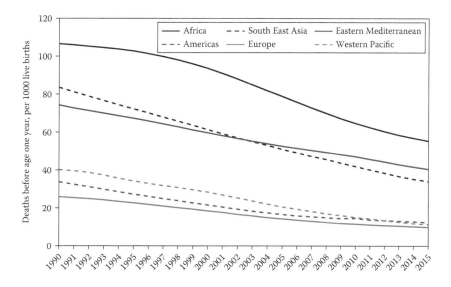

Figure 8.1 Infant mortality rate by world region.

Source: UNICEF, WHO, World Bank, and UN Population Division. *Levels and Trends in Child Mortality 2015.* New York: UNICEF, 2015. With permission.

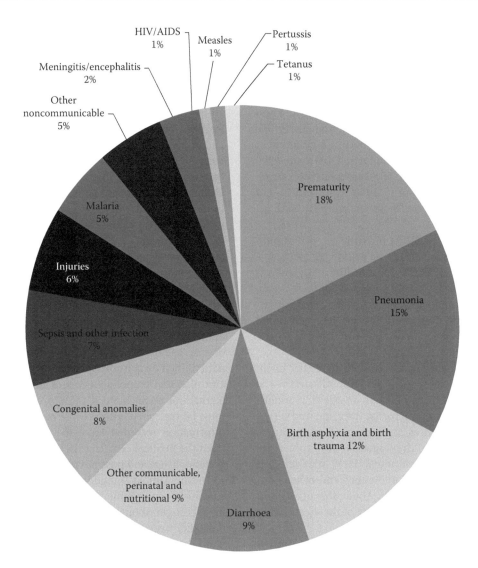

Figure 8.2 Causes of death among children aged under 5 years globally, 2015.

Source: World Health Organization. With permission.

the incidence of such diseases has declined very markedly, and non-communicable diseases are now responsible for a much greater proportion of morbidity and mortality.

In 2015, there were 3147 stillbirths in the United Kingdom, equating to 4.5 stillbirths per 1000 total births. Although the rate has fallen by 1.8% since the beginning of the twenty-first century, the fall is lower than in some other European countries, such as Poland. The stillbirth rate in Britain is one of the worst in the developed world. It is entirely unclear why this is. Possible explanations include suboptimal antenatal care, with services particularly failing to act quickly enough when issues arise; under-investigation of stillbirths, so that lessons are not learned; and insufficient awareness of the risk factors among parents and clinicians. Health inequalities are clear – women from the most deprived areas suffer the highest rates of stillbirth (Figure 8.3). Increasing attention is being paid to the need to monitor fetal health more closely and to raise clinical awareness that fetal growth failure raises the risk of subsequent stillbirth. Some coding inconsistencies

between countries make it difficult to directly compare stillbirth rates. Nonetheless, there is a need for improvement in the United Kingdom.

In the first half of the 1990s, there was a notable fall in mortality attributed to *sudden infant death syndrome* (SIDS), when the Department of Health's *Back to Sleep* campaign advocated putting babies to sleep on their backs. The origins of this highly successful public health campaign are described in Chapter 2.

Low birthweight is the single most important risk factor for perinatal death. The main factors associated with low birthweight are congenital malformations, multiple pregnancies, maternal smoking, consumption of alcohol, poor nutrition, low socio-economic status and teenage pregnancy. Many factors associated with low birthweight and perinatal mortality are interrelated, so assessing their independent contribution is difficult. Low birthweight is reducing, albeit gradually. Survival of babies with very low birthweight has improved over the last 40 years, partly

Index of multiple deprivation quintiles

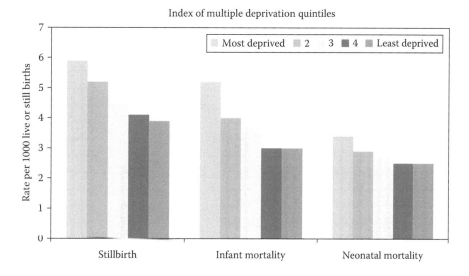

Figure 8.3 Stillbirth, neonatal and infant mortality rate by deprivation, England 2012.

Source: Office for National Statistics.

because of technological advances and the wider availability of intensive care facilities.

Survival of premature babies has also improved. Babies born between 32 and 36 weeks' gestation are described as *moderate to late preterm*; between 28 and 31 weeks 6 days, as *very preterm*; and less than 28 weeks, as *extremely preterm*. The more premature a baby is, the poorer its chance of survival. In 2010, a baby born at 25 weeks and admitted to a neonatal intensive care unit had a 70% chance of survival with intended care, up from 44% in 1997. Around half who survive suffer from long-term sequelae, including cerebral palsy, learning difficulties, behavioural problems and respiratory problems such as asthma. Although survival has improved, the proportion of surviving premature babies who suffer major long-term complications has not. There is therefore an increasing number of children with such complications, which represents an increased burden for families and for health and related services. Rates of very preterm birth (between 28 and 32 weeks' gestation) in the United Kingdom are higher than those in other European countries, but lower than those in the United States.

Twenty years ago, children under 19 years had a mortality rate in the United Kingdom similar to that in the rest of Europe. The rate has fallen over the last 20 years, but not as rapidly as elsewhere in Europe. As a result, the United Kingdom's rate is now one of the highest. The problem is most marked for children under the age of four years, whose death rates have fallen from the top to the bottom quartile.

The Royal College of Paediatrics and Child Health has estimated that if Sweden's child mortality rate (the lowest in Europe) was equalled in the United Kingdom, the lives of 1950 additional children would be saved every year. In other words, the United Kingdom currently has five excess child deaths a day, beyond the level found in Sweden.

The United Kingdom has performed relatively well in reducing injury-related mortality, but childhood cancer survival rates and diabetic control markers in children are worse than those in other comparable countries. Factors contributing to the United Kingdom's relatively poor performance likely include the quality of healthcare services, particularly for chronic disorders; the degree of health inequalities; and a high rate of preterm births and low-birthweight babies.

Every year, around 6000 children between the ages of 0 and 19 years die in the United Kingdom. Two-thirds are aged less than one year (Figure 8.4). After infancy, the next highest risk of death is among adolescents, for whom death rates have not improved over the last half a century.

Injury is the main cause of mortality for children over one year in the United Kingdom, and is a major cause of morbidity also. Intentional injuries most frequently include assault and self-harm, often due to maltreatment in preschool children and violence in adolescence. Unintentional injuries are more widespread than intentional injuries. They are most often due to accidents at home, including drowning, poisoning, falls and burns. An estimated 60 children under the age of five years die in England each year from unintentional injuries, which are also responsible for 450,000 visits to accident and emergency departments and 40,000 emergency hospital admissions. The types of unintentional injury that cause death vary by age group. The five main causes of unintentional injuries among the under-fives are choking, suffocation and strangulation; falls; poisoning; burns and scalds; and drowning.

In England, children living in the most deprived areas are 13 times more likely to die from poisoning and injury than those living in the least deprived areas. The rate of hospital admissions for unintentional injury is 45% higher in the most deprived areas than in the least deprived.

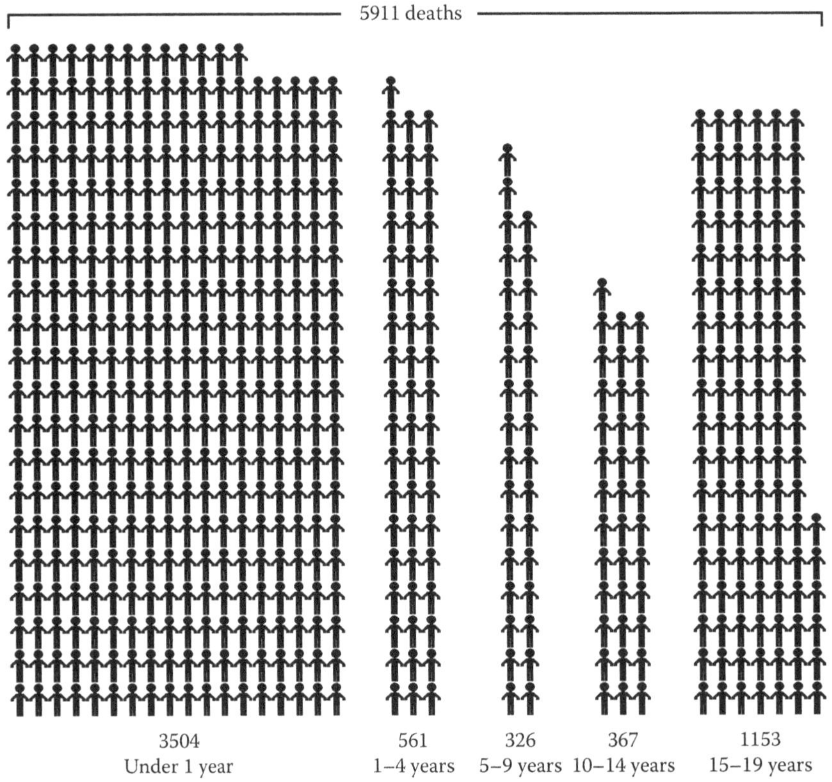

Figure 8.4 Deaths of children aged under 15 years, United Kingdom, 2012.

Source: Royal College of Paediatrics and Child Health and National Children's Bureau. With permission.

Several strands of action are needed to reduce the number and severity of injuries. These include legislation, regulation, modification of products and environments, education, health promotion and hazard surveillance. The Royal Society for the Prevention of Accidents (ROSPA) has run a number of successful campaigns, including on drink-driving legislation, compulsory seat belt wearing and blind cord safety. A number of initiatives have been introduced to reduce deaths from road traffic accidents in England, including the introduction of 20 mph speed limits. Mortality and morbidity rates for child pedestrians are improving and are now among the lowest in Europe.

FERTILITY AND FAMILY PLANNING

The everyday meaning of *fertility* is the ability of individuals and their partners to conceive children; technically, the more correct word for that is *fecundity*. The term fertility is also used to describe how many children a population produces, and to make comparisons between areas, and over time. Many factors influence this:

- Levels of affluence and poverty
- Women's status within a society
- Education and employment rates
- Women's and men's health
- Individuals' physiology

- Lifestyle choices
- Religion
- Societal expectations
- The law
- Availability and use of contraception
- Patterns of marriage and cohabitation

In England and Wales, fertility patterns have changed since the mid-1960s. Fertility generally increased after World War II, the so-called baby boom generation, to reach a peak, and then fell so that by 1977 it had returned to the level that it was at in 1933. Since then, fertility rates have remained fairly stable.

The fall in fertility between the mid-1960s and the late-1970s was influenced by many factors. One was the availability of effective contraceptive methods. The oral contraceptive pill, introduced to Britain in the early 1960s, gave women the ability to control their reproductive lives effectively and simply for the first time. This is not the whole explanation, though, because fertility fell in the 1930s, and in the late 1960s in other industrialized nations where family planning services were much less well developed. Income levels and attitudes about future prosperity may well have played a role; both were times of major economic recession. Also, an increasing number of women of childbearing age were entering the workforce, and therefore restricting family size to progress in their careers. However, the increase in married women working was just as steep in the 1960s as it was in the 1970s. In short, fertility rates are the product of multiple factors.

Childbearing has changed in other ways over the last 70 years too. There are more childless women. An increasing proportion of births are outside marriage: 48% in 2012 compared with 4% in 1938. The age of childbearing is also changing, with the greatest live birth rate now among 30- to 34-year-old women (Figure 8.5). In 1971, by sharp contrast, the birth rate among women aged 20–25 years was more than double that of women aged 30–34 years.

In a population, fertility is described numerically by a number of important indices (Table 8.4). In addition, a population's *replacement fertility rate* is the total fertility rate at which a population remains precisely stable, because women have exactly enough children to replace themselves and their partner. The replacement fertility rate depends on female mortality and the birth sex ratio, as well as on fertility. Obviously, it is around 2, but must be slightly greater than this to compensate for women who die before or during the childbearing years, and for the unbalanced birth sex ratio. In Europe, it is 2.10, and in Africa, it is 2.70. In the United Kingdom, it is falling as mortality rates fall among young women.

Infertility

Infertility and subfertility are usually due to the inability to produce sperm or ovulate or a blockage in either the vas deferens or the fallopian tubes. Approximately 35%–40% of infertility problems relate to the male partner and 35%–40% to the female, with no apparent cause in the remainder of cases. In women, infections such as gonorrhoea, chlamydia and other pelvic inflammatory conditions can lead to scarring or blockage of the fallopian tubes, causing acquired infertility. Acquired infertility in men is less well understood and harder to treat. Female fertility declines with age, while the effect of age on male fertility is less well understood. Obesity and smoking are likely to reduce fertility in both sexes.

Formerly, adoption was the only solution for infertile couples. As effective contraception became widespread and abortion was legalized, the number of babies offered for adoption reduced markedly. This has, to some extent, been countered by the development of assisted reproduction methods such as *in vitro fertilization* (IVF), which is regulated by the Human Fertilisation and Embryology Authority. With treatment, about a third of infertile couples achieve a successful pregnancy, although success rates vary

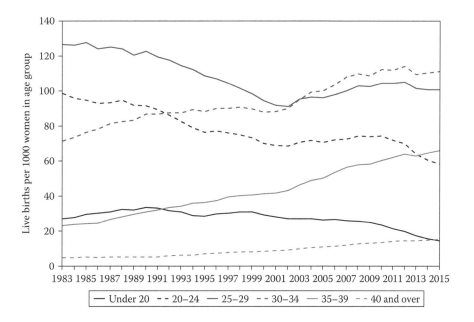

Figure 8.5 Age-specific fertility rates in England and Wales.

Source: Office for National Statistics.

Table 8.4 Important fertility indices

Crude birth rate	The number of live births in one year per 1000 total population
General fertility rate	The number of live births per 1000 women in the population of child-bearing age (15–44 years)
Age-specific fertility rates	The number of live births in women of a certain age per 1000 women in the population of that age
Total fertility rate	Sum of all age-specific fertility rates expressed as live births, equating to the average number of children born to a woman over her lifetime if she were to live to the end of her reproductive years.

according to the woman's age, clinical factors and service performance. *In vitro* fertilization has led to an increase in multiple births. This may create longer-term health problems, as many are of low birthweight. In recent years, surrogacy has also become possible. This involves a woman carrying and bearing a child – either through straight (or traditional) surrogacy, in which the baby is conceived using the surrogate's egg, or by host (or gestational) surrogacy, in which *in vitro* fertilization is used and the egg is either from the intended mother or from another donor egg. The legal aspects of surrogacy vary between countries.

Contraceptive methods

Ancient methods of contraception include *coitus interruptus*, which is still used; the natural family planning method, which involves understanding the timing of fertility in a woman's cycle; and various acidic or alkaline substances inserted into the vagina. Effective male and female barrier methods of contraception were introduced in the nineteenth century. Condoms in particular are still an effective method of contraception, and also protect against sexually transmitted infections. Since the 1960s, the oral contraceptive pill has dominated contraceptive methods, but is increasingly being replaced by new hormonal delivery systems and the intrauterine device. Sterilization for males or females is a permanent method of contraception. There are two methods of emergency contraception: hormonal (levonorgestrel) treatment or the insertion of an intrauterine device. The hormonal method can be used up to 72 hours after sex and the intrauterine device up to 5 days later. While the insertion of an intrauterine device requires professional involvement, the emergency contraceptive pill can be easily obtained, including in most pharmacies.

The efficacy of the various methods of contraception varies. Typically, the proportion of women experiencing an unintended pregnancy within the first year of use of contraceptive pill is 8%, and 15% for the male condom. These are higher figures than many people realize, and reflect a significant degree of user failure. Used correctly, the failure rate falls to less than 1% for the pill and 2% for the condom. Failure rates fall as user experience increases. Some methods, such as sterilization and implants, have much lower failure rates and, by their nature, little variation between users: 0.05% for the long-acting implant and 0.5% for female sterilization. Risks related to the combined pill include breast cancer, thrombosis and stroke. However, the benefits include a reduction in endometrial and ovarian cancer risk. Media stories about the safety of hormonal contraception have stopped women from using it at different times, and rises in abortion rates in the years that followed have been attributed to the concerns. Women's health advocates argue that side effects of hormonal treatments, such as emotional well-being, weight gain, menstrual bleeding and headaches, are often ignored by researchers. All women, providing they are not at risk of acquiring an infection, can use intrauterine devices. Sterilization involves a one-time risk associated with surgery.

Family planning services in Britain are provided in three main ways: by general practitioners, in the community through specialized family planning and sexual health clinics and in obstetrics and gynaecology departments in local hospitals.

Abortion

Globally, the World Health Organization estimates that 42 million pregnancies are voluntarily terminated in a year. Of these, an estimated 22 million are terminated safely and 20 million unsafely. These figures are rough estimates and are not updated every year. The World Health Organization defines an unsafe abortion as 'a procedure carried out either by persons lacking the necessary skills or in an environment that does not conform to minimal medical standards or both'. It identifies a range of factors likely to lead to unsafe abortion:

- No pre-abortion counselling and advice.
- Abortion is induced by an unskilled provider, frequently in unhygienic conditions, or by a health practitioner outside official or adequate health facilities.
- Abortion is provoked by insertion of an object into the uterus by the woman herself or by a traditional practitioner, or by a violent abdominal massage.
- A medical abortion is prescribed incorrectly or medication is issued by a pharmacist with no or inadequate instructions and no follow-up.
- Abortion is self-induced by ingestion of traditional medication or hazardous substances.
- The lack of immediate intervention if severe bleeding or other emergency develops during the procedure.
- Failure to provide postabortion check-up and care, including no contraceptive counselling to prevent repeat abortion.
- The reluctance of a woman to seek timely medical care in case of complications because of legal restrictions and social and cultural beliefs linked to induced abortion.

Unsafe abortions were common in the United Kingdom before the *Abortion Act 1967*. The act covers England, Scotland and Wales but not Northern Ireland, where abortion remains illegal. The current requirements are that two registered medical practitioners certify that certain defined indications for abortion have been met, that the abortion is performed by a registered medical practitioner and that the procedure is undertaken in a National Health Service (NHS) hospital or other approved premises. The abortion regulations require any termination to be notified within 14 days to the chief medical officer according to where the termination takes place. Abortion is legally defined as 'the emptying of a pregnant uterus up to the 24th week of pregnancy'. A termination of pregnancy is the legal ending of a pregnancy. Spontaneous abortion or miscarriage occurs in an estimated 9%–15% of recognized pregnancies – usually for unknown reasons.

Overall, the proportion of conceptions that end in termination of pregnancy is around 22%, although this varies by age. The highest rates in 2014 were among 22-year-old women. The figure for the older group reflects terminations undertaken as a result of screening for congenital anomalies – Down's syndrome in particular. The abortion rate fell in the lowest age groups between 2009 and 2014, but it remains higher than the average of European member states (Figure 8.6).

Since abortion became legal, the abortion rate has generally risen. In 2014, there were 15.9 abortions per 1000 women resident in England and Wales aged 15–44 years. This was the lowest rate for 17 years, but is three times greater than the rate of 5.2 in 1969, the first full year of the act's operation.

Teenage pregnancy

Teenage pregnancy (sometimes called *adolescent pregnancy*) is defined as pregnancy in a female aged less than 18 years; international comparisons are usually made using rates for the under-15s and the under-18s. It is an important societal and public health issue in many countries of the world. The World Health Organization estimates that 16 million girls each year become pregnant. In poorer countries, it is often associated with child marriage; for example, in Niger one in three girls are married before they are 15 years old. There is a similar position in some other countries. The United Nations has focused on the problem of motherhood in childhood and estimates that there are seven million teenage pregnancies in low-income countries, 2 million in girls aged 14 years or younger.

Girls who become pregnant at a young age are harmed physically and mentally; they are disempowered and lose opportunities available to other women; they are at higher risk of mortality and other complications of pregnancy (this is particularly so for girls in rural and isolated locations). United Nations Fund for Population Activities (UNFPA) executive director Babatunde Osotimehin has said, 'Adolescent pregnancy is intertwined with the issue of human rights. A pregnant girl who is pressured or forced to leave school, for example, is denied her right to education'.

In the United Kingdom, around three-quarters of teenage pregnancies are unplanned, and half end in abortion. There can be negative sequelae for both mother and baby. Compared with older women, teenage mothers have worse antenatal health, poorer mental health (including a greater risk of postnatal depression), higher rates of smoking during pregnancy and lower rates of breastfeeding. Teenage mothers are also more likely to end up as single parents and to bring up their children in poverty, and are less likely to finish their education or find a good job. Their babies are more likely to die, and to have a low birthweight, poorer health, and lower educational attainment. They are more likely to be unemployed, and to become teenage parents themselves. The young people most likely to become teenage parents are those with below-average achievement levels and low socio-economic status.

Rates of teenage pregnancy have decreased in most industrialized countries since the 1960s. In the United Kingdom, the rate fell by 40% between 1998 and 2012 but remains high in comparison with other member states of the European Union (Figure 8.7).

The UK government has developed various initiatives to reduce teenage pregnancy rates. A national strategy implemented from the end of the 1990s seems to have been particularly effective. Under-18-years' conception rates are a key priority and monitored carefully.

Effective methods to reduce teenage pregnancy include working with health, education, social and youth services, and the voluntary sector; effective, well-publicized, young people-centred contraceptive and sexual health advice services; giving high priority to personal, social and health

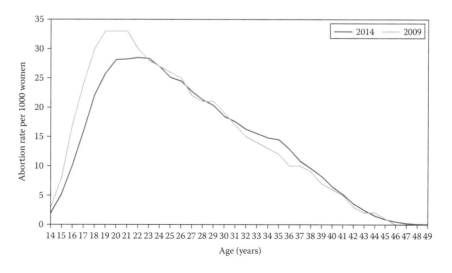

Figure 8.6 Abortion rate by age, England and Wales, 2009 versus 2014.

Source: Office for National Statistics.

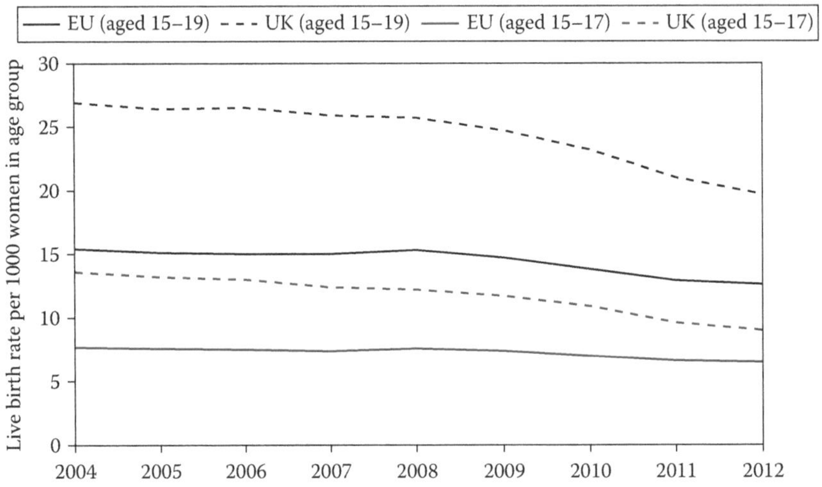

Figure 8.7 Live birth rate to teenagers in United Kingdom and European Union.

Source: Office for National Statistics.

education in schools; easier access to contraception; wider availability of counselling and support services; targeted interventions with young people at high risk; and availability of sex and relationships education training for professionals.

ANTENATAL CARE

A strong system of antenatal care gives mothers and babies a greater chance of a positive outcome of pregnancy. In low- and middle-income countries, attention has been focused on creating access to antenatal care, initially with a goal of at least one visit (in the poorest parts of the world). This goal has been extended in recognition that the full life-saving benefits of antenatal care are best realized through four visits. In 2012, 55 million pregnant women in low- and middle-income countries did not receive the four antenatal visits. Although the benchmark of four visits is helpful, the content of the antenatal care given is vital. Essential measures include recognizing and dealing with complications of pregnancy, such as pre-eclampsia; giving tetanus toxoid immunization and intermittent preventive treatment for malaria; and identifying and managing infections such as HIV, syphilis and chlamydia. Good antenatal care can enable the promotion of the use of skilled attendance at birth and breastfeeding, as well as planning postnatal care and pregnancy spacing. In a review of antenatal care in 41 low- and middle-income countries, the delivery of necessary interventions was below what was needed (Figure 8.8).

In the United Kingdom, comprehensive antenatal care encompasses lifestyle advice (smoking, alcohol, drugs and diet); screening for maternal illness (hypertensive disease, diabetes and infection); recognition and treatment of anomalies in pregnancy; assessment of fetal size, development and well-being; psychological preparation for delivery (including antenatal classes); and education about breastfeeding and parenting. In clinic and in classes, women are

encouraged to think about pregnancy even before conception, including discussion about lifestyle, timing of conception and the value of taking folate supplements to prevent neural tube defects. Most women want to do the best for their baby, and so antenatal care is a good time to promote health for the woman, child and whole family.

The most common model of antenatal care in the United Kingdom involves a shared approach between the midwife, the general practitioner and the hospital obstetrics and gynaecology department. Midwives are involved in a woman's care from identification of pregnancy through labour and birth, and until 28 days after the baby is born. They work both in the community and in hospitals.

Some women's health places their babies at higher risk of fetal anomaly. Women with diabetes, for example, require preconceptual care and monitoring of the pregnancy and delivery. Drugs prescribed in pregnancy can cause fetal anomalies, so women on long-term medication (such as for epilepsy) need preconceptual advice and possibly changes to their medication regime. Low birthweight, which is a risk factor for adverse long-term health and developmental outcomes, occurs more commonly to women who are very young, or much older.

The main modifiable risk factors during pregnancy are smoking, illicit drug use, obesity, mental illness, psychosocial stress and undernutrition. Many cluster together in the same women, and some women are more susceptible to the effects than others. Undernutrition has been associated with heart disease in the future adult, lower birth rate and congenital abnormalities. The association between smoking and low birthweight, first documented in the mid-1950s, persists, and maternal smoking also raises the risk of miscarriage, stillbirth, sudden infant death syndrome and neonatal death. Heavy alcohol consumption, particularly early in pregnancy, can lead to *fetal alcohol syndrome*. This is characterized by retarded growth and anomalies of the face and nervous system, as well as abnormal behaviour of the baby.

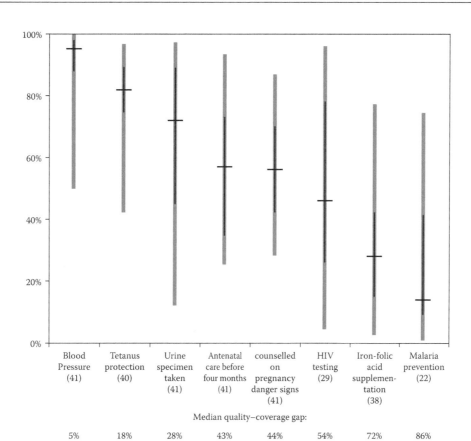

Figure 8.8 Coverage of key antenatal services amongst pregnant women receiving four or more antenatal care visits in 41 countries.

Source: Hodgins S, D'Agostino A. The quality–coverage gap in antenatal care: toward better measurement of effective coverage. *Global Health: Science and Practice* 2014;2(2):173–81.

Vitamin D deficiency is common in the United Kingdom, affecting an estimated two-thirds of women in some urban areas. This can lead to poor bone health and an increased risk of infection, such as tuberculosis, in the baby.

There is a great deal of public health advice about what women should and should not eat and drink during pregnancy. Most official sources advise pregnant women to avoid certain soft and blue cheeses; pâté; raw or undercooked eggs and meat; cold-cured meat; liver; certain fish, such as shark or swordfish or excess oily fish and tuna; and raw shellfish. It is also recommended that they restrict caffeine and alcohol intake.

In the United Kingdom, pregnant women are offered tests, antenatally, to identify risks to the mother or the child. These include blood tests (full blood count, blood group, rhesus D status, random blood sugar, sickle cell disease, thalassemia, HIV, hepatitis B, syphilis and rubella) and midstream urine tests (protein, glucose and bacteriuria). Women also have a fetal anomaly scan at 18–20 weeks' gestation. Women at high risk may be offered screening for psychiatric illness or genetic diseases.

In the first trimester, pregnant women are also offered screening for Down's syndrome. Down's syndrome affects approximately 1 birth per 1000. Information from maternal serum marker results is combined with maternal age and the ultrasound measurement of nuchal thickness (fluid at the back of the fetal neck) to estimate the risk that the baby will have Down's syndrome. Depending on the results, parents can choose either chorionic villus sampling or amniocentesis, depending on the gestational age. Parents can then be counselled according to the results. A new noninvasive diagnostic test for Down's syndrome currently in clinical trials involves a maternal blood test to check fetal DNA.

The National Screening Committee keeps the content of this antenatal screening programme under review, updating it as needed. As for any diagnostic or screening test, it is important that the woman fully understands the possible outcomes of the process and gives informed consent. Some test results raise the possibility of terminating the pregnancy. In such cases, parents can be counselled, and potentially offered this, based on the results and on the stage that the pregnancy has reached.

HEALTHCARE AFTER BIRTH IN THE UNITED KINGDOM

Most neonates are given a dose of vitamin K immediately after birth. Vitamin K is required for blood clotting and therefore reduces the risk of bleeding. This dose is particularly important for premature or unwell babies and poor feeders. Immediately after birth, a spot of blood is taken from the neonate via a heel prick. This is tested for cystic fibrosis, sickle cell disease, congenital hypothyroidism and inherited metabolic diseases (phenylketonuria and medium-chain Acyl-CoA dehydrogenase deficiency [MCADD]) and four further inherited metabolic diseases (maple syrup disease, isovaleric acidaemia, glutaric aciduria type 1 and homocystinuria).

Within 72 hours of birth, and again at six to eight weeks of age, all babies have a comprehensive physical examination. Commonly referred to as the *baby check*, this is formally the NHS Newborn and Infant Physical Examination Programme. Eyes are examined for cataracts and retinoblastoma (found in 2–3 babies per 10,000 live births). Hips are examined for developmental dysplasia (incidence of cases requiring an operation is between 1 and 2 in every 1000 live births). Boys are examined for undescended testes (found in 2% at birth). The heart is examined for any murmurs suggestive of congenital heart disease (which affects around 8 of every 1000 live births).

After birth, the family is given the personal child health record (*Red Book*), in which immunizations, weight, height and developmental checks are recorded. The Red Book also signposts parents to information that they might need. The record is given to parents, rather than being retained by medical staff, with the aim of empowering parents and encouraging partnership between them and medical staff. An electronic version of the Red Book will likely soon be introduced, although the paper book will still be given to parents so that they have choice of access to information. The six- to eight-week check also includes a developmental review and the opportunity for health promotion, principally promoting breastfeeding, immunizations and safety at home. On each occasion, babies are also generally examined, and their weight and length measured.

The final element of the standard screening programme for newborns and neonates is a hearing test within the first three months – either an automated otoacoustic emissions test or an attenuated auditory brainstem response test.

The majority of neonates can be discharged home within 24 hours of birth, but some require medical care in hospital. Neonatal care is categorized into three levels. *Level 1* neonatal units provide special care, but no high-dependency or intensive care. They may or may not have resident medical staff. *Level 2* units provide high-dependency care and some short-term intensive care. *Level 3* units provide the whole range of medical neonatal care. The outcome for very small and very preterm babies is better if they are treated in higher-level units. Some neonates require additional specialist services – such as surgery – that are available at a subset of level 3 units.

BREASTFEEDING

Breastfeeding has important health benefits for mother and baby. For the baby, there is evidence that it lowers neonatal mortality risk, reduces long-term obesity, protects against some infections through the immunoglobulins passed from mother to child in breast milk and may enhance cognitive development. Some studies suggest that it also reduces the incidence of gastrointestinal, respiratory and ear infections; dermatitis; inflammatory bowel disease; coeliac disease; and the long-term risk of diabetes, asthma, heart disease, atopy and leukaemia. For the mother, it increases her connectivity to the baby, promotes weight loss and reduces the risk of ovarian and breast cancer. Breastfeeding can also be more convenient, cheaper and less prone to error than the use of powdered milks.

The World Health Organization recommends initiation of breastfeeding within one hour of birth, exclusive breastfeeding for the first six months of life and introduction of nutritionally adequate and safe complementary (solid) foods at six months, together with continued breastfeeding up to two years of age or beyond.

The United Kingdom has one of the lowest rates of breastfeeding in Europe, although it has increased in recent years. At six to eight weeks, the prevalence of breastfeeding is less than 50%. In Norway, 90% of babies are breastfed. There is also a great deal of variation in breastfeeding uptake between areas, with initiation generally lower in more disadvantaged areas of the United Kingdom. Some reasons that women give for not breastfeeding are fear of not producing enough milk to sustain the baby's necessary weight gain, social restrictions for feeding in public, reliance on them for feeding and lack of knowledge and support. Regular initiatives and campaigns are undertaken in the United Kingdom to increase the uptake of breastfeeding.

MATERNAL MENTAL HEALTH

Postnatal depression affects 10%–15% of women. It usually begins one to two months after a baby is born, but can start at any time during pregnancy or within the first year. Symptoms, which must last for two weeks for a diagnosis of postnatal depression to be made, include persistent low mood, irritability, anxiety and lack of sleep. Baby blues affects half of mothers, occurring around 3–10 days after childbirth and involving milder symptoms, such as mood swings and irritability. Postpartum puerperal psychosis is not common (0.1%–0.2% of women after childbirth) but is a severe mental illness, with symptoms such as delusions and hallucinations. Women with a history of bipolar disorder are at higher risk of postpartum puerperal psychosis. Other mental disorders, such as generalized anxiety states, can also occur during and after pregnancy.

Depression and psychosis around the time of birth can have serious consequences for the mother, baby and family unit, when most women expect to be happy. Very few women harm their babies. There may be risks to the baby associated with a mother taking antidepressants during pregnancy or breastfeeding, which must be weighed against the risks to the mother and baby of not giving such treatment. The National Institute for Health and Care Excellence

(NICE) advises that risk factors and symptoms of postnatal depression should be checked at the various contacts a woman has during her pregnancy and in the first year after birth, and that women judged at risk of mental illness should have additional support.

CHILDREN'S SERVICES IN THE UNITED KINGDOM

A wide range of public services are available to help and support children and families, some provided by the NHS, others by local authorities and still others by nongovernmental bodies (e.g. the National Society for the Prevention of Cruelty to Children [NSPCC]).

Healthy and unhealthy behaviour

Children's health is influenced by many different factors: their genetics, their physical and socio-economic environment, their family, their peers, the health services available to them and, more broadly, the cultural and political context in which they grow up. The same is true for adult health, but childhood is a particularly important time. As described in Chapter 5, the early years have a major influence over health throughout the rest of life.

Each of the six major risk factors for ill health in adulthood has firm foundations in childhood or adolescence. Damage starts to accumulate even before birth, and habits established in the early years are powerful. In England, more than a fifth of reception age schoolchildren and more than a third of year 6 children are obese or overweight. Many children eat food that is deficient in essential vitamins and minerals, and high in sugar. England consumes more sugary drinks per person than anywhere else in Europe. Teenagers in the United Kingdom report more heavy drinking than their counterparts in Europe, while more than a quarter of deaths among people aged 16–24 years are attributable to alcohol consumption. Only a quarter of children eat five or more portions of fruit and vegetables every day. One quarter of children in the United Kingdom are thought to be vitamin D deficient.

One in six children aged 11–15 years has taken drugs at least once before. Cannabis is the most commonly used drug, with side effects that include bronchitis, lung damage, depression, anxiety and schizophrenia. Use of class A drugs and volatile substances is rarer. The precise agents change all the time; for example, in the second decade of the twenty-first century, the use of legal highs increased greatly – these are chemical substances that are not sold for human consumption (e.g. as incense, bath salts and plant food), but they are bought and used for a psychoactive effect. They are banned but not covered by drug misuse legislation. Alterations to their chemical composition allow them to remain legal. For example, a product called *herbal haze*, sold legally in 2014, contained laboratory-designed cannabinoid approximately 100 times stronger than naturally occurring cannabis. There are considerable overlaps between those drinking alcohol, using drugs and smoking.

More than a quarter of children aged below 19 years are in, or at risk of, poverty or social exclusion. The adverse health impacts of poverty include:

- Psychosocial effects, including stress, poor self-esteem and poor parenting
- Environmental effects, such as damp or poor housing and exposure to pollutants
- Direct effects of low income, such as not having enough or sufficiently nutritious food
- Difficulty in accessing health services

As is discussed in Chapter 9, on mental health, 1 in 10 children between the ages of 5 and 16 years suffers from a mental health disorder, which is now the most common cause of childhood disability in the developed world. The most common are conduct disorders, emotional disorders (such as anxiety and depression) and attention deficit hyperactivity disorder (ADHD). Many more children have wider emotional and behavioural problems. Adolescents are at risk of personality disorders, depression and anxiety, all of which may be exacerbated by substance misuse. As well as causing distress, poor mental health impacts on a young person's physical health, educational achievement, social relationships and future mental health. Services for young people with mental health disorders are provided through Child and Adolescent Mental Health Services (CAMHS). They should be accessible in primary care, hospitals, schools and the community, although in reality, Child and Adolescent Mental Health Services are regularly criticized for a major shortfall in provision. In 2014, the House of Commons Health Select Committee published a hard-hitting report in which it found 'serious and deeply ingrained problems with the commissioning and provision of children's and adolescents' mental health services. These run through the whole system from prevention and early intervention through to inpatient services for the most vulnerable young people'.

There is a two-way relationship between health and schooling. Pupils with better health and well-being do better academically. In turn, the school environment influences the health and well-being of pupils quite substantially. School is a large part of life for children and young people. It is the backdrop to a number of positive health factors, including school nurses and physical, social, health and economic (PSHE) education, and more negative factors, like bullying and poor educational attainment. Around 35%–45% of British children experience bullying, which can impair mental health in both the short term and long term. There are two important transitions within the school years: at age 4–5 years, when most young children start school, and at age 11 years, when children move to secondary school. These periods can be challenging and stressful for children, especially for those from deprived backgrounds and vulnerable groups, but are also an opportunity to build resilience. Positive experiences of transition can mean good engagement with school and learning, and improved self-esteem. Successful transitions are associated with good health.

The Healthy Schools Programme in England has four core themes: personal, social and health education; physical activity; healthy eating; and emotional health and well-being. The programme has been successful in focusing schools on a whole-school approach to health and well-being, and there is evidence that this type of approach works best to improve exercise and nutrition in young people. School nurses lead the Healthy Child Programme for school-aged children, and promote healthy behaviours in schools. However, there are only around 1200 school nurses in England. This equates to one nurse for 7000 children. Young people say that they want better access to school nurses with guaranteed, confidential appointments. School nurses are very important for children with complex conditions and needs, who regularly have to miss school for hospital appointments and appreciate the benefit of having a nurse's support at school. Physical, social, health and economic education is another resource for young people at school, although Ofsted (the school standards inspectorate) has judged it as either needing improvement or inadequate in 40% of schools in England.

Adolescents and young people

Over the last 50 years in the United Kingdom, 10- to 19-year-olds have had the least health improvement of any age group. Indeed, in many countries, adolescent mortality is now greater than mortality at all other ages in childhood after the neonatal period. The main causes of death among adolescents are potentially preventable. The World Health Organization defines adolescents as young people aged 10–19 years, and the United Nations defines young people as those up to the age of 24 years.

Adolescence has also become more prominent because it is increasingly recognized that many chronic conditions have their origins in this stage of life. For example, 75% of adult mental health problems start in those under 18 years, and five of the top 10 risk factors for all ill health are influenced or shaped by adolescence. Adolescence is the time when children are making their own lifestyle choices, which may include unsafe sex, substance abuse (most commonly alcohol) and smoking. Children who drink early are at a greater risk of becoming alcohol dependent as adults. Adolescence is when young people with long-term disorders start to manage their own diseases for the first time. Good practice can pave the way for good disease management throughout life. Adolescence is a time not just of major physical and hormonal changes, but also of important brain development, including increases in white matter volume.

The main causes of death in adolescence are injuries (both intentional and nonintentional) and non-communicable diseases, particularly cancer. Sexually transmitted infections and poor mental health are important causes of morbidity. Sexual practices have changed over the last century, so that young people are having sex earlier, and often with more than one partner. This has led to higher rates of sexually transmitted infections.

The most common mental health problems in adolescence are conduct disorders in males and emotional disorders in females, including anxiety and self-harm. Girls are more likely to self-harm than boys. A World Health Organization 2013–14 study found that a fifth of 15-year-olds in England reported hurting themselves in the last year. Hospital admissions related to self-harm among children and young people have increased by nearly 70% over the last decade. Many adolescent mental health problems are never reported, so rates may be much higher than estimates suggest. Among people aged 15–29 years, the suicide rate in 2011 was 13.3 per 100,000 for males and 4 per 100,000 for females. These rates have largely remained stable over the last decade.

Health services are not sufficiently responsive to the needs of adolescents. Few services are targeted specifically for them, and people aged 16–24 years report the worst NHS experience of any age group. Young people feel particularly strongly about the need for better transition from child to adult services. Teenagers are often grouped either with very young children or with adults on the wards, both of which can be inappropriate. Many service users and mental health charities feel that Child and Adolescent Mental Health Services are currently inadequate in the United Kingdom, particularly due to a lack of funding. There is evidence that adolescent hospital wards with targeted services can lead to better outcomes, and keep young people within the health system. The World Health Organization and UNICEF stress the need for a holistic and developmental approach to care for young people.

Universal and targeted support for families

All families with children aged less than five years should have a health visitor. The role of a health visitor is to improve and promote the health of children. Some families receive additional targeted support, such as lone parents, teenage parents, disabled children, children with other additional needs and low birthweight babies. In the United Kingdom, this support is provided through additional health visitor time, or through specialized services such as the Family Nurse Partnership and Troubled Families programmes.

The Family Nurse Partnership Programme is a preventive maternal and early childhood health programme for first-time young parents, aged 19 years and under. It was modelled on a similar programme in the United States, and involves structured home visiting by trained family nurses from early pregnancy until the child is two years old. The goals are to improve pregnancy outcomes, promote child health, enhance development and boost future school achievement. The aim is to do so by enabling parents to provide competent and sensitive care for their babies, and to improve parents' own ongoing development and economic self-sufficiency. The family nurses do this by developing strong therapeutic relationships with young families. They guide them to make informed choices and adapt to the behaviours required for parenthood, and so adopt healthier lifestyles for themselves and their babies.

The Troubled Families Programme was launched in 2012, in the wake of the London riots. It initially aimed to turn around the lives of 120,000 troubled families through the efforts of a family support worker; this target was later extended to include 400,000 additional families. The expanded programme defines a troubled family as one with at least two of the following: parents and children involved in crime or antisocial behaviour, children regularly truanting, an adult on out-of-work benefits or a young person at risk of worklessness, domestic violence, vulnerable children identified as being in need or on a child protection plan, and mental or physical health problems. An *intervention worker* helps families that are part of the programme to get better control of their lives and to reduce the level of crisis, drawing on other services as required.

Healthcare

The model for children's healthcare services in the United Kingdom closely parallels that for adults. Community child health services are offered locally through primary care, through general practitioners and their surgeries. They can refer children onward to secondary care for hospital, outpatient or day care. Tertiary care is provided by specialized wards in acute hospitals, and by children's hospitals.

Unlike in some other European countries, general practitioners in the United Kingdom do not work alongside community paediatricians. General practitioners might not have had any specific training in paediatrics beyond their undergraduate training. The ideal model of integrated care is that all health professionals involved in a child's care are coordinated, with the child at the centre. In England, clinical commissioning groups are now responsible for primary and secondary healthcare services

for children and some of the Child and Adolescent Mental Health Services, although NHS England commissions other aspects. Local authorities, guided by health and well-being boards, are responsible for public health budgets, including health promotion and smoking services.

Children see general practitioners and use emergency departments more than adults do. Children represent 30% of the English population, but 40% of general practice consultations and 37% of emergency department visits. They use inpatient and outpatient services less than adults do, with 19% and 18% use, respectively.

Children's use of health resources is increasing. This reflects a change in the way that parents use the system more than any change in the underlying patterns of ill health. Over the last decade, hospital admissions for children aged under 15 years have increased by almost 30%. Acute hospital admissions through the emergency department have increased more than threefold for adolescents over the same period. Emergency department attendance is particularly high in very young children. Every year, more than half of all children aged under one year visit an emergency department and one in three of these are admitted.

Strong primary care is particularly important for children. Half of all children subsequently found to have meningococcal infection are sent home from a first primary care consultation. This does not suggest suboptimal care in all these instances, though – the illness often has nonspecific features in its early stages. However, it is estimated that 75% of asthma admissions among children could be avoided with optimal primary care. Getting young people to use health services appropriately is important, in part because it shapes their future use as adults.

The central government Department of Health in England identifies 10 topic areas to help providers and commissioners improve services for young people. The Healthy Child Programme sets out a framework of services to promote health and development from conception until the age of 19 years (Figure 8.9). In practice, recipients do not see these services as being part of a programme. The purpose of setting them out as a programme is to establish

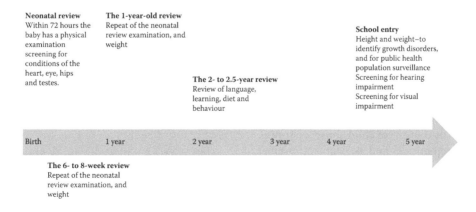

Neonatal review
Within 72 hours the baby has a physical examination screening for conditions of the heart, eye, hips and testes.

The 1-year-old review
Repeat of the neonatal review examination, and weight

The 2- to 2.5-year review
Review of language, learning, diet and behaviour

School entry
Height and weight–to identify growth disorders, and for public health population surveillance
Screening for hearing impairment
Screening for visual impairment

Birth   1 year   2 year   3 year   4 year   5 year

The 6- to 8-week review
Repeat of the neonatal review examination, and weight

Figure 8.9 Structured health assessments in childhood in the United Kingdom.

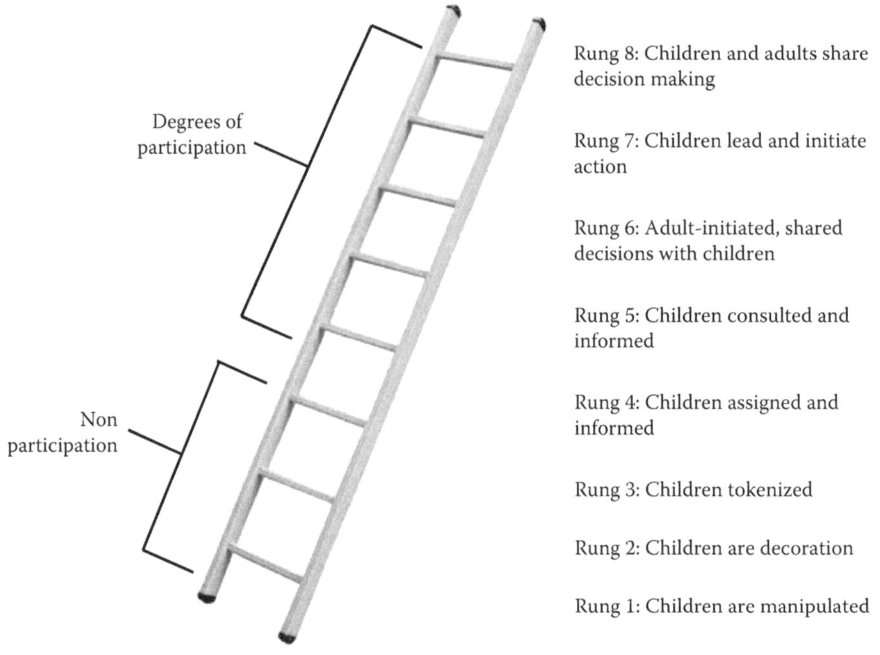

Figure 8.10 Roger Hart's ladder of participation.

Source: Hart RA, *Children's Participation: From Tokenism to Citizenship.* Florence: UNICEF International Child Development Centre, 1992.

clear standards for health professionals, commissioners and service providers, for what every child should receive. The Healthy Child Programme puts particular focus on prevention and early intervention. Its parts are delivered by, among others, general practitioners, midwives, health visitors and children centres.

There has been a move over recent years, in the United Kingdom and elsewhere, to encourage patients of all age groups to more fully contribute to decisions about their own healthcare, and also to participate in developing new healthcare services and in developing health policy. This should be no different for children and young people (Figure 8.10).

Children's participatory rights have become increasingly recognized in UK healthcare over the last decade with the appointment of Children's Commissioners as a formal, high-level advocate for children's rights. Progress has been made, but many health organizations still have much farther to go in involving children and young people fully.

Safeguarding children

The traditional concept of child protection today tends to be subsumed within the wider idea of *safeguarding*. In addition to the long-established forms of child abuse – physical, sexual, psychological, emotional and neglect – a number of other phenomena place children at risk; they include exploitation, trafficking, grooming, cyber abuse and bullying. Areas of the world in conflict lead to children crossing borders, sometimes completely alone, and some arrive in the United Kingdom.

In the United Kingdom, there was growing attention, public and professional, on child abuse after the first papers were written on the 'battered baby syndrome' in the 1960s. This terminology is outmoded. Policy responses by the governments of the day have been driven by tragic occurrences in which children have been killed or seriously harmed by adults. An enquiry into the death of seven-year-old Maria Colwell in 1974 uncovered serious deficiencies in professional practice and service response. It led to the establishment of stronger procedures to identify and manage risk to children.

Not all child abuse is physical. It can be sexual and emotional. Neglect is the most common form of child abuse in England. The World Health Organizations defines child maltreatment as:

abuse and neglect that occurs to children under 18 years of age. It includes all types of physical and/or emotional ill-treatment, sexual abuse, neglect, negligence and commercial or other exploitation, which results in actual or potential harm to the child's health, survival, development or dignity in the context of a relationship of responsibility, trust or power.

Between 1 in 10 and 1 in 25 children are maltreated. Rates of child maltreatment have remained constant over the last 30 years. Some trends have been positive. Children's rights are now better protected, and parents are less likely to physically punish their children. There is also greater willingness to report neglect and abuse.

Child maltreatment can cause profound physical, mental and emotional harm and suffering. This often has a long-term component. Adults who have been abused as children generally have poorer health behaviours, and are more likely to be obese, have high-risk sexual behaviour and depression, and to be a perpetrator or a victim of violence. There is also an economic impact that includes the costs of hospitalization, mental health treatment and child welfare, as well as longer-term health costs. Children at most risk of abuse are those with special needs, those aged under four or over 10 years and those whose parents are criminals or substance abusers, or have financial difficulties. A toxic trio of substance misuse, parental mental health problems and domestic violence stood out as the most common features in a retrospective review of serious cases in families where children had been seriously harmed. Preventing child abuse requires multidisciplinary coordination between health services, local authorities, social services, voluntary sectors and police.

The *Children Act 1989* built on a background of several enquiries into physical abuse that had occurred in the 1970s and 1980s. The Act established the principle that the welfare of the child is paramount, but it also emphasizes the need to care for children whenever possible within their families and to seek to avoid court orders unless absolutely necessary. The Act acknowledges the inherent tension between the need to protect children and the importance of their family to them.

In England and Wales, more than 60% of murdered children are less than five years old. In two-thirds of cases, the parent is the main perpetrator. Another very serious form of abuse is child sexual exploitation. The perpetrators of this range from young people to gangs of adults, and may be one-time or multiple offenders. The National Society for the Prevention of Cruelty to Children has estimated that between 5% and 16% of children under 16 years old in the United Kingdom are sexually abused. Typically, it takes about seven years for a young person who is interviewed to disclose his or her sexual abuse. The victims of sexual exploitation are most commonly girls aged 10–14 years, and are already vulnerable or living in care.

Deaths of children from abuse and neglect continue to occur. Public outrage is fuelled by subsequent enquiries that show that services had failed to detect and prevent the tragedy. Victoria Climbie was an eight-year-old girl murdered by her guardians in London in 2000. An enquiry resulted in major changes to how children's services operate. The policy direction was established under the title *Every Child Matters*. Its key thrust was to integrate children's services to ensure that children would be protected and cared for. In August 2007, 17-month-old Peter Connelly ('Baby P') died after suffering severe physical and sexual abuse at the hands of three adults, including his mother and her boyfriend. He had a child protection plan and was seen by a number of professionals in the run-up to his death. He lived in Haringey, the same childcare authority as Victoria Climbie. For these reasons, as well as the harrowing circumstances, his death received very high-profile attention.

Child protection is not only about preventing individual tragedies. It must also protect whole groups of vulnerable children. In Rotherham, South Yorkshire, an estimated 1400 children – some girls as young as 11 years – were sexually abused by gangs of men. They suffered rape and torture, and were trafficked for sex. This was the finding of an independent enquiry report, published in August 2014. The Rotherham independent enquiry found a series of collective failures of political and officer leadership within the police service and that 'the seriousness of the problem was underplayed by senior managers … regarding many child victims with contempt and failing to act on their abuse as a crime'. Similarly, in 2012, a group of nine men was convicted of grooming girls, sex trafficking, sexual assault and child exploitation in Rochdale. The 2014 independent report about this, *Real Voices*, by Ann Coffey, highlighted the volume of crimes, the degree of underconviction and concern that 'in some neighbourhoods, child sexual exploitation had become the new social norm'. Cases of child sexual exploitation have also come to light in Oldham, Stockport, Derby, Oxford and Peterborough.

The *Children Acts* of 1989 and 2004 provide the legislative basis, and framework, for the child protection system. Nationally, child protection is the responsibility of the Department for Education. The *Children Act 2004* created a wide-ranging legal duty to safeguard children, and sought to tackle the problems of communication and cooperation often found in many serious child protection failures. The 2004 act created local safeguarding children boards to 'co-ordinate and quality assure the safeguarding children activities of member agencies'. These are composed of local authorities, police, health professionals and the voluntary sector. They also review the circumstances of any child death, and investigate allegations against individuals or services. Their reviews of child deaths should not just identify the circumstances, but also any public health or safety concerns that arise from individual deaths or from a pattern of deaths in the area. The *Children and Families Act 2014* further protects children who are vulnerable, including improved support for those with parents who are separating, children in care and children with special educational needs and disabilities. It also introduced changes to the adoption system, and assistance for parents to balance family and work life.

Child protection services are planned and provided by local authorities. Public or professional concern about a child is passed to the local authority child protection team. That team, or the police, assess the child's safety. Immediate steps can include an *emergency protection order* to remove the child to a place of safety or an *exclusion order* to remove the abuser from the home. Following a full risk assessment, there may be no further action, or a range of options is available if action is necessary: designation of the child as a *child in need*, further social services support or a plan to gather more information about the situation, perhaps through a *Section 47* enquiry. If a child has been harmed, or is considered at risk, a child protection conference makes the decision about whether to initiate a child protection plan. The parents are allowed to attend this conference. A *child protection plan* outlines provisions for care and monitoring, including how to reduce the child's risk, how best to support the family, how social services will be involved and how the case will be monitored and evaluated. It may require removal of a child from his or her family if he or she is at continuing risk. A series of case conferences take place, continuing until the child is no longer at risk. More and more children in the United Kingdom are on child protection registers and protection plans. If a child dies or suffers significant harm, a *serious case review* takes place, aiming to learn lessons.

The nature of children's vulnerability changes over time. Unheard of as a threat to children's well-being 20 years ago, up to one-third of young people, particularly girls, now experience cyber bullying. Targeted action on social media and Internet chatroom website abuse has led to distress and even suicide. One-fifth of children have seen online material that they are worried about or have found nasty or offensive. Pornography and sexual exploitation through the Internet is also a danger, especially for young and vulnerable children. There is now specific UK legislation to protect children from online grooming by sex offenders.

Looked-after children

In England, more than 1 in every 200 children (60,000 in total) is in the care of a local authority, under the supervision of a social worker, away from their families. *Looked-after* children may have been abused, abandoned or neglected; they may have severe behavioural or emotional disturbance; their parents may not be able to cope, or may be incapacitated. Two-thirds remain in care for at least two and a half years. Depending on the circumstances, children may be placed into care through voluntary agreement between the local authority and the parents, or through a care order. If the former, parents can retain responsibility. If the latter, responsibility is taken over by, or shared with, the local authority.

There are many types of care settings – from fostering to residential care to secure institutions. Any child being considered for care should be fully assessed, and his or her preferences understood. The aim of care is to improve children's life chances and to ensure that they are protected. Children looked after by local authorities are vulnerable. They tend to have worse health, poorer educational attainment and more negative social outcomes than other children. When they leave care, looked-after children are known to be at risk of becoming homeless and of prostitution, drug addiction and criminal behaviour.

OTHER SOURCES OF HARM

Domestic violence

One in three women and one in six men will be a victim of domestic violence during their lives, although many more cases go unreported. Two women are killed every week by a current or previous partner. Approximately 30%–40% of sexual abuse is familial. The Home Office defines domestic violence as 'any incident or pattern of incidents of controlling, coercive or threatening behaviour, violence or abuse between those aged 16 or over who are or have been intimate partners or family members regardless of gender or sexuality. This can encompass but is not limited to the following types of abuse: psychological, physical, sexual, financial or emotional'.

Domestic violence is associated with depression, suicide, alcohol and drug abuse and death. It often starts, or becomes worse, during pregnancy. This can potentially lead to miscarriage or fetal death. Women with mental health disorders such as depression and anxiety are at increased risk of domestic violence. A Home Office strategy and action plan, *A Call to End Violence against Women and Girls* (the risks to men and boys are not covered), has four areas of focus: preventing violence, providing support, working in partnership and ensuring that perpetrators are brought to justice.

Female genital mutilation

Worldwide, more than 125 million females alive today have undergone female genital mutilation (FGM), defined by the World Health Organization as 'all procedures that involve partial or total removal of the external female genitalia, or other injury to the female genital organs for non-medical reasons'. Most of the girls affected live in Africa and the Middle East. The practice is also followed in the United Kingdom, though. In September 2014, when reporting first became mandatory, 1279 historic cases and 467 new cases were uncovered in England, more than half of them in London. It is primarily performed on those aged less than 15 years. Short- and long-term complications include bleeding, infection, tissue damage, urinary problems, infertility, cysts, complications in childbirth and a higher risk of perinatal and neonatal death.

Successive UK governments have taken a strong position on the subject of female genital mutilation. The practice was made illegal in 1985. The main focus has been to enact legislation, to ensure that it is enforced and to educate communities. Further legislation in 2003 (2005 in Scotland) made it illegal for UK nationals or permanent residents to have any role in the procedure, whether in the United Kingdom or abroad. In 2010, the World Health Organization published *Global Strategy to Stop Health-Care Providers from Performing FGM*, and in 2012, the United Nations General Assembly adopted a resolution on its elimination.

CONCLUSIONS

During the twentieth century, there were great improvements in maternal and child survival, that in turn improved adult health and life expectancy. In the United Kingdom and similar countries, the surge forward came in the middle decades of the twentieth century. It is now being echoed in the poorest countries of the world, where maternal and child death rates are now plummeting.

Children's health, not just their survival, has also improved in most respects. Childhood is now well recognized as the foundation of a healthy life. The importance of the early years is clear – today's most prominent public health issues, including obesity and poor mental health, have their roots in childhood.

The United Kingdom, like many other countries, clearly still has farther to go. Stillbirth rates remain high. Too many children are still dying from preventable and treatable causes, particularly injuries. Over the last half century, adolescents have had less health improvement than any other age group in the country. And there remain disturbing inequalities between the children born into privilege and those born into relative deprivation. Each of these is a rallying cry for the growing number of public health professionals interested specifically in child health – and for the growing number of child health professionals broadening this perspective to public health.

CHAPTER 9

Mental health

INTRODUCTION

Mental disorders rank very highly in the overall burden of disease compared with many other causes of ill health and disability, although this is not widely appreciated by policymakers and health system managers. Their economic impact on governments and societies is also very substantial. Despite this relatively high level of need for treatment and care, around three-quarters of those with mental health needs in low- and middle-income countries do not receive adequate evidence-based treatment or have no access at all. Even in a rich country like the United States, more than half of those with very serious mental disorder are not in receipt of services. Only 10% of people with mental disorder in the European Union receive 'notionally adequate' treatment. While 30% of the disease burden in the United Kingdom is due to mental disorder, only 11% of the National Health Service (NHS) budget is spent on it.

At the end of 2014, a group of more than 70 international healthcare policy experts, practitioners and service users met at a Salzburg Global Seminar event. They issued a declaration calling for a renewed global commitment to mental health. They made a strong case that improving mental health should be a global priority, given:

1. The global prevalence of mental disorders and psychosocial disabilities, with one in four people experiencing mental disorder in their lifetime.
2. The excessive treatment gap in low- and middle-income countries, where often more than 90% of people with mental disorders receive no effective treatment.
3. The global underfinancing of the mental health sector, and the critical shortage of mental health services.
4. The breach of the universal right to health for up to 600 million people with mental disorders across the world each year.
5. The growing global impact of mental disorders and psychosocial disabilities, which contribute 23% of the total global burden of disease.

6. The often long-lasting disability caused by mental disorders and psychosocial disabilities, and the high impact of the excess mortality, and suicide.
7. The global crisis of human rights violations, social exclusion, stigma and discrimination of persons with mental disorders and psychosocial disabilities.

This seven-point rationale for global action starkly illustrates the scale of mental disorder; the lamentable lack of care; the need to reorientate towards the underlying determinants of poor mental health; the major impact of mental disorders in social, economic and human terms; and the dimensions of ethics, human rights and social justice. Mental disorder is vastly underfunded, relative to the burden of disease that it represents (Figure 9.1). It is consistently associated with low income, unemployment, deprivation and poorer physical health. People with mental disorders die some 15–20 years earlier than those without. Health risk behaviour (e.g. smoking) arises at a similar time to mental disorder and is the largest cause of premature mortality in people with mental disorder.

There is very clear evidence that people with mental disorder experience discrimination. There is significant stigma, although the extent of this seems to be decreasing; in England, two-thirds of those with a mental disorder still feel the need to conceal it. Tellingly, euphemistic language is often used, such as 'mental health issues', in contrast to most physical illnesses, which are given a medical name.

To address these important themes is profoundly challenging. Change on the required scale will need strong political will from global leaders, with sustained advocacy by people who suffer from poor mental health, the organizations that represent them and experts.

The concept of parity of esteem means according the same priority to high-quality treatment for mental health as for physical health. Mental health is not just the absence of mental disorder. It is a state in which a person is able to fulfil an active, functioning role in society, interacting with others and overcoming difficulties without suffering major distress. For too long, health policymakers and health service managers have taken an imbalanced approach. Their emphasis

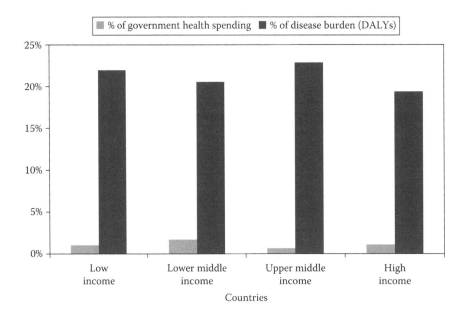

Figure 9.1 Government spending on mental health relative to the burden of disease, 2013.

Source: Institute for Health Metrics & Evaluation (burden); World Health Organization (spending).

has been on reacting to the needs and demands of those with mental disorder. This is essential, but it needs to be matched with equal commitment to preventing mental disorders and promoting mental well-being. There are effective actions and interventions to do this also, but few are being used. This represents major lost human potential and a cost to the economy of the United Kingdom and to the economies of nations around the world.

The term *public mental health* is increasingly used. This correctly implies that the tenets of public health can be helpfully applied to improving mental health in populations. Too often, as with physical disease, policymakers and health service managers take a narrow approach, which centres on improving the services available to those who have mental disorders. Although this is clearly important, a fuller approach to improving public mental health also involves:

- Assessing the burden of poor mental health and mental disorder
- Identifying risk factors and protective measures for poor mental well-being, and for specific mental disorders (some risk factors are common to all mental disorders)
- Appropriate interventions to promote well-being, prevent mental disorders and treat them early
- Assessing the intervention gap in a population for treatment, prevention and mental health promotion
- Tackling the health inequalities that are strongly related to the occurrence of poor mental health, and the extent to which disadvantaged people are unable to access the services that they need
- Understanding and reducing the extent to which mental ill health and physical ill health are interlinked
- Promoting mental well-being and preventing mental disorder

BURDEN OF POOR MENTAL HEALTH

In 2014, the World Health Organization estimated that the burden of years lost to disability due to mental disorder was nearly 23% of the entire global disease burden. The figure for the United Kingdom was even higher, estimated at 30%. The true burden is likely to be higher still, as the methodology for arriving at these estimates excludes certain mental disorders.

These figures have a dramatic impact when worked through in economic terms. In England, for example, the annual cost of mental disorder is around £100 billion, the cost of depression is nearly £8 billion and that of dementia is nearly £15 billion. There are many areas where there is an economic impact beyond the costs of treatment and care of particular conditions. For example, the annual cost of crime associated with those who had behavioural and conduct disorders earlier in life is estimated at £60 billion for England and Wales.

About half of lifetime mental illness (excluding dementia) starts by the age of 14 years, and three-quarters by the mid-20s. This is a very different natural history to chronic physical illnesses that generally begin in middle age or later and is highly relevant to the design of mental health policies and programmes. The need is for public mental health interventions earlier in life; currently, this is a weak feature of many health systems around the world.

Describing the size and nature of mental disorder in the population and the range of needs of people who experience it is essential to proper planning and commissioning of public mental health services. In England, work supported by the Joint Commissioning Panel for Mental Health means that estimates are available for the prevalence and numbers affected by different mental disorders. International

Table 9.1 Impact of public mental health intelligence

- Transparency and accountability
- Facilitates whole system approach
- Informs strategy, prioritization and commissioning
- Facilitates investment in and use of public mental health interventions
- Prioritise mental health across sectors
- Supports evaluation of interventions

Source: Campion J. Personal communication.

comparisons are more difficult because of variation between psychiatrists in the use of disease labels. However, internationally agreed diagnostic criteria are established and supported by assessment tools. Assembling data on the pattern and frequency of mental disorders is also essential for assessing needs for services at the local level. Good mental health intelligence has great advantages (Table 9.1).

Researchers commissioned by the government have carried out a series of major population (household) surveys of adult mental illness in England on a seven-year cycle. These surveys have provided valuable insights into the pattern of mental disorder, yielding results such as:

- 17.6% of adults had at least one chronic mental disorder.
- 0.4% of adults had a psychotic illness.
- 5.4% of men and 3.4% of women had an established personality disorder.
- 33.2% of men's and 15.7% of women's alcohol intake was at a hazardous level.
- 20% of women aged 16–24 years screened positive for an eating disorder.
- 5.6% of people had attempted suicide and 4.9% had engaged in self-harm.
- 4.5% of men and 2.3% of women were classified as dependent on drugs, mainly cannabis.

A similar survey has demonstrated that 10% of children and young people have a mental disorder. Another source of information is the use of a standardized and well-validated 12-item questionnaire (GHQ 12) as part of the Health Survey for England. This asks about factors such as general level of happiness, depression, anxiety, self-confidence and sleep disturbance. It identifies people who are likely to have a mental illness in general, rather than applying a particular psychiatric diagnosis. A score of four or more on the General Health Questionnaire suggests probable mental illness. In England, 18% of women and 12% of men in the population fell into this category. The prevalence of probable mental illness (i.e. a score of four or more) was highest among those in the lowest fifth of disposable income (27% of women, 24% of men) and those rating their health as 'very bad' (75% of women, 61% of men).

The admission to hospital of people with mental disorder is a poor proxy for the population burden of disease. It may simply reflect the availability of facilities, the policy for admission, the social stigma attached to mental illness in general or to a particular institution for its treatment, or the tolerance of the community towards abnormal behaviour. The extent to which mental health services rely on hospital admission to provide care varies greatly around the world.

Suicide is a rare outcome of mental illness but demands attention because it is catastrophic. The epidemiology of suicide has also been extensively studied, and evidence on it is available from official death statistics. In the immediate postwar period, suicides in England and Wales increased to a peak in the mid-1960s and then fell until the mid-1970s. Thereafter, suicides increased to a peak in the early 1980s among women and in the late 1980s among men. From then until the late 1990s, suicide rates in both sexes fell (more so in women than men). These overall trends conceal contrasts between the age and sex groups. Since 2000, suicide rates have fallen further, reaching their lowest historical rate in 2007 (Figure 9.2). The highest rates of suicides are among men aged 35–49 years and older men aged 75 years and above. Across all age groups, three times as many men kill themselves as women. Overall, men kill themselves more often by hanging and suffocation, while women most often use drug-related poisoning (Figure 9.3). The majority of people who commit suicide had a mental disorder – since the majority of people with mental disorder receive no treatment, improved awareness, detection and treatment coverage are important elements of preventing suicide.

When things go wrong in mental health services, they tend to attract considerable media attention. This is particularly so in the case of homicides committed by people with mental illness. This all too easily fuels an impression that homicide related to mental illness is far more common than it actually is. Such incidents do happen, though, and are analysed by the National Confidential Inquiry into Suicide and Homicide by People with Mental Illness in the United Kingdom and its constituent countries. It found that the average annual number of people convicted of homicides over the last decade was 546, while the number of offenders who had been in contact with mental health services over the previous year was on average 52 per year.

RISK AND PROTECTIVE FACTORS

Mental disorders and poor mental health occur throughout the course of life. In childhood and adolescence, certain groups are at higher risk: children being looked after by the state; those with learning disabilities; children from the lowest socio-economic groups; those whose parents themselves have mental disorders; children who have suffered physical, sexual or emotional abuse; and young offenders (particularly those in custody, who are greatly at risk of suicide). Mental disorder in childhood and adolescence is associated with a range of poor adult outcomes, including ongoing mental disorder, self-harm, suicide and health risk-taking behaviour. Childhood adversity accounts for 30% of adult mental disorder – the more severe the adversity, the greater the risk.

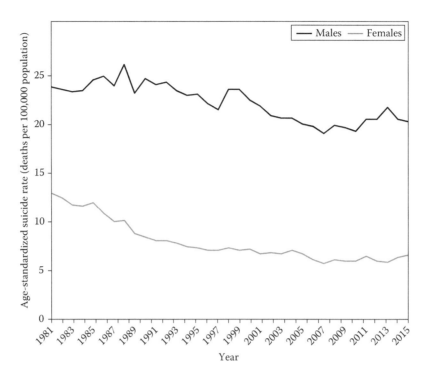

Figure 9.2 Suicide rates in the United Kingdom.

Source: Office for National Statistics.

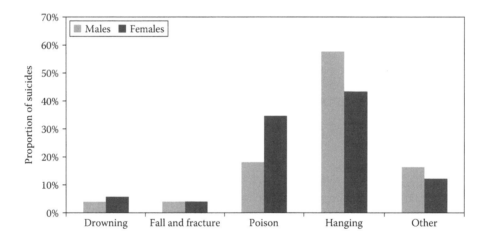

Figure 9.3 Method of suicide in the United Kingdom, 2015.

Source: Office for National Statistics.

Worklessness increases the risk of mental disorder, and mental disorder in turn increases the risk of worklessness. This can result in a vicious cycle – one of several that is often seen in mental disorder. The others include homelessness and crime. A study of the mental health of prisoners carried out at the end of the 1990s found, starkly, that 90% of them had one or more of five mental disorders: psychosis, neurosis, personality disorder, hazardous drinking and drug dependence. Most observers would say that little has changed.

The epidemiology of some specific mental disorders is well established. Schizophrenia is one of the mental disorders that has been most extensively studied. There are some

26 million people worldwide who are affected by it, while 9 in 10 people with untreated schizophrenia live in low- and middle-income countries. Studies of risk factors have yielded many influences on the frequency of the disease (Table 9.2). The systematic reviews used in the study shown in Table 9.2 suggest a lifetime risk of schizophrenia of 7 individuals per 1000. Familial risk is now well established, and a great deal of subsequent work has been done to elucidate whether this is due to genetic or environmental causes. The greatest interest in causation pathways and potential novel treatment agents currently lies in the field of epigenetics (study of genes at the molecular level, particularly what activates and

Table 9.2 Influences on the distribution of estimates from the systematic reviews of schizophrenia incidence, prevalence and mortality

	Sex	Migrant status	Urban status	Secular trend	Economic status	Latitude
Incidence: core	Males > females	Migrant > native born	Urban > mixed urban and rural	Falling over time	No significant difference	High latitude > lower latitude (males only)
Prevalence: combined estimates	Males = females	Migrant > native born	No significant difference	Stable	Developed > least developed	High latitude > lower latitude
Standardized mortality ratio: all cause	Males = females	Not available	Not available	Rising over time	No significant difference	Not available

Source: McGrath J, Saha S, Chant D, Welham J. Schizophrenia: a concise overview of incidence, prevalence, and mortality. *Epidemiologic Reviews* 2008;30(1):67-76. With permission.

deactivates them). It now appears that the chemical components of DNA and surrounding proteins remain labile enough to be modified by environmental and other external factors. This work starts to suggest a molecular pathway for a gene–environment interaction that triggers the onset of schizophrenia. Meta-analysis of studies examining the impact of abuse in childhood strongly suggests that sexual, physical and emotional abuse, as well as other sources of psychological trauma, put a child at between two and a half and three times higher risk of developing schizophrenia (Table 9.3). Sociodemographic risk factors for schizophrenia have been classified into mutable (e.g. marital status) and immutable (e.g. ethnic origin).

The annual incidence of suicidal thoughts is 4% (3% in men and 5% in women). Risk factors for onset of suicidal thoughts include age (10% of 24-year-olds reported onset of suicidal thoughts); being single, separated or divorced; living alone; lower educational attainment; lower social class; unemployment; being long-term disabled; having several stressful life events; smoking; and illicit drug use. However, the strongest risk factor is a high-baseline psychiatric symptom score (2% of people who score 0–5 symptoms reported onset of suicidal thoughts, compared with 23% of those with

Table 9.3 The effect of adverse childhood experience on risk of psychosis

Adverse childhood experience	Odds ratio of psychosis (with 95% confidence interval)
Sexual abuse	2.38 (1.98–2.87)
Physical abuse	2.95 (2.25–3.88)
Emotional abuse	3.40 (2.06–5.62)
Bullying	2.39 (1.81–3.11)
Parental death	1.70 (0.82–3.53)
Neglect	2.90 (1.71–4.92)

Source: Varese F, Smeets F, Drukker M, et al. Childhood adversities increase the risk of psychosis: a meta-analysis of patient-control, prospective-and cross-sectional cohort studies. *Schizophrenia Bulletin* 2012; 38(4):661–71.

a score of 18 symptoms and above). Prisoners, mental health inpatients and those in contact with mental health services are at heightened risk of suicide. People who attempt suicide are 100 times more likely than average to kill themselves in the succeeding year, so people who have previously harmed themselves are regarded as being at increased risk of suicide. Careful risk assessment and management of such individuals is needed, but this is very difficult. The vast majority of people who self-harm do not go on to commit suicide, and many people who commit suicide did not previously self-harm.

MENTAL HEALTH INEQUALITIES

Socio-economic disadvantage increases the prevalence of mental disorders. So too do income inequalities. The additional illness generated by these two drivers leads to greater health inequalities because mental disorders themselves heighten social and economic disadvantage due to incapacity and increased risk of physical illness and premature death. Mental disorder thus results in a further range of inequalities that can be prevented by prompt treatment of mental disorder, early intervention for health risk behaviours, effective diagnosis and treatment of physical illness and targeted well-being promotion to facilitate recovery (Table 9.4).

The World Health Organization European Office has set out five high-level conditions that would reduce inequalities in mental health:

1. Employment opportunities and workplace pay and conditions that promote and protect mental health
2. Social, cultural and economic conditions that support family life
3. Education that equips children to flourish both economically and emotionally
4. Partnerships between health and other sectors to address social and economic problems that are a catalyst for psychological distress
5. Reducing policy and environmental barriers to social contact

Table 9.4 Inequality and mental disorders

- Income inequality in rich countries increases risk of mental disorder
- Economic disadvantage means greater likelihood of mental disorder
- Economic downturns widen income inequalities
- Only 0.03% of NHS mental health budget spent on adult mental health promotion
- Addressing inequalities that lead to, and arise from, mental disorders is vital for sustainable mental health strategies.

Source: Derived from Campion J, Bhugra D, Bailey S, Marmot M. Inequality and mental disorders: opportunities for action. *Lancet* 2013;382(9888):183.

Table 9.5 Smoking and mental disorders

- Smoking is the largest avoidable cause of premature death and health inequality in those with mental disorders who die 10–20 years early
- Adults with mental disorders disproportionately experience tobacco-related harm
- Smoking cessation improves mental and physical health and reduces the risk of death
- Impact of smoking cessation on mood and anxiety disorders is as great as antidepressants
- Smoking increases the metabolism of some psychotropic drugs (doses need to be reduced during smoking cessation to prevent toxicity)

Source: Campion J, Shiers D, Britton J, Gilbody S, Bradshaw T. *Primary Care Guidance on Smoking and Mental Disorders – 2014 update.* London: Royal College of General Practitioners & Royal College of Psychiatrists, 2014.

MENTAL HEALTH AND PHYSICAL HEALTH

Poor mental health increases a person's risk of having one or more physical illnesses, including cardiovascular disease and cancer, and of dying prematurely. In contrast, a state of well-being lowers the risk of developing serious physical illness. Physical illness increases the risk of mental disorder (e.g. leading to a sevenfold increased risk of depression in people with two or more long-term conditions). Mental disorders are also an underlying cause of a range of behaviours that are established risk factors for physical illness. Smoking is a good example of this. An estimated 42% of adult tobacco consumption in England is by those with mental disorders, while 43% of smokers aged under 17 years old have either an emotional or a conduct disorder. People with mental disorders are also much more likely to adopt other risk behaviours, such as alcohol and drug misuse, sexual risk-taking, low physical activity and unhealthy eating patterns. This strong association of key risk factors with mental disorder raises the question of why more is not being done to target health promotion and preventive action at these groups within the population. The evidence suggests, for example, that there would be considerable gains if smoking cessation programmes were tailored to those with mental disorder (Table 9.5).

The presence of mental disorder increases the likelihood of premature death. This is so for both severe and enduring mental disorders, as well others. Particular diagnoses are associated with greatly increased mortality. Depression increases mortality from all diseases by 50%, schizophrenia reduces life expectancy for men by 20.5 years and for women by 16.4 years, and opioid-use disorders lead to a reduction in life expectancy for men of 9 years and for women of 17.3 years.

The relationship between mental and physical health has other strands, including the emergence of evidence of mechanisms mediated through inflammation (this is described in more detail in Chapter 5). People with mental illness are much less likely to have their physical illnesses recognized, and even when they are, the illnesses are likely to be less well managed. Mental and physical illnesses commonly coexist among people with multimorbidities, making their care more complex. At a clinical level, the interrelationship between physical health and mental health needs to be much better understood, particularly by health service staff in primary care and in non-mental health areas of service provision. Simple actions need to become routine, such as checking people with mental illness for physical illnesses and risk factors for chronic disease. Early interventions, including public health measures, to address the key drivers of physical illness can do much to improve mental health and reduce their risk of premature death. In turn, exploring the psychological health of people with disease like cancer, diabetes, heart disease and arthritis can uncover depression and other mental health conditions that may be having a major impact on the person's life and his or her ability to cope with his or her illness.

MENTAL HEALTH PROMOTION AND PREVENTION OF MENTAL DISORDERS

The factors that influence positive mental health can be thought of in three key categories:

1. *Structural* – good living environments, housing, employment, transport, education and a supportive political structure.
2. *Community* – a sense of belonging, social integration, social support, a sense of citizenship and participation in society.
3. *Individual* – the ability to deal with thoughts and feelings, to manage life, emotional resilience and the ability to cope with stressful or adverse circumstances.

Mental health promotion is to do with improving mental health by addressing these conditions. This involves undertaking a range of interventions and programmes. Different agencies may be tackling just one factor, so public health bodies and their leaders have an important role to

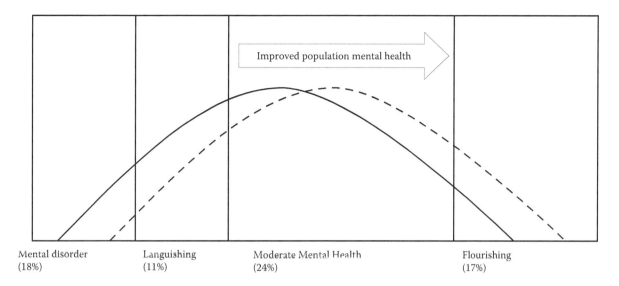

Figure 9.4 Spectrum of population mental health.

Source: Friedli L. *Mental Health, Resilience and Inequalities.* Copenhagen: WHO Regional Office for Europe, 2009. With permission.

coordinate activities between them. The aim is not simply to reduce the burden of mental illness, but to improve the state of mental health across a whole population (Figure 9.4). It is also important to target mental health promotion towards people with the lowest well-being; the largest single group with poor well-being is those with mental disorder.

Belonging to a social or neighbourhood network, involving communication and supportive relationships, is protective of good health and positive well-being; strong links between social support and mental health have been found in studies of both positive mental health and mental disorder. Protective social factors for mental well-being include a culture of cooperation and tolerance between individuals, institutions and diverse groups in a society; a sense of belonging to family, school, workplace and community; and a good network of supportive relationships.

In contrast, social exclusion damages both physical and mental health. For example, racial discrimination is a significant factor in the poor health of ethnic minorities, over and above the contribution of socio-economic factors. Populations at most risk from social exclusion include those with limited opportunities for employment, particularly women; racial and ethnic minority groups; refugees and sex workers; people living with disabilities, addictions or chronic illnesses; homeless people; the long-term unemployed; school leavers; and older people living on reduced income. Research on social capital has specifically pointed to important influences on mental health by community cohesion, involving levels of trust, reciprocity and participation. Emotional well-being is a strong predictor of physical health and longevity. Physical exercise has a well-documented beneficial effect on mental health and on reducing depressive symptoms.

Good mental health is vital in influencing children's life chances (Table 9.6). Deprivation or social disadvantage early

in life can have a profound effect on the individual's adult mental health.

Work and workplaces are particularly important to mental health. Positive employment substantially improves mental health for most people. There is a vicious cycle in which worklessness worsens mental health, and mental illness increases the risk of worklessness. Employment legislation, and the action of employers, can have a profound impact on population mental health.

A policy commitment, and strong programmes of action, to promote mental well-being within a population opens up a wide range of potential benefits, ranging from improved educational attainment and outcomes to greater economic productivity (Table 9.7).

As well as policies that seek to promote mental health, an important set of policies target the prevention of mental disorders and improvement of their outcomes. Suicide has long been an important target. The UK government has a suicide prevention strategy with the following key elements: targeted action at high-risk groups; tailored mental health provision

Table 9.6 Mental health for children and young people

- Capacity to enter into and sustain mutually satisfying and sustaining personal relationships.
- Progression of psychological development.
- Ability to play and learn so that attainments are appropriate for age and intellectual level.
- A developing sense of right and wrong.
- Capacity to deal with normal psychological distress and maladaptive behaviour consistent with age and context.

Source: NHS Advisory Service. *Together We Stand: The Commissioning, Role and Management of Child and Adolescent Mental Health Services.* London: NHS Advisory Service, 1995.

Table 9.7 Benefits of positive mental health

- Improved educational outcomes
- Greater work productivity
- Better physical health
- Lower premature mortality
- Increased social participation
- Reduced suicide risk
- Less risk-taking behaviour
- Resilience against adversity

Source: Adapted from Campion J, Bhui K, Bhugra D. European Psychiatric Association guidance on prevention of mental disorders. *European Psychiatry* 2012;27(2):68–80.

for vulnerable groups, for example, abused children, veterans, those with untreated depression and ethnic minority groups; reduction in access to the means of suicide; better information and support for those affected by suicide; and encouraging more sensitive media coverage of suicide.

Once mental disorder has developed, even the best evidence-based treatment can currently only reduce the burden of disease by 30%. This means that preventing mental disorder from developing in the first place is valuable, and illustrates that the relative lack of interest by policymakers and health programme managers in developing strategies to promote well-being and prevent mental disorders is very short-sighted. Many of the risk factors for mental disorder and protective factors for mental well-being are outside the health sector, so that public health leaders have a key role in focusing attention on it and coordinating multisectoral action.

MENTAL HEALTH SERVICES

The design of mental health services and the component parts of the system of care vary greatly around the world. Western countries have developed models of care built on specialist care and with heavy emphasis on medication. Historically, many mental disorders were treated in hospitals, in effect asylums. In Britain, the mental hospital, a closed community, often situated in a remote locality, served a predominantly custodial role, with little attempt to treat mental illness or forge links with the wider world. The discovery of psychotropic drugs helped to support a reduction of psychiatric hospital inpatient admissions. The modern era of policy on care of those with serious mental illness in Britain can be traced back to the famous speech by Enoch Powell in the 1960s when, as minister for health, he declared that the 'water tower' hospitals for those with mental illness had had their day and should be replaced with modern forms of local comprehensive care.

It was similar in the United States and many other industrialized countries. This more optimistic outlook in treatment led to changing attitudes to mental illness among professionals and the public. Locked doors were opened, and many more patients left hospital to live in the community, where local authorities began to provide an increasing

quantity of supportive services. Not all service designs around the world are enlightened. Many parts still rely on hospitals, together with overemphasis on drug treatment.

An important aim of mental health services is recovery. For many people, this does not mean complete recovery, free of mental disorder. Instead, recovery is about building a capability for mental well-being, as well as controlling the symptoms of mental disorder. Recovery is generally considered to have three elements: agency, opportunity and hope. Agency is to do with gaining a sense of control over one's life, with meaning and a positive sense of self. Opportunity is to do with building a life beyond illness. Hope lies in a belief that one can still pursue hopes and dreams, even with ongoing illness. Helping patients to achieve these central aims in life requires mental health services not only to provide diagnosis and medical treatment, but also to provide practical support in areas such as getting patients back into work.

The precise pattern of mental healthcare varies throughout the United Kingdom because different models of service have developed according to local circumstances. A number of key principles should govern the approach to mental health. The emphasis should be on moving upstream to prevent as much mental disorder as possible and to promote mental well-being. Services and models of care should be integrated between health and social care and be focused on giving individuals with mental disorders, and also their families and carers, as much control as possible.

Services can be regarded in a tiered way:

- *Mental health promotion* – for the general population, as well as targeted at groups with poor mental well-being (such as people with mental disorder).
- *Mental disorder prevention* – targeting higher-risk groups.
- *Primary care* – where most people should be detected, receive treatment and be referred from.
- *Secondary care* – inpatient and community services that can refer on to more specialist tertiary care.

A major breakthrough in creating a template for comprehensive modern mental health services in the United Kingdom came with the establishment of a National Service Framework for Mental Health in 1999. This set clear standards, described models of care and allowed local services to be developed in a consistent way, aiming for high quality across the board. It involved the shift of treatment for more severe illness from hospital to the community. For the first time, mental health became a national priority, alongside cancer and heart disease. This National Service Framework was superseded, after 10 years, by new strategies and frameworks; the most recent was *No Health Without Mental Health*.

More than 1.7 million people use NHS mental health services annually. The great majority of mental healthcare is delivered outside of hospitals. Only 3% spend time as an inpatient. Those who do so have a median stay of 23 days. Around 40% of them are subject to the *Mental Health Act*

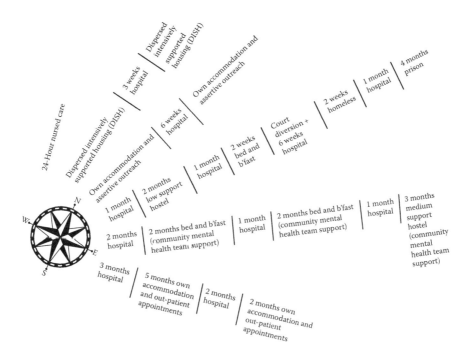

Figure 9.5 Examples of the diversity in pathways of care for people with mental illness.

Source: Sainsbury Centre for Mental Health. *Keys to Engagement: A Review of Care for People with Severe Mental Illness Who Are Hard to Engage with Services.* London: Sainsbury Centre for Mental Health, 1998. With permission.

(so-called sectioning). Individuals with chronic mental disorder can have quite complex pathways of care over their lifetime (Figure 9.5).

Primary care

The most common mental disorders are mild to moderate in nature, comprise a number of disorders and affect one in six adults. About half are depression, anxiety or these two conditions together. The majority of mild-to-moderate mental disorders can be managed in primary care. General practitioners assess patients and may initiate drug treatment and/or refer for counselling, cognitive behavioural therapy or other psychological therapies (often termed the talking therapies). In more severe, or complex, mental disorders, general practitioners commonly refer the patient to specialist mental health services, often via a community mental health team. Many patients with chronic mental disorder will receive continuing support from members of the primary care team, often alongside a specialist community-based team. Close integration is a particularly important component of good mental healthcare: between primary care services, specialist mental health services and other agencies (both statutory and voluntary) that provide care, help and support.

Secondary care

A minority of people who access secondary mental health services will get admitted to hospital. The development of primary care and various models of community mental health teams (CMHTs) has meant that many past reasons for admitting people with mental illness to hospital are now averted. Some people still do need to be admitted to hospital when they cannot be managed in the community because of the complexity, intensity or volatility of their illness. They may have an acute illness that needs a short stay for intensive treatment and support. Or, they may have severe and enduring mental disorders that has relapsed and periodically requires care in an acute inpatient unit. Many such inpatient units also have small psychiatric intensive care units (PICUs) as part of their range of services.

Team-based specialist community care

Different types of community teams focus on different groups with the more severe types of mental disorder. Some are doing secondary prevention by focusing on early intervention for a first episode of psychosis or prodrome (a set of symptoms that can precede the onset of a mental disorder).

Community mental health teams are drawn from a wide range of local agencies. They have been developed to serve the needs of local communities. They deal predominantly with people who have more severe or complex mental illness. The precise model of service varies. The very best are made up of staff from all relevant local agencies, who deliver multidisciplinary care in a way that is seamless as far as the user is concerned. Teams can comprise psychiatrists, community psychiatric nurses, social workers, clinical psychologists, specialist social workers, psychotherapists, counsellors, occupational therapists and welfare rights and benefits advisers. Their strength is that they enable users of services to be helped through a single point of delivery, avoiding some of the fragmentation and lack of coordination of the past. They take referrals from, and liaise closely with, primary care services; they carry out assessments, as well as providing continuing care.

Within this framework of local, community-based specialists, other teams have been configured to provide particular functions. For example, *assertive outreach teams* aim to manage the care of people with severe mental illness while enabling them to continue living in the community. This is particularly valuable for patients that have lapsed in their contact with mental health services but still have major health needs. They try to be flexible in where they see the person; they can visit at home or in any other place where the individual feels comfortable. They have an important role in reconnecting people with severe mental illness to specialist services, as well as mobilizing support from other key agencies and organizations in a locality (such as housing associations, police, local authorities, leisure facilities and employment offices) so that they are able to address a wide range of an individual's needs. The teams work best when there is good leadership that is stable over a period of years and when team members retain a clinical role rather than purely working in an organizational or management capacity. It is also important that teams do not take on too large a caseload. Risk management is particularly important, since failure in this area would undermine the credibility of, and public and professional confidence in, the assertive outreach model of care.

Other examples of team configurations include *assessment and brief intervention teams* that can see people quickly, assess them and organize short courses of treatment (e.g. talking therapies) or referral; *early intervention for psychosis teams*, which usually focus on first-episode psychosis and result in estimated net savings of £18 for each pound spent over usual care; *crisis resolution and home treatment teams*; and those covering a wide range of other needs – children and young people, dementia, eating disorders and perinatal illnesses.

Certain groups at higher risk of mental disorder require particular attention if services are to be truly comprehensive. Local commissioning of services needs to focus on key information to fully understand population needs (Table 9.8). In certain of the inner city areas of Britain that tend to have a larger than average proportion of homeless people, specialist multidisciplinary teams have been established to maintain contact and thus to attempt to prevent a crisis. More generally, the provision of adequate housing for previously homeless patients discharged from acute psychiatric care is a key issue in maintaining future mental health. Projects that bring together local authority housing departments, housing associations, social services and the NHS are particularly important.

Making services appropriate for, and acceptable to, minority ethnic communities is also a challenge. Issues such as varying cultural norms of what constitutes acceptable behaviour may have contributed to the overrepresentation of people from certain minority ethnic groups within those groups that are diagnosed as suffering from mental illnesses and those groups that have a greater than average proportion of their admissions to hospital being subject to the compulsion of law (as opposed to voluntary). The focused effort of the statutory mental health services working in conjunction with local minority communities is essential if services are to be fully effective.

Half of lifetime mental disorder has arisen by the age of 14 years. Prevention of – and early intervention in – child and adolescent emotional problems, symptoms of mental disorder and abusive environments represents a huge opportunity for public mental health to reduce the burden of adult disease. Despite evidence-based interventions such as the National Institute for Health and Care Excellence (NICE) recommendation of first-line parenting interventions for 5- to 16-year-olds with conduct disorder or attention deficit hyperactivity disorder (ADHD), NHS levels of provision are very poor. This results in a range of adverse outcomes, including higher rates of adult mental disorder and crime.

Children's mental disorders can manifest in ways different from those of adults. For this reason, and because they need different care, there are specialist services for children and adolescents who have mental illnesses. Child and Adolescent Mental Health Services (CAMHS) teams usually include child and adolescent psychiatrists, child psychologists, child psychotherapists, family therapists and nurses. There is a need for a wider range of agencies to be involved in child and adolescent mental health. Of these, the most notable is the education services, in whose settings disruptive or disturbed behaviour is often first noticed and who have a statutory duty to provide education to the child throughout his or her illness – with little support from commissioned Child and Adolescent Mental Health Services, in many places. Other involved services include education welfare services, special educational services (including special schooling for children with severe emotional and behavioural difficulties who cannot be managed within the mainstream) and (where appropriate) the input of the probation service (often through specialist youth offending teams) and the voluntary sector.

Table 9.8 Public mental health intelligence: Key information for local commissioning

- Local levels of mental disorder and well-being, including in higher-risk groups
- Local levels of risk and protective factors
- Impact of mental disorder and poor well-being
- Proportion of the population receiving public mental health interventions, including those with mental disorder

Source: Campion J. Public mental health: the local tangibles. *The Psychiatrist* 2013;37: 238–243.

Hospital care

The aim of hospital inpatient care for people with mental illness is to create a safe environment for assessment, treatment and therapeutic activity. Most people can then be returned to the community with ongoing support from their primary care provider and the local community mental health team or other specialist mental health team. The physical environment of care is important in mental healthcare, even more so than in the treatment of physical illness. Wherever possible, there should be separate accommodation for men and women. Other features, such as outdoor space and natural light, are not just desirable but also can be therapeutic.

In some parts of the country, there are day hospitals and crisis houses. These can be a valuable alternative to inpatient admission. They can also meet the needs of people who could have solely been treated at home, but lack family or other support to make this feasible.

Liaison psychiatry services have been developed to provide a bridge between general hospital services and mental health services. The teams providing liaison psychiatry (sometimes called liaison mental health services) are made up of a psychiatrist and other specialist mental health professionals. They are usually based in a teaching hospital, general hospital or a group of hospitals. Much of their work will be done in the emergency department and admission wards. They will assess patients, provide advice on diagnosis and treatment, evaluate risk, initiate treatments (such as cognitive behavioural therapy), make referrals to mental health services, organize community mental healthcare and generally promote awareness about mental disorders among health service staff dealing with physical illness.

A small group of people with severe mental disorders are a danger to themselves or the population at large. They need secure provision and sometimes the expertise of forensic psychiatrists. This is available with a range of levels of security, which are dependent on the degree of risk posed by the patient. At the lower end of the spectrum are locked wards within mental health units. If more security is required (e.g. for patients with offending behaviour), medium-secure care (within what were previously called regional secure units) is available. The small number of patients deemed extremely dangerous can be cared for in high-secure hospitals.

Residential care

Many types of residential care exist for people who would in the past have been in long-stay psychiatric hospitals. Services and projects vary. Some provide specialist staff (such as nurses) living with residents, and others provide a measure of independent living with backup support. The range needs to include capacity for intensive support in order for it to be provided over the longer term as well as around the clock if necessary.

People with severe and enduring mental disorders are sometimes described as the *new long stay*, and although they are a relatively small group (a few thousand in England), they can end up occupying acute inpatient beds inappropriately. They need access to 24-hour care and support and recognition of the fact that they are chronically ill. The concept of 24-hour staffed accommodation is not new and is a key component of effective comprehensive mental health services.

Continuing care facilities will always be needed for those people whose illnesses are too severe in impact and chronic in nature to allow them to live on their own. Rather than being provided in traditional hospital wards, these services should be available in more intimate and community-based care settings, such as hostels, group homes and supported lodgings. Services provided in this way not only reduce the dislocation of the individual from society but also, when provided in a comprehensive network, allow easier progression to more independent forms of accommodation as the person's condition permits.

The spectrum of residential care for people with mental illness living in the community is wide. It ranges from independent living accommodation (e.g. single flats in shared accommodation), to shared group accommodation (with or without support), to living as part of a family (including fostering), to hostels and staffed housing schemes.

Care for offenders with mental disorders

The mental health of people who come into contact with the criminal justice system has been a long running concern in the United Kingdom. The same is true in many other countries of the world.

The Prison Reform Trust has published statistics on the prevalence of various types of mental disorder among prisoners. Overall, a tenth of male prisoners and nearly a third of women had a previous psychiatric admission before being sent to prison. Around 25% of women and 15% of men in prison reported symptoms suggesting psychosis. Personality disorders are particularly common among people in prison: 62% of male and 57% of female sentenced prisoners have one. A Ministry of Justice study found that 49% of women and 23% of male prisoners were suffering from anxiety and depression. This is much higher than the prevalence of these disorders in the general population. Nearly half of women prisoners and a fifth of male prisoners admitted having attempted suicide at some point in their lives.

Successive Her Majesty's Inspectors of Prisons have expressed serious concern about the mental health of prisoners. A report by one was entitled *Patient or Prisoner?* This rather aptly captured the essence of the problem. Many consider prison not to be the best place for someone with severe mental disorder. Indeed, the environment can worsen the person's condition, sometimes culminating in suicide. A positive move was the mid-2000s transfer of responsibility for prison health out of the prison service to local NHS bodies.

There is a strong need to act on the link between conduct disorder in childhood and crime, with the opportunity to prevent a large proportion of crime through provision of treatment for conduct disorder. Another area for improvement is the plight of the people who become embroiled in the criminal justice system as a result of their poor state of mental health. It has for some years been recognized that many of those who commit crimes as a result of mental disorder should receive care rather than custody. Although many mentally disordered offenders still end up in the prison system due to the still patchy nature of services, there has been a considerable growth in services to divert them away from the criminal justice system. Such initiatives include education and training for police officers, lawyers and those involved in administering criminal justice within the courts. This enables the recognition of mental disorders and hence referral to teams of mental health specialists who can formally diagnose whether a mental disorder is present and arrange for an admission to hospital. It is likely that there will be further growth in such initiatives, as well as still greater liaison and cooperation between agencies such as the police, probation, social services and mental health services.

Engagement of users and carers

All services for people with mental disorder must share the aim of allowing maximum autonomy. It is increasingly recognized that people should have influence over the care that they receive and that when this is encouraged by services, a positive outcome from treatment is more likely. Mechanisms like patients' councils have been established to facilitate this process. Advocacy and other schemes to involve users can help people with mental illness express their views on services. User-led services are an increasingly common development.

Mental disorder, particularly when it first develops in an acute form, can be extraordinarily stressful and difficult for families and friends of the affected person. As with other groups with special needs, the role of informal providers of care is of fundamental importance in the planning and delivery of services. Needs assessments of people with mental disorder must also include an appraisal of their carers' needs. Statutory services must seek to involve carers in planning the patient's care, and also provide support to the carer. The absence of such support can lead to the collapse of the informal caring arrangement and the consequent admission of the patient to the statutory service.

Quality of mental health services

The quality of mental health services is not easy to assess. There are clear internationally agreed criteria that enable the diagnosis of different mental disorders. However, there is need for appropriate education of both health professionals and the public about the symptoms of these different mental disorders. There are few campaigns in the mental health field that compare with those that aim to educate the public about symptoms of cancer, heart disease or stroke.

The National Institute for Health and Care Excellence distils the available evidence, as it does for physical illness. There is guidance for many mental disorders and clear treatment recommendations. However, only a minority of people with mental disorder receive any treatment, and probably a large proportion of people who do receive treatment do not receive a version consistent with the guidance.

The quality of mental health services tends to be formally assessed mainly by inspections and reviews by the main health and social care regulator; in England, this is the Care Quality Commission (a number of reports in the public domain were produced by one of its predecessor bodies, the Healthcare Commission).

In the NHS in England, specialist providers of mental health services for adults and commissioners of services are required to collect and submit information to NHS Digital, which maintains the Mental Health Minimum Data Set. Detailed data are collected on each spell of care, and there is linkage to national mortality information through the Office for National Statistics. The idea is that this should create rich data for service managers, commissioners of care, users and carers, as well as researchers. The data set is extremely useful, and on the whole, the data are of good quality. It can enable benchmarking against comparator local authorities, trusts and deprivation to inform commissioning.

In the mid-1990s, the Royal College of Psychiatrists was commissioned to develop a scale to rate the level of health and social functioning of people with severe mental illness. The scale was initially intended to assess progress towards a target set in the *The Health of the Nation* public health White Paper: 'to improve significantly the health and social functioning of mentally ill people'. Over time, this has broadened; the scale is now used for a wider range of purposes: assessment of need, evaluating care and treatment interventions, resource allocation and planning of care and services more generally. There are now 12 areas, with each rated for the severity of the patient's problem. There are a number of versions covering different groups, such as working-age adults (HoNOS), people with learning disabilities (HoNOS-LD) and people who have had brain injuries (HoNOS-ABI). The Health of the Nation Outcome Scales are part of the Mental Health Minimum Data Set. There are other important routine sources of data on outcomes that contain mental health elements, for example, the NHS Outcomes Framework, the Adult Social Care Outcomes Framework, the Public Health Outcomes Framework and a range of other measures.

Public Health England organizes the Mental Health Intelligence Network that brings together data on mental health that have been collected from different sources. These cover:

- Indicators relating to the determinants of resilience and positive mental health
- The prevalence and risks of developing mental health problems
- Promotion and prevention, including social factors
- Early intervention

- Access and waiting times for services
- Treatment standards
- Service-level and patient outcomes

Individual services can assess their quality in a variety of ways, for example, through using the Health of the Nation Outcome Scales, through taking account of user and carer views and experience or through examining outcomes of care. International bodies have drawn together more global indicators of service performance. An example in Table 9.9 was produced by international consensus under the auspices of the Organisation for Economic Cooperation and Development (OECD). As the table shows, though, such key data are simply not available in many countries.

The Quality and Outcomes Framework (QOF) for general practice is described in Chapter 6. It provides a set of evidence-based clinical indicators for different groups of patients and conditions. General practices score points based on their achievement of these indicators and then are paid on their scoring. As part of this system, information on the prevalence of different mental disorders and various process measures is held in registers by all practices.

Emerging models of mental healthcare

As many low- and middle-income countries have started to develop mental health services for their populations, often with a poor level of existing provision, experts and commentators have urged a rejection of the Western model that they regard as expensive, fragmented and ineffective. They advocate instead an approach based on integration; more community-based, non-medicalized interventions; greater cultural sensitivity; and stronger engagement with patients and families.

At any time, in any part of the world, services will be responding to mental health needs using models of care that are very different to the traditional types of care. It is impossible to summarize these in a simple description because they have often been developed to reflect a local or cultural context. They can very much be bottom up, derived from discussions between agencies providing care, local communities and users of services. Alternatively, they can be centrally driven and designed, based on evidence from research or evaluation. By and large, the most successful innovations in mental health integrate the primary, social and specialist care sectors of a health system; they involve users and carers in the design, and they engage a wide range of agencies. The very best, in addition, build in a core element of public mental health.

A special expert group established by the World Health Organization – the Mental Health Gap Action Programme – has produced extensive evidence-based tools to enable key mental disorders to be addressed in non-specialized healthcare settings. Their work covers areas such as depression, psychosis, bipolar disorders, dementia, self-harm and suicide. The programme also addresses certain neurological and behavioural conditions, as well as drug and alcohol problems. Its tools and guidance encourage the management of these disorders in non-specialized settings, particularly in low- and middle-income countries.

Information technology can be used to good effect. Cognitive behavioural therapy is usually delivered by a therapist, often one to one. Computerized cognitive behavioural therapy allows those who can benefit from this type of therapy to do so at a much reduced cost, and therefore makes it available within populations where healthcare resources are severely limited. Telepsychiatry allows specialist psychiatric services to penetrate into remote areas, providing consultations through videoconferencing.

Table 9.9 A set of indicators of mental healthcare quality

Area	Indicator name	% of OECD countries where data are readily available
Continuity of care	Timely ambulatory follow-up after mental health hospitalization	28
	Continuity of visits after hospitalization for dual psychiatric/substance related conditions	33
	Racial/ethnic disparities in mental health follow-up rates	17
	Continuity of visits after mental health-related hospitalization	33
Coordination of care	Case management for severe psychiatric disorders	28
Treatment	Visits during acute phase treatment of depression	17
	Hospital readmissions for psychiatric patients	72
	Length of treatment for substance-related disorders	67
	Use of anti-cholinergic anti-depressant drugs among elderly patients	50
	Continuous anti-depressant medication treatment in acute phase	22
	Continuous anti-depressant medication treatment in continuation phase	22
Patient outcomes	Mortality for persons with severe psychiatric disorders	72

Source: Organisation for Economic Cooperation & Development (OECD), 2014.

MENTAL HEALTH LEGISLATION IN THE UNITED KINGDOM

The *Mental Health Act 1959* introduced a more liberal approach to mental health than under earlier legislation. This act was based on the report of a royal commission and embodied the basic principles of its recommendations, which were that the mentally disordered should be treated in the same way as those suffering from physical illness, and that compulsory admission and detention should be used as infrequently as possible. The procedures became a mainly medical, rather than a judicial, affair. *The Mental Health Act 1983* consolidated the *Mental Health Act 1959*. It principally concerned the grounds for detaining patients in hospital or placing them under guardianship, and aimed to improve patients' rights and protect staff in a variety of ways. A code of practice under Section 118 of the *Mental Health Act 1983* is prepared from time to time for the guidance of professional staff in the implementation of the Act.

In the late 1990s, the government decided to review the *Mental Health Act 1983* to ensure that the current legislation was updated to support the effective delivery of modern patterns of care for people with mental disorders. This review aimed to ensure an appropriate balance of safety of communities against the rights of individual patients and the wider community. However, amendments to the *Mental Health Act 1983* were made in the *Mental Health Act 2007*, which came fully into force in November 2008. The key changes made to the 2003 act by the 2007 act were:

- A new simple definition of mental disorder, renaming previous separate categories
- New criteria for detention on the basis of an 'appropriate medical treatment' test
- Broadening of professional roles
- Supervised community treatment after detention
- Suitable environment for the under-18s
- Advocacy arrangements

CONCLUSIONS

The World Health Organization states that 'there can be no health without mental health'. This mission statement for universal access to high-quality mental health services has been a powerful rallying call, endorsed by a wide range of other international and national mental health bodies. Despite this, the funding and attention that mental health and mental disorders receive still lags substantially behind that given to physical health and illness. Moreover, the United Nation's omission of mental disorder from priority noncommunicable diseases, despite being the single largest cause of burden of disease, is strikingly inconsistent.

Mental health services in the United Kingdom have changed very substantially over recent decades, with much more emphasis on primary care and community-based teams rather than hospital care. The big missed opportunity is still to drive forward on all the strands of public mental health – including prevention.

There is a big gap between what could, and should, be done to treat those with mental disorder and what is currently done. There is an established evidence base of effective treatments, but the majority of sufferers do not receive them. Society would not accept such a situation for physical illness. Public health also has a key role in highlighting the size and impact of this gap and facilitating improved coverage. Similarly, there is a chasm between what could be done to improve population mental health and the current norm. Jonathan Campion, professor of population mental health at University College London, has been a particularly important champion of the need for governments and health system leaders to take action to close the gap between need for care and access to effective treatment, and to realize the equally important gains that would be made if action on risk factors for mental disorder and promotion of positive mental health were truly embraced. He has said this about the present situation: 'It represents a systematic contravention of rights to health and huge lost human potential'.

CHAPTER 10

Disability

INTRODUCTION

Many people have a narrow concept of disability. They associate the word with wheelchairs, and with causes of serious physical disability, such as paraplegia and cerebral palsy. In reality, the spectrum of disability is vast. Common chronic diseases, such as diabetes and chronic obstructive airway disease, disable a large number of people – often mildly. By some definitions, 15% of the population have some form of disability. Disability comes from not just physical impairments, but also sensory impairments (most notably hearing loss and sight loss) and intellectual impairments (usually known as learning disabilities). Many also consider mental health conditions within the spectrum of disabilities, but these are discussed separately in Chapter 9. Over time, a person's disability may worsen, improve, stay stable or fluctuate greatly.

The very concept of disability is contested. There are many different ways in which disabilities can be prevented. Disabled people have particular health needs, often including rehabilitation. Many disabilities are associated with barriers to healthcare. Two important groups of people deserve close consideration – those with sensory impairment and those with learning disabilities. To the greatest extent possible, disabled people should be able to live independently, be educated fully and be gainfully employed. There have been improvements in these areas in the United Kingdom over recent decades, but substantially more remains to be done. Each of these aspects is essential to a rounded view of disability. In short, disability is a wide-ranging and complex subject.

DISABILITY WITHIN THE POPULATION

One billion of the world's 7 billion people are disabled. Four-fifths live in low- and middle-income countries. The prevalence of disability is rising – because of the shift from communicable to noncommunicable diseases, population ageing and improvements in survival for people with impairments.

The major causes of disability are musculoskeletal, particularly arthritis and rheumatism. This accounts for about 30% of all disability in Europe. Depression is also a major cause of disability. It ranks third in the United Kingdom and second globally, in the *years lived with disability* measure. One in five working-age adults have a mental disorder. A similar proportion of adults experience long-term pain, and 8% have an impairment of mobility.

In the United Kingdom, sight loss affects about 2 million people, including 25,000 children and 80,000 working-age adults. The prevalence of visual impairment increases with age. In the United Kingdom, it affects 20% of people aged over 75 years and 50% over age 90 years. Similarly, 55% of people over 60 years and 90% of patients over 81 years have hearing loss.

Learning disability is less common, affecting around 2% of the population. Conditions like Down's syndrome, Fragile X and autism are common diagnoses in learning disabilities, but the majority of them are of unknown origin.

In the United Kingdom, the British General Household Survey finds that 18% of people (9 million people in England) describe themselves as having a limiting long-standing illness. Whether or not people say this depends not just on the illness itself, but also on the social, environmental and psychological factors that contribute to whether they feel limited by the illness.

There is a steep age gradient in the prevalence of disability (Figure 10.1). A small minority (around 2%–3%) of disabled people are born with their impairment. The prevalence of disability is 5% in children, 10% in working-age adults and more than two-thirds in those aged over 85 years. The number of older people in the population is rising, and so the prevalence of disability in the population is rising with it. At the end of the first decade of the twenty-first century, it was predicted that there would be 86% more disabled people aged 65 years and above by 2026. Increasingly, disabled people have more than one medical condition. The range of impairments suffered by disabled people is wide, but it is essential to understand which areas of function are limited (Table 10.1).

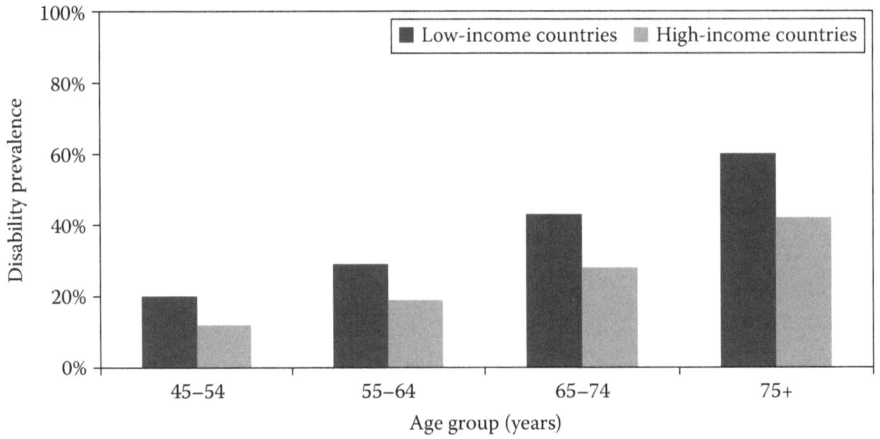

Figure 10.1 Disability prevalence worldwide.

Source: World Health Organization (WHO) and World Bank. *World Report on Disability.* Geneva: WHO, 2011. With permission.

Table 10.1 The prevalence of impairments, United Kingdom, 2012

Difficulty with	People affected
Mobility	6.5 million
Lifting and carrying	6.3 million
Manual dexterity	2.8 million
Continence	1.8 million
Communication	2.2 million
Memory, concentration or learning	2.5 million
Recognizing when in danger	0.8 million
Physical coordination	2.7 million
Other	4.1 million

Source: UK Government Office for Disability Issues.

The prevalence of disability is higher in lower socio-economic groups. The poorest 10% of the population are more than twice as likely to become disabled as the richest 10% (Figure 10.2). Disability is more prevalent in the north of England and in Wales than in the south of England, and in poorer local authority areas (35% in Port Talbot vs. 15% in London). Children with special educational needs, caused by learning difficulties, are more likely to be from poorer families.

Around a third of Pakistani or Bangladeshi people in the United Kingdom are covered by the disability provisions of the *Equality Act 2010*, compared with around a quarter of white, Indian and black people. Moderate and severe learning difficulties are more common among children from traveller and Roma communities. Profound multiple learning difficulties are more common among children of Pakistani or Bangladeshi descent.

Research and data collection use varying definitions and thresholds, and these have changed over time. Studies obtain different results depending on whether they rely on self-reporting or on clinical diagnosis. Some ask about specific health conditions, while some measure general functioning. There are efforts to standardize data collection and achieve comparability of national and international disability data.

CONCEPTS OF DISABILITY

Disability is a complex phenomenon. There has been substantial controversy about its nature and definition. Historically, the term has referred to the functional limitations of body or mind that an individual experiences as a result of illness or impairment. This is a narrow, medical perspective. Disability also involves a societal phenomenon. Disabled people often experience discrimination and prejudice, such as being denied access to employment or becoming victims of abuse or violence. People with mobility and sensory limitations frequently experience access barriers. Many disability rights advocates express the view that people are more disabled by these environmental factors within society than by their illnesses or impairments. They argue that illness and impairment need not disable people if society makes proper adjustments and allowances.

These two views are often called the *medical model* and the *social model*. They have been a matter of fierce debate. As in many controversial matters, choice of language is very important. Advocates of the medical model prefer the term *people with disabilities* rather than *disabled people*. This reflects the preference of talking about 'people with' diabetes, asthma or depression – rather than diabetics, asthmatics or depressed people – to avoid implying that a person is wholly defined by his or her disability, diabetes, asthma or depression. Those who favour the social model prefer the term *disabled people* to emphasize that people are disabled by factors external to them.

The medical model and the social model are each valid. Most people, including most disabled people, think that disability is a combination of individual aspects of health and

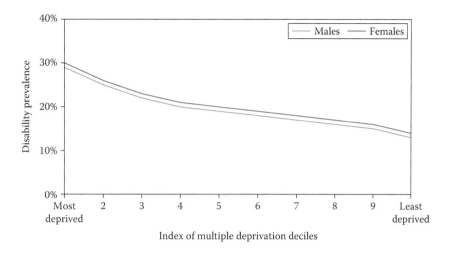

Figure 10.2 Disability prevalence in England by deprivation decile (age-standardized), 2011.

Source: Office for National Statistics.

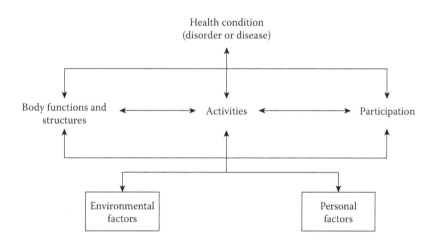

Figure 10.3 International classification of functioning, disability and health: key concepts.

Source: World Health Organization (WHO). *Towards a Common Language for Functioning, Disability and Health.* Geneva: WHO, 2002. With permission.

functioning, and societal problems of discrimination and barriers. There is also a relevant psychological element, particularly in understanding how some people with disabling health conditions are motivated to overcome obstacles, while others are less so.

At the beginning of the twenty-first century, the World Health Organization launched the *International Classification of Functioning, Disability and Health* (Figure 10.3). This developed over a long period of time, through discussion and consultation with a wide range of individuals and groups from the academic, policymaking and clinical worlds and, importantly, with disabled people and their representative organizations. It superseded a previous international classification, which encapsulated the concepts of impairment, disability and handicap. The new classification conceptualized the field very differently, and sees problems with human functioning as three

interconnecting strands: *impairments* (problems in body function or alterations in body structure), *activity limitations* (difficulties in executing activities) and *participation restrictions* (problems with involvement in society and life as a whole).

The classification attempts to synthesize the best elements of the medical and social models, and so to capture the complexity of disability instead of describing just one of its aspects. It sets out how people are disabled when they have a health condition, and that this is influenced by personal factors and environmental factors. The classification acknowledges that personal factors are critical to how an individual participates in society. Such factors include self-esteem, motivation, educational level, race, gender, age and coping style. The classification does not specify personal factors in detail, because they vary widely between cultures. The term *environmental factors* in the classification suggests a rather narrow and physical dimension, but in fact, the elaboration of this concept makes it clear that it is wide ranging, encompassing products and technology, the natural and built environment, support and relationships, attitudes and services, systems and policies.

The *International Classification of Functioning, Disability and Health* also distinguishes between *capacity* and *performance*. Capacity is what somebody can achieve in an ideal situation – for example, a physiotherapy gym. Performance is how he or she functions in everyday life. This distinction allows the impact of assistive devices or environments to be measured. The international classification is therefore an important enabler for research, for rehabilitation science and for barrier removal. It also emphasizes that disability is a question of degree, not a binary matter of disabled versus able-bodied. Finally, it highlights that everybody can become disabled, temporarily or permanently, through disease, injury or the ageing process.

Disabled people are often marginalized. The United Nations has outlined a human rights approach to disability. This echoes national legislation that has been introduced by many countries, beginning with the *Americans with Disabilities Act 1990*. The *United Nations Convention on the Rights of Persons with Disabilities* refers to 'those who have long-term physical, mental, intellectual or sensory impairments which in interaction with various barriers may hinder their full and effective participation in society on an equal basis with others'. This human rights approach treats disability in the same way as gender, race/ethnicity and sexuality, as a matter of equal opportunities and social justice. The onus is on society to remove barriers and provide services, enabling disabled people to achieve the same goals as everybody else.

The United Kingdom has passed a stream of legislation to enact these principles. The *Equality Act 2010* superseded the *Disability Discrimination Acts* of 1995 and 2005. The rights of disabled people have been expanded with each successive act. The *Equality Act 2010* defines a disabled person as someone with 'a physical or mental impairment which has a substantial and long-term adverse effect on his ability to carry out normal day-to-day activities'. Individuals have the right to be protected from discrimination in education, employment, access to goods and services and other areas. Discrimination may take the form of direct discrimination, failure to make reasonable adjustments, disability-related discrimination and victimization. When courts interpret this legislation, they consider two things: (1) whether a complainant can be defined as disabled and (2) whether he or she has been unfairly treated. Public sector bodies, such as the National Health Service (NHS) and local authorities, have a duty to *eliminate* discrimination, promote equality and foster good relations between people.

The human rights philosophy can apply to every area of life, including healthcare. The *United Nations Convention on the Rights of Persons with Disabilities* emphasizes that access to good-quality healthcare is a human rights issue. Unless basic needs for health and rehabilitation are met,

children and adults with disabilities cannot enjoy their other rights – such as attending school, participating in the community and getting a job. Interventions – even those as basic as the provision of an appropriate wheelchair – can make the difference between a person being included and that person being left on the margins.

It is important for health professionals and researchers to understand the disability rights agenda. In particular, professionals need to adopt the human rights principles of respect, dignity, equality and nondiscrimination in their interactions with disabled people. Equally, advocates of disability rights need to acknowledge the value of medical and rehabilitation interventions.

PREVENTION OF DISABILITY

The prevention of disability is complex and controversial. With increasing emphasis on equality for disabled people, it could appear inconsistent to try to prevent people becoming disabled. Simplistic messages risk being disparaging to disabled people – when they portray disability as a tragedy, for example. Sensitivity is required to reduce the incidence of preventable impairment while also promoting disability rights and equality. Prevention cannot simply focus on reducing the incidence of disabling impairment or illness. It must also focus on reducing the societal disabling barriers.

Spinal cord injury illustrates how effective prevention is multifaceted. Road traffic injury and falls are the main traumatic causes of spinal cord injury. Violence is a third major cause in some parts of the world, and sports and recreational injuries are also important contributors. All these causes can be tackled. The means of doing so include safe traffic systems, occupational safety measures, gun control and changing the rules of sports such as rugby and diving. In low-income countries, people can suffer spinal cord injury as a result of carrying heavy loads on the head. A simple wheelbarrow can reduce this. The main nontraumatic causes of spinal cord injury are tuberculosis, HIV and cancer. Here too, prevention can reduce the overall burden.

The World Health Organization has estimated that 285 million people globally are visually impaired, of whom 39 million are blind. The great majority (perhaps four-fifths) of this visual impairment is avoidable. Globally, cataracts cause a full third of visual impairment, but simple surgery can treat them effectively. The leading infective cause of blindness is trachoma, affecting 8 million people, yet its impact can be reduced by a combination of environmental improvements, hygiene, antibiotics and, in the advanced stages of the disease, surgery.

In Canada, adding folate to flour has halved the incidence of neural tube defects from 1.13 to 0.58 per 1000 pregnancies. Some learning disabilities result from fetal alcohol syndrome, which can be reduced by tackling alcohol misuse through maternal education and measures such as alcohol pricing. Screening in early life is also important. If hearing loss is identified early, supportive measures can be put in place to minimize or prevent developmental delay.

Newborn screening can identify cases of phenylketonuria, enabling dietary modifications to be taken to avoid the risk of learning disabilities.

Prenatal diagnosis through ultrasound, serum screening and amniocentesis or chorionic villus sampling allows an increasing number of conditions to be detected, including Down's syndrome and neural tube defects. The majority of mothers or parents opt for termination of pregnancy – in more than 90% of Down's syndrome–affected pregnancies, for example. Preconception counselling and carrier screening can help families with inherited conditions (like Tay–Sachs disease, cystic fibrosis and mitochondrial disease) to make informed decisions. Prenatal screening does raise psychological concerns and ethical debate. It is important to provide support and balanced information, and to ensure informed consent.

More generally, disability is strongly associated with many social conditions that it should be possible to change – poverty, poor living conditions, tobacco, alcohol, unhealthy diet, and unsafe work.

HEALTH NEEDS OF DISABLED PEOPLE

Disabled people have particular needs, both in health terms and otherwise (Table 10.2). Their health is not only affected by the disease that causes their disability. They are also at greater risk of *secondary impairments*. People with spinal cord injury, for example, develop pressure sores and urinary tract infection. Similarly, Down's syndrome is associated with congenital heart disease, impaired hearing and early-onset dementia.

Disabled people are also at higher risk of multimorbidity. Nearly a third of people with a long-term physical condition also have a mental health condition such as anxiety or depression. Conversely, people disabled by mental health conditions are at increased risk of obesity, high blood pressure, diabetes and cardiovascular and respiratory disease.

Evidence from the UK Learning Disability Observatory suggests that: people with learning disabilities are much more likely to be underweight or obese than the general population, less than 10% of adults living in supported accommodation eat a balanced diet, and carers generally have poor knowledge of what constitutes a healthy diet. Partly as a consequence, mortality rates among people with moderate to severe learning disabilities are three times higher than in the general population. Mortality is particularly high for young adults, women and people with Down's syndrome. This is not simply caused by health impairment, but also by standards of care for people with learning disabilities.

Disabled people are 50% more likely than nondisabled people to experience violence. This figure is 200% for disabled children and for people with mental health conditions. Disabled people also tend to be at higher risk of unintentional injuries, such as falls and road traffic injury. The causal pathways are not straightforward. For example, the association between disability and ill health may be partially explained by people from socially marginalized groups being more likely to be disabled. Similarly, adverse health behaviours may lead to disability.

All these aspects of disabled people's health must be taken into account to ensure that their health needs are understood and met.

Barriers to healthcare

Disabled people face a range of barriers in society, including within healthcare services. Some are physical, such as the design of transport, buildings and even examination couches. Some are attitudinal, such as when bus drivers or healthcare workers do not see the need to make appropriate allowances. Difficulty in accessing information can be a barrier for people who are blind or deaf, while those with cognitive limitations may be unable to process it.

Table 10.2 Some key areas of need for disabled people

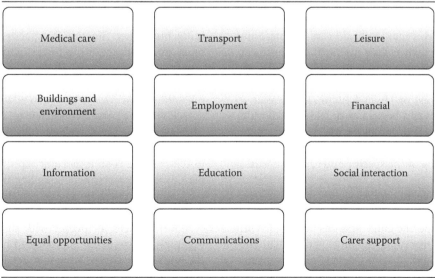

Medical care	Transport	Leisure
Buildings and environment	Employment	Financial
Information	Education	Social interaction
Equal opportunities	Communications	Carer support

Less tangible are systemic barriers that arise from particular education policies or benefit regulations. The important common thread is that all these environmental factors can be reduced or mitigated. Disability equality legislation has led to major improvements, particularly in the accessibility of buildings and transport.

The World Health Organization *World Report on Disability* highlighted barriers that disabled people encounter in healthcare worldwide. They are twice as likely as nondisabled people to find healthcare provider skills or equipment inadequate, three times as likely to be denied care and four times as likely to be treated badly. The same report showed that access to rehabilitation is often inadequate due to a shortage of trained doctors and therapists, and also because rehabilitation services are often not well integrated into primary healthcare.

In the United Kingdom, despite the general ease of access to healthcare in the free-at-the-point-of-use NHS, it has repeatedly been demonstrated that disabled people have worse health outcomes. The reasons for this include ill-informed and negative attitudes among healthcare staff. Too many health professionals fail to communicate adequately with the disabled patient directly – seeking consent for procedures from a carer or relative, for example. People with visual impairment may have problems reading information, and may make errors taking medications if they misread labels. A person with hearing loss may have difficulty making an appointment or may mishear vital information.

Diagnostic overshadowing is a strikingly consistent phenomenon. It occurs when healthcare professionals concentrate too much on a person's most obvious condition, rather than on his or her other health problems. For example, people with learning disabilities who develop cancer are less likely to be informed of their diagnosis and prognosis, less likely to be given pain relief and less likely to receive palliative care. Disabled people are less likely to benefit from screening and other preventive interventions. These include vision and hearing assessments, dental care, cervical smears, breast self-examination and mammography. This particularly applies to people with learning disabilities.

To overcome barriers to healthcare requires action on several fronts. It involves making healthcare premises and facilities accessible to wheelchair users. It means meeting the communication needs of people who are visually impaired or have hearing loss or learning disabilities. For example, better contrast or larger fonts make it easier to read labels, and letters can be sent as digital or audio files rather than on paper. Training of healthcare workers can both challenge negative attitudes and assumptions and improve understanding of the specific and general needs of disabled people.

Most mainstream healthcare services can be provided to disabled people, but some targeted interventions may be needed – such as specific clinic sessions for people with learning disabilities. Overall, as with other patients, enhancing the health literacy of disabled people and their family members can improve self-management and promote healthy lifestyles. Equality legislation promotes the principle of 'reasonable adjustments'. This means that necessary changes must be made to facilitate accessibility, as long as making these changes does not impose a disproportionate burden on a service.

Rehabilitation

Rehabilitation is often neglected. Yet, it can prevent loss of function, slow or stop further loss of function, improve function or compensate for lost function. The term *habilitation* is often used in reference to children born with impairments, since *rehabilitation* implies return towards a level of functioning that the individual previously had.

Rehabilitation services have historically been a strong feature of care in the aftermath of conflict, including both World Wars, the Vietnam War and the Middle Eastern conflicts of the twenty-first century. Many survivors of serious war injury have considerable residual disability. Their function is often greatly improved by intensive rehabilitation, including provision of wheelchairs, prosthetics and orthotics. After the Vietnam War, the development of the disabled person's Independent Living Movement in the United States was a major force in the growth of rehabilitation and disability services in that country. More recently, there has been a revival of interest in military medicine (and with it, rehabilitation techniques) as a result of the twenty-first century wars in Iraq and Afghanistan.

In the first half of the twentieth century, the average life expectancy of people with spinal cord injury was just one or two years. Life expectancy for people with paraplegia has now risen to approximately 90% of that of nondisabled people. Much of the gain has come from reducing mortality from urinary tract infections and pressure sores, through better equipment and nursing care. Specialist surgery can have an important role to play in correcting, or at least improving, functioning – particularly of the musculoskeletal and urinary systems.

Rehabilitation services have a number of functions. They start with a full assessment of the disabled person, ideally in their home or other place of residence. This involves examining his or her functional capacity and identifying the scope for lost functions to be restored and new skills to be acquired. Assessment also identifies if equipment is needed, or if adaptation to the home environment is required. The rehabilitation service should then establish a clear care plan, agreed with the person concerned and any carers. Disabled people tend to experience better health if they are partners in their own rehabilitation. Supporting and educating them to self-manage is an important aspect of the rehabilitation plan. With the assessment complete and a plan agreed, services and other measures to deliver the care plan can be set in train.

Local services for people with disability must take an organized, team-based approach to rehabilitation. Within the NHS in the United Kingdom, rehabilitation medicine is growing as a medical specialty. Consultants in rehabilitation medicine are core members of local rehabilitation teams, and also provide specialist advice to consultants in other disciplines (e.g. neurology, geriatric medicine, orthopaedics and rheumatology) in which conditions that give rise to disability are commonly seen. Rehabilitation is predominantly delivered by a range of therapists, particularly physiotherapists, occupational therapists and speech and language therapists. It also involves people who are specialists in assistive technology, such as wheelchairs, hearing aids and assisted communication.

The diversity of disability means that people's needs for rehabilitation vary greatly. In some cases, rehabilitation begins after an acute hospital admission – because of stroke or traumatic injury, for example. In others, rehabilitation services may be offered to somebody who has had a long-standing condition, like multiple sclerosis, but has not previously had help of this sort. Disabled people often have long-term care needs that will continue to benefit from rehabilitation services – the notion that it is a single course of therapy is outmoded.

Rehabilitation is needed in acute inpatient facilities, in outpatient settings and in the community. Many hospitals have specialist inpatient units (stroke units are common, but more general disability units are also developing). Community teams provide a link to the hospital-based service. Some of these community teams cover the full range of rehabilitation services and deal with all conditions. Others are more specialized (such as community multiple sclerosis teams and stroke early discharge teams). Local rehabilitation teams are multiprofessional, using skills such as physiotherapy, occupational therapy and speech and language therapy, in addition to those of medicine and nursing.

Three groups of people require particularly specialist rehabilitation: those with acute traumatic spinal cord injury, those with disabling head injuries and those who have had a stroke. All have profound physical, psychological, social and financial consequences, which require the tailored provision of services for affected individuals.

Globally, access to rehabilitation services is often very limited. Many sub-Saharan African countries, for example, have one or two occupational therapists or speech and language therapists for the entire population. Less than 15% of people who need wheelchairs have one that is appropriate to their requirements. Without rehabilitation, some people who are born or become disabled cannot participate in school or in work, and so remain dependent. Death rates from problems such as pressure sores and urinary tract infections are very high.

INDEPENDENT LIVING

Disabled people face barriers to participation in a number of different aspects of society (Figure 10.4). Since the 1970s, disabled people have been organizing themselves to challenge social exclusion. They have formed disability rights groups, coalitions and self-advocacy groups to strive for better services, barrier removal and antidiscrimination legislation. They have given the disability community a greater voice in the planning and provision of services, and in health and social research.

Community care reforms in the 1980s in the United Kingdom resulted in many disabled people leaving residential institutions to live in the community. Although originally founded to campaign for inclusion, disabled people's organizations increasingly also became providers of advice and support services.

The disability rights community pioneered the concept of 'personal assistance'. In this model of support, a person's needs are assessed by local authority social workers, and they are then given the money to pay for their own support workers or personal assistants directly. At first, this was managed by the Independent Living Fund charity, and then later direct payments to individuals became legal and are now the preferred method of support. This is far from universal, though. Many people, particularly older people, still receive home care that is funded by the local authority and

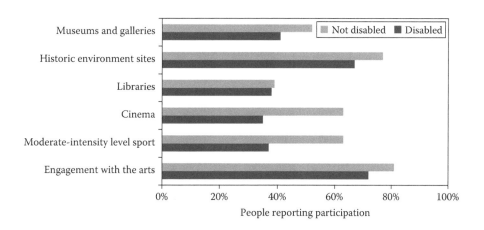

Figure 10.4 Participation in cultural, leisure and sporting activities in the United Kingdom, 2012.

Source: Office for National Statistics.

delivered sometimes by local authority staff, but more often by private agencies.

Claims for the success of personal assistance have been controversial. Personal budgets involve an individual receiving funds to pay for the services that he or she chooses. In the past, such individuals would have received a place at a day centre or other services. This is intended to increase people's control over their lives. Policy critics claim that it may be motivated as much by a need to reduce the costs of social care as by a wish to enhance the lives of disabled people.

Disabled people can be at risk when they live in the community. Social housing is often in deprived neighbourhoods, where they may be isolated. In the United Kingdom, disability hate crimes were officially recorded and counted for the first time in the first decade of the twenty-first century. Around 2000, such crimes are reported every year, but there is thought to be a much greater incidence of bullying and harassment that goes unreported.

The United Kingdom is one of the world leaders for disabled access, second only to the United States. Buses, trains and airports are almost all accessible, and major cities have accessible taxis. In other areas of life, barriers remain.

EDUCATION AND EMPLOYMENT

A fundamental determinant of whether a person achieves his or her full potential is the extent to which his or her educational needs are met in childhood. In all countries that have been studied around the world, this is an area of concern – not just in the content of education, but in access to it (Figure 10.5).

In the United Kingdom, many disabled children attend special schools, despite having rights to be educated in the mainstream system. Overall, 90% of children with moderate learning difficulty, 27% of children with severe learning difficulty and 18% of children with profound multiple learning difficulty are educated in mainstream schools in England. Advocates of special schools say that the small class sizes and specialist provision allow children with complex needs

to receive the support they need. Disability rights activists claim that this is a form of segregation that violates human rights. They argue that properly supported inclusion, with classroom assistants and adjusted curriculum, can help disabled children grow up feeling less abnormal, and help nondisabled children grow up with a better understanding of disability and diversity. Many disabled young people leave school with no qualifications or inferior ones, and they are less likely to transition to tertiary education.

Employment is an arena where disabled people remain disadvantaged. This is partly a direct consequence of disabling health conditions – one-third of disabled people in work (and two-thirds of disabled people out of work) say that their health condition has an impact on their ability to work. However, it is also to do with social factors. People can face discrimination in getting a job if they have a disability, and in keeping a job if they become disabled. Disabled people are 50% more likely than nondisabled people to experience unfairness, discrimination, bullying or harassment at work. Access barriers can limit transport to a workplace and movement within a workplace. As a result, there is still a large gap in the employment rate between disabled and nondisabled people. Just under half of working-age disabled people are employed. People with mental health conditions are among the most disadvantaged, with an employment rate of less than 15%. Worse, just 6% of people with learning difficulties are employed. Traditionally, efforts to reduce the employment gap have consisted of sheltered employment services and sheltered workshops. These have been criticized as a form of segregation, and also because so few people made the transition to working in the open labour market. Supported employment is now more favoured, in which a person works in the mainstream, but receives additional support, such as coaching, specialized training or assistive technology. In the United Kingdom, the *Access to Work* scheme helps disabled people and their employers meet costs, such as travel and technology, in the workplace. Vocational rehabilitation is the process of trying to enable people who become disabled to return to work. The previously favoured model was 'train and place'. Now the favoured approach is 'place and train'.

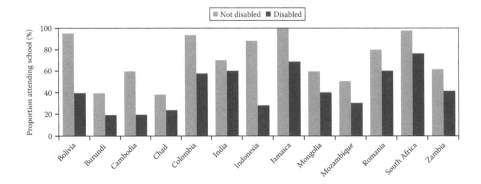

Figure 10.5 Proportion of children aged 6-11 years who are in school.

Source: World Health Organization (WHO). *World Disability Report.* Geneva: WHO, 2010. With permission.

Flexible working – including in working hours, schedules, tasks and environments – can make it easier for a disabled person to work.

Within work, disabled people can experience a glass ceiling like other disadvantaged groups. They are overrepresented in lower occupational roles, and much less likely to be in managerial and professional roles. They are 14% more likely to work part-time than nondisabled people, and far more likely to retire early than nondisabled people. In sum, this means that their incomes tend to be lower. In recent years, in the United Kingdom, eligibility for the main welfare benefits has been tightened to reduce public spending. Many people still do not claim benefits to which they may be entitled. Specialist advice and support help gain access to entitlements, particularly because some people only receive benefits on appeal after the initial rejection of their applications.

SENSORY IMPAIRMENTS

The three principal groups with sensory impairments are: people with blindness, people with deafness and people who are both deaf and blind. There are various definitions of blindness and deafness in use. The *National Assistance Act 1948* defines blindness as 'that a person should be so blind as to be unable to perform any work for which eyesight is essential'. Although there is no statutory definition of partial sight, in practice this refers to those who, although not blind within the meaning of this act, are substantially and permanently disabled by defective vision caused by congenital defect, illness or injury.

The UK government measures rates of preventable sight loss. The principal aim of doing so is to focus attention on improving care for people with glaucoma, age-related macular degeneration and diabetic retinopathy. When an ophthalmologist assesses vision as falling below the threshold, a certificate of visual impairment is completed. This serves the dual purpose of alerting local authority social services and contributing to national monitoring. People can be registered as *severely sight impaired* (previously referred to as blind) or as *sight impaired* (previously referred to as partially sighted). Severe sight impairment is defined as central visual acuity of less than 3/60 with normal fields of vision, or gross visual field restriction; 3/60 means that a person

cannot see at 3 m what a normally sighted person sees at 60 m. *Sight impairment* is defined as central visual acuity between 3/60 and 6/60 – in other words, the person can see at 3 m, but not at 6 m, what a normally sighted person sees at 60 m.

Social services authorities are required to maintain registers of people in their areas who are sight impaired. Individuals are not obliged to register in order to access social services, although some concessions provided by other agencies are available only to people who are registered. The concessions available for blind people (such as the blind person's income tax allowance) are generally more significant than those available to partially sighted people, so there is a stronger incentive for blind people than for partially sighted people to register. Even so, it is thought that registers significantly underrecord the prevalence of blindness.

Hearing loss affects 10 million people in the United Kingdom. There are four different levels of hearing loss (Table 10.3). The prevalence is predicted to increase steeply as the population ages. Many people are slow to have their problem assessed and seek hearing aids, which are the simplest intervention for those with mild and moderate hearing loss. In the most severe forms of deafness, as with disability, deafness is politically contested. Many deaf people who use sign language (most of whom have been deaf since childhood) reject the concept of disability and consider themselves as part of a linguistic minority. This is signalled by using a capital *D* for *Deaf*. Among this group, cochlear implantation is controversial because it is seen as a threat to sign language and thus to Deaf culture.

Other terms are used in describing deafness:

- *Deaf* (often written with a capital D): People who are born deaf or who become profoundly deaf in childhood and whose preferred language is British Sign Language (BSL).
- *Deafened*: Those who become profoundly deaf after acquiring spoken language in the usual way and who identify mainly with hearing people.
- *Deafblind*: Those who have a severe degree of both visual and hearing impairment. This is not precisely defined, but does not necessarily imply that a person is completely blind or completely deaf. It has been

Table 10.3 Levels of hearing loss

Category	Nature	Quietest sound heard (Decibels)	Proportion of over 50-year olds affected in the United Kingdom
Mild hearing loss	Difficulty following speech	25–39	21.6%
Moderate hearing loss	Difficulty following any speech without hearing aid	40–69	16.8%
Severe hearing loss	Rely on lip reading and may use sign language	70–94	2.7%
Profound deafness	Usually need to lip read or use sign language	95 or more	0.6%

Source: Action for Hearing Loss (formerly Royal National Institute for the Deaf), 2015.

estimated that 40 people in every 100,000 are deafblind. People aged over 65 years are thought to account for more than half of those who are deafblind, and the incidence of deafblindness increases sharply after the age of 75 years.

Causes of deafblindness vary, as does the point in life when a person becomes deafblind. Until recently, the most common cause of deafblindness among newborn babies was rubella contracted by the mother during pregnancy. Vaccination has reduced the incidence of rubella, but congenital deafblindness can also result from premature birth and birth trauma. Many of those who are deafblind from birth also have other disabilities, particularly learning disabilities. Some genetic conditions mean that people will become deafblind by the time they are young adults. Usher's syndrome, for example, results in deafness from birth and gradual loss of sight in late childhood. As the population ages, the number of people who are deafblind because of age-related visual and hearing impairment is growing.

There is no separate register of people who are deafblind, although social services authorities may be able to provide some figures on the number of people in the area whom they know to be deafblind. The needs of deafblind people can often not be met by services that have been designed for people who are either visually or hearing impaired, as these often assume that visually impaired people have unimpaired hearing, and vice versa.

LEARNING DISABILITIES

The definition of learning disability in the United Kingdom has four elements and is 'a significantly reduced ability to understand new or complex information, to learn new skills (impaired intelligence), with a reduced ability to cope independently (impaired social functioning), which started before adulthood, with a lasting effect on development'.

This definition encompasses a wide range. Mild learning disability, for example, is usually defined as two standard deviations below average IQ: such people might be able to live independently, get married and do a job. By contrast, people with profound learning disability may be unable to study, speak, work or take care of themselves, and hence require extensive support.

Running through the modern approach to care is the concept of normalization. As far as possible, the person with learning disability is given the same rights and entitlements as other members of society, and leads a life as close to the ordinary as possible.

In the United Kingdom, national policy on learning disability has moved a long way over recent decades. A 2001 White Paper entitled *Valuing People* set out a philosophy of care and a range of commitments for the care and support of people with learning disabilities. It aimed to achieve equality of citizenship, advocacy and person-centred care for this important group of the population, so often neglected and shunned. In 2008, this was updated with the publication of *Valuing People Now*.

There have been a number of major failings in the standards of care for people with learning disabilities. The Healthcare Commission (one of the predecessor bodies to the Care Quality Commission) investigated concerns about poor standards of care and abuse of people with learning disability in the Cornwall Partnership NHS Trust in 2006. It found poor practice, an unacceptable care environment and physical abuse of people with learning disabilities. A year later, the learning disabilities charity Mencap publicized six case studies of avoidable death. It alleged that these pointed to institutionalized discrimination against people with learning disabilities in the NHS. This led to *Healthcare for All*, an independent enquiry into access to healthcare. Its report recommended some actions for implementation throughout the NHS to ensure that the *Equality Act* is not breached and that 'reasonable adjustments' (as required under the *Equality Act*) are made so that people with learning disabilities can have equal access to healthcare services. Reasonable adjustments for people with learning disabilities include the use of pictorial information and the provision of liaison nursing staff in acute hospitals. Learning Disability Partnership Boards are the vehicle for coordinating delivery of services for this population.

In England, there are around 150,000 working-age people with learning disabilities. Both children and adults with a learning disability can successfully live in their own home or in their family home, only being admitted to residential or hospital care when serious problems develop with their health or behaviour.

Support for parents

Parents of a child with a learning disability often need a great deal of counselling and practical support to help them come to terms with the birth of an affected baby. As the child grows older, many continue to require emotional support, advice and practical help, including with welfare benefits. The presence of a person with a learning disability can give rise to particular challenges in a family.

Day services and respite care can provide parents with a break from the demands of raising a child with a learning disability. Some schemes place carers in the family home, allowing parents to get away for a short time. Families can also be supported by health visitors, community learning disability nurses, social workers or voluntary workers. Parents often find it helpful to be in contact with others who are in a similar situation. Support groups such as Down's Syndrome Association and Contact a Family provide advice, and a network for both parents and disabled people themselves. Parents often value practical assistance with transport or workload. Provision of suitable housing can help ease the challenges of caring for a person who has a learning disability.

Parents frequently voice concern about the future for their son or daughter after they themselves die. Some voluntary sector initiatives attempt to help, running trustee schemes. Families need help in considering the future and their options for continuing support needs.

Community teams

In England, most health localities have at least one multidisciplinary community team for people with learning disabilities. These are usually managed by social services. Most teams include a social worker, a community learning disability nurse, a psychiatrist, a psychologist and therapists (physiotherapists, occupational therapists and speech and language therapists).

Teams provide a domiciliary service to people with learning disabilities and their families. Core team members make routine visits to clients' homes. They provide advice and assistance with current day-to-day problems. They also advise on welfare benefits, arrange respite care and advise on or assist with any problem behaviours. They can be helpful in breaking down the organizational barriers that sometimes exist between agencies, and in improving the coordination between different services.

There is a wide range of services available to people with learning disabilities who no longer live in their family home. These services vary across the country. Supported living arrangements enable people to live in their own home, or with a peer or a small group. These are developing, increasingly with the help of direct payments (individual budgets).

Challenging behaviour

Some people with learning disability exhibit very disturbed behaviour. If this behaviour seriously jeopardizes the physical safety of the person or others, the term *challenging behaviour* is used. The same term is also used if an individual's behaviour makes the use of community facilities impractical. The most common challenging behaviours are aggression and self-injury. Some hold the view that people demonstrating seriously aggressive or self-injurious behaviours should be cared for, wherever possible, by specialists visiting them in their own homes. Another view is that challenging behaviour units should be planned for a health locality (or on a shared basis between several health localities). Such units can operate as part of an assessment and treatment unit, with the hope that individualized care plans can enable people to return to community living once the reasons for their behaviour have been understood.

People with a moderate or severe learning disability who have committed crimes (such as arson, assault or rape) may be admitted to one of the special hospitals in England, or to a regionally based secure unit for treatment. There is a

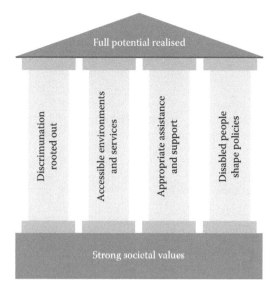

Figure 10.6 Disability: the four pillars.

general view that this group should be treated in specialized units, not within the general forensic psychiatric services.

CONCLUSIONS

A just society for disabled people removes barriers to participation, and meets the additional needs of those who cannot flourish in the mainstream (Figure 10.6). Health services and health professionals have an important role in improving the lives of disabled people. They should help to fulfil the human rights of disabled people, and provide reasonable adaptations to ensure that needs are met and dignity is respected.

Assessing need at both the individual and the population level is a key prerequisite to providing appropriate services. To do so, high-quality information needs to be gathered and maintained. Services for disabled people are strongest when they are based on such needs assessment. They are also most effective when founded on teamwork – at the individual level (doctors, nurses, therapists and social workers) and at the organizational level (health authorities, local authorities and nongovernmental organizations). Above all, there needs to be partnership between professionals and service users. As with all areas of public health, the health of disabled people cannot be examined in narrow terms or in isolation. Education, employment and independent living significantly improve quality of life.

The prevalence of disability in the population is increasing. Taking a holistic view of both disability and health, much has improved over the last 50 years. Yet, no country in the world is close to realizing the true equality of right and opportunity for disabled people to which so many now aspire.

CHAPTER 11

Health in later life

INTRODUCTION

Most babies born in the year 2000 in such countries as Japan, Italy, Denmark, Sweden, France, Germany, Canada and the United Kingdom will probably live to celebrate a 100th birthday. Life expectancy has been linearly increasing by three months a year over the last two centuries. There are no signs of a slowdown (Figure 11.1). A postulated 85-year ceiling for life expectancy was broken by Japanese women in 2007, making it obvious that human life expectancy has not reached its limit. Average life expectancy is rising in most high-income countries of the world, predicted to reach 96.4 years in 2050. This extraordinary gain in longevity is humankind's greatest achievement. It has brought with it, though, enormous challenges for modern societies. As people live longer, the question is how to ensure that those extra years are spent in health and not burdened by disease, disability and dependency on others.

Population ageing is a global phenomenon. In high-income countries, the number of people aged over 60 years will increase by 45%, from 287 million in the middle of the second decade of the twenty-first century to 417 million by the beginning of the sixth decade of the century. In poorer countries, the population will age at an even faster pace: there, the pool of over-60s is expected to expand from 554 million to 1.6 billion over the same period. By 2100, globally, there will be close to 3 billion people aged 60 years or older. Another characteristic of this greying of the planet will be a faster growth of the higher age groups. Whereas by 2100 the number of over-60s will have more than tripled, those aged 80 years and over will have risen sevenfold to 830 million. This remarkable increase is due to a complex interplay between reduced mortality in early and late life because of advances in human development (economy, living conditions, education, nutrition, medicine and public policy) and decreased fertility rates.

Advanced age is the biggest risk factor for most clinical conditions. This helps to perpetuate negative stereotypes about ageing while consolidating the misconception that there is uniformity in the older age groups. Ageing is multifaceted, driven by a gradual and lifelong accumulation of molecular and cellular damage leading to progressive loss of function in cells and tissues, and increased risk of disease, disability and death. Ageing occurs at different rates in different tissues. It varies greatly within and between individuals, implying heterogeneity in the ageing experience.

Human ageing is a malleable process, as changing world demographics over the last 200 years have confirmed. It occurs over the life course and, biologically, is not confined to a decline and accumulation of losses in later life, but starts gradually in utero. Ageing is not a synonym for disease and infirmity. Human ageing and longevity are affected by genetic, environmental and lifestyle factors. Twin studies have shown that 25%–50% of individual variability in longevity is due to genes and the rest to nongenetic factors (e.g. diet, smoking, excess alcohol, low physical activity and infections). So, ageing is a complex process driven by multiple causal mechanisms and pathways that often overlap with those of age-related diseases; it also shows great plasticity and heterogeneity.

Researchers and policymakers have repeatedly warned that increases in life expectancy will drive big rises in healthcare and social care costs. This is based on the assumption that advanced age is necessarily associated with declining health and function. But how strong is the link between chronological age and health?

Advanced age is certainly associated with more illness and disability, but different people experience different health trajectories. Some have multiple diseases by their 60s; others have good health and lead active lives into their 70s, 80s and 90s. The ageing process has different impacts on health, influenced by multiple factors, including race, gender, income, education, lifestyle and environment.

Today, the concept of an old person is much more fluid than before. Chronological age and various cut-offs used to categorize older age groups, although necessary for administrative purposes and record-keeping, are not good markers of a person's functional and biological status. The line between middle age and old age is ever more indistinct.

Decades ago, gerontologists invented the terms *young-old*, *old-old*, *very old* and *oldest-old* to emphasize functional status over chronological age. The emergence of highly

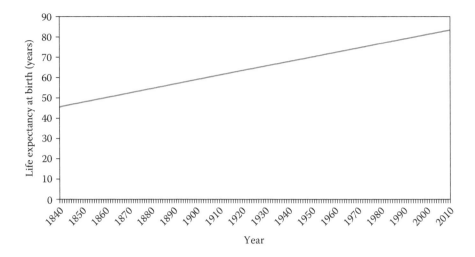

Figure 11.1 Human life expectancy has increased linearly over the last 150 years.

Source: Oeppen J, Vaupel JW. Broken limits to life expectancy. *Science* 2002;296(5570):1029–31.

functional subgroups of older adults with low demands for health and social care reflects a very dynamic relationship between chronological age and health. Health outcomes vary between and within age groups in later life. For those who have aged well, and experienced few limitations in late life, chronological age has little meaning.

Figure 11.2 shows this heterogeneity. Across eight age groups, health and functioning decline gradually with advancing age. However, within this overall pattern, substantial proportions of older adults are in good health and living independently very late in life, while some people in their 50s have serious health limitations. Looked at for likely costs for healthcare and social care, both high and low consumers are present in all age groups.

Another way to characterize the fluidity of age groups is the social life cycle, or four-age framework (Table 11.1). The conventional version sees the third age as a time of

retirement, a period of life free from formal structures and constraints of full-time work and career building. It is also an empty nesting time, without responsibilities for dependent children. The fourth age is then the final period of life traditionally associated with decline, disability and disease.

There is now an alternative way of viewing this classification. The third age can be depicted as a time of transition, refinement and fulfilment. It becomes full of opportunities for self-growth, learning and renewal. New careers, interests and life portfolios can be developed. It can encompass preretirement as well as retirement. The fourth age can then be redesigned as a period of successful or healthy ageing.

CONCEPTS OF HEALTHY AGEING

With populations ageing steadily around the world, the main challenge for nations is to increase years of

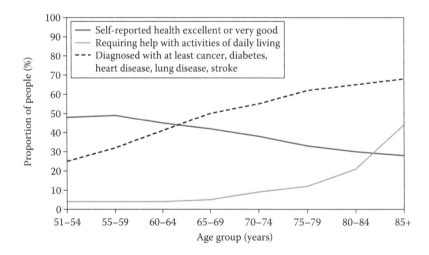

Figure 11.2 Changing health status with increasing age.

Source: Lowsky DJ, Olshansky SJ, Bhattacharya J, Goldman DP. Heterogeneity in healthy aging. *The Journals of Gerontology* 2013:glt162.

Table 11.1 The Four Age Framework and Ageing

	Conventional description	New understanding
First age	The period of childhood and socialisation	Preparation
Second age	The period of work and family raising	Achievement
Third age	The period free of the formal structures of full-time work and dependent children	Fulfilment
Fourth age	The period of eventual dependency and disability	Successful ageing

Source: Derived from Carnegie Institute. *Life, Work and Livelihood in the Third Age: Final Report of the Carnegie Inquiry into the Third Age.* Pittsburgh: Carnegie Institute, 1993.

healthy life. There is no real consensus on nomenclature or definitions of healthy ageing; several models have been relied on (Table 11.2).

Successful ageing embodies (1) absence of chronic disease and disability, (2) high cognitive and physical functioning and (3) active engagement with life. Although widely used, this model is seen by some as too biomedical, too concerned with physiological function and too narrow. In addition, it overlooks any subjective evaluation of the optimal ageing experience. Studies have shown that up to 90% of older adults consider themselves as ageing successfully even if they have diseases and disabilities. Critics have argued that the model represents ageing as being totally within the control of older adults who, by adopting specific lifestyles and behaviours, can change its course. Social, economic and cultural context and inequality in life chances are ignored. The best definition of successful or healthy ageing should be acceptable to researchers, clinicians and older adults and would not place emphasis on avoidance of disease and disability or negative outcomes.

The concept of *optimal ageing* views successful ageing as a diverse process with multiple outcomes. It is a balance between gains and losses. In later life, losses outweigh gains, but older adults can compensate for the losses and still be satisfied with their lives – especially if they choose domains in life that are important to them, and optimize available resources to ensure success and compensate for losses. Stressors, such as declining health (e.g. hearing loss and reduced mobility), may increase and resources decrease in later life. The process of selection, optimization and compensation become increasingly important for maintaining a positive balance between losses and gains. Because resources are scarce or lost, personal domains and goals must be carefully selected. Resources are further optimized so that goals can be achieved, and compensation strategies become essential. An older adult may

compensate by using new technology (e.g. hearing aid) or learn a new skill (e.g. to walk with an assistive device). This model essentially describes the process through which older adults actively cope with changes associated with ageing. It implies that successful ageing is not about avoiding all losses, but instead dealing with negative changes in the best way possible and selecting achievable personal goals. The model is strong in emphasizing the process of reacting to multiple age-associated changes; it is weak in failing to identify preventive strategies to avoid or ameliorate losses.

The World Health Organization has called for a paradigm shift to a positive vision of ageing. The model of *healthy and active ageing* is a lifelong process of seizing opportunities to improve and preserve health; physical, social and mental wellness; independence; and quality of life. The European Union has a key political framework to ease the impact of ageing demographics. The model of active ageing encourages activity in later life within a supportive social environment. Healthy ageing is directly affected by social policies designed to prevent poverty in later life, which is still prevalent in many parts of Europe.

DEMOGRAPHICS OF AGEING: TRENDS, PROJECTIONS AND CHALLENGES

A combination of low fertility and even lower mortality, especially in older age groups, has produced the population ageing patterns of many countries today. However, looking back over the last 200 years, increases in life expectancy have not been driven by uniform reductions in early-life and late-life mortality. Socio-economic development and advances in living conditions (sanitation and nutrition) and access to healthcare (vaccinations, antibiotics and breakthroughs in biomedical sciences) have played important roles. Until the 1920s, improvements in life expectancy were due mainly

Table 11.2 Health-related models of ageing

Model	Definition
Successful ageing	A three-part model encompassing low probability of disease and disability, high physical and cognitive functioning and active engagement with life
Optimal ageing	Ageing as a changing balance between gains and losses over the lifespan
Healthy, active ageing	Process of optimising opportunities for health, participation and security to enhance quality of life

Table 11.3 Stages of demographic transition

Fertility	Mortality	Population
1. High birth rate	High mortality in early life	Predominantly young
2. High birth rate	Mortality falls in early life	Still predominantly young
3. Birth rate falls	Mortality falls further	Proportion of adults increases
4. Birth rate low	Mortality falls across all ages	Proportion of older adults sharply increases
5. Birth rate low	Mortality falls further, especially in late life	Proportion of very old adults increases

to decreases in infant and child mortality. When early-life mortality rates started to fall, more children survived into adulthood, and young age groups were predominant in the population. As mortality rates fell further and fertility rates started to decline during the twentieth century, gains in life expectancy were driven by reduction in late-life mortality. As a result, the older age groups began to make up a much greater part of the population than ever before. This gradual process – in which a society moves from high fertility and mortality rates to low rates of fertility and mortality – is termed *demographic transition* (Table 11.3).

In countries with long-lived residents, including the United Kingdom, the probability of dying between ages 80 and 90 years has halved for both women and men over the last five decades. This extraordinary reduction in old-age mortality is predicted to continue through the twenty-first century. A baby born in 2007 in Canada, France, Italy and the United States has about 50% chance of celebrating a 104th birthday. A Japanese baby will live to 107.

Population pyramid becoming a rectangle

Demographers use several indicators to estimate and predict population dynamics. Fertility rates are, in most countries, the primary determinant of population ageing. The age structure is often shown graphically as a population pyramid. In the high-income countries, for much of the twentieth century, age structures did indeed resemble a pyramid. Most, if not all, had a large portion of the population under the age of 15 years and a narrow pyramid shape, with a few people on the top reaching very old age.

This long pyramid base characterized the population structure of many developing countries in the 1980s; this did not change much even by the beginning of the twenty-first century (Figure 11.3). Since then, further demographic transition has caused the younger age groups to move into working age and older age. Since fertility rates remained below the population replacement rate of 2.1 live births per woman (as in most high-income nations today), the proportion of older people increased. The population structure changed from the dominance of younger age

groups into middle and older, and the pyramid became rectangular.

If projected low fertility rates remain until 2040, the population pyramid will eventually invert, with a wider top compared with the bottom. The number of very old people (aged 80 years and over) will outnumber children younger than five years. Additionally, by 2040 many high-income countries will experience simultaneous population ageing and overall population decline.

United Kingdom: Reasons for demographic transition

The demographic transition in the United Kingdom started to gather pace, as in other industrialized countries, during the late nineteenth century and the first half of the twentieth century. In 1901, there were 1.8 million people over the age of 65 years out of a population of 38.2 million – representing 4.7% of the total. There were only half a million people 75 years and older, or 1.3% of the total population. By the middle of the first decade of the twenty-first century, the population structure had changed dramatically: an estimated 16% of the population were aged 65 years and over, and 8% were aged 75 years and over.

Taking a long view of human history, it is striking that there was relatively little improvement in mortality from the sixteenth century through to the latter part of the nineteenth century. For most of the period of several hundred years before 1850, average life expectancy at birth was about 35 years. Fluctuations coincided with periods of famine and epidemics of infectious diseases. Improved methods of agriculture and food distribution during the eighteenth century enabled better nutrition for more people. Action on public health and social conditions made the major impact on mortality during the late nineteenth century. Proper disposal of sewage, purer water supplies and less crowded, higher-quality housing all helped to reduce the incidence, spread and consequences of the major infectious diseases of the day. This resulted in big reductions in mortality rates in infancy and childhood. By the beginning of the twentieth century, an average life expectancy at birth for a male child was 48 years.

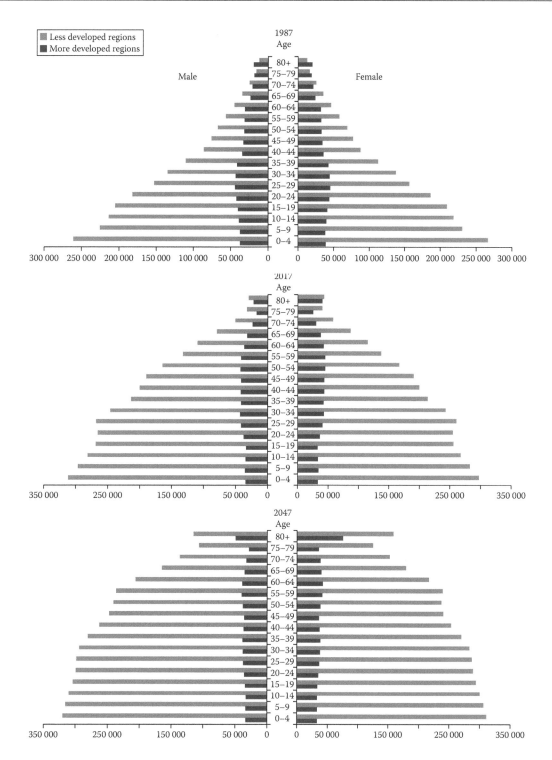

Figure 11.3 Past, current and projected population pyramids in more and less developed regions of the world.

Source: United Nations Population Division.

On average, women currently outlive men by almost four years. This is a result of a complex relationship between behavioural, social, environmental, economic and genetically linked factors. The excess male-over-female mortality can be largely accounted for by higher mortality for men from some non-communicable diseases (e.g. coronary heart disease, lung cancer and cirrhosis of the liver) and fatal accidents in industry and on the roads.

Life expectancy for people who have already lived to the middle and later years of their lives has also increased since the beginning of the twentieth century. A man aged 60 years in 1901 lived an average of 13 more years. By the end of the

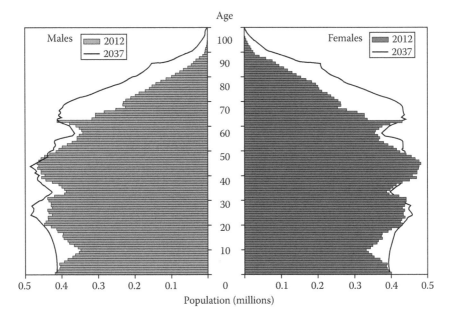

Figure 11.4 Age structure of the United Kingdom population: 2012 (estimated) and 2037 (projected).

Source: Office for National Statistics.

first decade of the twenty-first century, the comparable figure was almost 19 years for men and more than 21 years for women. The major changes in the age structure of the UK population in the twentieth century were due to falling birth rates and improvements in mortality. Recent additional ageing of the population is due to falling mortality rates in old age. Thus, when a population is already ageing but has relatively low fertility and low mortality rates, changes in death rates in the older age groups are the major determinants of further population ageing.

Estimates indicate that the population will increase from 63.7 million in 2012 to 73.3 million in 2037 in the United Kingdom (Figure 11.4). Of this increase, 5.4 million (57%) will be due to a positive population replacement rate (more births than deaths) and 4.2 million (43%) will be due to immigration. Unlike Japan, the UK population is ageing but not decreasing. The UK population will continue ageing, with the average age rising from 39.7 years in 2012 to 40.6 in mid-2022 and 42.8 by mid-2037.

Global ageing trends and projections

The world's older population has been increasing steadily over the last two centuries, but each country is at a different stage and is experiencing the population shift at a different rate. For most countries, the rise of the 65-years-and-over age group from approximately 7% to 14% of the total population took between 45 and 115 years to happen. The growth of older populations in countries that previously had a very young age structure is occurring at a much higher pace. It will take a country such as Brazil about 20 years to double its population of over-65s compared with, say, Sweden, which took 85 years for the same to occur.

The demographic transition that occurred in many developing countries in the late nineteenth century (and is still occurring) has had slightly different origins. Social, public health and economic improvements have been important. These populations have also benefited from immunization programmes in childhood, modern birth control methods and more advanced medical care. None of these technological influences was available to assist the speed of the demographic transition in Victorian and Edwardian Britain or the other industrialized countries of the northern hemisphere.

Europe will remain the region of the world with the highest percentage of older adults. By 2040, one in four European adults will be 65 years and older, and most likely one in seven will be aged 75 years and over. North America will have one in five adults aged over 65 years. Sub-Saharan Africa will still be the youngest region because of high fertility rates and the continuing impact of AIDS on life expectancy.

Life expectancy at birth varies greatly among countries and world regions (Table 11.4). There is a difference of 20 or more years between high- and low-income countries across the northern hemisphere. Female advantage is almost universal – it starts at birth and continues as women age. Although the male–female gap has recently narrowed in some high-income countries, it exceeds 12 years in many countries of the former Soviet Union. The gender gap in life expectancy at birth is predicted to widen in many low-income countries as increases in alcohol intake, tobacco consumption and road and industrial accidents make a differential impact on male death rates.

The life expectancy for people who have reached the age of 60 years in high-income countries is increasing twice as fast as in the poorer countries of the world, and three times

Table 11.4 Life expectancy at birth, by country

	Life expectancy (years)
Japan	84
United Kingdom	81
United States of America	79
South Africa	63
Somalia	55
Central African Republic	53

Source: World Health Organization (WHO). *World Health Statistics.* Geneva: WHO, 2016. With permission.

faster than in sub-Saharan Africa. At any older age, female mortality rates are lower and age-specific life expectancy is greater (with some regional variations). Importantly, many high-income countries are experiencing mortality improvements in older age groups (e.g. aged 70–74 and 80–84 years), which will greatly affect the proportion of exceptionally old people.

Retirement and work in later life

Population ageing puts great pressure on a nation's ability to fund such public services as education and social security benefits, as well as on the level of health and social care provisions, especially when the number of working-age people declines and the old-age population grows. Population ageing also reduces the base of people who can be taxed on their employment income and reduces the funds coming into government. These trends have prompted moves by the governments of a number of European countries to increase the retirement age.

An important demographic indicator of societal support is the older dependency ratio. This is the number of people 65 years and over per 100 people aged 20–64 years. Japan and some western European countries have the highest ratios. An older dependency ratio above 30 means that fewer than three working-age adults support (notionally, not literally) one adult aged 65 years and over. This statistic is not as universally accepted as it once was; for example, it rigidly implies that all people 65 years and over do not work and need support, while all adults aged 20–64 years do work and provide support to older members of society.

Labour force participation rates for older adults decline nearer to retirement age, more so for women. The employment rate of older workers (aged 65 years and over) varies across regions and is generally higher in low- and middle-income countries. In most of Europe, fewer than 10% of older people aged 65 years and over are working, compared with the 33% or more who are in the labour force in the less affluent parts of the world. Part-time work is often used as a transitional phase between full-time job and retirement (phased or gradual retirement) but is also a function of health, economy, the scarcity of career

opportunities for older workers and favourable pension and annuity schemes.

The number of older workers of, and above, the state pension age employed in the United Kingdom almost doubled in the first two decades of the twenty-first century. Better health, a wish to remain active in society and the desire, or need, to maintain income at a level above their pension are some of the drivers away from the traditional approach of entirely stopping work at a fixed age.

The UK population pyramid shows an increase in the age group of 64 and 65 years as a result of the post–World War II so-called baby boom generation (born in 1946–47). As the boomers approach retirement age, many countries will be hit by shortages in skilled and experienced workers, coupled with an increased financial burden due to loss of taxable income and increases in tax-funded services. Many national governments are already implementing policies geared to promote longer labour force participation of boomers and of the cohorts that preceded them (e.g. changes in the national pension system, removal of compulsory retirement age and increase in early retirement age) to ensure sustainability of state-funded pensions.

Population ageing and informal caregiving

Adult children, spouses and other family members are the major source of informal (unpaid) care and support for older people in most countries, regardless of wealth and an available formal (paid) care structure and welfare regime. With the changing demography, the societal challenge is how to secure an adequate pool of potential informal caregivers and economically active people to sustain the needs of older adults.

Except for the period of baby boom (1946–64), family size fell sharply in most high-income countries during the twentieth century, resulting in smaller support systems available for older adults' care. In most European countries, informal care comes primarily from a spouse and secondarily from an adult child if the spouse dies. While there are some differences across Europe, many older adults live alone, but most are geographically close to an adult child, which indicates their wish to remain independent but have opportunities for contact with children and grandchildren. Older adults without children generally have less potential source of support and informal care.

Although childlessness was low in cohorts born between the two World Wars, analysis of the boomers' attitudes and behaviour shows an increase in voluntary childlessness in western Europe and the United Kingdom. This has been associated with women's participation in the labour force and building of full careers, education, birth control and societal acceptance of divorce. Boomers who have divorced (whether or not they have remarried) may have more complex family relationships, which can weaken their capacity and commitment in providing tangible support to their older parents. On the other hand, complex family structures associated with divorce create new extended family networks, and sometimes a bigger source of informal care emerges.

Increased geographical mobility also affects the pool of potential supporters of older people. Following retirement, some older people migrate to more rural locations or to coastal communities with favourable amenities and warmer climate. For example, many northern Europeans move to the Mediterranean, and older Americans migrate from northern states to the South. Today, there are more than 1 million older British citizens who have moved to continental Europe, particularly to Spain and France. This has put a strain on care services in these countries and has reduced access to family caregiving networks.

Looking at population ageing globally, China is an important country to understand. China implemented a national family planning policy (one child per couple) in the 1970s to slow population growth. Although the policy was amended in later years, fertility rates remained below the population replacement rate. This is causing rapid population ageing and change in population structure. Decreased family size and continuous migration of young workers to the cities will further overburden the traditional family support system in coming decades. Without siblings to share the care for older parents, a young couple born during the one-child policy will support two sets of older parents. If this policy of family planning continues, children in China will reach adulthood only to face major future care responsibilities, for both parents and grandparents.

HEALTHY LIFE EXPECTANCY

The number of additional years older adults are expected to live gives a snapshot of survival patterns in a population. Life expectancy at age 60 years continues to rise globally in both men and women, more so in the higher-income countries. This indicates that mortality is being compressed further into later life. Such forecasts are useful for planning future pensions, healthcare and social care. However, these quantitative data give little insight into quality of life after age 60 years. The statistic does not separate healthy (active) years from those spent with diseases and disabilities.

Advancing age is the strongest risk factor for diseases, disabilities and frailty, and therefore of needs for health and social services. However, even at very old age, adults exhibit a greater heterogeneity in health, abilities and needs than is often appreciated. Adding qualitative data to mortality numbers allows for a clearer picture of the health and social needs of the older population. No single measure or source of data can be relied on to assess the health and social status of an older population and the extent to which this translates into needs. To determine population health in later life, various indicators of health and functioning and models of pattern of change in mortality, diseases and disabilities have been developed.

Along with demographic transition from high fertility and high mortality to low fertility and low mortality, most countries have also experienced an epidemiologic transition. As more children have survived into old age and fertility has declined, the morbidity (sickness) profile and causes of death in such populations have shifted towards non-communicable disease in later life.

The level of independence that older people can maintain, their physical and social well-being, together with the strength of their social networks and interactions, is very strongly linked with what is sometimes called functional capacity. This is measured by a person's ability to perform activities of daily living (Table 11.5). Methods of assessing this vary greatly across studies and countries.

The European Union introduced a structural health indicator called *healthy life years* to monitor health expectancy trends annually across its member states. The main purpose of this index is to determine which pattern of population health is accompanying increases in life expectancy across Europe: decrease in unhealthy years (compression of morbidity), increase in unhealthy years (expansion of morbidity) or decrease in levels of severity of unhealthy years (dynamic equilibrium).

The European Union uses the global activity limitation index to factor in disability; this assesses self-reported,

Table 11.5 Activities of daily living

Basic activities of daily living	Instrumental activities of daily living	Additional mobility items
Feeding oneself	Preparing meals	Walking from room to room
Toileting	Taking medication	Climbing a flight of stairs
Dressing	Using a telephone	Walking outside one's home
Grooming	Managing finances	
Bathing	Doing laundry	
Transferring from bed to chair	Doing housework	
Moving about one's home	Shopping	
	Using transportation	

Source: Adapted from Gill TM. Assessment of function and disability in longitudinal studies. *Journal of the American Geriatrics Society* 2010;58(s2):S308–12.

long-term limitation (over six months) in usual daily activities in three levels of poor health. There is great variation across Europe. For example, in 2005, an older adult in Sweden had 20 more healthy years at the age of 50, but an older adult in Hungary had only 11 additional years without disabilities.

Monitoring the trends in an index like this is important not only for allocation of resources to healthcare and social care but also for European Commission and member states' policies on the extension of working life years and decreasing health inequalities.

Over the past 20 years, life expectancy in the United Kingdom has increased by about four years for both women and men – but only two were healthy years. The Office for National Statistics publishes regular updates about healthy life expectancy at birth (based on self-rated health) in the United Kingdom. It investigates factors that influence variations in length and quality of life across different residential areas. Although women live longer than men, deprivation significantly affects gender inequality in healthy years of life.

ETHNIC MINORITY OLDER ADULTS

In the last few years of the twentieth century, ethnic minority communities made up about 7% of Britain's population. The proportion was much higher in certain conurbations. The relatively young age structure of these communities reflects a high birth rate in some groups and the waves of immigration that occurred in the 1960s and early 1970s and for those who came from Caribbean countries in earlier years still. Between 1991 and 2011, the nonwhite minorities in England and Wales doubled to almost 8 million, or 14% of the population.

While the proportion of older people belonging to ethnic minority groups is as yet small, compared with the older population identifying as British white, their numbers are expected to increase across all age groups.

Compared with the British white population, most ethnic minority groups have shorter life expectancy at birth and shorter life spent without disabilities (Figure 11.5). In all ethnic groups, women live longer than men do but spend shorter periods of their lives disability-free.

It is important not to fall into stereotypic assumptions about the needs of this group of older adults. For example, it is widely believed that old age is a greatly revered state in some ethnic minority communities within Britain. Hence, it is assumed that an older person will enjoy the warmth, support and care of an extended family, so little attention should be given by formal care services to meeting their health and care needs. While this may be the ideal shared by people in some ethnic minority communities themselves, patterns of geographical mobility and other factors will mean that it is unlikely always to be realized. Contrasts between this cultural ideal and the social reality may give rise to problems for older ethnic minorities, as well as leading to false assumptions among those responsible for providing services.

In responding to the needs of older people from ethnic minority communities, it is especially important for health services to ensure that they are aware of and work with varying cultural norms. Knowledge of and sensitivity to such issues as diet, religious practice and observance and the role of the older person in his or her own community are of particular significance.

COMMON FEATURES OF ILL HEALTH IN LATER LIFE

Many of the health problems of later life pose special challenges for the older adults themselves, their families and the

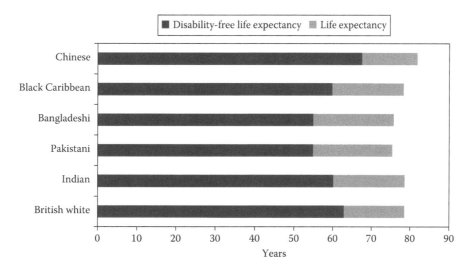

Figure 11.5 Life expectancy and disability-free life expectancy in England and Wales for selected ethnic groups.

Source: Wohland P, Rees P, Nazroo J, Jagger C. Inequalities in healthy life expectancy between ethnic groups in England and Wales in 2001. *Ethnicity & Health* 2015;20(4):341–53.

agencies responsible for planning and providing health and social care services.

Multimorbidity

As any organism ages, the risk of impairment, disease or death is greater. In most, including human beings, the risk of death fluctuates during the early years of life before rising progressively with time.

The ageing process relates to disease in three main ways:

1. *Altered response to disease:* Some diseases are overcome less easily in older people than they are in younger people, such as pneumonia and fractures.
2. *Increased risk with ageing:* Many diseases occur much more commonly when old age is reached (such as many types of cancer).
3. *Diseases associated with ageing:* Some disease processes are so closely associated with ageing that they occur to some extent in all individuals as they age. The best example of this is arteriosclerosis.

The hallmark of disease in older people is the presence of more than one disease or condition, so-called multimorbidity. Some of these diseases surface for the first time in old age, whereas others are carried over from middle age. Other properties of ill health in later life are important when designing medical care responses (Table 11.6). Many very old people have impaired adaptability to disease, so their health problems show up in atypical ways, with symptoms such as falls and confusion, making them difficult to diagnose. Rapid deterioration and a relatively high incidence of complications are also features of disease in very old age. The importance of rehabilitation in recovery is much more important than it is in younger age groups. So is the environment in which care is provided.

Older people's health needs can be seen in three broad categories: (1) those who, regardless of chronological age, remain in reasonably good health and require few services, other than preventive activities such as vaccination and cancer screening; (2) those at the other end of the spectrum, the minority who are frail or have one of the major disabling illnesses, such as dementia or stroke (they are major users of acute hospital services and of long-term residential and domiciliary care); and (3) the largest group, those starting to experience age-related health problems, including early

Table 11.6 Important aspects of illness and ageing

- Multi-morbidity
- Risk of dependency
- Presentation of problems often not typical
- Side effects and complications frequent
- Limited resilience and decreased physiological reserve
- Care environment important
- Multidisciplinary care essential

memory loss and sensory deficits, that put them at risk of feeling permanently unwell and losing independence.

As pathological processes and disease burden interfere with older adults' level of functioning and produce disability, assessment of their ability to perform activities of daily living is frequently used to determine the unmet needs and gaps in care and services at both the individual and population level. It gives a focus for a multidisciplinary approach to care for older adults and case management through integrated locally based teams in the community. Population-level assessments of functional capacity provide a common currency that enables the aggregation of data so that it is possible, for example, to describe the proportion of an older population with dementia at a national or local level, and then organize an appropriate service response.

Polypharmacy

About 20% of those aged 70 years and over take, on average, five or more medications. Some conditions, such as heart disease and diabetes, require multiple medications for treatment and prophylaxis. They can be life-saving and improve the quality of life of an old person. However, overtreatment and adverse drug reactions among older patients are major problems. Polypharmacy is usually defined as concurrent use of five or more medications. Inappropriate polypharmacy, on the other hand, has been described as the use of more medications than clinically necessary, which could pose harm and outweigh the benefits of the treatment.

The risk of adverse drug reaction increases with age because of changes in body composition and weight (lower body water and fat-free mass), decrease in drug clearance in liver and kidneys and overall depletion of physiological reserve. These processes cause changes in pharmacodynamics and kinetics of drugs and may lead to drug–drug and drug–disease interactions. For example, many drugs that affect the central nervous system have an exaggerated response in older adults. Older adults are particularly sensitive to adverse effects of antipsychotics, which cause an increased sedative effect, postural sway and risk of falls. Some prescription medicines can precipitate confusion and acute delirium, especially in the very frail. Older adults can have great difficulty adhering to their medication regime, particularly if they also take two or three over-the-counter drugs for minor complaints. To warrant safety and quality of prescribing for older patients with multiple chronic diseases, several structured decision tools have been created, and regular medication reviews and adjustments are recommended.

Frailty

Frailty is a multidimensional condition that puts an older person at increased risk of adverse health outcomes, including falls, delirium, disability, morbidity and death. Frail older adults are vulnerable to stressors and lack adequate physiological response to cope with these stressors.

Frailty is a better descriptor than biological age of a person and is used in both clinical practice and research to identify at-risk older adults. Clinically, frail older adults have limited functional reserve, so even a minor illness can have catastrophic consequences. It can result in disability, failure to thrive and inability to recover from stressors.

There are two main concepts of frailty. The *frailty phenotype* sees frailty as a biological syndrome affecting multiple body systems. This phenotype comprises several health deficits (e.g. extreme fatigue, slowness, weakness, low energy expenditure and unexplained weight loss). Other deficits in health as a part of the frailty syndrome may include adverse changes in mental health in both affect and cognition. Conversely, the *frailty index* uses a cumulative deficit approach. Frailty is interpreted as a multidimensional risk state. It combines symptoms, diseases and disabilities to predict different degrees of frailty. Within clinical settings, various stages of frailty and fitness of older people require different care plans and supportive services (Table 11.7).

Several frailty scales – including the Edmonton Frail Scale, the Groningen Frailty Indicator and the Tilburg Frailty Indicator – are in use. They mostly show that in community populations of older adults, frailty increases with ageing and mortality risk increases with frailty. Women have higher frailty scores, on average, than men, who live longer with the same degree of frailty. Understanding and harmonizing frailty scales across various care settings is important for clinical care, research and policy planning.

Falls

Every year, about 33% of adults aged 65 years and over and about 50% aged 80 years and over fall. Falls in hospital are one of the most common reasons for patient safety incident reports. Falls are a leading cause of hospital and long-term care facilities admission. Falls are strongly associated with advancing age, frailty, disability and death. Strategies to prevent falls among older adults include recognizing risk factors that precipitate falls (problems with balance, muscle weakness, visual impairment, medication causing postural sway, physical barriers and tripping hazards at home) and implementing activities and programmes that improve physical strength and well-being.

The propensity of older people to fall over has long been recognized. Many falls in older adults result in no injuries. However, partly because of the increased fragility of bones in old age (osteoporosis), a fracture is a common outcome of a fall. Fracture of the neck of the femur is a particularly serious example that can result from seemingly quite trivial falls. Even with the modern approach of immediate operation – to pin the fracture or replace the hip joint – and early mobilization, case fatality can still be as high as 25%. The management of hip fracture in very old adults is especially difficult because of comorbidities and a higher incidence of dementia and delirium. A less serious fracture, such as Colles' fracture of the wrist, may still be a considerable handicap for an older woman attempting to cook her meals and do her housework with an arm immobilized in plaster.

An older woman is more likely to die from the complications of a hip fracture than from breast cancer. Accidents are a common cause of death, disability and hospital admission in later life. Falls are the single most important cause of accidental death in older people, the remainder resulting from road traffic accidents, burns and a variety of other causes. The economic costs are high, with fractured hips alone estimated to account for nearly £2 billion of expenditure in the health and social care system in the United Kingdom.

The types of falls have been classified into three categories:

1. *Intrinsic:* In most older people who have fallen, there were underlying causes, such as disorders of vision, disorders of balance (e.g. vestibular disorders), neurological problems (e.g. Parkinson's disease) and cardiovascular disorders (e.g. carotid sinus syndrome).

Table 11.7 Degrees of frailty

Stage	Description and needs
Very fit	Fit, robust, exercise regularly
Well	No symptoms, but less active and exercise only occasionally
Managing well	Have symptoms, but well-managed on appropriate medication. Not regularly active beyond walking
Vulnerable	Feel fatigued and slowed up. Limited activity but no daily help required
Mildly frail	Further slowed up. Need help with instrumental activities of daily living
Moderately frail	All outside activities problematic. Unable to manage a household. Need assistance with such activities as bathing and dressing
Severely frail	Completely dependent on others for all activities of daily living. However, symptoms stable and not at risk of dying within next six months
Very severely frail	Completely dependent on others and approaching the end of life
Terminally ill	Life expectancy less than six months

Source: Rockwood K, Song X, MacKnight C, et al. A global clinical measure of fitness and frailty in elderly people. *Canadian Medical Association Journal* 2005;173(5):489–95.

2. *Drug induced:* About 7% of acute hospital admissions among older people are related to drug side effects, the most common of which is drug-induced falls. Drugs that are particularly dangerous include sedatives and drugs with anticholinergic properties, including some antidepressants, which induce postural hypotension.
3. *Extrinsic:* Environmental factors, such as poor lighting and loose rugs, are thought to contribute to about 40% of falls.

In the general population, throughout life, increasing the level of exercise, particularly weight-bearing activity, reduces the risk of falls and fractures in later life. In primary care, many older people report a history of a fall. It is not possible to offer everyone a full multidisciplinary assessment and treatment programme, nor is there evidence that this would be cost-effective. Nevertheless, older people who have fallen should be reviewed to encourage weight-bearing exercise, check vision, enquire about the home environment and take stock of medication regimes. Older people who suffer recurrent falls and those who have been in hospital with a major fall should also be reviewed by a multidisciplinary falls and bone health service. There is good evidence for the cost-effectiveness of screening for and treatment of osteoporosis in people who have had fragility fractures. The approach to reducing the impact of falls in hospital is improving with the use of evidence-based care bundles.

Urinary incontinence

Urinary incontinence commonly occurs among older men and women. Estimates suggest that the overall prevalence is around 30% in community-dwelling older adults, and about 50% among those in care homes and other institutions. It is perhaps the most embarrassing, distressing and ultimately humiliating problem of old age. Its onset is often the reason why an older person is judged as no longer fit to remain in his or her home, ejected from a family or friend's home or considered an unsuitable candidate for certain forms of residential care. Urinary incontinence is defined by the International Continence Society as 'the involuntary loss of urine which is objectively demonstrable and is a social or hygienic problem'. The Society recognizes three main subtypes of urinary incontinence: *urgency,* involuntary loss of urine associated with urgency, *stress,* involuntary loss of urine upon physical effort, exertion, sneezing or coughing; and *mixed,* involuntary loss of urine due to combined effects of urgency, effort, exertion, sneezing or coughing.

In addition to identifying the type or pattern of urinary incontinence, it is important to assess its severity (amount and frequency of volume loss) in older adults. Older women with a small volume loss due to stress incontinence may employ various coping mechanisms and not seek medical advice. But if faced with an episode of a large volume loss, most are more willing to seek professional help.

The causes are many and may arise from local factors, for example, bladder neck obstruction (most often due to prostatic enlargement), stress incontinence (usually due to weakening of pelvic floor musculature following childbirth), overactive bladder or urinary tract infections. General factors in older adults that may lead to incontinence are often multiple and not clear-cut. A common reason for urinary incontinence is loss of inhibition of need to void when the bladder is partly full. When this occurs mainly at night, it is known as nocturia. Bereavement, accidents or illnesses can give rise to incontinence of either a transient or a permanent nature. Confusion from organic cerebral disease, including stroke, or side effects of sedatives or psychotropic drugs can also lead to incontinence. Other drugs, such as rapidly acting diuretics, may also contribute. Incontinence may be a feature of limitation of mobility, with the older person being unable to reach the toilet in time to avoid an accident.

Urinary incontinence degrades the quality of life of older adults. It has been associated with reduced physical activity, social isolation, depression, disability, poor self-rated health and increased caregiver burden.

For continence of urine to be maintained, five factors need to be fulfilled. Approaches to management need to identify which of these factors is contributing to the loss of continence in the individual concerned and then address the problem. The following factors are necessary to maintain urinary continence:

- Adequate function of the lower urinary tract to store and empty urine
- Adequate cognitive function to recognize the need to urinate and to find the appropriate place
- Adequate physical mobility and dexterity to get to a toilet and use it
- Motivation to be continent
- Absence of environmental barriers to continence

The cornerstone of management of urinary incontinence in older adults is correctly diagnosing the cause, together with a sympathetic and understanding attitude of caregivers. This means good assessment by, for example, a continence adviser with expertise and experience in this field. Incontinence is seldom the result of a single underlying cause. It cannot be overemphasized that the presence of incontinence is a deeply emotional issue, both for the older people who have it and for relatives, friends and neighbours who are in contact with them.

In some cases, operative treatment of an enlarged prostate or of a gynaecological disorder, treatment of an underlying urinary tract infection or review of a long-standing drug regime may solve the problem. Aside from these measures, probably the most important step in treating urinary incontinence is bladder training. For patients already in an institutional setting, episodes of incontinence must be recorded on a fluid chart, and staff should ensure regular toileting to re-educate the bladder. Such bladder training may be supplemented by physiotherapy to strengthen pelvic floor muscles.

A wide variety of support is possible for older people with incontinence in the community. Specialized continence advisers can visit, make assessments and provide help to those whose problem has been diagnosed. The use of specialized underclothes and pads is an important adjunct to specific interventions and therapies.

Depression

Mental illness in later life can take many forms. Its impact on the well-being of older adults is greater because of the presence of comorbid physical problems. Finding a workable medication regime for both can be challenging.

Depression is the most common mental health disorder in later life and affects approximately 10%–15% of the population aged 65 years and over. It is often difficult to differentiate depression from nonspecific symptoms related to ageing. Depression in later life can be precipitated by any of the major life events common in this age group, for example, loss of a spouse, retirement, decreasing social support or physical illness associated with pain. Depression will be the greatest contributor to disease burden in older adults living in high-income countries by 2030. The manifestations of depression can be quite wide ranging and include apathy, social withdrawal, neglect of personal appearance, tearfulness, sleep disorders, loss of appetite and suicide. For many older people, an episode of depression may resolve with professional help and medication, but in others, the condition becomes chronic. Depression in later life significantly increases the risk of stroke, myocardial infarction, dementia, disability, polypharmacy, hospital admissions and mortality. Additionally, depression remains the strongest risk factor for suicides in later life.

A number of approaches for the management of comorbid depression in older adults have been used: antidepressant therapy and psychological interventions (cognitive behavioural therapy, problem-solving therapy and life reviews therapy) and collaborative care models. Collaborative care models recognize the recurrent and chronic nature of depression in later life and emphasize the importance of a structured management plan and interdisciplinary approach through primary care in treatment of depression in later life.

Dementia

Dementia is an umbrella term that describes several disorders of brain functioning that lead to deterioration in the capacity of the mind. It affects memory, planning, decision-making, understanding and the use of language. Older adults with dementia can also have disturbances of normal behaviour that lead them to wander, to sleep irregularly and fitfully and to exhibit disruptive and antisocial behaviour. Progressive loss of function is an important feature of the disease. Dementia varies in its impact on mental, physical and social functioning of any individual older person (Table 11.8).

Minor degrees of memory impairment and temporary confusion may not necessarily threaten an independent existence. However, more severe and sustained problems of this kind, especially when coupled with disturbed or erratic behaviour and an inability to perform basic activities of daily living, will lead rapidly to dependency.

Advancing age is the strongest risk factor for dementia. Dementia prevalence doubles every five years, from 2%–5% in people aged 65 years and over to close to 40% in those aged 90 and over (Figure 11.6). The leading charity, Alzheimer's Disease International, has estimated the worldwide dementia prevalence at more than 35 million cases, with a predicted rise to more than 67 million cases by 2030.

Currently, 800,000 people in the United Kingdom have dementia, and this number will double in the next 40 years. Two population-based surveys of older adults aged 65 years and over in England and Wales showed a decrease in age-specific dementia prevalence in two recent decades (Figure 11.6). This is in line with reductions in other high-income countries, especially western European countries, which have been explained by improvements in education of younger cohorts of older adults and prevention

Table 11.8 Features of dementia

Progressive impairment of intellectual functioning	Example
Memory problems	Unable to remember recent events and access new memories
Loss of sense of time	Unable to tell time, day or season
Loss of sense of place	Unable to recognise familiar places
Loss of sense of self	Unable to recognise one's image in mirror or photo
Language difficulties	Losing words and inability to follow a conversation
Personality and behavioural changes	Paranoia
Neglect of personal care and hygiene	Forgetting to bathe and change clothes
Incontinence	Forgetting how to use toilet
Emotional instability	Frequent and abrupt mood swings
Loss of social inhibitions	Inappropriate outbursts

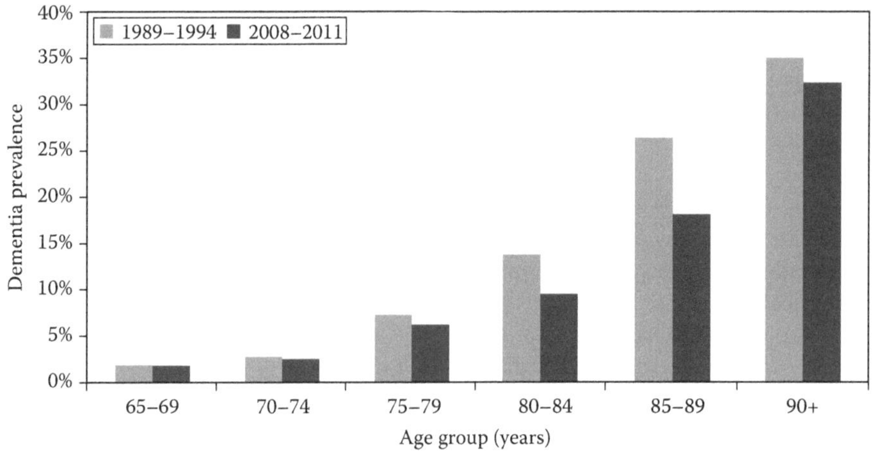

Figure 11.6 Two-decade comparison of age-specific dementia prevalence in women in England and Wales, 1989–94 and 2008–11.

Source: Matthews FE, Arthur A, Barnes LE, et al. Medical Research Council Cognitive Function and Ageing Collaboration. A two-decade comparison of prevalence of dementia in individuals aged 65 years and older from three geographical areas of England: results of the Cognitive Function and Ageing Study I and II. Lancet 2013;382(9902):1405–12.

and treatment of diseases that can cause dementia, such as hypertension and stroke. Despite decreasing age-specific rates, the number of people with dementia is rising rapidly due to population ageing.

Alzheimer's disease and vascular dementia are the most common types of dementia. Other less common forms include Lewy body dementia, frontotemporal dementia (including Pick's disease) and dementia associated with neurodegenerative disorders (such as Huntington's chorea, Parkinson's disease and Creutzfeldt–Jakob disease). The symptoms and signs of dementia can also be produced by vitamin B12 deficiency, cerebral tumours, thyroid disease and chronic alcoholism.

Alzheimer's disease is a complex, progressive neurodegenerative disorder characterized by loss and severe abnormalities of nerve cells and their processes. In particular, nerve cells that produce important chemical substances for brain activities are lost. The brain pathology of the disease consists of two main toxic proteins: the amyloid-beta peptide, the main constituent of senile plaques that accumulate outside the cells, and abnormal protein tau, which collects inside the cells. Together, they contribute to nerve cell loss and brain degeneration. Alzheimer's disease accounts for about 50% of all cases of dementia among the over-65s. Dementia is much less common in middle age and early old age, but when it does occur here, Alzheimer's disease is often the reason, and is linked to several genetic mutations.

Anticholinesterase inhibitor drugs are moderately effective in delaying decline in mental function for people with Alzheimer's disease of moderate severity. Reduction in cardiovascular risk factors reduces the incidence of Alzheimer's disease. Extensive investigation by the pharmaceutical industry into the pathophysiology of Alzheimer's disease is likely to yield more effective approaches to detection and treatment.

Vascular dementia, on the other hand, is a disease of the arteries of the brain, causing death of small or large areas of brain tissue due to oxygen and nutrient deprivation. It can be precipitated by a major stroke, or it can develop over time from small recurrent strokes. Unlike Alzheimer's disease, vascular dementia tends to progress in a stepwise fashion with periods of stability, depending on the severity and frequency of strokes.

Among older people admitted to hospital for treatment of acute medical, surgical or orthopaedic conditions, delirium (confusion) is common. Unlike dementia, it is an acute, reversible disorder of attention and cognition. Delirium in older adults with a diagnosis of dementia is a frequent problem. It is associated with worsening of dementia symptoms, physical decline and prolonged hospitalization. Many people can be managed clinically if they are identified at an early stage and underlying factors are treated. Delirium in acute hospital settings is still underdiagnosed.

Hypothermia and excess winter deaths

Accidental hypothermia is present if the core body temperature is below 35°C. The term *accidental* is used to distinguish this type of hypothermia from that induced deliberately for therapeutic purposes. The diagnosis of hypothermia is confirmed with a special low-reading thermometer inserted rectally. Such instruments are becoming an increasingly common part of the equipment of doctors and nurses working in the community. It is estimated that 3%–4% of people aged 65 years and over who are admitted to hospital have a core body temperature below 35°C. More than 90% of cases of accidental hypothermia occur indoors.

Older people with hypothermia do not usually shiver or complain of being cold. They have an impaired perception

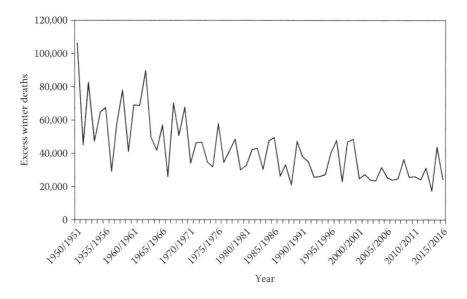

Figure 11.7 Trend in excess winter deaths in England and Wales.

Source: Office for National Statistics.

of temperature change. Pale, cold skin is a warning sign. So is clouded consciousness with drowsiness and disordered thought and speech. Coma is more likely the lower the body temperature becomes. Movement and reflexes are sluggish. Speech may be slurred. Respiratory rate is often too slow, and there may be characteristic changes in an electrocardiograph. Blood pressure may fall. Some patients with hypothermia may become agitated and restless. If sedation is given, this can complicate and conceal their serious condition. Fatality is high. Treatment, usually in hospital, consists of gradual rewarming (if conducted too rapidly, this may be fatal) and other supportive measures, such as administration of oxygen, intravenous fluids and broad-spectrum antibiotics.

The main causes of accidental hypothermia are defective thermoregulatory mechanisms (a consequence of ageing) and exposure to cold through low environmental temperature. Other factors – such as immobility due to general infirmity, mental impairment, strokes, falls, effects of medicines or certain illness (e.g. infections and endocrine disorders) – may be superimposed.

Reducing the occurrence of accidental hypothermia in later life is through community programmes directed at the homes of older people, particularly those living alone. Health education advice to older people should emphasize moving around, if possible, to increase body heat by metabolic activity, and ensuring adequate nutrition and clothing. Financial support through the benefits system for heating, insulation and cold weather payments is particularly important.

Measuring mortality in the winter months (usually December to March) as a proportion of mortality at other times of the year yields a measure called *excess winter deaths*. The excess winter mortality index is calculated as the number of excess winter deaths divided by the average

nonwinter deaths, and is expressed as a percentage. The excess mortality is due to circulatory illness (ischaemic heart disease and stroke), respiratory disease (particularly influenza), accidents and violence (including hypothermia) and a range of other causes. The excess winter mortality rate rises sharply with age in the older age groups and is worse in years with influenza epidemics. The number of excess winter deaths in Britain has fluctuated year to year but generally has decreased over the decades (Figure 11.7).

Heat waves and excess summer deaths

Until recently, the effect of weather and environmental temperatures on the health of older people was always a matter of exposure to the cold. Summer weather patterns attributed to climate change in western Europe have raised the risks of extreme heat. This came to prominence in France in August 2003, when very high temperatures led to nearly 15,000 excess deaths. The majority were women aged 75 years or older. There were major recriminations for the French government. A satellite image of Paris in the summer of 2003 revealed a temperature difference of 1°C–2°C between the inner city and a rural suburb. However, this small difference resulted in twice the mortality risk between urban and rural dwellers.

In the United Kingdom, there is now a heat wave plan that provides advice and contingency plans to protect older and vulnerable people. The plan is triggered by particular ambient temperature thresholds.

Isolation in later life

Loneliness can be a major factor in the health and social problems of later life. It can cause apathy, lack of interest, malnutrition, hypothermia and general self-neglect.

Older people's social networks are a vital determinant of whether they need care as they age. An older person living alone is not always socially isolated, but the nature of his or her social contacts, not just the number, is important in the lives of older people. The potential impact of social and demographic changes related to these issues was discussed earlier in the chapter. Much less is known about the extent to which other societal changes have influenced older people's own perceptions of the importance of social networks. For example, an old person living alone in an inner-city area who enjoys regular social contact with relatives and friends may be so fearful of personal attack that she would much rather reside in a sheltered housing scheme than remain in her own home any longer.

The social networks of older people are based heavily on relatives, but friends and neighbours are also important. The number of social contacts that people maintain in later life varies and depends on their social and educational background, their ethnic group, the type of community they live in and their personal attitudes and outlook. There is some research evidence suggesting that health and mortality in later life are both affected by the strength of older people's social networks.

Changes in the position of older people in society are also closely related to the economic effects of growing old. In the United Kingdom, retired people who are mainly dependent on a state pension and pension credit have lower income than other groups. State pensions and other welfare benefits provide the main source of income for older people. However, 10% of older adults with private pensions live in poverty, defined as living in a household below 60% of the median income, after deducting household costs. Older people spend a higher proportion of their income on basics – housing, fuel and food – than do younger people. Recent trends also suggest that as the share of working-age people occupying low-income jobs or living in work-less households in poverty increases, the risk of poverty for older retirees with only state pensions is much greater.

CARE IN LATER LIFE

For some considerable time, the central objective of policy for care in old age in the United Kingdom has been to enable older adults to remain in the community for as long as possible. For many people in later life, their ability to reside in their own home is a potent symbol of autonomy, independence and self-determination.

Contrary to popular belief, most older adults do in fact lead an independent existence in their own home. Between 30% and 40% of those aged 80 years and over rate their health as very good or excellent. About 60%–80% of people in this age group receive no help with activities of daily living.

Measures to promote health and prevent disease earlier in life can help to improve health in later life by delaying the onset of some of the chronic diseases mentioned. However, action in old age itself can also have an impact. The World Health Organization has estimated that about 50% of the burden of disease in older adults could be eliminated by adopting the healthy lifestyles associated with preventing the major non-communicable diseases. However, with advancing age and the impact of the negative forces of old age, their independence can be compromised and less easily maintained. Several key features particularly determine health needs in later life (Table 11.9). When older people are no longer able to manage on their own, a wide range of services may be available to provide help, support and advice.

A shift to preventive and proactive care centred on older people's homes and communities can embed physical and mental well-being and quality of life in a model of integrated care that also provides chronic disease management in primary care and the investigation and treatment of acute illness in hospital. Such an approach is not well established across the United Kingdom but is a goal that must continue to be at the forefront of the thinking of policymakers and planners. Without a comprehensively designed system of care centred on the needs of older people (and their caregivers), as well as on the ideal of healthy ageing, the problems and concerns about the capacity, capability and appropriateness of services will continue.

One way of viewing integrated care is through the 10 components set out in Figure 11.8. This model uses a whole-person, life-course approach. The main goal of the first component of care could be accomplished by adapting a life-course approach for health and well-being and by promoting healthy lifestyles throughout life (including later in life), combating social isolation and loneliness, implementing screening programmes, vaccination and hot and cold weather planning. The second is based on continuity of care, care management and coordination delivered through community-based teams. The third care component recognizes the importance of frailty risk assessment to identify frail older adults promptly. Other elements include prevention of falls, addressing inappropriate medication regimes and providing support for people with dementia. The fourth emphasizes the importance of being ready to respond well to crisis situations. The fifth care component addresses acute (hospital) care and the need for it to involve comprehensive, interdisciplinary assessment of older patients, specialist elderly care units and wards, and dignified person-centred care to minimize the harms of hospitalization. The sixth

Table 11.9 Key features that determine health needs in later life

- Social networks and support
- Income level
- Presence of disease and illness
- Mobility and capacity for self-care
- Housing quality and neighbourhood environment
- Sensory impairment
- Personal security
- Access to services and health information

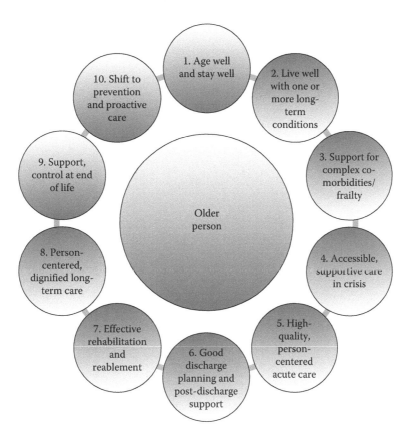

Figure 11.8 Ten components of high-quality, person-centred care of older people.

Source: From Oliver D, Foot C, Humphries R. *Making Our Health and Care Systems Fit for an Ageing Population.* London: The King's Fund, 2014.

makes clear that when an older person is in hospital, good discharge planning and postdischarge support are also vital; this should involve older adults and/or their carers in decision-making. The seventh care component covers the frequently neglected subject of rehabilitation to ensure that it is firmly rooted in a vision of high-quality integrated care. The eighth covers the type of provision needed when all alternatives to preserve independence have been exhausted. Nursing and residential care are areas where there have been many concerns within the United Kingdom about variable quality, neglect of elderly residents and serious failures in standards. In this sector, care must be safe, holistic, person centred and dignified. End-of-life care, the ninth care component, should be approached as a natural, last phase of life. It should be dignified and planned whenever possible so that older adults have choice and control over life decisions (particularly over areas such as place of dying, pain relief, treatment options and do not resuscitate notices). All these care components should be integrated into one continuum to ensure quality of care of older adults and support for their families and carers. The tenth component emphasizes the value of focusing on preventive and proactive care, which is frequently neglected in the last stages of life.

CONCLUSIONS

Many older people will enjoy exceptionally long lives. But is the price for these longer lives a much increased risk that the extra years will be scarred by disease and disability? The global response to population ageing and increased longevity needs to be based on the concept of healthy or successful ageing.

An ageing population inevitably brings with it increasing need for help and support from society – medical, social, emotional and financial. The ultimate aim of public health is to increase the period of later life that is free of poor health, disability and dependency, and to ensure that adequate policies, services and support are in place for healthy ageing of older populations. This will be achieved by promoting healthy lifestyles and preventing disease earlier in life and by action taken in old age itself.

For people who have become frail, the key is to assess individual need on a multidisciplinary, multi-agency basis, and then organize an appropriate response. Improved systems of anticipatory care planning and end-of-life care are important for ensuring choice, control and dignity for frail older people.

CHAPTER 12

Environment and health

INTRODUCTION

The publication of Rachel Carson's seminal book *Silent Spring* in the early 1960s is viewed by many as the moment of awakening for modern concern about the importance of the environment to life on the planet. It dealt primarily with the role of chemicals (in particular DDT) as toxins. Alerted to the death of large numbers of birds after widespread spraying with DDT, Carson began her meticulous scientific documentation of the chemical's effects. She showed how it poisoned plant and animal life, and how readily it entered the human food chain. One of the most powerful chapters, 'A Fable for Tomorrow', describes an imaginary American town where plant, animal and human life fall silent. Carson died of breast cancer in 1964 but left behind one of the truly great books of the twentieth century; it continues to inspire the fight for healthy, life-enhancing and sustainable environments.

Today, 50 years on, the understanding of the relationship between environment and health is much more extensive. Concerns about environmental risks to health are still dominated by polluted water, inadequate sanitation and poor air quality, particularly in low- and middle-income countries. Large-scale, complex environmental shifts, such as climate change and urbanization, also receive a great deal of focus. Distributional injustice and inequity are core phenomena in environmental health – the poorest parts of the world and societies are the worst affected by environmental risks.

According to the World Health Organization, between a fifth and a quarter of the global disease burden is attributable to environmental factors. The proportion is much higher in children and in poorer countries. Figure 12.1 illustrates the contribution of environmental factors to particular diseases.

The environment affects health in many different ways, and at a range of scales. Very local conditions impact on individuals. Broader environmental conditions affect whole societies, or indeed the whole world. Housing quality, for example, affects the health of individuals and families, while climate change is global in its reach. Environmental effects (both positive and negative) are not only felt at their source. For example, air pollution may originate in one region but spread to cause health problems in neighbouring regions; how far and in what direction the pollutants are spread depends on many factors, including the type of pollutant, land characteristics and local weather.

As societies develop economically, the threats to health from the environment change. This is called *environmental risk transition*. Traditional risks include unsafe water, lack of sanitation, indoor air pollution and food contamination. Today, these are still the predominant elements in low-income countries. In the more advanced economies of middle- and high-income countries, modern risks come from increased industrialization and economic development, and include urban air pollution from transport or industry and water pollution from intensive agriculture. If development and urbanization are managed poorly and inequitably, populations can be faced with both traditional and modern risks.

CONCEPT OF ENVIRONMENTAL HEALTH: DEFINITIONS AND FRAMEWORKS

Basic definitions of environmental health describe the physical, chemical and biological environmental factors that affect health. Broader definitions also embrace social and cultural conditions. The World Health Organization's definition is:

> Environmental health addresses all the physical, chemical, and biological factors external to a person, and all the related factors impacting behaviours. It encompasses the assessment and control of those environmental factors that can potentially affect health. It is targeted towards preventing disease and creating health-supportive environments. This definition excludes behaviour not related to environment, as well as behaviour related to the social and cultural environment, and genetics.

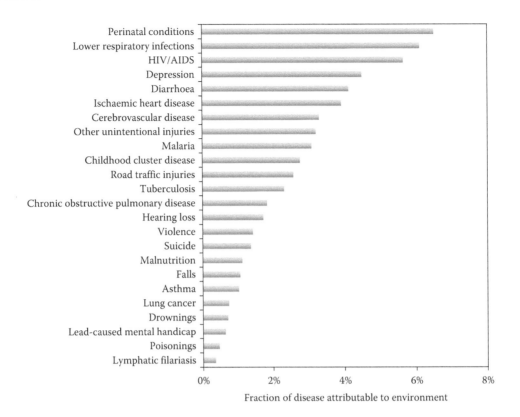

Figure 12.1 Diseases for which there is an important environmental contribution to causation.

Source: World Health Organization (WHO). Preventing Disease through Healthy Environments: Towards an Estimate of the Environmental Burden of Disease. Geneva: WHO, 2006. With permission.

The relationship between environmental factors and health is often highly complex. The World Health Organization's Driving Force–Pressure–State–Exposure–Effect–Action (DPSEEA) framework (Figure 12.2) helpfully elucidates the interactions that are involved. Understanding this helps in the selection of targets to improve health.

Driving forces are upstream factors that affect society. They include population growth, technological change and economic development. Government policies also act as driving forces, in diverse fields including the economy, energy, agriculture and trade. These driving forces can exert *pressures* on the environment – the *P* in the abbreviation. For example, population growth increases demand for power, which worsens air pollution if fossil fuels are used. The extent to which the driving force of population growth results in the pressure of reduced air quality is not fixed, but is amenable to modification. It can be improved, for example, by policies on fuel provision and on the energy efficiency of buildings.

The *S* of DPSEEA refers to *state* – the quality of aspects of the environment. The state of the air, for example, reflects the amount and types of air pollutants. State is directly related to *exposures*. The extent to which these exposures result in health *effects* (the second *E*) depends on the proportion of the population exposed, the level of exposure, the dose–response relationship and the route of exposure (inhaled, absorbed or consumed). The health effects can be acute or chronic, and immediate or delayed.

Lastly, the *A* of the DPSEEA framework stands for *action*. The action taken depends on the level of actual or perceived risk. Whether policies are created to control a hazard depends on cultural, social and economic considerations, as well as their relative importance to governments and populations.

It is not possible to absolutely eliminate environmental health risks, but actions to mitigate them can be applied through any or all aspects of the DPSEEA framework – from modifying the upstream driving forces to introducing policies that limit the health effects of exposure.

SUSTAINABILITY

The concept of sustainability emerged through recognition that development of all kinds must occur in a way that preserves natural resources and does not damage the environment. Sustainable development is progress without compromising the environment, explicitly recognizing the interdependence of people and their environment. In 1992, the United Nations Conference on Environment and Development, also known as the Earth Summit, was held in Rio de Janeiro, Brazil. One hundred heads of government were there, the largest-ever gathering of world leaders. The action plan, Agenda 21, recommended that every country produce a sustainable development strategy. Current international commitment to sustainability is demonstrated

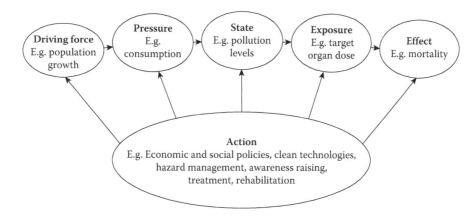

Figure 12.2 The World Health Organization DPSEEA framework.

Source: World Health Organization (WHO). *Preventing Disease through Healthy Environments: Towards an Estimate of the Environmental Burden of Disease.* Geneva: WHO, 2006. With permission.

Table 12.1 Sustainable development

Sustainable development is development that meets the needs of the present without compromising the ability of future generations to meet their own needs

Source: United Nations. *Report of the World Commission on Environment and Development (the Brundtland Commission).* New York: United Nations, 1987.

through the Sustainable Development Goals (which supersede the Millennium Development Goals).

A United Nations commission formally defined sustainability in the 1980s (Table 12.1). The definition embraced a wider idea of securing the health of the planet in the long term, with an underpinning moral requirement for current generations to preserve its natural resources for those not yet born. The three most often described themes of sustainability, the so-called three pillars, are economic development, social development and environmental protection. The Institute for Sustainability at Newcastle University in the United Kingdom has produced a particularly succinct and memorable definition of sustainability: 'Enough, for all, forever'.

The field of sustainability has become a very active area of research that is richly interdisciplinary. In policy terms, large numbers of public and private organizations have debated and produced their own definitions of sustainability, their own strategies and their own programmes of action. The idea of sustainability is applied in very diverse ways even within health policy and practice, and it goes beyond the relationship between the environment and health. For example, the financial sustainability of a country's healthcare system is a complex matter of profound importance. The extent to which people's ways of life promote their health will partly determine the burden of preventable chronic disease, and so this too is relevant to sustainable healthcare. Sometimes, the concept can be used in quite a circumscribed and local way, say, redesigning

patient flows to and from a hospital emergency department to make intolerable demand and workload pressures manageable for the long term.

The most direct application of sustainability thinking to healthcare lies with the carbon footprint of the health system itself. Looking at the health and social care system in England from this perspective yields dramatic statistics. It produces 32 million tonnes of carbon dioxide equivalent in a year. This equates to the whole output of some medium-sized countries. The sources of this carbon consumption fall into three broad groups: procurement and services (72%), building energy (15%) and travel (13%). A large single category within the carbon footprint of the National Health Service (NHS) is pharmaceuticals, accounting for a fifth of the service's carbon consumption. Assessing their impact means looking at them in very broad terms, taking account of manufacture, packaging, distribution, clinical practice and waste. Analysis highlights some striking features; for example, more than 70 million inhalers are disposed of in the NHS each year, over half into landfill sites. Simple recycling schemes can produce a big carbon reduction gain when such large numbers are involved.

Any healthcare system can make a big impact on its carbon footprint if it addresses the challenges comprehensively, including making reductions in carbon in every aspect of the procurement process; reducing unnecessary energy usage, using energy more efficiently and introducing low-carbon forms of energy; reducing waste; promoting greener transport policy; and redesigning plants and facilities.

PLANETARY BOUNDARIES

The big picture in sustainability is, of course, the health of planet Earth itself, although even this broader focus has many ramifications for human health, both directly and indirectly. The science of sustainability has been applied to develop the concept of planetary boundaries. The work of nearly 30 scientists, coordinated by a group in Stockholm,

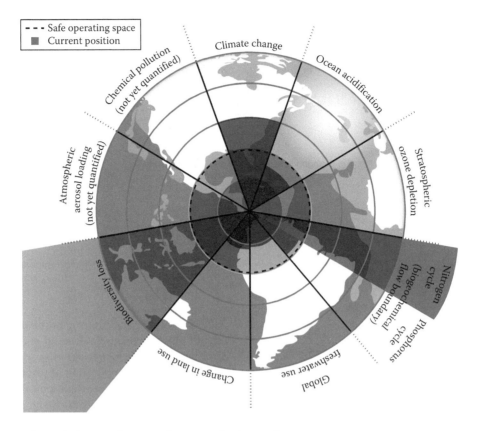

Figure 12.3 Planetary boundaries: a safe operating space for humanity.

Source: Rockström J, Steffen W, Noone K, et al. A safe operating space for humanity. *Nature* 2009;461(7263):472–5.

Sweden, has established nine boundaries within which human activity can take place safely. Alternatively, breaching the boundaries is likely to lead to abrupt and nonlinear changes that might not be reversible. Exceeding one boundary may disturb others since many of the areas are interconnected. A sustainable world would mean everyone being committed to the action necessary, no matter how radical and inconvenient, to introduce the resilience currently missing to create a healthy planet Earth: one whose citizens and their representatives respected, and lived, within its boundaries.

The nine boundaries are climate change, ocean acidification, stratospheric ozone depletion, perturbed nutrient flows, global freshwater use, biological diversity loss, land use change, chemical pollution and atmospheric aerosol loading. Scientists have determined upper limits for the first seven of these but not yet for the last two (Figure 12.3).

CLIMATE CHANGE

The earth's climate has fluctuated substantially in the past. There have been ice ages, and there was a medieval warm period. They were tumultuous periods in the planet's evolution. There is increasing concern about today's climate change and the future challenges it will pose.

The *weather* is the day-to-day variation in wind flows, temperature, humidity and precipitation. Some environmental studies focus on the direct effect of weather-related variables (such as temperature) on health outcomes. *Climate* is the average weather in a region. It is variable over the short term and caused by a number of different natural phenomena. By contrast, *climate change* is the shift in those properties of the climate that lasts for decades or longer.

The broad scientific consensus, based on review of historical scientific data, is that climate change over the twentieth and twenty-first centuries, including global warming, is highly likely to have been caused by human activities. Burning of fossil fuels (coal, oil and others) has been the main contributor, increasing carbon dioxide concentration in the atmosphere and the oceans. Carbon dioxide is the main greenhouse gas, stopping the flow of heat from the planet and causing it to warm. It is of greatest concern because, once produced, it can take many decades to dissipate. There are other greenhouse gases (e.g. methane, nitrous oxide, fluorinated gases and water vapour) arising from industry, agriculture, transport and domestic consumption. Such gases also absorb and hold infrared radiation. The importance of particular gases is determined by how much they are present in the environment, how long they stay around and how much heat they absorb and thus trap in the atmosphere. This varies greatly; for example, the substance sulphuryl fluoride was characterized as recently as 2009. It is used as an insecticide and makes up a very small proportion of the total greenhouse gases. Yet, it has a life of 40 years and is more than 4000 times as efficient as carbon dioxide in trapping heat. Increasingly, all greenhouse gases are being expressed as carbon dioxide equivalents, so that a single number (made up of the amount of carbon dioxide plus other gases) can be used to monitor trends and assess the impact of interventions. Forests and other vegetation are important because they absorb carbon dioxide. Deforestation for commercial purposes, greater land use, fires and other activities that reduce the green area of the planet contribute to the vicious cycle of excess carbon dioxide production.

Another key dimension of the impact of humankind on the natural environment is the health of the *ozone layer*. This occurs naturally and forms a protective boundary around the planet about 10–35 km above the Earth. It absorbs radiation from the sun and helps to prevent too much solar radiation getting through. It particularly stops excess ultraviolet B radiation from reaching the planet's surface. When excessive amounts of ultraviolet B radiation reach the ground, they affect human health, increasing the incidence of diseases such as skin cancer and cataracts, as well as damaging the immune system. This form of radiation also harms plant life and disrupts aquatic ecosystems, including damage to algae.

The ozone layer constantly passes through natural cycles. At some periods, it thins only then to replenish itself. In the last 30 years, much scientific attention has focused on so-called ozone-depleting substances that destroy the ozone layer to the extent that natural processes cannot heal it. Chief among these are chlorofluorocarbons (CFCs), but there are many others. They had become firmly established in products that were highly successful adjuncts to modern living, such as refrigerator coolants, aerosols and some other solvents. Ultraviolet light interacts with these products and chlorine atoms are released. There is then no natural process to break them down as they drive up into the stratosphere. One chlorine atom destroys 100,000 molecules of ozone. Most concern has been concentrated on the Antarctic, where a so-called 'hole' in the ozone layer developed. The low temperatures in this region speed up the conversion of chlorofluorocarbons to chlorine atoms. The hole is not a true gap in the ozone layer, but rather a substantial reduction in its thickness. International agreements, such as the Montreal Protocol, have sought to phase out chlorofluorocarbon-based products. This has been a successful demonstration of collaborative international action – so much so that scientists monitoring the ozone layer report some recovery of the previous damage, but estimate a further 50 years for it to be made good, provided that there is no reversal.

The Intergovernmental Panel on Climate Change (IPCC) has released a series of assessment reports, the most recent in 2014. The Panel's view is clear – atmospheric and oceanic warming has occurred since 1950 at rates unprecedented in the historical record, and it is extremely likely that human activity has been the main cause of this. The panel estimated that the climate has warmed by about 0.8°C over the last 100 years, and that the last 30 years have been the warmest period for 1400 years. By the end of this century, the panel estimates that global surface temperatures are likely to warm by at least a further 0.7°C. Some of the scenarios considered feasible by the panel project increases of up to 4°C. Extremes of hot and cold temperatures are also expected to occur more frequently in most regions of the world.

Climate change remains a controversial subject – a minority of scientists, commentators and political figures are highly sceptical. Professor David MacKay, Regius Professor of Engineering at the University of Cambridge in England, addressed the sceptics of man-made climate change. He said, 'Some sceptics have asserted that the recent increase in CO_2 concentration is a natural phenomenon. Don't you think that something may have happened between 1800 AD and 2000 AD? Something that was not part of the natural processes present in the preceding thousand years?' MacKay's point is related to the sharp increase in atmospheric carbon dioxide that occurred in the late eighteenth century (Figure 12.4). His proposition is that this was started by James Watts's patenting of the steam engine in 1769 – this was a key driver of the Industrial Revolution.

Temperature-related changes are not the only effect that climate change is predicted to have. Land, water and atmosphere systems are highly connected. Changes in precipitation will lead to more floods and greater risk of drought, as well as changes in arctic ice and sea levels.

The main predictions of the Intergovernmental Panel on Climate Change are that:

- Changes in the water cycle will not be uniform, but the contrast in rainfall between wet and dry seasons will generally increase.
- The global ocean will continue to warm. Increased temperatures from the surface water will affect the deep ocean levels, altering ocean circulation.
- Arctic sea ice is very likely to continue to melt, and glacier volume will decrease globally.
- Mean sea level will continue to rise globally – very likely at a faster rate than has been observed over the last 40 years – due to the increased ocean temperatures and glacial melt.
- Carbon cycle processes will be altered by climate change, leading to a further increase in atmospheric carbon dioxide concentration.

The Intergovernmental Panel on Climate Change issued its first assessment report in 1990. The most recent, in 2014, was its fifth. With each report, growing evidence has increased the panel's degree of certainty in its conclusions. With each, its view about the action required has become increasingly urgent. The current report makes clear that human activity has affected carbon dioxide concentrations so substantially that climate change will continue even if carbon dioxide emissions were now cut. It urges action now, highlighting that delay will only make it more difficult and expensive.

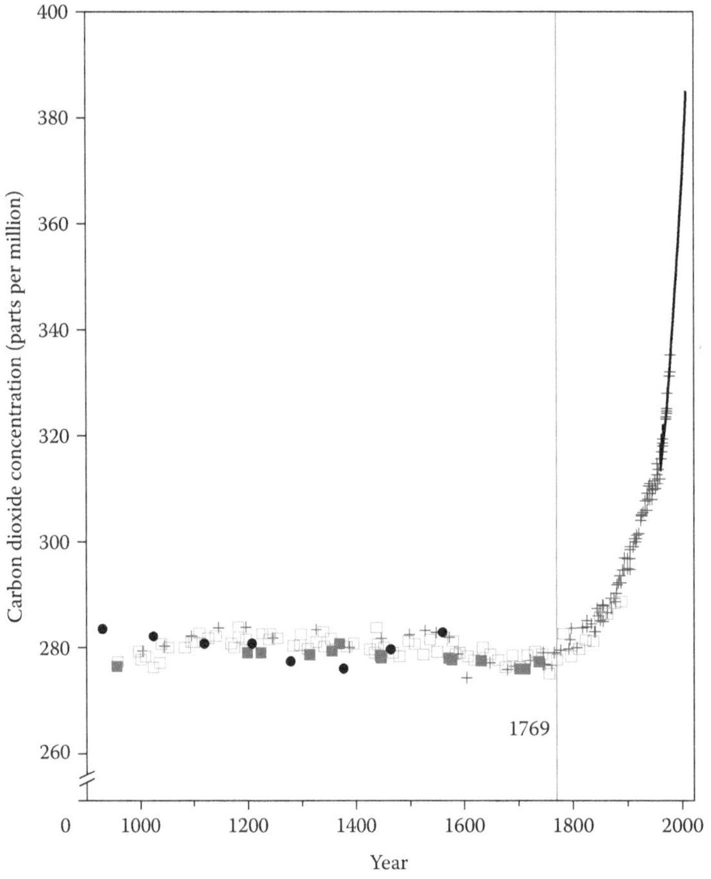

Figure 12.4 Atmospheric carbon dioxide concentration over the last thousand years.

Source: MacKay DJC. *Sustainable Energy without the Hot Air.* Cambridge: UIT, 2008.

Climate change will affect which crops can grow where – through direct temperature effects, water shortages and droughts; it influences the distribution of pests and plant diseases that decrease crop yield. The anticipated hazards of climate change vary between world regions. The specific risks and their potential impacts depend on the underlying vulnerability and adaptive capacity of communities. Areas that lack the infrastructure and socio-economic capacity to effectively adapt will be most affected. In short, the poorest communities are those at most risk.

The health impacts of the changing climate can be modelled by applying the known associations between climatic factors and health outcomes to future climate and socio-economic scenarios. As with most modelling, there is considerable uncertainty. Typically, a number of scenarios, which take into account different trajectories, are used to give alternative projections. The uncertainties do not mean that the information from scenario-based modelling is not useful, but just that the uncertainties and assumptions need to be understood by those using the information.

Epidemiological studies can contribute to understanding the risks of climate change. They can, for example, study the impact of past extreme events or climatic factors (e.g. heat waves) on health outcomes, and help understand the current associations between climatic factors and health. They can also examine interventions that might reduce risk or vulnerability.

The effects that climate change might have on health are direct or indirect. Direct threats include those posed by heat waves and weather-related disasters. Indirect threats include a wide range of influences interacting in a complex way (Figure 12.5).

There are clear examples of weather affecting health in the United Kingdom. Prominent examples include the 2003 heat wave, which is thought to have caused at least 2000 excess deaths in England and Wales. Every year, both hot and cold air temperatures result in some increased risk of hot- or cold-related mortality. The floods of 2007 and 2014 demonstrated that a number of regions and homes are vulnerable to natural extreme weather events.

The Climate Change Act 2008 gives a legally binding framework to cut the United Kingdom's greenhouse gas emissions and a framework for the country to adapt to changing climate. A five-yearly assessment of risks and opportunities is required, the most recent carried out in 2017. Risk will occur because of increased high temperatures and heat waves, changes in air pollution, aeroallergens, vector-borne diseases, ultraviolet radiation and

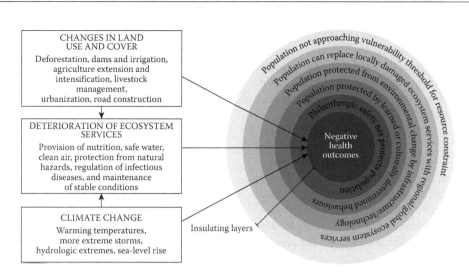

Figure 12.5 Altered environment, climate change and human health.

Source: Myers SS, Bernstein A. The coming health crisis: Indirect health effects of global climate change. *F1000 Biology Reports* 2011;3(1):3. With permission.

Table 12.2 Actions with co-benefits for public health and climate change

Action	Positive effect on climate change	Positive benefit for health
Less motorised transport use, more 'active transport' (walking, cycling)	Reduction in greenhouse gas emissions from vehicle production and fuel use	More people achieving recommended exercise levels. Less obesity, heart disease and stroke. Greater mental well-being
Less use of fossil fuels for energy generation	Alternative energy source generating fewer greenhouse gas emissions	Alternative energy sources generating less air pollution, reducing illnesses and deaths from heart and lung disease
Fewer animal products in the diet	Reduction in the substantial greenhouse gas emissions produced by livestock farming	Less saturated fat in the diet. Less obesity, heart disease and diabetes
Improvements to household ventilation and insulation	Enhanced energy efficiency	Insulation reduces cold-related illness and death. Ventilation provided cleaner air, cutting respiratory disease including lung cancer

Source: Department of Health (DH). 2009 *Annual Report of the Chief Medical Officer.* London: DH, 2010.

the indoor environment. International agreements on greenhouse gas reduction targets have proved difficult to negotiate and implement. The most recent Paris Agreement in 2015 was signed up to by 195 countries.

Broadly, there are two approaches to reduce climate change risk – *mitigation* and *adaptation*. Mitigation involves reducing the amount of greenhouse gases released in the atmosphere – by decreasing production or by sequestration. Production can be decreased by reduced consumption of fossil fuels for power, relying more on sustainable or renewable energy sources, strengthening building insulation and improving the efficiency of power production and power appliances. Action must also include prevention of deforestation. Adaptation involves reducing the harmful impacts of climate change, and maximizing any benefits of a change in climate. Actions

include planning for extreme weather events, improving public services' ability to anticipate them and looking for all opportunities to minimize their impact.

Some mitigation and adaptive strategies have cobenefits for public health (Table 12.2). For example, encouraging cycling both decreases fuel use and increases physical activity. There are also negative consequences of adaptive and mitigation strategies. For example, although air conditioning is an adaption to increased temperatures, and can prevent heat-related deaths among older people, air conditioning units increase power consumption. Unless that power is derived from sustainable sources, it exacerbates emissions. Also, the poorest in society may not be able to afford air conditioning, and so relying on this as an adaptation strategy may exacerbate health inequalities.

Climate change has profound ethical and political dimensions. High-income countries have released most of the emissions that have contributed to climate change so far, yet their negative effects will fall most heavily on low-income countries. Those living today are leaving a large environmental, economic and health legacy for future generations.

WATER

Water is a fundamental requirement for life, sanitation and hygiene. It is vital for the food supply chain, from agriculture and fisheries to food transport and preparation. Lack of access to safe water and sanitation is a leading cause of illness, disease and premature death. The absence of this most basic of human needs is responsible for millions of cases of diarrhoeal disease around the world and is particularly associated with high death rates among the under-fives. There are many individual infectious diseases and chemical pollutants producing harm through unclean water. Improving access to water and basic sanitation was one of the Millennium Development Goals. The goal was to decrease by half the number of people without sustainable access to safe water. Access is defined as the source being less than a kilometre from where it is used, and an adequate amount is 20 L per person per day. The World Health Organization sets guidelines for what constitutes safe water; this has microbial, chemical and physical aspects. Access may be through a direct household connection, or from a borehole, well, public standpipe or rainwater collector.

It is far better for people to have ready access to water, instead of having to walk long distances to collect it. Beyond the direct health benefits, ready access frees people's time and energy for other activities, such as education or work. It may also improve personal safety, by reducing the need for potentially dangerous journeys.

According to the United Nations, the water access Millennium Development Goal was met by 2010. Profound geographical and socio-economic inequalities remain, though – particularly between rural and urban areas, but also between formal and informal urban settlements. To measure progress, community surveys ask about improved sources of water, but this does not necessarily mean clean or risk-free. Even if it is clean at the source, water can be contaminated through transport or during storage. Globally, 750 million people still use unimproved water sources, 178 million use surface water and a full 1.8 billion drink water from a source that is faecally contaminated. The availability of water differs greatly between countries. Per capita water use varies with availability, level of development and affluence.

By 2025, it is estimated that half the global population will live in water-stressed areas. The pressures come from population growth, increasing urbanization and intensification of agriculture. As in most adverse aspects of global health, the absence of safe, clean water is most strongly linked to poverty. Finding solutions (again in common with other global health areas) not only is about resources and infrastructure but also involves the complex mix of political, social, economic and cultural factors that determine how policy decisions are taken and how progress and development occur. Climate change is also an important part of the water health dynamic. Its precise points of impact are difficult to predict, because its effects on precipitation and the hydrological cycle are complex, but it will cause severe water shortages in some regions of the world. There are well-documented areas of water conflict, where disputes arise over water as a resource for both domestic use and irrigation.

Although the greatest burden of disease from inadequate water and hygiene falls in low-income countries, outbreaks still occur in high-income countries because of water quality deficiency. In recent years, water sources in the United Kingdom have been implicated in outbreaks of *Cryptosporidium, Campylobacter, Giardia, Escherichia coli* O157 and *Astrovirus*. In the United Kingdom, surface water is the main source of public supply. As water flows over the ground (in rivers and lakes), it dissolves minerals and can carry suspended matter, bacteria, viruses, protozoa, algae and various other plant and animal products. About 35% of drinking water comes from upland surface water in natural lakes and man-made reservoirs. This is relatively free from contamination by human and animal waste. Lowland rivers, which supply about 30% of drinking water, become more polluted as they flow from their source to the sea. Some parts of the United Kingdom have to draw on sources from the lower reaches of rivers, which may necessitate full purification treatment.

Underground water from deep wells and boreholes needs only minimal treatment, being of good quality and almost always free from contamination. This source contributes about one-third of the public water supply. Purification treatment aims to remove pathogenic bacteria, harmful chemicals, suspended matter and any substance causing colour, odour or undesirable taste. Water purification methods include coagulation filtration, disinfection with chlorine and the use of ozone and activated charcoal. In general, underground water needs less treatment than river water.

In the United Kingdom, the Drinking Water Inspectorate (the Drinking Water Quality Regulator in Scotland) is responsible for monitoring drinking water standards. The quality of drinking water has improved markedly since its establishment in 1990. A chief inspector for the Drinking Water Inspectorate produces an annual report for the government, which is made public.

In England, the average person uses 150 L of water a day – a figure that has been growing by 1% a year since 1930. This only refers to the water that is used directly – in drinking, bathing, cooking and toilet flushing. The water used to manufacture all the food and other products consumed by a typical person on an average day is vast – an additional 3200 L. Appropriately managing all this wastewater is vitally important to health. The key concern is to prevent wastewater from contaminating the reservoirs and pipes through which drinking water is delivered.

Wastewater is thought of in three main categories, each of which is potentially hazardous to health. These are domestic sewage, industrial wastewater and agricultural wastewater. Domestic sewage contains a large number of intestinal organisms. Industrial and agricultural wastewater may contain toxic chemicals, and sometimes run into public sewers or directly into rivers.

Typically, sewage treatment has three main stages. Primary treatment involves separating solid from liquid waste. A system of mechanical grills and settlement channels removes large materials, such as rags, sanitary products, stones and grit. Smaller solids then settle out in sedimentation tanks, as solid sewage sludge. This sludge is a major by-product of the sewage treatment process. In the United Kingdom, most is disposed of on farmland (until the late 1990s, it was often dumped at sea). With the solids separated out, the liquid then proceeds to secondary treatment. In this stage, aerobic action turns dissolved organic material into solids, which are then removed. The remaining liquid goes on to tertiary treatment, which is disinfection. A variety of chemical or biological approaches can be used, readying the water for discharge into the sea or watercourse. Sewage treatment is now highly developed in the United Kingdom and other high-income countries. However, there are still places in which full treatment does not take place. There are also many where in conditions such as heavy rain, sewage can bypass the treatment system entirely and pollute waterways.

There is increasing public and research interest in *micropollutants*. The term is applied to both inorganic and organic substances present in low concentrations in natural water, drinking water and wastewater. Inorganic micropollutants are mainly metals. Some are naturally occurring and important for maintaining normal body functions. Others result from industrial processes and can be harmful to human health and aquatic life (e.g. lead, cadmium and mercury). Organic micropollutants include pesticides (herbicides, fungicides, insecticides, rodenticides, soil sterilants, wood preservatives and surface biocides), hormones and medication residues. People are exposed to pesticides not only in water but also through air and food. The health effects of acute exposure to a high dose of pesticides are well documented. Illness usually follows either accidental or deliberate ingestion, or skin contamination following careless handling. Symptoms develop quickly, and in most cases, there is complete recovery without long-term complications. UK and European legislation precisely defines specific pesticide substances. Risk assessment requires the establishment of *acceptable daily intakes* and *maximum residue levels* for particular pesticides. Maximum residue levels are not 'safe' levels but are simply the upper limit of the concentrations of pesticide that would be found if they were used according to their authorization. It also sets out the controls that govern their sale, storage and

use – to protect people, animals and plants; to protect the environment; and to make information available to the public. Pesticide manufacturers must go through a formal process of approval, as must importers and distributors. Farmers and growers are not required to tell members of the public what pesticides they are using. Industry is, however, required to take all reasonable precautions to protect human and environmental well-being. There is considerable scepticism on the part of some sections of the media and environmentalists about the concept of safe levels. This has been exacerbated by the growing capability of modern methods of biochemical assay to detect smaller concentrations of pollutants.

A two-tier system of regulation of pesticides operates. At the European level, products are assessed and, if accepted, are placed on an official approved list of active substances. They are then assessed and approved by the regulatory bodies of individual European Union member states. The UK Expert Committee on Pesticides provides independent scientific advice to the government officials and ministers on matters relating to the effective control of pests, including advice on the approval and authorization of pesticides. The Department for Environment, Food and Rural Affairs (DEFRA) Expert Committee on Pesticide Residues in Food advises the government on this aspect of pesticides. The levels in both home-produced and imported food are monitored. Policy on pesticide use is one of the most controversial areas in the environment and health field. There is heavy media coverage of studies showing apparent risks to human health, while any suggestion that government is suppressing or interfering with independent scientific advice is guaranteed to be widely publicized. The latter is illustrated by a report in the *Guardian* newspaper in 2015: 'UK government gags advisers in bees and pesticides row: Expert Committee on Pesticides told to postpone publication of minutes after refusing to back farmers' request to use banned neonicotinoids on oil seed rape'.

AIR QUALITY

The World Health Organization estimates that 7 million deaths annually are caused by indoor and outdoor air pollution. More than half are attributed to coronary heart disease and stroke, and most of the remainder to respiratory disease. In public health in the past, most attention in the field of air quality has been given to outdoor pollution – such as that which caused the great smog of London in 1952, killing thousands of people (Figure 12.6). Today, there is equal concern about the impact on health of poor air quality in dwellings and other buildings. In low-income countries, indoor air pollution is a major contributor to the burden of disease (Figure 12.7). Indoor air pollution comes from biomass fuels used for cooking, emissions from curing food and other sources, including tobacco smoke, household products and pesticides. Of these, the most important is biomass, which more than half of the world's people still use for cooking. Particularly when combined

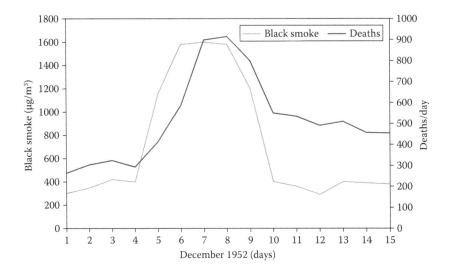

Figure 12.6 The Great London smog, 1952.

Source: Wilkins ET. Air pollution and the London fog of December 1952. *Journal of the Royal Sanitary Institute* 1954;74(1):1–21.

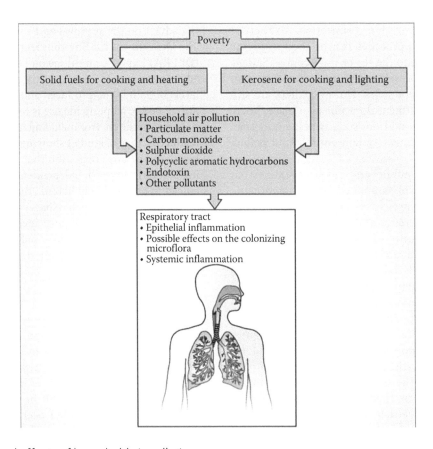

Figure 12.7 Causes and effects of household air pollution.

Source: Gordon SB, Bruce NG, Grigg J, et al. Respiratory risks from household air pollution in low and middle income countries. *Lancet Respiratory Medicine* 2014;2(10):823–60.

with inadequate ventilation, this fuel produces a large variety of pollutants, including sulphur dioxide, nitrogen dioxide, particulate matter and heavy metals. The risk is particularly high for women and children. Indoor air pollution has been linked to acute respiratory infections, lung cancer, chronic obstructive airway disease, low birthweight and ischaemic heart disease.

Three groups of interventions are effective. First, alternative cleaner fuels and better stoves reduce the production of the pollutants. The main alternative fuels are electricity, solar power and liquid petroleum. Stoves are safer if they have better combustion and faster cooking times. Second, improving ventilation of the living environment reduces exposure. Third, some interventions aim to change behaviour when using stoves (such as drying wood before use, and keeping young children outside the polluted environment).

Historically, poor outdoor air quality has been caused by local industrial output. The local concentration of a given air pollutant depends on the emission source, local geography, weather (e.g. wind direction and precipitation) and properties of the pollutant itself. This highlights the epidemiological challenge of studying air pollution – concentrations vary in time and space, so it is very difficult to accurately measure and assign exposure. Techniques such as time-series regression and case-crossover studies can help examine short-term associations between levels of air pollution and health outcomes.

Air pollutants are any dusts, gases, fumes or odours that are harmful to human health or that cause discomfort. They can be primary (directly emitted from a source) or secondary (formed in the atmosphere by physical or chemical reactions between precursors). Not all pollutants come from human activity (*anthropogenic pollutants*). Some, such as volcanic gases and dust from deserts, are natural (*biogenic pollutants*). Air pollutants can also be classified by their physical form – gases or particles – and, finally, by how they are regulated legally.

There are many different air pollutants, including ozone, carbon monoxide, lead, arsenic and sulphur dioxide. The two most important are particulate matter and the oxides of nitrogen. Particulate matter (Figure 12.8) comprises a range of different substances that have the common feature of circulating as tiny particles. Particulate matter smaller than 10 μm (PM_{10}) is readily drawn into the lungs. The smallest of the particles (those less than 2.5 μm, known as $PM_{2.5}$) are drawn deeper into the lungs and can enter the bloodstream. They therefore cause the greatest damage. Road transport, industrial emissions, and (in some parts of the world) sand- or dust storms are the major sources of particulate matter.

The oxides of nitrogen are nitrogen monoxide and nitrogen dioxide. They are described together because their sources and effects are similar. They principally arise from road transport (particularly from diesel), industry and gas use (both domestic and industrial). Nitrogen dioxide is the greater concern. Particulate matter and nitrogen dioxide can combine in the atmosphere to produce ozone, a powerful pollutant and greenhouse gas.

The sources and health effects of ambient air pollutants are wide ranging. The effects can be from acute or chronic exposure. The acute effects of particulate matter include respiratory illness and increased risk of myocardial infarction. Some pollutants increase the long-term risk of cancer. Exposure to pollution is often associated with socio-economic status (e.g. living in a poorer neighbourhood and occupation type).

Air pollution, depending on its particulate and chemical composition, produces a wide range of health effects, both short-term and long-term. The impact on the respiratory system is the most obvious, with increased risk of asthma, chronic lung disease and cancer. In areas with persistently high levels of air pollution, heart attacks are more common and mortality rates from cardiovascular disease and stroke are higher. The International Agency for Cancer Research, based in Lyon, France, considers outdoor air pollution to be the most widespread environmental cause of cancer. These effects can be assessed through epidemiological, toxicological, animal and controlled human exposure studies. Although the magnitude of risk for a given health outcome

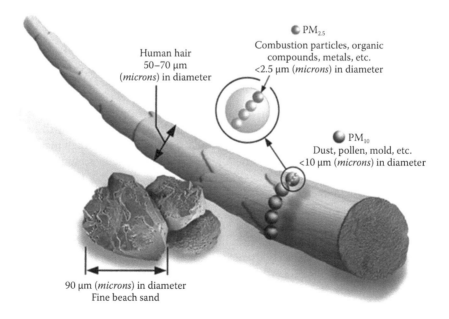

Figure 12.8 Particulate matter.

Source: U.S. Environmental Protection Agency.

may be small, because of the large number of people exposed, the burden of disease from ambient pollution is large.

In the United Kingdom, the policy backdrop for managing and improving air quality comes from a European Union directive and the Committee on the Medical Effects of Air Pollutants has been set up to advise on the health effects of air pollutants. In England, local authorities are responsible for monitoring air pollution and taking action to achieve reductions. In other parts of the United Kingdom, this responsibility has been passed to the devolved assemblies and parliaments. Action and monitoring is led and coordinated by the UK central government department, the Department for Environment, Food and Rural Affairs. Monitoring is based on a range of automated or staffed monitoring stations around the country. The *Daily Air Quality Index* (on a scale of 1–10) is produced, and interactive maps are publicly available showing pollution levels in different parts of the country. London is the worst place in the country for air pollution. A monitoring station on Marylebone Road records a higher concentration of nitrogen dioxide than all but three such stations across Europe.

The documented negative effects of air pollution on health, along with the large number of people exposed, have led to a variety of approaches to improving air quality. These range from interventions to limit the pollution released, such as the use of scrubbers at coal-fired power stations and the prohibition of lead additives to petrol, to regulations or recommendations about the maximum amount of air pollutants allowed. Because the same air pollutants come from many different industries and from transport, multisectoral working and policymaking is essential. Multinational action may be required when pollution is widely dispersed. With increasing industrialization, large-scale production and the proliferation of transport, the effects of pollution from one location can now be felt far from the source.

HOUSING

Living accommodations should provide shelter, security, privacy and comfort. In reality, the standard and permanency of housing varies widely within and between towns, cities and countries. Poor-quality housing can negatively affect occupants' health to a very significant degree, while a safe and clean environment helps to maintain health. In the United Kingdom, the health effects of poor housing cost the NHS around £600 million per year.

Poor housing puts occupants at an increased risk of injury. Nearly half of all accidents occur in the home. Factors such as poor lighting, worn carpets, steep staircases and a lack of appropriate stair rails substantially increase the risk of falls, particularly among older people and young children.

Cold housing is a major contributor to the excess deaths that occur every winter, by increasing the risk of respiratory and cardiovascular disease. Respiratory problems are twice as common among children living in cold homes than those in warm homes. Cold housing also increases the level of minor illness, such as colds. In the United

Kingdom, political attention in recent years has focused on fuel poverty, and ensuring that older people can afford to adequately heat their homes. Given the financial and environmental cost of fuel use, improving homes' insulation is also important, and this too has been the subject of government initiatives. The government's *Standard Assessment Procedure* assesses the energy performance of buildings. It quantifies a dwelling's energy use per unit floor area and provides an energy efficiency rating and an environmental impact rating. All homes sold in the United Kingdom must be tested in this way, and the results reported to potential buyers. New-build homes are subject to increasingly stringent fuel efficiency requirements.

There is an important association between damp dwellings and respiratory symptoms, particularly in children. Damp causes condensation, which can lead to fungal spores. There is a dose–response relationship between the level of damp in a home and the severity of asthma.

Overcrowding increases the risk of stress and sleep deprivation. For children, an overcrowded home is not conducive to study and can impair educational achievement. In England, a home is said to be overcrowded if it does not meet the official bedroom standard of having a separate bedroom for each married or cohabiting couple, each single person aged 21 years or over, each pair of adolescents aged 10–20 years of the same sex and each pair of children under 10 years whatever their sex.

Poor housing can also adversely affect mental health in other ways. Particularly for disabled and frail people, accessibility is important. A home with treacherous steps leading to the front door, or on a high floor without a lift, risks such people staying at home and becoming socially isolated. Poor housing can also fail to insulate its inhabitants from noise in the surrounding area, which has harmful health effects that are discussed later.

The Housing Act 2004 introduced a Housing Health and Safety Rating System (Table 12.3). This is a tool used during house inspections to assess the risks posed by a home. It covers 29 physiological, psychological, accident and infection hazards. As this list makes clear, a vast range of housing factors can and do affect health in a very major way.

Housing inspectors use the tool to rate a home's hazards for the likelihood that they will cause harm, and the potential severity of harm. They make this assessment based on the most vulnerable person who might live in, or visit, the home. The purpose of the assessment is to highlight areas for potential improvement in all homes, not solely to ensure compliance with a particular level. However, the statutory minimum requirement is that a home should not exceed a score of 1000. Homes that do are categorized as having Category 1 hazards, and the local authority has a duty to act.

There are 26.7 million households in the United Kingdom. Two-thirds of these are owner occupied. One-third are rented – half through the private sector and half through the social housing sector. In England, the Department for Communities and Local Government runs the English Housing Survey on a continuous basis. The survey records a

Table 12.3 Housing hazards

Physiological hazards	Accident hazards
Damp or mould	Falls associated with bathrooms
Excessive cold	Falls on the level
Excessive heat	Falls associated with stairs and steps
Asbestos	Falls between levels
Carbon monoxide and fuel combustion products	Poor electrical wiring
Lead	Fire risks
Radiation (e.g. radon)	Hot surfaces and materials
Uncombusted fuel gas	Collision and entrapment risks
Volatile organic compounds	Explosion risk
	Poor position and operability of amenities
	Risk of structural collapse and falling elements
Psychological hazards	**Infection hazards**
Overcrowding	Poor domestic hygiene and/or pests
Entry by intruders	Poor sanitation and drainage
Poor lighting	Poor water supply for domestic purposes
Excess noise	Poor facilities for food safety

Source: The Parliamentary Office of Science and Technology. *Housing Health and Regulation System.* London: The Parliamentary Office of Science and Technology, 2011. Box 3, p. 3. Contains Parliamentary information licensed under the Open Parliament Licence v3.0. With permission.

number of measures, including whether houses are *decent*. A decent home is defined as one that meets the statutory requirements set out by the Housing Health and Safety Rating System, is in a reasonable state of repair, has reasonably modern facilities and services and provides a reasonable degree of thermal comfort. Each of these criteria is precisely defined.

The English Housing Survey in 2015 showed that almost 5 million homes – 19% of all homes in England – were rated as *nondecent*. Although a high number, this represents a significant reduction over recent years – in 2006, 35% of homes were nondecent. The proportion of nondecent homes is highest in the private rented sector (28%), and lower but still significant in owner-occupied homes (18%) and the social rented sector (13%). The English Housing Survey also found that 678,000 homes – 3% of the total – are overcrowded.

Environmental hazards and pollutants close to housing can also have an adverse effect. Heavy traffic, waste disposal sites, factories and sewage works tend to be near cheaper housing. Those who cannot afford housing elsewhere are more likely to live in areas prone to natural hazards, such as floods or landslides that may threaten the permanency of their dwellings.

NOISE AND LIGHT POLLUTION

Noise is unwanted sound that causes discomfort to the listener. It is an important public health problem. Sound is a product of vibrant modern life – of travel, entertainment, work, socializing, construction and industry. As more and more people live in cities and population density increases worldwide, noise is a growing concern.

Noise is linked to acute and chronic hearing loss, poor school performance, hypertension, ischaemic heart disease, stress, annoyance, and a range of general physiological and psychological measures. The World Health Organization's European Regional Office has calculated that noise pollution is the second greatest environmental public health problem after air pollution. It estimates that 1 million healthy years of life are lost every year in western Europe as a result.

Noise is measured by its level, frequency, loudness and time. Workers have a high risk of noise-induced deafness in environments with noise levels equivalent to a continuous sound of 90 decibels or more. In the United Kingdom, employers are required under the Control of Noise at Work Regulations to act when average noise exposure exceeds 80 decibels, and to take more stringent action if it reaches 85 decibels.

Noise at night has a range of adverse effects on health and well-being, many of which occur because of sleep disturbance. Noise can disturb sleep even if people do not recall being awoken. A number of the effects of sleep disturbance are metabolic. Sleep loss has been found to increase the blood concentration of C-reactive protein, an inflammatory marker associated with cardiovascular disease risk. It also reduces leptin concentration, increasing the risk of weight gain and impaired glucose tolerance. Night-time noise comes particularly from roads, noisy neighbours and aircraft. Road noise can be mitigated by interventions such as speed restrictions, installation of noise barriers and low-noise road surfacing.

The European Environmental Noise Directive of 2002 required countries to create noise maps that show people's exposure to environmental noise. These were most recently updated in 2014. They are used to identify noise hot spots, and action plans are put in place to deal with them. England's Public Health Outcomes Framework includes a measure of the percentage of the population affected by noise.

In the United Kingdom, local authorities have a range of regulatory powers in relation to noise, based particularly on the *Environmental Protection Act 1990*. If they identify a source of noise that is a nuisance or harmful to health, they must serve an abatement notice on the person responsible. If the person does not comply with this notice, he or she can be prosecuted. Local authorities are responsible for licencing entertainment premises, and noise is an important consideration in this.

Light pollution is a more recently established field of environmental pollution. It is defined in various ways but essentially addresses sources of direct illumination and so-called sky glow (the more diffuse light within the environment). The problem is not restricted to larger towns and cities but is most prominent there. Hong Kong is frequently cited as the worst offender, although people who live there probably do not see it so negatively.

Concerns about the adverse impact of light pollution are varied. Many campaign against it for aesthetic reasons, pointing to the beauty and wonder of a dark, starry sky. Closely linked to this is the importance of purely natural light to the scientific field of astronomy. There is limited evidence of health effects. Light exposure at night does disrupt normal physiological processes, including circadian rhythm. At its simplest, this can affect sleep duration and patterns leading to fatigue and stress. Light pollution also disrupts ecosystems and, through that, indirectly threatens human health. In the United Kingdom, an act of Parliament, the *Clean Neighbourhood and Environment Act 2005*, defines light pollution under certain conditions as a statutory nuisance.

CONSUMPTION AND WASTE

The scale of human consumption is vast and ever growing. The average household now has more than 2000 items within it. People expect to constantly update their wardrobes and their electronic goods. Per head of population, the amount of food, services and industrial production grows year-on-year. Every year in the United Kingdom, 330 million tonnes of waste requires disposal. Consumption is part of modern society, and is a crucial part of the sustainability story told earlier in this chapter. The health dimensions of consumption are not all to do with climate change; some relate to production and waste handling directly.

The strategies for dealing with waste are: reducing the types of consumption that lead to waste production, reusing and recycling materials, recovering energy from waste and, finally, disposal. The public health effects of waste management depend on the type of waste and method of disposal, and can often be difficult to assess.

Waste can be classified according to where it is produced (household, institutional, industrial or commercial) or by its state (gaseous, liquid or solid). Separately, some waste is also classified as hazardous, in which case specific regulations govern its disposal.

Only a quarter of waste is from households and businesses. The bulk comes from sewage works, the construction industry, agriculture and the extractive industries. The most common means of disposal is landfills, although their use is in decline – partly due to shortage of capacity. Landfill sites produce methane, a greenhouse gas, and can adversely affect the health of local populations. The effects depend on local geography and on characteristics of the disposed waste, such as how easily it leeches into soil or is emitted into the air. Investigating the relationship between a landfill site (a spatially determined hazard) and health outcomes is very complex.

One alternative to landfills is incineration. Approximately 10% of UK waste is incinerated. This proportion is lower than most of Europe, but has grown in recent years. The main health concern is that incineration produces air pollutants. A better alternative, likely to be increasingly used, is combined heat and power plants, in which electricity is generated from the heat of burning waste.

There is a stringent regulatory framework regarding waste disposal. This has been strengthened in recent years, in response to public concern about both health and environmental pollution. The United Kingdom's approach to waste management is governed by the European Union Waste Framework Directive, which covers collection, transport, recovery and disposal of waste. Additionally, the European Directive on Integrated Pollution Prevention and Control requires operators of new facilities (such as incinerators) to apply for a permit. The directive takes a *best available techniques* approach to environmental protection, and mandates efficient use of energy. To achieve the goals of the directive, the Environmental Permitting (England and Wales) Regulations came into force in 2008. These introduced a simplified system of environmental permits for waste disposal companies.

The amount of household waste in the United Kingdom is actually decreasing – slowly – year-on-year, particularly as a result of increasing public interest and measures to reduce packaging. The proportion of household waste that is recycled is increasing. It currently stands at around 45%. The target set by the European Union is to achieve 50% by 2020.

Low- and middle-income countries tend to have substantially less developed waste reduction and management systems. Those that are undergoing rapid economic development particularly struggle with the increases in consumption and waste that they experience as a result.

RADIATION

Radiation is the emission of energy as electromagnetic waves or moving subatomic particles. Across the electromagnetic spectrum are a range of radiation forms, measured

Table 12.4 Five sources of radiation exposure: millisieverts (mSv)

Eating 100 g of Brazil nuts	0.01 mSv
Chest x-ray	0.014 mSv
Annual average radon dose to people in Cornwall	7.8 mSv
Air-crew annual polar route	9.8 mSv
Full-body CT scan	10.0 mSv

by wavelength and frequency. Radiation occurs naturally, but can also be man-made (Table 12.4). Some natural elements, such as radium and uranium, have no stable form and are said to be radioactive, emitting radiation from their nuclei as they move towards a more stable configuration. Radioactive forms of stable elements can also be produced artificially – by bombarding them with neutrons, for example – and are used in industry, and in medicine for imaging and therapies. Most radiation exposure is external – deposited on skin or clothes. Internal radiation exposure happens through inhalation or consumption of radionucleotides. For public health purposes, the most useful distinction is between ionizing and nonionizing radiation. Most major health effects are caused by ionizing radiation.

Radiation exposure is managed using the ALARA principle. This is the concept that doses should be kept *as low as reasonably achievable*. The term *reasonably achievable* allows for the social and economic context to be taken into account when setting policy. The established dose limits should not be exceeded by any individual. In the United Kingdom, there are limits for occupational exposure and guidelines on exposure from medical procedures.

IONIZING RADIATION

Radiation is said to be *ionizing* if it has enough energy to break the molecular bonds within cells that are exposed to it. This gives rise to ions and free radicals, damages cells and has both acute and chronic health effects. DNA is particularly vulnerable to damage.

There are three main sources of public exposure to ionizing radiation: natural background radiation, medical procedures and discharges from the nuclear industry. The naturally occurring sources include cosmic rays (to which those living at higher altitude are more exposed), radon gas from the rock and soil in some places (including Cornwall, where levels of radon exposure are monitored and adequate home ventilation is important) and radionucleotides that occur naturally in living cells, such as the unstable potassium-40 found in bananas.

Some occupations involve exposure to radiation beyond the normal background levels – medical radiography, the nuclear power industry, the airline industry and the uranium mining industry, for example. In high-income countries, their employees are regularly monitored and there are strict guidelines on maximum exposures. In some countries, however, the regulations are less well enforced, and adequate monitoring equipment may not be available.

There are three principal types of ionizing radiation. *Alpha particles* give up energy easily, and so are said to be densely ionizing. They have very low penetrating power (being stopped by a sheet of paper or dead layers of skin) and so usually only damage health if ingested or inhaled. *Beta particles* penetrate further than alpha particles, up to a centimetre of tissue. *Gamma rays*, like X-rays, have very high penetration, and are typically only stopped by materials such as thick aluminium, lead or concrete.

Large doses of ionizing radiation can cause health effects immediately. In a nuclear accident, for example, a whole-body radiation dose of 5 Gy damages the gastrointestinal, haemopoietic, pulmonary and central nervous systems, and is likely to be fatal. Whole-body doses of about 1–3 Gy may cause acute radiation sickness. The symptoms depend on dose and develop over time.

Radiation exposure also has a number of later effects on health. The two most important are induction of malignant disease and damage to developing embryos. The impact of radiation on embryo development depends on time of exposure and dose, but may include reduced IQ and increased risk of leukaemia and other cancers. These effects follow exposure to high doses of radiation over a short period of time. This is relatively rare. It is more common for people to be exposed to relatively small doses over longer periods. Various cohort studies have followed exposed workers and populations to examine the effects of such exposure. There is no agreed threshold below which there are thought to be no effects. A small dose can create a small additional risk for each exposed individual, which can be significant at the population level – causing additional deaths from cancer, for example.

NONIONIZING RADIATION

There are two broad types of nonionizing radiation: optical (ultraviolet, visible and infrared) and electromagnetic fields (microwave, radio frequency and extremely low frequency). Optical sources of radiation include solar radiation, infrared radiation and lasers. Electromagnetic fields are produced by electrical power lines and by electrical appliances at home and at work. In basic terms, optical and microwave radiation are packets of energy (photons), while radio frequency and extremely low-frequency fields are electric and magnetic fields moving in wave-like patterns.

Nonionizing radiation creates harmful effects of three main types: photochemical, thermal and electrical. Photochemical means chemical reactions in the body, caused by the absorption of photons. Solar ultraviolet radiation, for example, can cause sunburn and snow blindness. Ultraviolet radiation does not penetrate far into human tissue, so the eyes and skin are the organs most at risk. Ultraviolet radiation can cause skin cancer – both malignant and nonmalignant.

Malignant melanoma is less common than nonmalignant skin cancers, but of concern because it is serious and has increased rapidly in incidence over recent decades.

There has been much speculation about the delayed health effects of electromagnetic field exposure – in particular, whether it increases cancer risk. Mobile telephones and base stations have been of particular concern. There have been multiple epidemiological studies of occupational and population exposures to various electrical and magnetic sources. There is no persuasive evidence to date that electromagnetic field exposure influences any of the stages of cancer development.

URBANIZATION AND CITIES: THE BUILT ENVIRONMENT

More than half of the world's population lives in urban areas. This position has been reached because of a trend in which nations' populations have migrated from rural areas, driven by economic opportunity as jobs, services and education became concentrated within cities. Since 1940, more than half of the world's gross domestic product has been generated in industry and services, rather than in agriculture, mining and other rural-based economies.

There are health benefits to urban dwelling, referred to by some as the urban advantage. Urban dwellers generally have longer life expectancy than those in rural areas. In part, this is because cities usually have better healthcare facilities. The urban advantage is not the same for the urban poor, though. There are major health inequalities between and within cities. Wealthier areas tend to have better housing, more green space for recreation and lower air pollution levels. Communities in which low-income families live are more likely to contain environmental hazards and fewer opportunities for physical activity and cheap healthy food.

Rapid urbanization in low-income countries often involves the creation of informal settlements (more often known as slums). Many lack adequate clean water, sewage systems and robust housing structures. The health of urban dwellers in these areas may be worse than among comparative rural populations.

The built environment is a major health determinant. It can impede health or improve health, depending on how well it is planned and executed. Ideally, strong urban planning should benefit both health and the environment. There are many examples of this cobenefit. Provision of more green spaces encourages physical activity, improves mental health, reduces pollution and decreases urban heat island effects. Better house insulation reduces carbon emissions and mitigates the negative health risks of cold weather.

RISK ASSESSMENT AND MANAGEMENT

Risk assessment is the process of evaluating the risk that a specific exposure poses to a population. *Risk management* involves not just assessing the risk, but also examining the measures that are available to mitigate the given risk, and selecting and applying appropriate measures.

Risk is a crucial concept in environmental health. In traditional epidemiology, risk is expressed as the number of health outcomes (e.g. deaths) expected as a consequence of a given population exposure. Risk in environmental health can be seen as two elements – the chance of a certain event happening and the severity of that event.

Published in 1983, *Risk Assessment in the Federal Government* (known as the Red Book) first formalized the risk assessment process within environmental health. It divided risk assessment into four key stages. The discipline has evolved since then, but the essential elements remain the same. *Hazard identification*, the first stage, involves determining whether an environmental agent causes an adverse health outcome. This involves gathering evidence from available sources and study types (epidemiological, toxicological and animal), and then judging the strength of the evidence for causation. The hazard might be a single substance or a combination of environmental agents (e.g. air pollution) or processes (e.g. climate change). The hazard of interest needs to be precisely defined, as does the health effect (e.g. increased rate of cancer or death).

Dose–response assessment involves quantifying the relationship between a given dose of an agent and the health outcomes. A full dose–response assessment should not look for a single answer, but assess how the effect of the exposure varies between people – by age, for example.

Exposure assessment, the third stage, involves estimating the exposure that a defined population has had (or will have) to the hazard. Ideally, this will incorporate information on the magnitude, length and route of exposure. In practice, exposure can be difficult to assess because it is so dependent on behaviour (e.g. how long people were in a particular location when the exposure occurred).

Risk characterization draws together information from the three preceding stages, and summarizes it as an estimated effect of given exposures to a hazard within a defined population.

Risk assessment is not an exact science. Mostly, insufficient data are available to inform all stages of the process, creating uncertainty in the risk assessment. Judgement is then required. Scenarios and estimations are often used. The risk characterization, even with a paucity of data to make it, must provide a clear and fair presentation of the uncertainties of all estimations of risk.

Establishing an evidence base through research for the health impact of environmental exposures is difficult. Exposures often change over short time periods – temperatures and air pollution levels fluctuate hour by hour, for example. Specialized methods, such as time-series regression analysis and case-crossover studies, can be used to examine short-term associations between exposure and effect. In some environmental studies, it can be difficult to establish the amount of exposure to a given environmental factor. If a certain level of a substance is present in a location, it might be assumed that the population living in this area is exposed. In reality, of course, the population exposure, being made up of individual exposures, is affected by how long every person actually spends at home in that location, as opposed to at work or travelling. Unless exposure can be directly measured at the individual level, this can lead to misclassification of exposure.

Studying chronic risks is a particular challenge. It is unethical to expose populations to hazards in order to assess the effect. Studies often rely on naturally occurring exposed populations. Occasionally, it is possible to undertake a traditional cohort or case-control study – for example, if a cohort of workers is exposed to a certain type of radiation (particularly if the exposure was known in advance, as is the case for radiographers, and forms part of occupational health records).

Environmental hazards commonly vary geographically, and studies often use spatial epidemiology techniques. They can examine, for example, the health effects of living within a certain radius of a waste disposal unit. Studies of this nature may be instigated in response to public concern – such as if there seems to have been a high number of cancer cases around a certain waste disposal unit. If such a study finds a higher number of cases in this area than among the general population elsewhere, it remains difficult to determine whether this is due to chance alone, to the exposure or to another confounding factor present in the neighbourhood. This is not to say that clusters of disease should not be investigated. Such studies are important, but mainly to generate a hypothesis about environmental exposure and effect, rather than to prove a causal association.

Following risk assessment, risk management involves establishing options for reducing the risk, and then deciding which of these options would be most effective and appropriate. The process should consider the risk assessment alongside information about local social, economic, political and cultural circumstances. It should also consider the technical and legal feasibility of the different options. When all these considerations are balanced, the appropriate decision may be not to intervene. The risk posed by increased air pollution from the building of a new road, for example, must be balanced with the economic benefits of increasing transport to an area, and the social benefits of linking communities.

HEALTH IMPACT ASSESSMENT

Policymakers sometimes do not fully consider the impact of their policies on the environment or health. For example, for a long time, diesel was promoted over petrol as a greener fuel for cars, as it produced lower amounts of carbon dioxide and thus less greenhouse gas. Motorists were given incentives to buy cars with diesel engines. However, diesel exhaust fumes are particularly toxic, containing small particulate matter that easily enters the lungs and the cardiovascular system and causes damage. They also contain many hazardous chemicals, such as benzene and formaldehyde. Thirty years ago, diesel was positioned at the heart of the green agenda. Today, policymakers are rowing back, recognizing that it is very deleterious to air quality, particularly in major cities like London.

Many different areas of public policy have an impact on the environment and on health – from road building, to education, to waste disposal, to power generation, to constructing a new airport runway. Health impact assessment is a formal process of assessing the health consequences of a particular policy. It takes a broad view, attempting to explore the diverse health benefits and risks. These may range from communicable and non-communicable diseases, to mental health and nutritional effects, to wider social determinants of health. This broad view is in contrast to the narrower focus taken by the risk assessment process, which examines only specific health consequences of a particular hazard. The health impact assessment methodology draws on the longer-standing concept of environmental impact assessment, used to assess how new building developments will have an impact on the environment. The methodology uses both quantitative and qualitative methods to assess both overall effects on health and how these effects are distributed within the population. Ideally, health and environmental impact assessment would be integrated. This has been the approach taken in planning some major projects, such as a second runway at Manchester airport.

In the late 1990s, the UK government decided that major new government policies should have their health impact assessed. They also directed that this process should apply at the local government level – that local decision makers must examine what effects their decisions might have on health, including whether they might increase or reduce inequality.

The impact assessment process has continued to develop over recent years. In the United Kingdom, national and local government decisions are often accompanied by an *integrated impact assessment*, which attempts to set out a policy's impact by gender, race and disability. Health impact assessment is part of this.

CONCLUSIONS

Early writings about the relationship between environments and health particularly recognized that the risks to populations were maldistributed. They still are. Unclean water, poor sanitation and unsafe disposal of waste took millions of lives among the crowded, pestilential hovels of Britain's towns and cities during the Industrial Revolution. Today, in the slums, shantytowns and encampments of the poorest parts of the world, the struggle to survive is still determined by the absence of these most basic of human needs.

The march of human progress brought with it novel products, technologies and manufacturing processes. They enhanced quality of life for some, and wealth and affluence for some, but their hazardous qualities brought disease and sometimes death for others. The poor and disadvantaged were worst hit. As late as the twentieth century, there were stark reminders of what waits in the environmental shadows. In 1984, 700,000 people in Bhopal, India, were exposed to a toxic gas released by the Union Carbide pesticide factory. Several thousand perished immediately and many were made ill. Over the 30 years since, the cumulative death toll is variously estimated as 20,000–30,000. Many more have become chronically ill or disabled. The land and surface water around the factory remain contaminated. The populations living there still suffer through higher rates of cancer, birth defects, long-term ill health and disability. This, the worst environmental catastrophe of modern times, remains mired in controversy, secrecy and the absence of accountability. Sometimes environmental health disasters lead to major improvements. In the winter of 1952, a combination of thick fog and smoke from coal fires in homes and factories led to the Great London Smog that killed 12,000 and brought the capital to a standstill. The public and political aftershock swept in a suite of clean air legislation. This, and the advent of central heating, greatly reduced the chances of a similar event in the United Kingdom, although not in some other parts of the world. The Chernobyl nuclear disaster in the Ukraine in 1986 was caused by an explosion and fires in the nuclear reactor; they released a radioactive cloud that had potential implications worldwide. This severe accident led to some lessons being learned and subsequent redesign of new nuclear reactors.

The latter years of the twentieth century and the dawn of the twenty-first opened the door to the greatest concern of all: the health of the planet itself. Global warming, climate change, depletion of the ozone layer, deforestation and acid rain are terms that would not have been recognized by the champions of public health in the nineteenth century. Yet they are now not just the domain of health policymakers alone; they are part of the political, media and public discourse. They threaten the health of plant, animal, aquatic and human life. They already determine patterns of disease and death but, if left unchecked, ultimately will control the fate of planet Earth as a place where life can be sustained.

Whether traditional or novel, broad or narrow, direct or indirect, global or local, the influences of the environment on health should be high on the list of priorities of public health leaders, policymakers, practitioners and researchers far and wide.

CHAPTER 13

History of public health

INTRODUCTION

The history of public health in the United Kingdom is inexorably linked to the demographic, social and economic upheaval that characterized the eighteenth-century Industrial Revolution. As millions of people flocked from the fields of small rural towns and villages in search of work, they crossed the threshold of the seething industrial cities that pitted the Victorian landscape. Slums, grossly overcrowded dwellings, streets flowing with sewage, contaminated water supplies and factory pollutants destroyed any prospect of a civilized way of life – and indeed stole life from children and adults up and down the land. The grim reality was that the manufacture of disease itself, and vast amounts of it, was one of the principal products of the Industrial Revolution. Infectious diseases – although they were not recognized as such at the time – killed and debilitated. Epidemics of cholera, typhoid and typhus swept through the population, along with childhood fevers (such as measles, scarlet fever and diphtheria). Tuberculosis (consumption) was rampant, accounting for as many as a quarter of all deaths. Life itself was pitiably short. Levels of vaccination (introduced in 1853) were not adequate to protect against outbreaks of smallpox. Diseases of malnutrition – particularly rickets – were very common. As different trades and forms of manufacturing became established, they triggered their own specific diseases, as well as the risk of accidents. The evil of widespread child labour completed the harrowing picture.

The political and economic climate did nothing to resist these forces of death, degradation and human misery. Ideologically and ruthlessly hands off, the free market thinking initiated by Adam Smith's *The Wealth of Nations* ruled supreme. An individual's circumstances were seen as largely a matter of personal choice, and the invisible hand of the market would nurture the fortunes of those whose ingenuity and endeavour drove them on. The role of the state was to uphold the law of the land, with charity stepping in to provide for the most needy. A number of forces eroded this purist doctrine. First, while the poor suffered the most, it was clear that the affluent could not escape the risk and reality of the many pestilences that carried all before them

to graves and limepits. The death of Prince Albert from typhoid in 1861 was but the most publicly visible demonstration that the nation was all in it together, whatever the protestations of the free marketers. Second, a reform movement was growing in strength. Social reformers such as Charles Dickens, celebrities in their day, powerfully brought the plight of the urban poor and dispossessed into public and political consciousness, in which it became irrevocably embedded. Third, high-ranking officials and doctors began to collect data and gather individual testimony so as to map out the burden of death and disease and create an evidence-based, irrefutable case for reform.

While Victorian England has been a favourite focus for public health historians, the long view takes in a wide sweep of health and diseases, enlightened civic authorities, pioneering individuals, policies, scientific developments, inspiring stories and laws. These build a bridge to modern times, where transformations sit alongside continuing challenges.

EARLY DEVELOPMENTS

The writings and teachings of Hippocrates (460–377 BC) had an impact far beyond his lifetime, which began on the island of Cos, near the Ionian coast of Asia Minor, about 460 BC and ended (legend has it) when bees swarmed on his grave, producing a special honey: the cure for stomatitis in infants. Many regard Hippocrates as the father of medicine, although it was practised before his time. Indeed, writings on such matters date back to the earliest civilizations.

One of the main contributions of the Hippocratic school lay in focusing intellectual attention on medicine in its own right, as a discipline founded on the observation of facts and the recording of clinical experiences. One of the major teachings was that the body contained four humours: blood, black bile, yellow bile and phlegm. In health, the humours mingled together and were in harmony or balance; in disease, there was a derangement of this mixture.

Hippocrates has relevance to the history of public health, not just to the foundations of clinical medicine. He was the

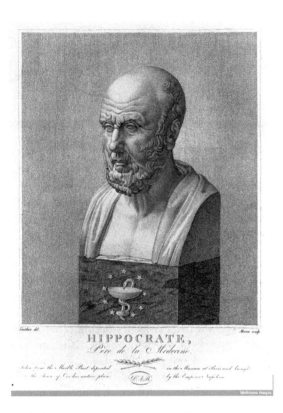

Marble bust of Hippocrates (460–377 BC). Engraving.

first to seek to explain the origins of disease, and in so doing, he put forward many observations that do not seem out of place even today. He distinguished between diseases that were endemic (always present in a given area) and those that at times become excessively common (epidemic). In suggesting a role for exercise, diet, climate, water and the seasons, he foreshadowed modern views of the importance of the interrelationship between people and their environment in the causation of disease.

Many of his aphorisms resonate with modern causal thinking, for example, 'Those naturally very fat are more liable to sudden death than the thin'.

During the time of the Roman Empire, which eclipsed its Greek predecessor, it is the name of another Greek, Galen (129–216), that stands out in the history of medicine. Galen is said to have cured the emperor Marcus Aurelius of abdominal pain. His observations on the nature and cause of disease added little to the Hippocratic writings, but he did advance knowledge in relation to anatomy and physiology. While Hippocrates had largely been an observer of Nature, Galen was mainly a theorist and a forceful one at that. Galen's writings and teachings established a medical doctrine that reigned for a thousand years. Even in the medieval period, centuries after Galen's death, it was heretical to criticize or doubt his work. This inhibited any intellectual challenge to the established view of the world.

Salerno, a coastal resort near Naples, became the seat of the first medical school in Europe. It flourished during the tenth to thirteenth centuries. Of particular interest to public health is a book produced there called *Regimen Sanitatis Salernitanum*. This was written in verse but was reprinted many times. It was the most widely read medical text right up until the beginning of the nineteenth century. The first English translation from the Latin original was by Sir John Harington, a member of the court of Queen Elizabeth I (see below).

Thomas Sydenham (1624–89) was an English physician who regarded experimental physiology, so much in vogue at the time, with contempt. His philosophy was to set aside all theory and begin by observing and recording symptoms and signs and their progression in the sufferer from the particular ailment. He is greatly revered for his classical descriptions of diseases such as gout, measles, scarlet fever and pneumonia. He is often called the 'English Hippocrates' because his observational method had many similarities with his distant Greek predecessor. Some of his views, which he subsequently discarded, seem bizarre for a man who was otherwise so rigorous in his work; for example, at one point he maintained that smallpox was a sign of physiological renewal of the blood. He was essentially a practical physician who espoused bedside medicine and had no time for theorizing, research or reading. Nevertheless, he was well connected to his professional peers and within the wider society of his day.

The organization of medical practice itself developed alongside the emergence of new schools of thought. By the early nineteenth century, it was emerging into three distinct strands. First, there were the physicians who were university educated; initially this was only at Oxford or Cambridge, where the medical content of their studies was not major and based largely on the teachings of Hippocrates and Galen. Second, the surgeons, evolving from the barber-surgeons, were taught in the increasing number of schools of anatomy (particularly in London) and apprenticed to senior surgeons. Third, the apothecaries, who prescribed, prepared and dispensed medicines and potions and provided general medical care at a cheaper rate than the physicians, were also apprenticed. For a time, there was a sizeable class of surgeon-apothecaries (more so outside of London – in London there were more pure surgeons). Gradually, these groups organized into a profession of medicine with medical education largely in hospitals and regulation of practice through the creation of a medical register in the first *Medical Act* of 1858.

THE GREAT EPIDEMICS

The terms used to describe the epidemics that swept through the populations of the ancient and medieval worlds were generally nonspecific or vague: plague, the sweats or, more often, simply the ague. Even when reference was made to the plague, it is doubtful if all the occurrences were truly bubonic plague. Histories and literature contain many accounts of the fear, devastation and death caused by the epidemic diseases that surged through populations, although the true causes were mysterious to those who wrote about them. Meteorological conditions, divine retribution, the flight path of owls and planetary movements were all confidently put forward as explanations. It was not until the scientific discoveries of the 1860s that the true mode of transmission of these devastating diseases became clear. Even looking back with modern scientific knowledge, the precise infectious agent responsible is difficult to discern from many of the historical accounts of the features of the conditions that caused so many deaths. Indeed, trying to surmise their causation is a field of academic study in its own right. While much historical attention has been given to the plague and cholera, diseases such as smallpox, typhoid, typhus, diphtheria and scarlet fever regularly took epidemic form and caused large amounts of illness and deaths.

In epidemiological terms, the medieval period is defined by the two most terrible pestilences that the world has ever seen: the *Plague of Justinian* in the sixth century and the *Black Death* in the fourteenth century. Both swept away millions in many countries in Europe and destroyed the fabric of societies.

Historical accounts of plagues and epidemics

There are many classic accounts of epidemic disease; some of the best known come from literature. Daniel Defoe (1661–1731) published, in 1722, *A Journal of the Plague Year, Being Observations or Memorials of the Most Remarkable Occurrences as well Publick as Private, Which Happened in London during the Last Great Visitation in 1665*. Long titles were the order of

the day in those times. It was written as if it were an eyewitness account, and such was the power and authenticity of the narrative that it was taken by some to be factual.

> The people of these parts had flattered themselves that they should escape; and how they were surprised when it came upon them as it did. For indeed, it came upon them like an armed man when it did come.

If his contemporaries were not convinced by the use of words that the work was that of a great artist rather than a humble chronicler, they only had to take note of Defoe's age in the year of the plague to realize it was fiction; he was six. Earlier, another great writer of prose, Giovanni Boccaccio (1313–1375) had published the *Decameron*, about the great plague that descended on Florence in 1348. He too had not been there, but his work of imagination was equally compelling and convincing: 'How many breakfasted in the morning with their kinfolk, comrades and friends and, that same night, supped with their ancestors in the other world'.

One of the earliest and most famous documented epidemics is the *Plague of Athens*. It struck the population around 430 BC. Thucydides (455–396 BC), the revered witness and chronicler of Ancient Greece (his *History of the Peloponnesian War* is considered by many authorities to be one of the greatest of all historical works), described it in great detail. Thucydides set out a faithful eyewitness account of the illness and its impact on the city's population. He described, in closely observed terms, the symptoms and

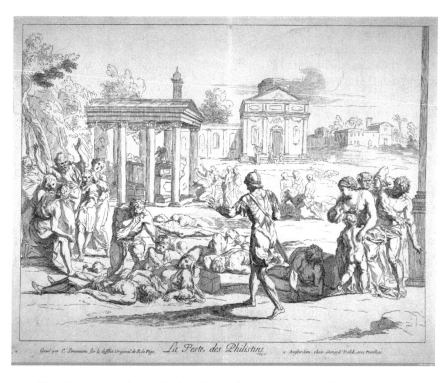

The plague at Ashdod. Etching by C. Simonneau, 1695 after R La Fage.

signs of the disease in those who contracted it. The description would not be out of place in an early twentieth-century textbook of medicine. He does not mention the buboes – the classic black swellings of the lymph glands – that are characteristic of the bubonic plague. This has led public health historians to speculate that the Plague of Athens might have been typhus or one of the other common epidemic infectious diseases active at the time.

In the Middle Ages, one of the most celebrated accounts of the plague, in this case affecting the inhabitants of Avignon, was written by a surgeon, Guy de Chauliac (1300–68). He was a man of great professional distinction, having written a widely read text on surgery, but his description of the plague at Avignon is pure public health. He discusses the geographical origins, distribution and spread of the disease and documents its key clinical features; crucially, he makes the distinction between the pneumonic and bubonic forms of the disease. In addition to its clinical objectivity, de Chauliac's account also has a lyrical side that emphasizes the helplessness of a population faced with a pestilence that killed three-quarters of their number: 'The father did not visit the son, nor the son his father. Charity was dead and hope destroyed'.

Eventually, though, he reverts from the recording of hard facts to asserting that the cause of this devastation was a consequence of the alignment of Saturn, Jupiter and Mars in the sign of Aquarius on 24 March 1345.

Plague of Justinian

After the fall of the Roman Empire to the Barbarians, the mainly Greek-speaking part to the east was based on the city of Byzantium, later known as Constantinople (and today Istanbul). Emperor Justinian the First (527–65) was the ruler. His goal was to reunite the old empire.

The disease that became known as the Justinian Plague first struck Constantinople in 541. Its course was savage. More than 10,000 deaths a day devastated the city, and it swept across the cities and towns of the Mediterranean and beyond, ebbing and flowing for more than 200 years. The total number of deaths has been estimated as 50 million. The historian Procopius (500–65) documented its spread. He wrote, 'The whole human race was near being exterminated'.

Modern genetic techniques seem to confirm that this was the bubonic plague, although its pneumonic and septicaemic forms must also have been present. It entered Constantinople on rats carried in grain boats from Egypt. Before that, the disease may have originated in China.

Black Death

The *Black Death* took a massive toll on medieval Europe. It entered England at the port of Melcombe Regis (now called Weymouth) in Dorset in early August 1348. It began to spread through the west country, depopulating as it went. It was in Bristol by 15 August, and after Oxford, it entered London on 1 November. Eventually, half the population of London died. It followed the trade routes of Europe. Estimates vary between 25% and 50% of Europe's population being fatal victims of the Black Death. The disease almost certainly originated in China and made its way to Europe through trade with China or countries in between.

Great Plague of London

Apart from the period following the entry of the Black Death into the country, London experienced other epidemics of the plague, particularly in 1563, 1603 and 1625. It is the visitation of 1665 that is referred to as the *Great Plague*. By that time, the population of London had increased, so many more people were at risk. In all, 100,000 died. Many wealthy people, and many physicians and clergy, fled the city, leaving the poor to become victims of a disease whose origins no one understood and that engendered mortal dread and panic. In the next few years, the country, and subsequently Europe as a whole, would be largely free of the plague. There are various theories as to why the plague receded in this way, but none can fully explain it.

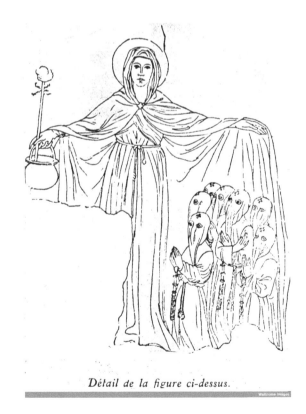

Détail de la figure ci-dessus.

St. Martha protecting under her cloak members of a brotherhood devoted to burying the bodies of plague victims; in the church of St. Martha at Carona, near Lugano. Line drawing from Aesculape, 1932.

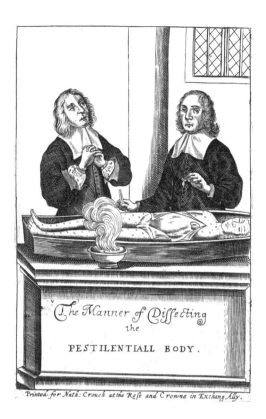

Two men dissecting a body with plague marks.
Incense burning to camouflage the stench.
Engraving, 1666.

Rise of King Cholera

Asiatic cholera was endemic in the delta region of the Ganges for centuries. It caused periodic epidemics, especially in India. It began to move westward in the first years of the nineteenth century, its progress enhanced by the easier transport of the steamboats and railways. Cholera first reached English shores in 1831 on a ship that docked in the port of Sunderland. The first person to die from it was a 12-year-old girl, Isabella Hazard, who showed first symptoms at midnight on 17 October 1831 and was dead by the next afternoon. She was famously depicted in a *Lancet* article as the Blue Girl (her moribund and fluid-depleted body in an advanced state of hypoxia). The number of countries infected increased, and now these waves of cholera in 1831, 1848 and 1854 are thought of as pandemics of the disease. The initial large numbers of cases were followed by years of local outbreaks.

For the public, cholera was a particularly terrifying disease. Since the departure of pandemic plague in the seventeenth century, there had been no disease that had struck such a note of fear and carried people to their deaths in such large numbers so swiftly.

THE LONG JOURNEY TO THE ESTABLISHMENT OF THE GERM THEORY

In the ancient and medieval worlds, thinking about the cause of epidemic diseases was not organized or directed

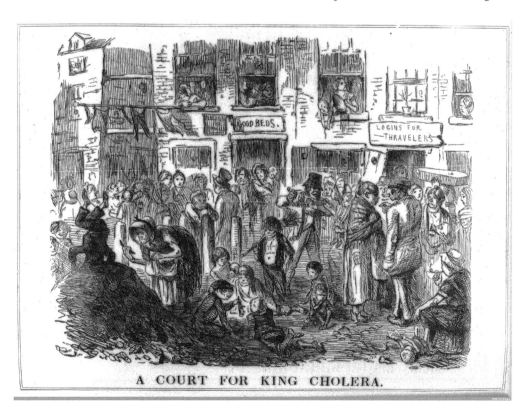

A court for King Cholera. Engraving. Punch, 1852.

towards discovery and enlightenment. Early death, illness and disability were accepted as an immutable part of life. Religion, astrology, superstition, prejudice and dogmatic assertion produced trenchant views and desperate adherence to beliefs that might be life sparing. For example, even in the 1600s, it was common to wear amulets to ward off the plague, the sapphire was held to be strongly protective and some people carried mathematical formulae written on scraps of paper. The clergy and even physicians recommended some of these actions.

From ancient times, there were three strongly held beliefs about the causation of what we now know as infections: *miasma*, *contagion* and *astral* forces.

Hippocrates wrote about the importance of air and climate, asserting that bad air was associated with outbreaks of disease. Galen strengthened this perspective by theorizing about a *miasmatic corruption* of air, implying that there were ingredients within it that caused plague and other epidemic diseases. This Galenic assertion continued to be accepted wisdom for a thousand years. The *miasma* was variously held to arise from decaying corpses, stagnant waters, rotting vegetation and other poisonous vapours. At times in history, it was mixed with superstition: it was held that the breath of gods or demons could cause a miasma. In *Timon of Athens*, William Shakespeare wrote,

> Be as a planetary plague, when Jove will o'er some high-viced city hang his poison in the sick air.

Even as great and revered a figure as the seventeenth-century physician Thomas Sydenham added little to the understanding of why people became ill. Because of his stature, his miasmic theory of the causation of disease – little more than a re-expression of earlier ideas – was much more influential

than it deserved to be. He believed that some febrile illnesses (e.g. plague and smallpox) were caused by atmospheric contact, while others were generated from within the body. As recently as the second half of the nineteenth century, many medical officers of health in their annual reports still related epidemics of infectious diseases to bad odours arising in a locality. Edwin Chadwick, a driving force of the sanitary revolution (see below) was a miasmist. Surprisingly, so was Florence Nightingale. The miasmic theory proved a good working assumption in guiding action because the solution was to flee the affected area to find purer air. This is what royalty, politicians and affluent people did – and it often seemed to work for them. Other methods of avoiding the supposedly affected air were also advocated and adopted, such as opening and closing windows according to the wind direction. In one period of the early seventeenth century, tobacco smoking was practised and even became policy to protect the boys of Eton School. There were also strategies to clean up the urban environment through whitewashing houses and emptying cesspits.

One observation that could have been an 'Aha' moment came from Fracastorius (1478–1553), a Veronese poet and physician, best remembered for writing a long poem about syphilis, or the 'French disease'. His views on the general nature and cause of infectious diseases were, however, remarkable and were expressed some 200 years before such ideas were embraced as new and revolutionary. In a stunning metaphor, Fracastorius compared contagion in disease to the putrefaction that passes from one fruit to another when it rots. Moreover, when he referred to the essential nature of infection, he suggested that minute particles or *seminaria* (seeds) were conveyed from person to person and propagated themselves.

As in many fields of scientific history, the path of discovery only seems linear in retrospect. Looking back,

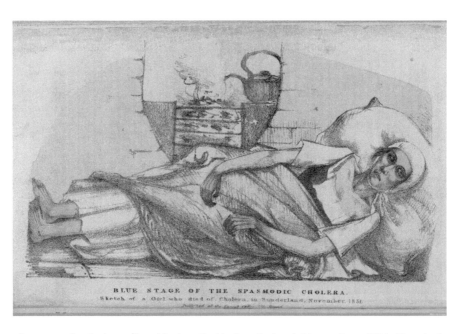

Blue stage of spasmodic cholera of a girl who died in Sunderland, November, 1831. Sketch. Lancet, 1832.

there are islands of enlightenment or flashes of insight that seem to be impossible to ignore, but somehow they fizzled out rather than igniting a new era of understanding. The first mention, by Fracastorius, of the possibility that diseases are caused by transmissible agents fell by the wayside. Indeed, he also had beliefs about the malign influence of alignment of the planets, seemingly at odds with his more 'scientific' views.

The invention of the microscope around 1670 had allowed living organisms, invisible to the naked eye, to be seen for the first time. Leeuwenhoek (1632–1723), a Dutch linen draper based in Delft, examined a range of materials, such as saliva, blood, water and faeces (although not from diseased people) and made drawings of micro-organisms, including what are now clearly recognizable as bacteria. He described them as *animalcula*, or little animals, and wrote a letter to the Royal Society in 1676. He made no apparent attempt to associate these living organisms with human disease. One person who did was a little known surgeon who lived in Red Lion Square in London, Benjamin Marten (c. 1690–1751). He published a number of pamphlets and booklets about disease for the public. In one, *A New Theory of Consumptions*, published in 1720, he put forward the idea that consumption (tuberculosis) was caused by an infective agent: 'the prime, essential, and hitherto unaccounted, inexplicable cause of consumption is a specific animalcule'. Marten went on to suggest that these 'wonderfully minute living creatures' might enter the body to cause other diseases. His writings attracted little attention because they were not of a scholarly nature, he was a minor figure in medicine and there was a mass of popular material making claims for causes and cures of the disease that were afflicting people in eighteenth-century England. Nevertheless, in retrospect, Marten's was a striking observation that preceded the acceptance of the germ theory of disease by 150 years. There were other minor figures like Marten in different parts of Europe who tentatively put forward similar ideas.

Essentially, the *miasma* theory was based on the idea that the disease threat came from the external world, in other words, from nature. In contrast, the theory of *contagion* held that the poison was generated from within the human body. It was then passed from person to person by direct contact or indirectly by their possessions, clothing and bedding. The more superstitious believed that catching the eye of an infected person (the evil eye) was enough. The actions flowing from the theory of contagion seem eminently sensible today. Quarantine on arrival of ships from infected areas was widely applied. Indeed, when the plague came into Europe in the fourteenth century, the Venetian authorities set up a sophisticated system to sift and deny entry to ships that might carry contagion; they also quarantined people and cargoes. Sustaining the miasmist rationale in response to this relatively effective contagionist control measure was the argument that ships carried air from the infected town in its hold so that it became released when the vessel docked

in a new area and its hold was opened. This microclimate idea seems particularly absurd in retrospect, but Galen's reach through the centuries was long.

Avoiding materials that were in contact with an infected person and isolation of the sick themselves were practised for centuries. One of the most poignant examples of blocking contagion is the way that lepers were cast out of their communities often after elaborate rituals and ceremonies in which they were rendered non-persons. Leprosy and societies' reactions to it feature at different points in the Bible. An extreme and noble act of isolation to prevent spread of a disease was the plague village in Eyam, Derbyshire. In 1665, a tailor from Eyam ordered a bale of cloth from London and unknowingly imported the bubonic plague that killed 260 villagers. The villagers sealed their borders to prevent the disease spreading. They acted selflessly to protect others.

The plague is the best illustration of how the two causal ideologies were split. The plague has three clinical manifestations: the *bubonic, pneumonic* and *septicaemic* forms. At times when the bubonic form was prevalent, the miasmists held sway since there was less evidence of person-to-person spread. We now know that the characteristic illness with black swellings (bubos) was caused by the bites of infected fleas travelling on rats. When the pneumonic plague was the predominant form, the heavily infected lung tissue led to coughing and excretions that readily produced infection after direct or indirect contact. This fit well with the theory of contagion.

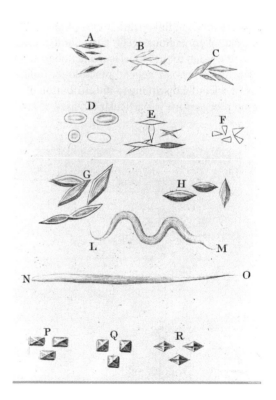

The microscopic animalcules seen in white vinegar.

Source: Hoole S. *The Select Works of Leeuwenhoek Containing his Microscopical Discoveries.* London: Fry, 1798–1799.

After more than a thousand years of argument, the true nature of communicable disease was revealed in the second half of the nineteenth century.

Two names stand out as transforming causal thinking and finally giving birth to the germ theory of disease that had been so slow in its gestation: Louis Pasteur (1822–95) and Robert Koch (1843–1910).

Pasteur firmly rejected the idea of spontaneous generation, a long-standing theory holding that tiny particles, which were present in the air, formed into living material. He believed that microorganisms came from the air and settled on the culture media in which they were found. To prove his theory, he conducted an experiment in which he filled two flasks with suitable culture medium. These flasks were then heated to kill any organisms that were likely to be present in the medium; one was covered and the other left open. Bacteria quickly appeared in the uncovered flask but not in the covered one, thus firmly refuting the idea of spontaneous generation.

Development of preparation and staining techniques allowed Robert Koch, a doctor working in the town of Wollstein, Germany, to isolate the tubercle bacillus in 1882 and the cholera vibrio in 1883. In a very short period of time, a wide range of organisms were identified and linked to human disease – *Bacillus anthracis* (anthrax), *Corynebacterium diphtheriae* (diphtheria), *Mycobacterium leprae* (leprosy) and *Salmonella typhi* (typhoid fever).

Such was the enthusiasm with which the medical establishment now embraced the germ theory of disease that attempts were made to link virtually every known disease to a specific causal contagious agent. Claim and counterclaim abounded. It was left to the Nobel laureate Robert Koch, who had begun his career as a general practitioner in Germany, to impose a scientific discipline to the attribution of a causal role for microorganisms in particular diseases.

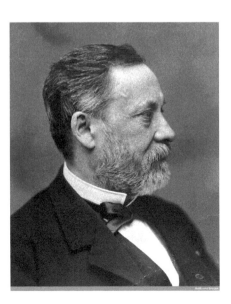

Portrait of Louis Pasteur (1822–1895). Photograph.

Koch's postulates, sometimes also referred to as the Henle–Koch postulates (Koch was Henle's pupil), can be summarized:

- Organism isolated in pure culture in each case
- Organism not present in any other disease as fortuitous and nonpathogenic finding
- Once isolated, must be grown in a series of cultures
- Culture should reproduce the disease on inoculation into an experimental animal

It is clear today that Koch's postulates, if interpreted literally, are too rigid and would exclude many viral diseases and also some bacterial diseases from having a proven causative agent. Nevertheless, they served as an important landmark at the time.

SOME CLASSIC INVESTIGATIONS

Some of the major discoveries of disease causation in public health in the nineteenth and early twentieth century came about through an inspired curious investigator studying a problem and gathering data to throw light on it. Looking back on these discoveries, they clearly pointed to a way to prevent or cure a disease that had hitherto been a mystery, and often they could save lives. Disappointingly, such discoveries were not seen as groundbreaking at the time and provoked hostility and denial as the medical, scientific and political establishments stood their ground in support of the prevailing paradigms. John Snow's clear demonstration that cholera was transmitted by polluted water failed to shake the causal beliefs of the miasmists, and he died without his theory being accepted. James Lind, in the first controlled trial, showed that citrus juice would prevent and cure scurvy and thus save thousands of lives that were being lost on long sea voyages. The Royal Navy did not adopt a policy of daily rations of juice for more than 40 years. Joseph Goldberger's discovery that the diet of poor sharecroppers, not infection, was causing so many deaths from pellagra in the United States provoked a furious political backlash at the idea that poverty could result in disease.

John Snow and the Broad Street Pump

There were serious outbreaks of cholera in London in the years after it entered the country. However, it is the one in Broad Street, Golden Square, Soho, London, that is the most famous. John Snow (1813–58), apprenticed as a doctor in Newcastle-upon-Tyne, could justifiably have settled for one claim to immortality when he became the first man to establish the scientific basis for the use of chloroform as an anaesthetic agent. He used chloroform in the delivery of two of Queen Victoria's children. His influential text *On Chloroform* was published shortly after his sudden death from a cerebral haemorrhage. Yet, it was his interest in cholera and his painstaking investigation of an outbreak of this disease that earned him a further place in medicine's hall of fame.

Snow's own words best describe the outbreak in 1854:

> The most terrible outbreak of cholera which ever occurred in this kingdom is probably that which took place in Broad Street, Golden Square and adjoining streets, a few weeks ago. Within two hundred and fifty yards of the spot where Cambridge Street joins Broad Street, there were upwards of five hundred fatal attacks of cholera in ten days. The mortality in this limited area probably equals any that was ever caused in this country, even by the plague; and it was much more sudden as the greater number of cases terminated in a few hours. The mortality would undoubtedly have been much greater had it not been for the flight of the population.

From May 1854, there was a rapid rise in cases, with London as a whole having a death rate of 45 per 10,000 people. In the late summer of that same year, the death rate in the area encompassing Golden Square, St James's, Soho from Wardour Street to Dean Street and part of the subdistrict of St James's Square was 440 per 10,000. Houses were densely clustered and very overcrowded, with some whole families living in a single room. By plotting the geographical location of each cholera case, Snow deduced that the deaths had occurred among people living in close proximity to the Broad Street pump (most families at this time had no water supply in their own homes, instead using

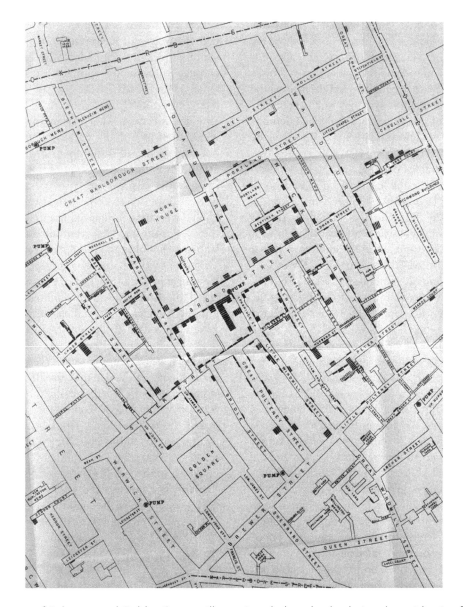

Street map of Soho, around Golden Square, illustrating cholera deaths during the epidemic of 1854.

Source: Snow J. *On the Mode of Transmission of Cholera.* London: Churchill, 1855.

a communal supply). There were one or two pieces of evidence, however, which did not at first seem to fit Snow's theory of the complicity of the pump. First, a workhouse with 535 inmates on a street very close to the Broad Street pump experienced only five deaths from cholera among its population. Second, a brewery on Broad Street itself had no fatalities among its workforce. Snow investigated these differences and found that the workhouse had its own pump on the premises (which drew its water from a different, uncontaminated, underground source), and the workers in the brewery never frequented the Broad Street pump. Finally, Snow turned his attention to a woman and her niece living at Hampstead, a considerable distance from Broad Street, who nevertheless died of cholera during the epidemic. As a result of his interview with neighbours and next of kin, Snow ascertained that the woman had a particular liking for the flavour of the water of the Broad Street pump and sent her son to it every day for a bottle to drink.

On completing his enquiries, Snow sought an interview with the Board of Guardians of St James's Parish (who were in charge of the pump), and as a result of his representations, the pump handle was removed and the epidemic, which was already declining, came to an end. The importance of the removal of the pump handle was symbolic of a new understanding of the nature of the disease, for Snow had demonstrated that disease can be conveyed by water and specifically that cholera is a waterborne disease. However, many powerful members of the establishment dismissed Snow's findings and reasserted the miasmic cause of cholera. A local clergyman, the assistant curate at St Luke's Church, Soho, Henry Whitehead (1825–96), who was initially a sceptic and miasmist, worked on a committee of investigation with Snow. They found that a cesspool drained into the well that supplied water to the Broad Street pump. The removal of the pump handle has immense symbolic importance, but the discovery that the well was contaminated by sewage was the true breakthrough. Even then, powerful forces discredited this wonderful epidemiological investigation.

Although Snow's cholera theory is almost universally linked to his investigation of the Broad Street pump, he had undertaken an earlier, less dramatic but similarly painstaking piece of epidemiology that was arguably even more compelling. In London at that time, a number of private companies supplied water to residents, and Londoners paid for their supply. Snow turned his attention to the water supplies of two of these companies: the Lambeth Waterworks Company and the Southwark and Vauxhall Water Company, which both supplied similar areas of London. In some cases, the pipes of both companies went down the same street, so it was possible to identify individual households supplied by one or the other. The death rate from cholera in the areas of London supplied by these two water companies was much higher than it was in places supplied by other companies. Both companies obtained their supply from the lower part of the Thames, which was the part most greatly contaminated by sewage.

A chance occurrence in 1852 had provided Snow with a marvellous opportunity for a natural experiment. In that year, the Lambeth water company changed its intake to another source, which was free from sewage. Snow obtained the addresses of all people dying of cholera and sought information on the source of the water supply to each household. During the epidemic in the year 1853, Snow found that there were 71 fatal attacks of cholera per 10,000 households supplied by the Southwark and Vauxhall company, compared with only 5 per 10,000 in those supplied by the Lambeth Company. In other words, people getting their water from the polluted part of the Thames had 14 times more fatal attacks of cholera than those getting their supply from the purer source.

Snow published *On the Mode of Communication of Cholera* in 1849. He considered that cholera was spread from person to person, from the sick to the healthy, rather than by contact with any miasma or similar substance. Moreover, he deduced that this spread took place via morbid material from the alimentary canal of the sufferer, which was then swallowed by other people and had the power of multiplication in the body of the person it attacked. Coincidentally, and with no apparent contact with Snow, another physician, William Budd (1811–1880), based in Bristol, in 1849 published a treatise entitled *Malignant Cholera: Its Mode of Propagation and Its Prevention*. In it, he maintained that the disease was caused by a living organism that bred in the human gut, and was transmitted by drinking water. He espoused a similar theory about typhoid. Budd's work had little impact. He was a minor provincial doctor whose views were not of interest to the London medical establishment. Later, he became influential in public health in Bristol and the west country. His eventual publication on mode of transmission of typhoid is a major landmark.

Snow's work, of course, was based in London, but even so clear an explanation backed by careful scientific observation failed to convince the many doubters who still categorically rejected the idea of a specific agent in the cause of disease. When Snow died at the age of 45 years in 1858, his theory of cholera transmission was not accepted wisdom and he did not have the satisfaction of seeing the flowering of the germ theory of disease and the flight of the miasmatists. When in 1992 the Northern and Yorkshire Regional Health Authority honoured Yorkshire's famous son by naming its headquarters 'John Snow House', they were taken to task by bureaucrats in the Department of Health for having the temerity to name an important government building after a cricketer. John Snow (1941–) was a distinguished Sussex and England fast bowler. The father of modern epidemiology may be forgotten in the corridors of power, but he remains a lasting hero to the public health service.

James Lind and Scurvy

James Lind (1716–94) was a surgeon in the Royal Navy at a time when long voyages were commonplace. The provisions taken on board were those that could withstand such voyages without perishing. Sailors were afflicted after a time at sea by a strange malady: lethargy and weakness, pain in the joints and limbs and swelling of the gums. This was scurvy, and it cost many thousands of lives on the great sailing ships of the time. In 1747, Lind performed an experiment on the ship on which he was appointed a naval surgeon: *HMS Salisbury.* He added different substances to the diet of 12 sailors on the voyage. He divided his subjects into six pairs and supplemented the diets of each pair with one of cider; elixir of vitriol; vinegar; seawater; a mixture of nutmeg, garlic, mustard and tamarind in barley water; or two oranges and one lemon daily. Only the sailors given oranges and lemons recovered. Today, this is regarded as the first controlled clinical trial in history. Thus, long before vitamin C was isolated, Lind had determined how to prevent scurvy. However, he returned to his medical studies in Edinburgh and did not write up his work until six years later; then, he published a 400-page treatise on scurvy. Surprisingly, given the clarity of Lind's argument, it had little impact and certainly did not change the Admirality's policy, although some captains and admirals adopted it for their ships. Although this seems strange in retrospect, the health of sailors was not seen as an important part of a successful navy. Lind's case was considerably weakened by his move from the simple pragmatism of his idea to elaborate and bizarre theories of the underlying pathophysiological basis of scurvy. He could not explain why the disease occurred within the prevailing framework for diseases. That was fatal to his case in the medical establishment of the day. Nor, ironically, did he ever accept that scurvy was a dietary deficiency disease, even though he had proven that fresh fruit could prevent and cure it. Lind went on to be in charge of the Royal Naval hospital at Haslar, where many cases of scurvy were admitted. He did not use this as an opportunity to strengthen his research and lost his focus, although he took his treatise through further editions. It fell to a naval surgeon of a different kind to win the day. Gilbert Blane (1749–1834) was appointed as a naval surgeon through his social connections; he did not come up through the ranks. He had the ear of powerful admirals and took an interest in the health of sailors, doing much to improve their situation and to keep many more fit to fight. He was convinced by Lind's work and after years of assembling data, using fresh fruit in the parts of the fleet where he was directly involved and using his social influence, he persuaded the Royal Navy to rule that all sailors on long voyages should have a daily ration of lemon juice. This largely eliminated scurvy. This official policy came in 48 years after Lind's original discovery on HMS *Salisbury.*

The use of limes as the fruit of choice on some ships led to the nickname *limeys* for British sailors.

Goldberger and Pellagra

In the first half of the twentieth century, in the United States, there were around 3 million cases of a disease called *pellagra* and some 100,000 deaths from it. It was more common

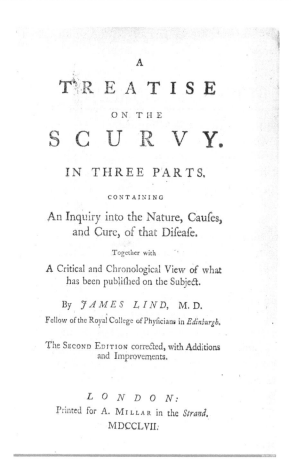

A

TREATISE

ON THE

SCURVY.

IN THREE PARTS.

CONTAINING

An Inquiry into the Nature, Caufes, and Cure, of that Difeafe.

Together with

A Critical and Chronological View of what has been publifhed on the Subjeft.

By *JAMES LIND,* M. D.

Fellow of the Royal College of Phyficians in *Edinburgh.*

The SECOND EDITION correfted, with Additions and Improvements.

LONDON:
Printed for A. MILLAR in the *Strand.*
MDCCLVII.

Title page of Lind's treatise on scurvy.

Source: Lind J. *A Treatise on the Scurvy.* London: Millar, 1757.

in the southern states. Some called it the *Sharecroppers' Disease.* In 1914, the U.S. Public Health Service assigned Joseph Goldberger (1874–1929) to investigate it. The symptoms of the disease were often summarized as the four D's: diarrhoea, dermatitis, dementia and death.

Goldberger surmised that the cause of the disease was dietary. He chose two orphanages and a mental hospital where pellagra was common among the residents. He fed them fresh meat, vegetables, eggs and milk instead of the prevalent corn-based diet. The disease was prevented and also reversed in those that had it. His next study was in a prison in Mississippi where inmates were offered a pardon if they would take part in an experiment in which they were given the diet of poor farmers. Those that participated developed the classic symptoms of pellagra. Goldberger's conclusions were highly controversial; not only did he reject the idea that the disease was infective in origin (as then believed), but by linking it to a deficient diet due to poverty, he wounded southern pride. It was also found that a similarly deficient diet fed to dogs caused a disease called 'black tongue'. The precise deficiency was later found to be niacin (vitamin B3).

By the mid-1930s, pellagra still caused 3500 deaths in the United States each year. Economic factors, food supplies and diet continued to precipitate the disease in the cotton workers and subsistence farmers in the south, albeit on a smaller scale than earlier in the century.

THE STORY OF VACCINATION

In parallel with the development of the concept of an infective agent causing infectious diseases, attention was also being directed to the capacity of a person to resist infection. It had been known since ancient times that people who had suffered from certain diseases and survived rarely contracted the same disease a second time. Before anything much was known about infection or immunity, this basic observation – and the devastating nature of some diseases – was causing people to experiment.

One practice – *variolation* – spread across Europe in the eighteenth century. Material was taken from smallpox pustules of sufferers and scratched into the skin, or veins, of healthy people. The theory was that this inoculation would induce only mild illness but protect against major infection in the future. It was a dangerous pursuit. Many inoculated in this way either caught full-blown smallpox (from which some died) or developed sepsis from the unhygienic administration of the pustular scrapings.

With an estimated 60 million people dying from smallpox in Europe alone, many were willing to take a chance that they might be spared by this uncertain method of protection. Estimates of death after variolation were 1 in 50, while as many as 1 in 5 who caught smallpox naturally died from it. The introduction of variolation to England is attributed to Lady Mary Wortley Montagu (1689–1762), a facially scarred smallpox survivor, who had seen it used in the Ottoman Empire where her husband was British Ambassador. Indeed, her children were inoculated and said to have had only a mild attack of smallpox with little scarring. Lady Montagu's enthusiasm and some successful tests on prisoners emboldened the royal family to risk variolation. There is earlier evidence of the practice being used in China and other parts of the ancient world centuries before.

Policy on variolation illuminates a moment in history. In 1776, American forces led by General George Washington failed to take Quebec because their ranks were decimated by smallpox; the smaller British Garrison, that had been variolated, held their position, and this played a part in keeping Canada in the British Empire.

Jenner: The country physician

Towards the end of the eighteenth century, Edward Jenner (1749–1823), a physician in Gloucestershire, decided to investigate a piece of local folklore relating to the disease. It was well known by country people that milkmaids often acquired, from infected cows, a disease called cowpox that gave rise to a pustule on the finger or crop of pustules on the body. It was believed that girls who contracted this mild disease would not contract smallpox when they were exposed to it. This observation is probably the origin of the following rhyme:

'Where are you going my pretty maid?'
'I'm going a-milking, Sir', she said.
'What is your fortune my pretty maid?'
'My face is my fortune, Sir', she said.

In 1779, Jenner took material from the sore of Sarah Nelmes, a milkmaid who had cowpox, and scratched it onto the arm of a boy, James Phipps. In an experiment that would be considered completely unethical today, the boy was later inoculated with smallpox. He did not develop the disease, and Jenner's experiment was repeated on others with similarly successful results. Thus, the practice of vaccination became widespread, although it was a very different procedure from that practised today. Material was scratched from arm to arm among vaccines without any antiseptic precautions, and complications were thus common.

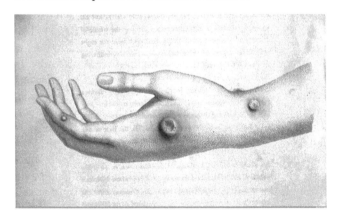

The hand of Sarah Nelmes infected with the cowpox.

Source: From Jenner, E. *An Inquiry into the Causes and Effects of the Variolae Vaccinae.* London: Low, 1798.

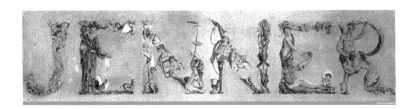

Aesculapius sending Hygeia to all parts of the globe Jenner's discovery of vaccination. Watercolour by Paytherus, 1815.

Despite its obvious historical importance and success in retrospect, Jenner's discovery was not universally accepted at the time. In many quarters of the medical establishment, he was bitterly denounced as a charlatan. Jenner had earlier been elected to the Royal Society as a Fellow following the publication of a treatise on the natural history of the cuckoo. Yet the Royal Society showed little interest in his cowpox discovery. It was many years before Jenner received his just professional and public acclaim for a discovery that became, and has remained, a principal weapon in the battle against disease in all corners of the world. Historical documents show that some years before Jenner advanced his theory, a Dorset farmer, Benjamin Jesty, had observed that milk-maids did not appear to get smallpox and had inoculated his own family with cowpox. Whatever the originality of Jenner's role in discovering the protective power of cowpox, he certainly wrote it up in a proper scientific account and history has accorded him the undisputed status as father of vaccination.

A statue of Jenner used to stand on the fourth plinth in Trafalgar Square in London. It was moved to Kensington Gardens, a less prominent place, where it still stands. Apparently, it was considered 'insufficiently militaristic'. It is a great irony that the person whose work has probably saved more lives than anyone else in human history should have such little public prominence.

Pasteur and the rabid dogs

Almost a century later, a further great advance was made in knowledge of how to protect the host against disease. Louis Pasteur (1822–1895) – who had developed techniques for immunization of animals against anthrax – turned his attention to rabies in humans. Rabies, frequently a disease of dogs, was one of the most feared diseases because of its universal fatality. At different periods in history, it had been attributed to the sun, the weather or the Dog Star. Although existing technology meant that he could not see or produce a free culture of the rabies virus, Pasteur reasoned that it existed in the saliva and nervous system of infected animals and was the mode of transmission of the disease. He attenuated material from infected animals by desiccation and then injected the material into other animals.

In July 1885, a mother from Alsace brought her nine-year-old son, Joseph Meister, to Pasteur's laboratory. The child, while walking to school alone, had been pounced on and bitten 14 times by a mad dog. Pasteur was a chemist, not a physician, and he consulted with his medical colleagues as to whether his success in the immunization of animals against rabies justified using it on a human being. It was decided that the child faced almost certain death, and thus a 10-day course of immunization was begun. The child survived, and Pasteur allowed himself the following excess of emotion when he wrote to his family: 'Perhaps one of the great medical facts of the century is going to take place; you would regret not having seen it!'

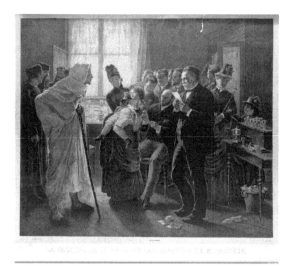

Rabies vaccination in Pasteur's clinic in Paris. Lithograph by F. Piroden after L-L Gsell, 1887.

Pasteur had further success with another celebrated case. A shepherd boy, Jean-Baptiste Jupille, had fought off a rabid dog that had been terrorizing a group of children. He had been badly mauled. Six days after the attack, Pasteur treated him with his new vaccine. The 14-year-old shepherd boy survived. Pasteur was the subject of criticism from many sections of the scientific and medical establishment who did not accept his claims. But as with Jenner, Pasteur's contribution to public health would turn out to be lasting and immense. A new era in preventive medicine had dawned.

Other developments

Jenner and Pasteur had used vaccines based on attenuated forms of live infective agents. Other researchers developed vaccines based on killed organisms. A leading figure in this work was Almroth Wright (1861–1947). He was appointed professor of pathology in the British Army Medical Services. He developed a killed vaccine against typhoid.

Another strand of research led to the treatment and prevention of diseases that involve toxins. The use of the antitoxin from the late nineteenth century onwards led to major reductions in the case fatality rate from diphtheria, and the later development of the toxoid-based vaccine began to prevent the disease. The approach to tetanus followed a similar pattern. Before the use of an antitoxin, the case fatality rate for tetanus was around 85%. The infection was a serious problem among injured troops, depending on the nature of the battlefield and the quality of surgical treatment of wounds. In the early months of the First World War, the incidence of tetanus in the British army was 8 cases per 1000 men; 85% died. Antitoxin became available, and by 1918, the incidence had fallen to 0.6 per 1000. The passive prophylaxis was important, but the real advance came through active immunization with toxoid. It was ready for use by the

Second World War; there were hardly any cases of tetanus in men who had been inoculated.

Other vaccines – live attenuated, killed and toxoid – were developed against a wide range of diseases throughout the twentieth century.

The importance of devices to deliver vaccines must not be overlooked. Alexander Wood (1817–84), a lecturer at Edinburgh University, pioneered the first hypodermic syringe in the United Kingdom. The importance of refrigeration in storing and transporting vaccines, particularly in tropical climates, was another vital development.

In 1853, vaccination of infants was made compulsory in the United Kingdom by an act of Parliament, with penalties for refusal. The 1867 *Vaccination Act* extended compulsory vaccination to the under-14s. Public attitudes began to turn negative, with large public protests against vaccination policy and the formation of the Anti-Vaccination League. A new act of Parliament in 1898 allowed refusal and the nonenforcement of penalties. This has parallels in modern antivaccine movements around the world and, in the United Kingdom, with the crisis of confidence in the MMR vaccine in the 1990s.

BEGINNING TO MEASURE HEALTH AND DISEASE

The 1830s was the period when interest in statistical description of the population began to surge. As the English historian George Young put it, 'It was the business of the [eighteen] thirties to transfer the treatment of affairs from a polemical to a statistical basis, from Humbug to Humdrum. In 1830, there were hardly any figures to work on. Even the census was far from perfect'.

The creation of statistical societies in London and other cities was inspired by the visit to Britain of Adolphe Quetelet (1796–1874), a Belgian astronomer and statistician, who spoke at a meeting of the British Association for the Advancement of Science in 1833.

John Graunt and the Bills of Mortality

The earliest systematic gathering of population statistics is largely due to the pioneering work of John Graunt (1620–74). He was 'a haberdasher of small wares' whose polymathic curiosity saw him elected a fellow of the Royal Society at the age of 43 years while remaining an important city tradesman. Graunt established a system of compiling data on the number of christenings, burials and causes of death under 60 categories. Information on the deaths was collected by 'searchers', who were often elderly women who would ask the attending doctor for cause of death information; if it was not forthcoming, they would ascribe it themselves. The Bills of Mortality were published and sold as broadsheets every week.

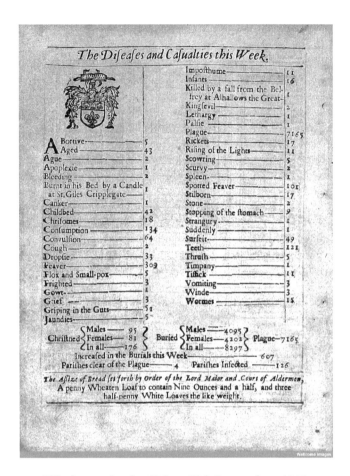

Bill of mortality for 12th to 19th September, 1665.

They listed, for the London parishes, the numbers and (in a crude fashion) causes of death. Well-to-do people purchased them to forewarn themselves of an outbreak of the plague and forsake the city for less hazardous surroundings. No age of death was recorded, nor was there any information on the size of the population. Many of the causes of death make curious reading; for example, in 1660, 249 deaths were attributed to 'Rising of the Lights', a condition that has no apparent modern disease equivalent.

Graunt was a friend and collaborator of another pioneering seventeenth-century statistician: William Petty (1623–87). He was a cabin boy, joined the Royal Navy, studied medicine and sought out the company of mathematicians. From this melting pot of experience and scholarship, Petty rose to be a professor of anatomy at Oxford University, a professor of music, an inventor and a landowner in Ireland where he did much of his work. He is credited as being one of the fathers of modern economics. He devised and used statistical indices to describe a country's economy.

William Farr and the General Register Office

From the seventeenth-century beginnings of vital statistics, William Farr (1807–83) took the concept to a new level when he was appointed as compiler of abstracts (in effect chief medical statistician) in the Registrar General's Office. Farr was the son of a Shropshire farm labourer. He went on to escape his poor upbringing largely due to the patronage of the man to whom he was apprenticed and who recognized his talent. He was given a medical education in Paris and London. In his national role, he built a lasting system of data collection of vital statistics amenable to epidemiological surveillance. His rigorous analyses were one of the engines of the great sanitary reforms in Victorian Britain. He produced regular reports highlighting the appalling levels of mortality, the health inequalities and some of the stark geographical and social variations in disease and death. His statistical techniques were not sophisticated by modern standards, but they galvanized attention on the problems they depicted. His letters that accompanied the *Annual Reports of the Registrar General* enabled him to get to the heart of the sanitary reform movement and influence change. He also introduced major improvements to government statistics, bringing a greater health dimension into the data gathered in the census, introducing a classification of occupations and devising a disease nosology that was the forerunner to the *International Classification of Diseases*. He was disappointed to be passed over when the Registrar General's post became vacant, retired and died three years later. William Farr's story does not have the romance of Snow's or the drama of Chadwick's, but he is without question one of the giants of public health history.

Florence Nightingale: The passionate statistician

Florence Nightingale (1820–1910) established a record-keeping system during her time in the Crimea that allowed her to calculate mortality rates in the hospitals. Later, she used these statistical data to create a polar area diagram (she called these Coxscombs) to depict mortality graphically during the Crimean War. One of the remarkable qualities of her multifaceted life was her ability to compile, analyse, interpret and use statistics in health. This was extraordinarily innovative for the time and made an impact on members of Parliament and civil servants who would not have bothered much with traditional statistical reports. When she returned from the Crimea, she sought out William Farr to provide help in the statistical basis of her campaign to improve the sanitary condition of the army and hospitals. They became firm and fast friends and worked together for the remainder of their lives. Miss Nightingale remained passionate about statistics until her death.

OCCUPATIONAL DISEASE

The possibility that factors in one's occupation could be a cause of illness and disease was largely ignored in ancient writings, despite the grim and inhuman working conditions that often prevailed, such as those endured in the quest for valuable metals in the mines of ancient Egypt, Greece or Rome. After the Renaissance, there emerged a man who

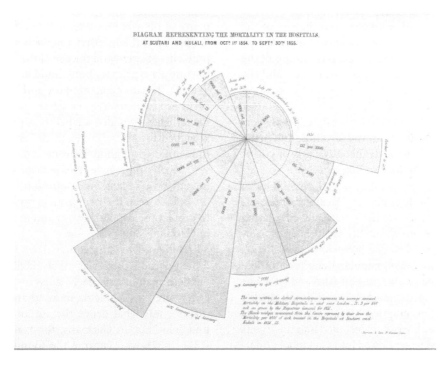

"Cocks-comb" diagram showing mortality in the hospitals at Scutari and Kulali 1854–1855.

Source: Nightingale F. A *Contribution to the Sanitary History of the British Army during the Late War with Russia*. London: Harrison, 1859.

is generally regarded as the father of occupational medicine: Bernardino Ramazzini (1633–1714). His *De Morbis Artificium*, published in about 1700, was a systematic study of diseases arising from occupational factors. When he recommended in his writings that, in addition to other questions and examinations, the doctor should ask the patient, 'What is your occupation?' he could scarcely have realized the enormous importance of his words.

Subsequently, occupational medicine has had a long and distinguished history. Discoveries such as Percival Pott's observation in 1775 of the occurrence of scrotal cancer in chimney sweeps as a result of persistent contact with soot, or of the cerebral effects of mercury poisoning in the hat-making trade (the basis of Lewis Carroll's Mad Hatter), opened new vistas when considering possible causes of disease.

SANITARY REFORM

Excavations of the ancient world show that several civilizations had developed systems of water supply and sanitation. Archaeologists have discovered drains and sewers, from 4000 years ago, in what is now northern India. In ancient Troy, there is evidence of sewers, as well as water pipes to homes. The Greeks firmly established sanitation as part of the infrastructure of their cities. With the Roman Empire came further advances, notably the network of aqueducts that carried piped water from more remote sources, avoiding nearby rivers that were heavily polluted. At the height of the empire, 14 aqueducts were functioning, supplying 100 gallons per head of population. Senior figures were appointed to oversee these projects, creating forerunners of the municipal officials of modern times.

With the fall of the Roman Empire, and the rise of the Barbarians, all of this disintegrated and it was more than a thousand years before there was any real recognition of the importance to health and longevity of clean water and the effective disposal of sewage and other waste. The sanitary successes and innovations of the Romans were dependent on a strong State or (in the case of cities) municipal authority identifying or stimulating technical advances and being able to implement them. Such advanced systems of governance disappeared with the Roman Empire.

Sir John Harington (1561–1612), a godson of Queen Elizabeth I, invented the first flushing lavatory. He was a courtier, periodically exiled by the Queen for circulating salacious poems. He wrote about his creation in *A New Discussion on a Stale Subject: The Metamorphosis of Ajax* (the last word a pun on 'jakes', popular slang for a toilet). He installed a prototype in his house in Bath and later one in the Queen's palace in Richmond. This did not quickly replace the chamber pot, emptied by the servants of the wealthy and the middle classes and decanted into the streets by the poor. The flushed water flowed into a cesspool underneath Harington's contraption. This prankster and mediocre poet deserves his place in this particularly English strand of public health history, but it was not until the emergence

of the S-bend that the contribution of lavatorial design to the advancement of sanitation took hold.

Considering the physical measures necessary to establish good sanitation is too narrow a focus for understanding the scope of the action required. It is the condition of the population that is so fundamental. A major figure in eighteenth-century public health was Johann Peter Frank (1745–1821). His influence in promoting understanding and the case for action is best exemplified by an extract from a lecture that he gave in 1790 at the University of Pavia, where he was professor of medicine and later dean:

> Starvation and sickness are pictured on the face of the entire labouring class. You recognize it at first sight. And whoever has seen it will certainly not call any one of these people a free man. The word has become meaningless. Before sunrise, after having eaten a little and always the same unfermented bread that appeases his hunger only half-way, the farmer gets ready for hard work. With emaciated body under the hot rays of the sun he plows a soil that is not his and cultivates a vine that for him alone has no reward. His arms fall down, his dry tongue sticks to the palate, hunger is consuming him.

Frank also held the post of director general of public health for his province and made extensive surveys of the health of the population and the distribution of facilities. He developed a groundbreaking five-year medical curriculum involving clinical attachments for students. He later moved to Vienna. Frank is not always seen as one of the key figures in the history of public health for a number of reasons: many of his writings were not translated, he came before the period of the Industrial Revolution and the acute health problems of cities, and the use of the German word *polizy* in the title of his primary book could be translated as 'policy' or 'police'. The latter conveyed the authoritarian idea of 'medical police', which was not representative of Frank's ideas but nevertheless provided a label to attribute to him. His book stretched to nine volumes in the end and was immensely influential throughout Europe. The breadth of his vision was deeply impressive. He describes in his autobiography how, as a young man, he saw his future goals as 'to teach rulers how to keep their subjects in good health, to draft laws to protect the people's health and to write a comprehensive book on the subject'.

As the nineteenth century dawned, and advanced to its fourth decade, there was an awakening to the significance of these matters and early steps towards reform. The fear engendered by cholera, more than any other epidemic disease, was what drove the authorities across Europe to find solutions. In Germany, for example, Rudolf Virchow (1821–1902), who became the founder of modern pathology, was in 1948 at the forefront of progressive thinking on the nation's state of health: 'Medicine is a social science', he said, 'and politics are nothing else than medicine on a large scale'. However, he was later a staunch opponent of the germ theory of disease.

In Britain, the conditions for the spread of disease were seen everywhere: poverty, overcrowded dwellings, polluted drinking water, streets flowing with sewage, domestic waste piling high and factories churning out noxious by-products. It took strong leadership, meticulous investigation and imaginative public reports to bring about change.

At the centre of this change was Edwin Chadwick (1800–90), a Victorian whose long life spanned the battle of Waterloo, the Corn Laws and the arrival of the Great Western Railway. Chadwick was a disciple of the high priest of utilitarianism, Jeremy Bentham, and acted as his secretary for a time. Chadwick had little regard for the individual and was a centralist, never happier than when manning the levers of command and control. As a junior civil servant, Chadwick had visited slums throughout England and seen for himself the conditions that people lived in; he had listened to and heard evidence gathered by those who shared his concerns. As a result, he strongly promoted the *sanitary idea*, though from a miasmatist standpoint. His efforts led to a Sanitary Commission in 1839, which reported in 1842. The report *The Sanitary Conditions of the Labouring Population of Great Britain* was a landmark in public health and – looking back – one of the most important documents in British history. It pointed to the importance of increasing the provision of a pure water supply, effective sanitation, drainage and disposal of sewage and improved standards of housing. Anthony Wohl, in his book on public health in Victorian England, memorably describes Chadwick's report: 'He skilfully wove the most lurid details, evocative descriptions, damning statistics, and damaging examples into a masterpiece of protest literature'.

One paragraph in the report stands out:

That for the general means necessary to prevent disease, it would be good economy to appoint

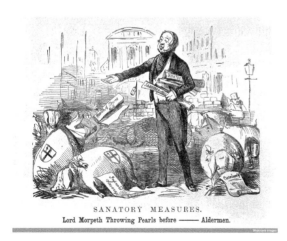

SANATORY MEASURES.
Lord Morpeth Throwing Pearls before —— Aldermen.

Cartoon of Lord Morpeth, mover of the Health of Towns Bill, throwing the bill before swine representing the Aldermen of the City of London. Engraving. Punch, 1848.

a district medical officer, independent of private practice, with the securities of special qualifications and responsibilities to initiate sanitary measures and reclaim the execution of the law.

This was the birth of the key post of medical officer of health. The first local authority to move on this was Liverpool. After a great deal of preparatory work, Parliament established the *Liverpool Sanitary Act 1846*, the first comprehensive sanitary act to come into law. It gave approval for the appointment of a medical officer of health. William Henry Duncan (1805–63) was appointed to this post. He worked with a very small department and confronted the major problems of filth, overcrowded dwellings and epidemic fevers with great determination. His work would not have been possible without two other new posts: the borough engineer (to design new municipal waterworks and sewerage systems) and the inspector of nuisances (to identify polluting houses and industries). As if these challenges were not enough, Duncan had to contend with the fallout from the Irish potato famine. Some 300,000 starving and destitute Irish people landed in Liverpool, placing intolerable pressure on slums already bursting at the seams. Duncan served for 16 years, eventually dying in office, and helped bring about improvements to the health of Liverpudlians. Like Chadwick, he remained firmly wedded to the causal influence of the miasma, but this did not detract from the appropriateness of the action that he recommended. William Henry Duncan set the standard for medical officers of health that were to follow him.

The *Public Health Act* of 1848 came next. It established a new national body, the General Board of Health, and permitted the establishment of local sanitary authorities. After the appointment of the country's first medical officer of health in Liverpool, in 1847, other local authorities followed suit. However, the 1848 act was fundamentally flawed because it was essentially permissive, with very few coercive powers. Many towns ignored this call for sanitary reform until forced to pay attention to it by the later Public Health Acts of 1872 and 1875. This included measures such as the municipalization of private water companies and the installation of sewers, public baths and wash houses.

Cholera, the malevolent driving force of sanitary reform, plunged the public health administration into virtual chaos during the devastating epidemic of 1848–49. In the earlier 1832 epidemic, the Privy Council had determined government policy and, with a contagionist philosophy, had placed heavy reliance on quarantine. With cholera sweeping through Europe in 1848, Chadwick was having none of this and focused his preparatory attention on filth, cesspools and sewers. He persuaded the government to transfer responsibility for the impending arrival of cholera on British shores from the Privy Council to the Board of Health. A 'cholera bill', the *Nuisances Removal Act*, was passed by Parliament and gave extraordinary powers to the Board. Tensions rose immediately; the *Lancet* called the Board 'a buccaneering piracy against medicine'. When the epidemic came,

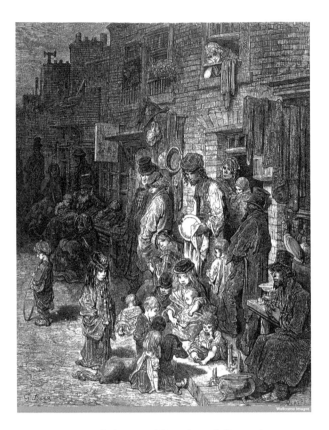

Wentworth Street, Whitechapel. Engraving. Gustave Dore, 1872.

the Board's preventive measures to remove filth had not been carried out in many local areas and the policy of house-to-house visits of cholera victims was largely abandoned by local Boards of Guardians. Chadwick made the disastrous decision to begin in March 1848 to flush out the sewers that drained into the Thames. The practice continued into the summer of 1849. Through this misguided miasmatist decision, he unleashed a waterborne disease on the population of London. Monthly mortality increased from 246 in June to 1952 in July to 4251 in August to 6644 in September. Still, there was no recognition of the true nature of the disease. Following through after the epidemic had passed, the Board of Health renewed its sanitary improvements, the right policy for the wrong reasons. The Board was soon abolished.

Chadwick was arguably the most important figure in the sanitary revolution. Fiercely determined, an unremitting advocate for reform, he was able to command and dominate this field of public policy. As his biographer S E Finer wrote, 'His religion was the public good'. Counterbalancing this ability to upend the status quo of an establishment firmly committed to maintaining it were deep character flaws that tragically became his undoing. Arrogant, egotistical and thin skinned, he was quick to form an opinion that immediately became unshakeable. Finer also said, 'Although when his mind was open, it was more open than most, it was never open for very long'. Chadwick was pensioned off in 1854 at the age of 54 years. In his long retirement (he died at the age of 90 years), he continued to write, speak, sit on committees

and preside over learned societies. Towards the end of his long life, he received many honours in recognition of the enormity of his contribution to public health and the health of the nation.

As Chadwick's influence was removed, the mantle of sanitary reform was taken on by others. Notable among them was Sir John Simon (1816–1904). He had been the first medical officer of health for the city of London. It was his appointment as medical officer to the General Board of Health in 1855 and shortly after as the first medical officer to the Privy Council that made him the country's first chief medical officer. Essentially, with Chadwick gone, he was the most senior public health figure in the country. Simon's determination to pursue the sanitary ideal was as strong as Chadwick's, but he had the ease of manner, the persuasive powers and the ability to work the political system that the former had lacked. He served for 21 years and oversaw the introduction and implementation of public health acts and a strong system of vaccination. In his early reports, he criticized the conditions of the female factory labourer and the difficulty she had in sustaining healthy motherhood. He spoke of 'Herodian' districts of the major industrial towns and cities where infant mortality was very high. He broadened and deepened the scope of national public health. Other chief medical officers were to follow, but Simon's health legacy for the country was immense.

The application of sanitary techniques to combat infection in clinical practice followed a similarly difficult path as sanitary reform had, in which pioneers were attacked and vilified. Ignaz Phillipp Semmelweis (1818–65) was a Hungarian obstetrician with an enquiring mind. He found himself as an assistant in the maternity wards at the Vienna General Hospital. He noticed the differences in rates of death due to puerperal sepsis in the ward purely used for training of midwives compared with the ward in which medical students were trained. The latter had much higher death rates. Semmelweis reasoned that the medical students coming from dissecting cadavers in the postmortem room were contaminating the women. He instituted a practice of ensuring that they cleaned their hands with chloride of lime and the death rate plummeted. Far from being lauded for saving lives, Semmelweis met a wall of hostility and denial from senior figures in the hospital, particularly his head of department. His assistantship was not renewed. He went back to his native Hungary where he became a director of service in Budapest. He instituted similar measures and achieved major reductions in deaths. He met with similar hostility and eventually was incarcerated in an asylum where he died at the age of 47 years. In fact, the American physician, poet and author Oliver Wendell Holmes (1809–94) had made a similar observation some years before Semmelweis. As a result, he read a paper, *The Contagiousness of Puerperal Fever*, before the Boston Society for Medical Improvement in 1843. He was also ridiculed, but Holmes was a major public figure through his writing and could not be crushed so easily. He lived to see his idea vindicated and also brought the contribution of Semmelweis to wide attention. Today, the two of them are recorded as the fathers of the hand hygiene movement.

Florence Nightingale (1820–1910) was not just the architect and inspiration of modern nursing but also became a major figure in public health and Victorian society. Her wider role stemmed from her time in the Scutari Hospital during the Crimean War where, through her nightly rounds, she was immortalized as the 'Lady with the Lamp'. She was asked to go to the Crimea by the British government as a result of a public outcry about the conditions of the wounded soldiers in the hospital. In 1854, she took a group of more than 30 nurses from England. What she encountered there was a seething cesspit, not worthy to be called a hospital. The building was overcrowded, men lay dying on straw-lined floors and basic supplies, such as sheets and medical equipment, were seriously lacking. There was no adequate ventilation. Standards of sanitation were appalling. The wounded soldiers arriving from the front line were emaciated, had infected wounds, were often infested with lice and suffering cholera or dysentery and were frostbitten. They died in large numbers due to these conditions, more than from the wounds that they had sustained in battle.

Women were set to work scrubbing floors and walls. A house at Scutari was converted to a laundry so that patients could have a clean shirt twice a week. Miss Nightingale introduced other practical measures, such as placing a screen around a patient being amputated to avoid distressing the soldier's comrades.

Conditions at the temporary barracks hospital were so lethal because of overcrowding, as well as defective sewers and lack of ventilation. A sanitary commission was sent by the British government to Scutari in March 1855, almost six months after she had arrived. It brought about flushing of the sewers and improvements to ventilation. Death rates were significantly reduced. During the war, Florence Nightingale was not completely convinced that poor hygiene was the predominant cause of death. She continued to believe the death rates were due to poor nutrition and supplies and overworking of the soldiers.

When she returned home and assessed the evidence, she came to believe that most of the soldiers at the hospital were killed by poor hygiene. Her change of thinking was heavily influenced by Dr William Farr, the superintendent of the Statistical Department of the Registrar General's Office. She advocated sanitary living conditions at every opportunity. As a result, she helped reduce deaths in the army during peacetime and turned her attention to the sanitary design of hospitals. Like Chadwick, though, she was a miasmatist. It was not until 1867 that she accepted that germs caused disease and renewed her championship of cleanliness and hygiene.

Once the germ theory had started to gain wider acceptance, the practical applications of the work were quickly realized. Joseph (later Lord) Lister (1827–1912) became Regius Professor of Surgery in Glasgow in 1860. Lister was greatly troubled by the high rates of septicaemia and death that were endemic to the surgical wards. The case fatality rate after operations on the limbs ranged from 25% to 50%. Gangrene was commonplace. Cleanliness was not a fundamental value of surgical practice at that time. Surgeons would not clean their hands between patients, instruments would be reused and wounds would be handled without gloves, gowns or masks. A professor of chemistry in the university drew Lister's attention to the work of Pasteur. Lister immediately recognized its importance. He used carbolic acid to clean dirty wounds and as a spray during his operations. He read a paper, *The Antiseptic Principle in Surgery*, to a meeting in 1867. He met criticism and resistance, but this was eventually overcome. Lister achieved remarkable reductions in mortality. His ideas founded the modern methods of antisepsis that transformed hospital wards from places where virtually every postoperative patient became septic and developed fever.

ORIGINS OF A SYSTEM OF HEALTHCARE

The development of services for the sick, aged and infirm in Britain is entangled with the attitudes of society towards the poor at various points in history. Sickness and old age are often strongly associated with poverty.

Much of the responsibility for the poor, aged and sick in medieval Britain fell on the church and on parishes.

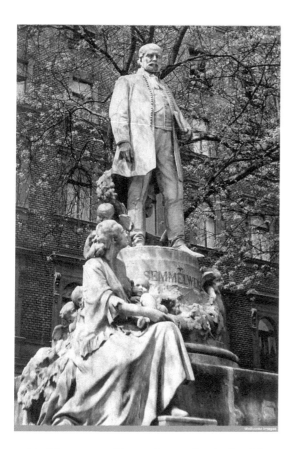

Marble statue of Ignaz Semmelweis. Strobl.

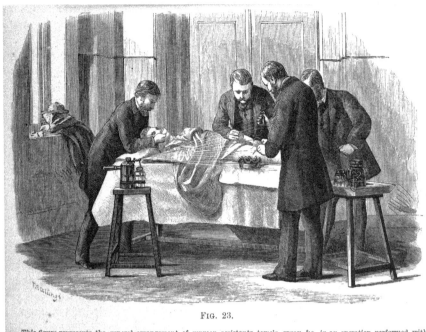

FIG. 23.

This figure represents the general arrangement of surgeon, assistants, towels, spray, &c., in an operation performed with complete aseptic precautions. The distance of the spray from the wound, the arrangement of the wet towels, the position of the trough containing the instruments, the position of the small dish with the lotion, the position of the house surgeon and dresser, so that the former always has his hands in the cloud of the spray, and the latter hands the instruments into the spray and various other points, are shown.

Use of the Lister carbolic spray.

Source: Cheyne WW. *Antiseptic Surgery: its Principles, Practice, History and Results.* London: Smith Elder and co, 1882.

They levied local taxes to provide relief. The dissolution of the monasteries and religious fraternities by Henry VIII meant severe hardship for large numbers of elderly and sick people who were left with no means of support. Many individual items of legislation passed during the reign of Elizabeth I were rationalized in 1601 with the passage of the Elizabethan Poor Law (most commonly referred to as the *Old Poor Law*). Under this law, parishes were responsible for ensuring that the impotent poor (e.g. the old or sick) were cared for in poorhouses or almshouses, while the able-bodied paupers were provided with work in houses of correction.

From the 1760s, purpose-built workhouses began to be provided, financed by the Poor Rate. Much of the responsibility for the administration of the Old Poor Law rested with individual local parishes in the form of parish overseers. While tyranny undoubtedly existed, there were also many examples of caring parishes, and by the early nineteenth century, the Poor Law was seen as the largest branch of public administration. Many parishes found it necessary to create some kind of organized system for the relief of the sick poor. Parishes tended to contract with surgeons and apothecaries to provide them with services.

Dissatisfaction with the Old Poor Law mounted for two main reasons. First, the law was proving an increasingly costly exercise. The system of *outdoor relief*, which gave payments in cash or kind to the poor, was becoming widespread in many parishes. However, because of the economic problems of the time, the size of the pool of such needy individuals and their families had grown. Second, some critics considered that the

regimes in houses of correction were too comfortable for their inmates. This climate of opinion led ultimately to the establishment of the Royal Commission of Inquiry into the Poor Law and to the subsequent *Poor Law Amendment Act 1834* (the *New Poor Law*). Edwin Chadwick was again at the centre of this reform and intimately involved in the framing and implementation of the legislation. Chadwick had made detailed calculations in the early nineteenth century of various costs of crime, disease and poverty that society had to bear. It was this economic motivation that helped to persuade Parliament of the need for legislation.

Given the belief in some political and ideological circles that the old system of poor relief and the condition of the houses of correction was actually encouraging idleness and pauperism, the New Poor Law of 1834 set out largely to do away with pauperism by measures based on deterrence. The system of outdoor relief for the poor was abolished. Those in need of support had to apply for it and were offered the workhouse. The workhouse regime was harsh and austere, deliberately designed to pose a very unattractive prospect for those applying for poor relief. By this central tenet of *less eligibility* (the person receiving poor relief could not be better off than the worst-paid independent worker), it was reasoned that only those who were truly needy would accept poor relief in the form of the workhouse. In short, the new law was designed to savagely reduce the number of claimants and so dramatically reduce costs. Under the New Poor Law, responsibility was taken out of the hands of some 15,000 individual parishes, which were instead grouped together as 643 Poor Law unions (administered by Boards of Guardians) and placed under the control of a central board headed by three Poor Law Commissioners. The aim was to introduce a uniform process of administration. Although separate provision was laid down for the sick and aged, in practice few unions allowed themselves the expensive luxury of separate workhouses, and in many mixed workhouses, the able-bodied pauper rubbed shoulders with the sick, the old and infirm, the disabled, children and the mentally ill.

Edwin Chadwick, by then secretary to the Poor Law Commissioners reviewed the impact of his supposed reforms and was shocked to find that far from poverty being a product of idleness, much of it arose from illness and disease. Public funding was then used to establish workhouse infirmaries. Although the Poor Law authorities stipulated that each union had to employ a properly qualified medical practitioner, they were poorly paid and under the control of the lay administrators, who decided on all applications for medical relief. Thus, it was in the interest of such relieving officers to turn down applications from sick paupers for relief and so save a doctor's fee. Initially, there were two types of medical officer: a district medical officer and a workhouse medical officer. Both provided services, and some of the remuneration was on an item of service basis. For example, a district medical officer could be paid £5 for the amputation of a leg, arm or foot, or for operating on a strangulated hernia. If the patient died within 36 hours, the fee was usually halved.

Standards within workhouses were pitifully inadequate, with overcrowding and insanitary conditions prevailing. Other inmates carried out much of the nursing. Moreover, the crux of the problem was still that the law implied poverty was a result of idleness or waywardness on the part of the individual. Florence Nightingale commented that these civilian hospitals were just as bad as, or worse than, the squalid military hospitals that she so strongly condemned in the Crimean War. Towards the end of the nineteenth century, conditions had become so appalling that Parliament authorized the building of separate infirmaries with trained medical and nursing staff.

Local authority hospitals

In addition to the Poor Law medical service, the major local authorities (county and borough councils) provided a separate publicly owned system of hospitals that had its origins in the isolation hospitals for infectious diseases constructed from the 1860s onwards and in the asylums for the mentally ill and handicapped. By the early part of the twentieth century, in many regions of the country, local authority (municipal) hospitals were also treating other, more general illnesses. Following the transfer of the powers and responsibilities of the Poor Law to local government by a further act of Parliament in 1929, the local authorities were allowed to take control of and administer the Poor Law infirmaries. The local authority hospitals fell mainly under the jurisdiction of the medical officer of health, who delegated responsibility

in each hospital to a medical superintendent. This achieved some degree of unity in hospital services, although many local authorities were slow to take up this opportunity.

Voluntary hospitals

The main alternative to the publicly owned hospital system was the voluntary hospital movement. Some of the earliest hospitals, such as St Thomas' Hospital in London, began life as religious institutions in the Middle Ages. However, there was a surge in hospital building from the middle of the eighteenth century, financed from donations, charitable funds and subscriptions. Mostly these were established to cater for the *deserving poor*, with the *undeserving poor* continuing to look to their local poorhouse for care. The bulk of medical care before the twentieth century took place outside institutions.

Over time, the size and function of the voluntary hospitals began to vary greatly as they became one of the main foci for medical practice. They often provided a standard of care that was far above that provided by the State, and indeed served as a model that the latter strove to attain. Each voluntary hospital had its own committee of lay governors, and originally they decided which patients deserved to be admitted. Visiting physicians and surgeons provided medical care; they were almost always in private practice and gave their services to the voluntary hospitals free of charge, as the prestige of a hospital affiliation enabled them to build up their practices.

The voluntary hospital system encompassed a wide variety of funding and administrative arrangements. Patients who could afford to pay were often asked to do so, while others provided themselves with some security for illness by making weekly payments to one of the hospital contributory schemes. As the involvement of the medical profession in the voluntary hospitals grew with the flourishing of teaching and research, so their function began to alter. Admission policies were selective, with an emphasis on patients with illnesses that were of a short term or acute in nature, thus ensuring a rapid turnover, or those with diseases that were of particular interest. There was little place for the elderly or chronically sick. Children, the mentally ill, those with infectious diseases and pregnant women were usually refused entry. Although some charitable specialist hospitals were formed in the late nineteenth century to meet these demands, the emphasis of traditional voluntary hospitals on acute medicine was partly responsible for the extension of the publicly owned hospital service to fill the gap.

Voluntary hospitals were hard hit by the economic depression of the period between World War I and World War II. Many were brought to the brink of insolvency by the increasing salaries paid to resident medical and nursing staff despite falling revenue and more demand for expensive services. Means testing for patients brought in some additional income, as did the Hospital Saturday and Sunday Funds. By the late 1930s, the voluntary hospitals were increasingly relying on income from treating patients funded by local authorities.

Hospitals became safer places in which to be treated following the introduction of anaesthesia and antiseptic practices in the nineteenth century. The development of new medical technology such as X-rays meant that middle- and upper-class patients were increasingly required to have their treatment in hospitals rather than in their homes. Many of the voluntary hospitals responded to this new demand by creating private beds, where patients paid fully for their treatment. By the interwar period, hospitals were beginning to lose the social stigma they once held and were increasingly seen as resources for the whole population.

Emergency medical service

As part of the preparation for the anticipated receipt of military and civilian casualties during World War II, a hospital service was created in 1938 to be administered directly by the Ministry of Health (which had been formed in 1919). The number of beds in some hospitals was increased, temporary buildings were erected, or premises extended, and some of the former Poor Law institutions were renovated or upgraded. Some centres were created with specialist facilities, such as rehabilitation, plastic surgery and neurosurgery, and the ministry laid down what the functions of the existing hospitals should be on a regional basis.

The emergency medical service is of considerable importance in the development of the National Health Service in Britain. Although its influence was short, in the context of the long period of evolution of the service it represented a watershed for hospitals. It resulted in the review and classification of all hospitals provided by the wide variety of agencies, and it brought their administration for the first time under a central authority, the Ministry of Health. This laid the foundation for the unified hospital service: the voluntary hospitals, the workhouse infirmaries and the various types of local authority hospital came together. When the National Health Service subsequently came into being in July 1948, three years after the war had ended, the unification of the hospitals held firm.

Primary care

Medical services for those who did not receive care in hospital were slower to evolve. Under the Poor Law, domiciliary care or treatment by the Poor Law medical officer existed in some parts of the country, but the standard was very variable and care generally very basic. Other forms of care were provided by a variety of other agencies, such as free dispensaries run on charitable lines or outpatient departments within voluntary hospitals. Dispensaries performed a vital medical service from the early nineteenth century. As well as dispensing medicines, they offered basic diagnostic and medical treatment for poorer people. The medical officers attached to dispensaries carried out home visits, and they were an important source of information on the prevalence of infectious diseases in communities. Other developments during the nineteenth century provided private panel

systems or clubs where, by paying a retention fee, the patient could claim the services of a doctor in time of need. Friendly societies and a few industries operated similar schemes.

The *National Health Insurance Act 1911 (the Lloyd George Act)* was the most influential development in primary care. The scheme was directed at relieving hardship among working men during periods of illness. When it was implemented in 1912, it was confined to workers earning less than £160 per year and it was based on contributions from the employee, the employer and the state. It entitled the insured man to choose his own general practitioner from a local panel of doctors (hence the term *panel system*) and to secure treatment (including prescribed drugs) and other consultations free of charge on demand. The exclusion of dependent wives and children from the scheme, together with the denial of the right of insured people to receive free hospital inpatient care, meant that considerable hardship was left untouched. Moreover, a sizeable proportion of the population still paid a fee to their general practitioner for advice or treatment.

This system continued (although the eligibility was subsequently increased) until the National Health Service was established in 1948. Until then, general practitioner services were administered throughout the country by a network of insurance committees responsible for making available these services for all insured people in their locality, representing almost half of the population.

Asylums and care of the mentally ill

In the Dark and Middle Ages, the treatment of mental illness was governed by ignorance and superstition. If the mentally ill had delusions of a religious nature, they were often revered; if their utterances were blasphemous, they were possessed by demons and treated, in the first instance, through exorcism by a priest or subjected to physical restraint, pain and degradation. In Britain alone, thousands of women and children, many of whom must have had mental illnesses, were subjected to the ducking stool or burned at the stake as witches. The last woman to meet her death in this way did so in Scotland in 1722.

In the early years of the eighteenth century, a number of singularly unpleasant fates could befall the person who was mentally ill, depending on the circumstances in which they found themselves. There was then no organized service to provide care for the mentally ill. If the manifestations of their illness led them into the trap of poverty, the pauper lunatic became subject to the conditions of the Poor Law. The law dealt with the vagrant very strictly, and thus the mentally ill who left their own homes to wander abroad as beggars would often find themselves in prison. Similarly, criminal insanity was not recognized. Hence, if a person's mental condition led him to commit a crime, he would be judged by penal law and usually find himself in one of the already crowded prisons. The deep shame attached to mental illness led many poor families, and well-to-do alike, to conceal its presence among their relatives. This led to the practice of keeping 'single lunatics' in remote places. It was not uncommon for a family member to be secured in a cellar like an animal for years at a time. The wealthy escaped the indignity of the workhouse or the prison cell, through one of the private madhouses that proliferated in England at the time. These were run for profit, and the fate of their inmates was scarcely better, and in many cases worse, than that of the pauper lunatic in the workhouse; shackling was commonplace.

Originally founded in 1247, as a priory by the Order of St Mary of Bethlehem, Bethlehem Royal Hospital in London was the largest, and for some time the only, public hospital in England devoted to the care of the insane. It existed largely on public subscriptions. The treatment meted out to inmates was as harsh as that in the private madhouses. The mentally ill were chained in confined surroundings and often subjected to bizarre and whimsical therapies, such as bleeding, purging or the induction of vomiting. Towards the end of the eighteenth century, the general public could be admitted to the hospital and for the fee of one penny amuse themselves by watching the antics of the inmates. The name of the hospital, corrupted in common parlance to *Bedlam*, gave the English language a new word that was synonymous with mindless disorder and chaos.

Discharged patients were given badges to allow them legitimately to exist as beggars without falling foul of the harsh vagrancy laws of the time. These *Toms O'Bedlam* soon found their ranks swelled by impostors who had forged their badges.

At the beginning of the nineteenth century, concern began to grow among a few enlightened reformers, and to a lesser extent in public opinion, about the appalling way in which the mentally ill were treated. In part, this came about through the existence of islands of compassion in the approach to mental illness. Outstanding in this respect was the Quaker, William Tuke (1732–1822), who founded the Retreat at York, where the mentally ill were not manacled and restrained but treated humanely. The success of this venture made a deep impression on attitudes to mental illness and its treatment.

Equally important were the findings of various parliamentary committees of the circumstances of those housed in public asylums and private madhouses. One of the best-known examples is the visit made by the Quaker philanthropist Edward Wakefield (1774–1854), to Bethlehem Hospital. During the visit, he discovered one of the inmates, William Norris, an American marine, who was half naked and chained to the wall in such a way that he could stand up or lie down but not sit. This wretched man had been kept in this way for nine years and by the time he became a *cause celebre* was in the terminal phase of tuberculosis.

Similar discoveries of conditions in private madhouses led to legislation bringing them under licence. Another important advance was the *County Asylums Act 1808,* which recommended that local authorities should build asylum to provide treatment for the mentally ill. The programme

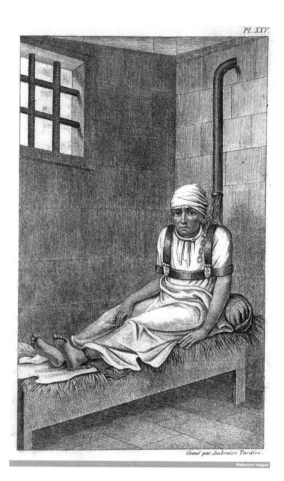

PL.XXV.

William Norris shackled sitting up on his bed at Bedlam. Engraving. Ambroise Tardieu.

Source: Esquirol JED. *Des Maladies Mentales.* Paris: Balliere, 1838.

was not compulsory, and consequently implementation was very slow in most parts of the country. It was designed to cater mainly for the pauper lunatic, who would otherwise have found himself in the workhouse.

The culmination of the reform movement was the passing by *Parliament of the Lunacy Act 1845.* In it, the power of the Lunacy Commissioners was greatly extended so that they were responsible for inspection, licencing and reporting on all places in which the mentally ill were housed or cared for. They were able to investigate and report the circumstances of the mentally ill in prisons and workhouses (which had previously been outside their jurisdiction), as well as in public hospitals, asylums, private madhouses and other licenced premises. Further measures introduced in the Act were the tightening up of procedures for certification of the mentally ill and the compulsory keeping of records by institutions treating them.

During the early years of the twentieth century, the mental hospital, closed and often situated in a remote locality, served a predominantly custodial role, with little attempt to treat mental illness or forge links with the community. One of the first rays of light on this depressing scene was the widespread establishment of psychiatric outpatient clinics, which together with the move towards voluntary admission were by-products of the enlightened *Mental Treatment Act 1930*.

In 1948, mental hospitals, along with other types of hospital, became part of the National Health Service and were no longer the responsibility of the local authorities.

Other local authority services

Although the Poor Law had provided a form of community health service (e.g. for expectant mothers and children), it was patchy and inadequate. During the first 20 years of the twentieth century, the health visitor system was developed and maternity and child welfare clinics were opened. This was welcomed at a time of increasing public and governmental concern about 'national deterioration' – the suggestion that the British were becoming unfit through inherited health conditions and lack of proper health education. It stemmed from a lack of physically fit men among recruits to the army at the time of the Boer War. These concerns were examined in the 1904 report from the government's Interdepartmental Committee on Physical Deterioration. Thus, by 1948, the local authorities not only had responsibility for a large part of the hospital service but also for a whole range of community services. When the National Health Service was established, it continued to be responsible for community services but lost responsibility for hospitals.

The personal social services, which were provided by the local authorities for groups such as the elderly, children and the physically and mentally handicapped, also had diverse origins. In a few cases, services arose from voluntary or charitable organizations; in most others, they arose from the structure of the Poor Law, with its strong orientation towards institutional care. The Liberal government that came into office in 1906 passed a number of important acts, which taken together can be seen as a 'welfare state in embryo'. Their innovations included free school meals and school medical inspections. Although local authorities subsequently assumed responsibility for certain services, it was not until the implementation of the *National Assistance Act 1948* that they became responsible for providing comprehensive welfare services.

CONCLUSIONS

The story of public health is closely intertwined with the history of the human race itself. From ancient times, through the Dark and Middle Ages, populations were ravaged by disease and pestilence: the plague, smallpox, diphtheria, tuberculosis, typhus, typhoid, cholera and leprosy are just some of the reasons that lifespan was so short and that millions of lives were lost. The causes of this misery were variously ascribed to divine or demonic intervention, atmospheric factors and astral influences. Later, the writings and ideas of Galen ossified intellectual progress, and for a thousand years, there was no coherent theory of disease causation that approached modern understanding. It was the Victorian era when the major breakthroughs were made: the germ theory of disease, major sanitary reform and the rudiments of a health service laid the foundations for the improved health and greater longevity that marked the twentieth century out from earlier times. Still to come were the epidemics of chronic illness, the so-called 'diseases of civilization' and the emergence of new and unanticipated communicable disease threats, some of which took pandemic form. Perhaps most sobering of all is the realization that some countries and regions of the world still face the same challenges that were prevalent in Victorian Britain more than 150 years ago. The lessons of public health history are strong and still relevant today.

Further readings

The content of each chapter is derived from extensive synthesis of existing sources and from our own knowledge and experience. For this reason, the text is not underpinned point by point with detailed individual references. Specific studies are fully referenced where they have been drawn on to devise or reproduce a table or figure. Extensive population data – both national and global – are now publicly available. We have referred to such data sources in general terms unless we have reproduced an analysis in a particular exact format. This section cites specific references and suggestions for further reading. We hope that this will be a starting point to explore subjects of interest in more depth. We have not provided individual web addresses because some rapidly go out of date and because Internet search engines provide a wider range of sources and raise awareness of contrasting perspectives on a subject.

CHAPTER 1: HEALTH IN A CHANGING WORLD

In the first part of the chapter, we describe and discuss some of the many initiatives taken by governments, country representatives and public health experts, often in meetings and conferences convened by the World Health Organization, to discuss health, health promotion and strategies for change. The following are good sources for further reading around this subject:

World Health Organization (WHO). *Primary Health Care: Report of the International Conference on Primary Health Care, Alma Ata, USSR.* Geneva: WHO, 1978.

World Health Organization (WHO). *Ottawa Charter for Health Promotion.* Geneva: WHO, 1986.

World Health Organization (WHO). *Budapest Declaration on Health Promoting Hospitals.* Copenhagen: WHO Regional Office for Europe, 1991.

World Health Organization (WHO). *Report of a WHO Expert Committee on Comprehensive School Health Education and Promotion. WHO Technical Report Series.* Geneva: WHO, 1997.

World Health Organization (WHO). *Intersectoral Action for Health: A Cornerstone for Health for all in the 21st Century.* Geneva: WHO, 1997.

World Health Organisation (WHO). *Shanghai Declaration on Promoting Health in the 2030 Agenda for Sustainable Development.* Geneva: WHO, 2016.

Nutbeam D. Evaluating health promotion: Progress, problems and solutions. *Health Promotion International* 1998; 13: 27–43.

The various approaches to defining health are surfaced in a conference report that we refer to in the text:

Huber M. *Invitational Conference: Is Health a State or an Ability? Towards a Dynamic Concept of Health.* The Hague: ZonMw, 2010.

Further study of the happiness aspect of population wellbeing should start with

Helliwell JF, Layard R, Sachs J (eds.). *World Happiness Report.* New York: Sustainable Development Solutions Network, 2015.

The refutation of a significant role for modern medicine in improving population health caused huge controversy in the 1970s, and the thinking can be found in

McKeown T. *The Role of Medicine: Dream, Mirage, or Nemesis?* London: Nuffield Provincial Hospitals Trust, 1976.

Further reading on areas of public health policy that we refer to in the chapter can be found in

Pan American Health Organization and World Health Organization (PAHO/WHO). *Public Health in the Americas: Conceptual Renewal, Performance Assessment and Bases for Action.* Washington, DC: PAHO/WHO, 2002.

Acheson ED. *Public health in England: The Report of the Committee of Inquiry into the Future Development of the Public Health Function.* Cm289. London: Her Majesty's Stationery Office, 1988.

The remarkable global improvement in mortality is discussed in

Peto R. Harveian oration 2012: Halving premature death. *Clinical Medicine* 2014; 14: 643–657.

Since the beginning of the twenty-first century, there has been a major growth of publications on global health in journals, by global institutions, by philanthropic organizations and in textbooks of global health. We cover global health in this chapter and also in all other chapters in the book. The content is synthesized from a wide range of places, as well as from the authors' knowledge and experience. Some sources are cited in individual figures and tables. A good overview of themes in global health can be found in

Jamison DT, Summers LH, Alleyne G, Arrow KJ. Global health 2035: A world converging within a generation. *Lancet* 2013; 382: 1898–1955.

CHAPTER 2: EPIDEMIOLOGY AND ITS USES

This is one of the larger chapters. It includes a substantial updating of content from the previous edition. The material is largely built up from the authors' knowledge and long-standing experience in teaching and explaining what are often complex and difficult concepts for someone encountering them for the first time. There are specific references cited in sources to figures and tables. They can be followed up if the reader wishes to find out more detail or is interested in the subject matter.

One of the challenges in preparing all past editions of the book is that some areas of the subject develop further after publication. In this chapter, that applies particularly to the section on routinely available data. With the move to more open government, with the power of modern computing and digital processes to extract data (so-called big data), and with the creation of new bodies to organize the collection and analysis of data and release of information, the situation is rapidly changing. That is why, for example, we explain the principles and purpose behind cancer registration but do not describe the National Health Service (NHS) Cancer Intelligence Network, which is the current organization that oversees and coordinates the registry function. A good overview of cancer statistics (not all of which are derived from cancer registries) is provided in

Public Health England (PHE). *National Cancer Intelligence Network: Cancer Statistics: Availability and Location.* London: PHE, 2015.

The chapter describes the classification systems that are used to aggregate data to enable within-country and international comparisons, as well as those over time. The most prominent classification is the International Classification of Diseases, now in its 10th revision:

World Health Organization (WHO). *International Classification of Diseases: ICD-10.* Geneva: WHO, 1994.

The process for upgrading each time is lengthy, widely consultative and very technical. An insight into the scope of the work is provided by one of the documents produced for the 11th revision, due to be released in 2018:

Roberts R, Greenberg M, Richardson H. *Report of ICD-11 Revision Review.* Geneva: World Health Organization, 2015.

This has been described as 'a balancing act between conservatism and innovation'. Conservatism is necessary because too much change prevents consistent comparisons with data compiled under the previous revision; too little innovation, and the classification will not meet the needs of users in the fast-changing world. The classification systems used in clinical care, especially in the era of the electronic medical record, are vital to the continuity and safety of care of individuals, but also to enable accurate aggregation of data and thus the ability to assess and evaluate services. A number of classifications of 'clinical terminologies' exist, but the NHS is adopting the SNOWMED system. Many papers and reports are available on this and can be found by an Internet search, but a good starting point is

International Health Terminology Standards Development Organisation (IHTSDO). *SNOWMED CT. Starter Guide.* Copenhagen: IHTSDO, 2014.

The use of NHS data, even in anonymized form, is an immensely publicly and politically sensitive area. A great deal has been written about it in the popular press and academic journals, and it is a continuing debate. A good starting point is the following article:

Hoeksma J. The NHS's care.data scheme: What are the risks to privacy? *BMJ* 2014; 348: g1547.

The concepts and methods of epidemiology are a major part of the content of this chapter. We draw upon classic studies to illustrate these, such as

Needleman HL, Gunnoe C, Leviton A, et al. Deficits in psychologic and classroom performance of children with elevated dentine lead levels. *New England Journal of Medicine* 1979; 300: 689–695

and others identifiable from the text. As with several other chapters in the book, this is the subject of whole books in its own right. Unlike some other fields, some of the older, classic textbooks still provide an excellent guide to epidemiology; some have been updated from their original editions. For anyone wishing to read these classics, here are some suggestions:

Schneider D, Lilienfeld DE. *Lilienfeld's Foundations of Epidemiology.* 4th ed. Oxford: Oxford University Press, 2015.

Susser M. *Causal Thinking in the Health Sciences. Concepts and Strategies in Epidemiology.* New York: Oxford University Press, 1973.

McMahon B, Pugh TF. *Epidemiology: Principles and Methods.* London: Little Brown, 1970.

Rose G, Barker DJP. *Epidemiology for the Uninitiated.* London: BMJ Books, 1986.

Bhopal RS. *Concepts of Epidemiology: Integrating Ideas, Theories, Principles and Methods of Epidemiology.* Oxford: Oxford University Press, 2008.

And the list could not be complete, of course, without Morris's seminal text:

Morris JN. *Uses of Epidemiology.* London: E & S Livingstone, 1957 and later editions.

We specifically describe in the chapter how this shaped thinking on the practical applications of epidemiology.

CHAPTER 3: COMMUNICABLE DISEASES

This is the largest chapter in the book. It is also one of the subject areas about which whole books have been written. We did not wish to write a textbook within a textbook, and so we made careful choices. First, we wanted to describe, as clearly as we could, the key concepts and principles of communicable disease transmission, prevention and control. We avoided too much technical detail to achieve greater clarity. This can be found in many specialist books on infectious or communicable diseases. Second, we wanted to tell the 'story' of the diseases. These are inherently very interesting, whether it is the mode of occurrence, the impact, the solutions that are used to control them or the political controversy that they generate. It is this description of communicable diseases 'in action', not the theoretical dimension, that sustains interest and is of practical relevance for the nonspecialist in this aspect of public health. Third, we wanted to strike a balance between communicable diseases that can cause infection in the United Kingdom, those that do or could cause imported infections, those that pose major global health problems and those that strongly emphasize aspects of the general principles of communicable disease transmission, prevention and control. For this reason, we have been selective in the actual diseases that we describe and discuss. Full-blown textbooks of communicable disease usually include more diseases but use more technical or specialist information when describing them.

The content of the chapter is synthesized from a very wide range of sources, draws on material from earlier editions of the book (where the information was not dated) and extensively uses the authors' own experience at the policy and the practical level. To read further, there are many good textbooks of communicable diseases, but an invaluable comprehensive field guide disease by disease is

Heymann DL. *Control of Communicable Diseases Manual.* 20th ed. Washington, DC: American Public Health Association, 2014.

A number of agencies (particularly the U.S. Centers for Disease Control and Prevention (CDC) in Atlanta, the World Health Organization, UNAIDS, the European Centre for Disease Prevention and Control and Public Health England) provide excellent up-to-date information on communicable diseases and give authoritative advice on the current geographical distribution of diseases, time trends, policies and the best control measures to use. Their websites

are the best place to start looking, where there will also be downloadable reports on many special topics, such as antimicrobial resistance.

CHAPTER 4: NONCOMMUNICABLE DISEASES

Over the last 50 years, the populations of all high-income countries have experienced a mounting increase in the numbers of people dying or suffering from chronic diseases like cancer, heart disease, stroke and obstructive pulmonary disease. Most governments of such countries have put in place strategies to try to combat these problems. Most have had limited success. Until recently, global health attention had been mainly focused on communicable disease threats, particularly those that took a high death toll in poorer countries, for example, AIDS, tuberculosis and malaria.

This chapter reflects a change of emphasis. Over the last decade and a half, all countries and global health agencies have begun to show heightened concern about the growth in chronic disease, although the term *noncommunicable disease* is more often used; it is the term that we have adopted for the title of the chapter. The reasons for this concern are several-fold: in most of the low- and middle-income countries of the world, noncommunicable diseases have become a dominant influence on overall population health; governments of most high-income countries are struggling to meet the costs of healthcare, due in large measure to the impact of these diseases on need and demand for care; and one problem in particular is causing great alarm among politicians and policymakers worldwide: obesity. This is because of its rapid rise and its ability to cause, relatively rapidly, large numbers of cases of diseases like diabetes, heart disease and cancer.

A good place to start to understand the trends, patterns and geographical distribution of the main noncommunicable diseases, as well as the global concerns and broad policy responses, is to study the reports of the main global health bodies on this subject, for example,

World Health Organization (WHO). *Global Status Report on Non-Communicable Diseases.* Geneva: WHO, 2014.
United Nations. *UN high-level meeting on NCDs: Summary Report of Discussions of the Round Tables.* New York: United Nations, 2011.
World Bank. *The Growing Danger of Non-Communicable Diseases: Acting Now to Reverse the Course.* Washington, DC: World Bank, 2011.

Many other bodies have produced reports or commentaries on the global state of noncommunicable disease; a nonofficial perspective is provided by a group of nongovernmental organizations (NGOs), the NCD Alliance; see, for example,

NCD Alliance. *Strategic Plan 2016–2020.* London: NCD Alliance, 2015.

The *Lancet* journal has regularly produced series of collected papers on noncommunicable diseases. An introduction to the 2013 series can be found at

Horton R. Non-communicable diseases 2015–2025. *Lancet* 2013; 381: 509–510.

from which the other papers in the series can also be accessed. Aspects of these reports and publications, at a general level, have helped to frame the content for this chapter.

The expert consensus and research evidence coalesce around a small number of risk factors that are responsible for generating the majority of noncommunicable diseases. A large part of the chapter is structured around these risk factors, their influences and the public health policy response to them. Given the large number of studies that have accumulated over the years to produce this consensus, we have not cited research in detail when summarizing the position in particular areas. We have highlighted a number of seminal studies and reports, and provide full references here. The Nurses' Health Study is the longest established study of women's health. It started in the United States in 1976 with a cohort of nurses whose lifestyle and health-related behaviour were assessed, and then they were followed up to monitor their disease experience. Later cohorts were added, and the range and nature of the data collected became more sophisticated. The findings of the studies have yielded a wealth of information on risks of disease. There have been a very large number of publications of these findings in medical and scientific journals. The Nurses' Health Study website provides an overview of the studies conducted, and links to the many publications that have arisen from them. A similar long-standing follow-up study of a population's health is the Framingham Study. We have not cited this specifically, but it has provided much of the evidence base for risks of cardiovascular disease. This started in 1948 by following a cohort of men in a town in New England to study cardiovascular disease. Over time, more participants were added, and today the diseases studied have expanded beyond cardiovascular disease. A good overview of the study is provided in

Mahmood SS, Levy D, Vasan RS, Wang TJ. *The Framingham Heart Study and the Epidemiology of Cardiovascular Disease: A historical Perspective.* Lancet 2014; 383: 999–1008.

The public health strategies for addressing the key areas of risk are discussed in the chapter. The common features are that no single intervention will succeed, but a combination of measures are required; the role of industries producing the products that can damage health will almost always seek to resist change that affects their profitability, and so regulation, and sometimes legislation, is necessary; price and access are important features in modifying unhealthy behaviour; multisector partnerships are usually essential to bring about real change; and bold public health action is usually politically contentious. In the chapter, we have concentrated on covering these themes and scoping the

action to address risk at a population level, giving practical examples. Given this, it has seldom been relevant to point to individual studies, but rather we have created these sections of the text by synthesis of many different sources and from our own observations and practical experience. However, in the field of tobacco control, it is important to be familiar with the groundbreaking reports of the Royal College of Physicians of London. An excellent overview of these can be found in

Britton J (ed.). *Fifty Years Since Smoking and Health: Progress, Lessons, and Priorities for a Smoke-Free UK.* London: Royal College of Physicians, 2012.

The politics of tobacco has been a long-running feature. We point to a specific example of where the British government came under pressure to slow action to combat the health effects of tobacco. This is described in a history of the chief medical officers of England:

Sheard S, Donaldson LJ. *The Nation's Doctor.* Oxford: Radcliffe, 2006.

The New Labour government's White Paper on tobacco control is an important landmark in the United Kingdom's public health policy,

Her Majesty's Government. *Smoking Kills.* London: The Stationery Office, 2006.

although even this was for a time mired in controversy because of allegations of delay at the behest of a party donor in introducing sponsorship of Formula 1 racing. The events and political manoeuvres surrounding the introduction of smoke-free public places in England, a recommendation to government by the then chief medical officer, gives another important insight into public health policymaking to combat noncommunicable disease in a political environment. This is analysed in

Institute for Government. *The Ban on Smoking in Public Places 2007.* London: Institute for Government, 2013.

The complexity of the web of causation underlying some noncommunicable diseases is well illustrated in the section on obesity in this chapter. For an excellent analysis of this, and the measures to combat the problem, the work of a group convened by the UK government's chief scientific adviser is the definitive source:

UK Government Foresight Programme. *Tackling Obesities: Future Choices.* London: Government Office for Science, 2007.

Policy on nutrition and health is not free of controversy, with debates running on the appropriateness of dietary guidelines, sugar taxes and the advertising of calorie-dense food to children. The challenges of tackling the global food industry in order to advance health are analysed in depth in a series of papers in a special issue of the journal *PLoS Medicine*, the introductory article of which can be found at

PLoS Medicine editors. *PLoS Medicine* series on big food: The food industry is ripe for scrutiny. *PLOS Medicine* 2012; 9(6):e1001246.

As the relevant section of the chapter demonstrates, underlying causation and policymaking are equally complex in relation to alcohol, with no credible strategy in place in the United Kingdom. A big debate has taken place on minimum pricing of units of alcohol, with a strong evidence-based policy recommendation arising from work by researchers at the University of Sheffield,

Holmes J, Meng Y, Meier PS, et al. Effects of minimum unit pricing for alcohol on different income and socio-economic groups: A modelling study. *Lancet* 2014; 383 (9929): 1655–1664.

failing to gain political traction in Downing Street.

The sections of the chapter on physical inactivity, high blood pressure and unintentional injury are referenced to sources in individual figures and tables. In the sections on prevention and screening, the quote from Deborah Small is based on her paper with colleagues:

Small DA, Loewenstein G, Slovic P. Sympathy and callousness: The impact of deliberative thought on donations to identifiable and statistical victims. *Organisational Behaviours and Human Decision Processes* 2007; 102: 143–153.

The original World Health Organization criteria to judge whether to introduce a population screening programme are still relevant even though they have been modified somewhat since their original publication. They were a major landmark in prevention.

Wilson JMG, Jungner G. *Principles and Practice of Screening for Disease.* Geneva: World Health Organization, 1968.

Much of the data on noncommunicable diseases in the chapter come from the Global Burden of Disease Study. Data are collected and analysed by more than 1000 researchers in more than 100 countries; the data capture premature death and disability from more than 300 diseases and injuries in 188 countries, allowing comparisons over time, across age groups and among populations. The study is a very widely cited source of information on noncommunicable diseases and is the first port of call for many who want to understand the context. In this chapter, we have drawn from this source for many of the statistics that we quote, but also from the World Health Organization and, for the United Kingdom, from the Office for National Statistics.

CHAPTER 5: SOCIAL DETERMINANTS OF HEALTH

A number of key publications and leading thinkers are mentioned in the chapter. They have dealt with the concept of health inequalities and set out the scope of their impact at the population level. The Black Report is the seminal publication that all modern studies of social determinants of health refer back to. Copies of the original report,

Black D. *Inequalities in health: report of a research working group.* London: Department of Health and Social Security, 1980.

are scarce. A later paperback book,

Townsend P, Davidson N (eds.). *Inequalities in Health: The Black Report.* London: Pelican, 1982.

although out of print, is more easily obtainable. The term *social determinants of health* is today used more widely internationally, but *health inequalities* is still used by the majority of researchers and policymakers in the United Kingdom. Modern thinking in this field is particularly associated with the work of Sir Michael Marmot. He and his research group have contributed a large number of scientific journal publications over the last three decades; they can be found through PubMed searches. The best overviews of the subject from Marmot's viewpoint are to be found in two of his books:

Marmot MG. *The Status Syndrome: How Your Social Standing Directly Affects Your Health and Life Expectancy.* London: Bloomsbury, 2004.
Marmot MG. *The Health Gap: The Challenge of an Unequal World.* London: Bloomsbury, 2015.

He also has led the production of reports for the British government and the World Health Organization that have provided analysis of patterns and trends in social determinants of health, as well as their impact, together with recommendations for action. They are referred to at various points in the chapter and provide excellent in-depth overviews of the subject. The full references for two of these reports are

The Marmot Review. *Fair society, Healthy Lives.* London: The Marmot Review, 2010.
Commission on Social Determinants of Health. *Closing the Gap in a Generation: Health Equity through Action on the Social Determinants of Health.* Geneva: World Health Organization, 2008.

The incoming Blair Labour government, in the late 1990s, commissioned a former chief medical officer to conduct a review of health inequalities and produce policy recommendations. This contains useful source material, as well as highlighting the challenges of formulating action to achieve major improvements:

Acheson ED. *Inequalities in Health: Report of an Independent Enquiry.* London: Her Majesty's Stationery Office, 1998.

At several points in the chapter, the work of the MacArthur Foundation's Research Network on socio-economic status and health is mentioned. This unique decade-long interdisciplinary scientific collaboration, sponsored by a U.S.-based philanthropic body, has produced an impressive breadth and depth of publications and reports on the social and economic determinants of health. A useful summary of the key themes can be found in

Adler NE, Stewart J (eds.). *Reaching for a Healthier Life: Facts on Socioeconomic Status and Health in the US*. Chicago: MacArthur Foundation, 2007.

In this chapter, we describe their work on subjective measures of social standing and neighbourhood factors that influence health. One section of the chapter describes emerging research on the biological pathways that mediate the impact of social deprivation on disease outcomes. The research network has memorably posed the question, how does socio-economic status get into the body? It addressed this by capturing an extensive review of research in this field in a publication:

Adler NE, Stewart J (eds.). *The Biology of Disadvantage: Socioeconomic Status and Health*. New York: Wiley-Blackwell, 2010.

To explore further the key concepts, influences and evidence base for health inequalities and social and economic determinants of health, a number of valuable sources not explicitly discussed in the chapter can be accessed. British epidemiologists, social scientists and economists have a strong track record in this field. Richard Wilkinson, for many years professor of social epidemiology at Nottingham University, has been a long-standing champion of the importance of income inequalities to a population's health status. He is an extremely important figure in this field. His book, written with his colleague,

Wilkinson RG, Pickett K. *The Spirit Level: Why More Equal Societies Almost Always Do Better*. London: Allen Lane, 2009.

is a brilliant and compelling analysis of the subject. Danny Dorling, a social geographer, who is a professor at Oxford University, is another leading thinker on health inequalities, and particularly their variation by place (e.g. the north–south divide in the United Kingdom). Two of his books scope the subject of health and social inequalities from his perspective superbly:

Dorling D. *Unequal Health*. Bristol: Policy Press, 2013.
Dorling D. *Injustice: Why Social Inequality Still Persists*. Bristol: Policy Press, 2015.

George Davey Smith is professor of clinical epidemiology at the University of Bristol. His group has researched and published extensively on health inequalities, especially in the following areas: understanding of the causes and alleviation of health inequalities, life-course epidemiology, systematic reviewing of evidence of effectiveness of healthcare and health policy interventions and population health contributions of the new genetics. Their work is a rich source of further exploration of the research evidence in the

inequalities field. Professor Dame Margaret Whitehead, who holds the chair of public health at Liverpool University, is another long-standing researcher in the field of health inequalities and social determinants, as well as a thought leader and adviser to governments and the World Health Organization. One of her coauthored papers in particular contains a conceptual diagram illustrating the rainbow of influences on the determinants of health in a population. It is extensively reproduced in other publications and teaching material and can be found in

Dahlgren G, Whitehead M. *Policies and Strategies to Promote Social Equity in Health*. Copenhagen: WHO Regional Office for Europe, 1992.

The *Barker hypothesis*, which proposes that nutrition in intrauterine and postneonatal life is a key determinant of health in adult life, is discussed in the chapter, is widely referred to and is an important concept in health inequalities thinking. Professor David Barker set out his thinking in the early 1990s, and the best place to start to understand his idea is in his book:

Barker DJP (ed.). *Fetal and Infant Origins of Adult Disease*. London: Wiley-Blackwell, 1992.

The theory has been developed and discussed by others since then and is now very well established, sometimes described as the Barker hypothesis but otherwise referred to as 'the thrifty phenotype' or 'the fetal programming hypothesis'. Barker consolidated his thinking with new evidence a decade later:

Hales CN, Barker DJP. The thrifty phenotype hypothesis. *British Medical Bulletin* 2001; 60: 5–20.

The section in the chapter on occupation-related stress highlights the work of Karaseck, who set out a model to explain workplace-related stress and its impact on health, particularly cardiovascular disease. It is determined by how demanding a person's job is and how much control he or she has over his or her work. An early description of the model can be found in

Karasek RA, Theorell T. *Healthy Work: Stress, Productivity and the Reconstruction of Working Life*. New York: Basic Books, 1990.

Many subsequent studies of health outcomes have tested Karasek's model, or other similar models, against the disease and mortality experiences of a workforce. Many such studies have found an association between lack of job control and cardiovascular events. The long-running study of British civil servants' health, the *Whitehall Study*, has explored this area. See, for example,

Bosma H, Peter R, Siegrist J, Marmot M. Two alternative job stress models and the risk of coronary heart disease. *American Journal of Public Health* 1998; 88: 68–74.

Other studies have found no relationship.

The section of the chapter on social mobility draws extensively on the work of the Organisation for Economic Cooperation and Development (OECD) and an independent Commission on Social Mobility and Child Poverty set up by the British government. The former, in a report on intergenerational mobility,

Organisation for Economic Cooperation and Development (OECD). *A Family Affair: Intergenerational Social Mobility Across OECD Countries.* Paris: OECD, 2010.

provides a striking analysis of the differences between countries, with the United Kingdom comparing badly with others.

Comparing health data for different social class groups (based on occupation) was the main way that health inequalities were demonstrated for the latter years of the nineteenth century and through most of the twentieth century. This was certainly a key feature of the analyses in the Black Report. Today, social class is less often used and has been replaced in British official statistics by a socio-economic classification. The introductory parts of the chapter give examples – both official and unofficial – for describing social position through various classifications. These sections of the chapter also illustrate some of the main ways in which geographical areas can be profiled in social and economic terms. The range of indicators of socio-economic position used in analysis of health data is reviewed in

Galobardes B, Shaw M, Lawlor D, Lynch JW, Davey Smith G. Indicators of socioeconomic position (part 1). *Journal of Epidemiology and Community Health* 2006; 60: 7–12.

At a number of points in the chapter, particularly insightful or apt quotations are given. These do not necessarily always come from published journal articles or reports. However, the job title and affiliation of each individual quoted are given so as to allow them to be explored further by Googling.

CHAPTER 6: HEALTH SYSTEMS

The chapter content covers the core principles, features and purposes of health systems; comparisons of different models of provision; and the development, current structure and functioning of the NHS in the United Kingdom.

Much of the material in the chapter is derived from the authors' knowledge and experience. Health systems, their importance, how they are designed and how they perform, is a very big subject, and interested readers may wish to pursue the subject matter further and in more depth.

Globally, much attention is being given to the goal of achieving universal health coverage. We deal with this in the chapter. Various bodies concerned with global health have produced reports and policy statements on it. A good document to provide orientation to the subject is

World Health Organization (WHO). *World Health Report: The Path to Universal Coverage.* Geneva: WHO, 2010.

An editorial by senior World Health Organization officials also frames the subject well:

Kieny MP, Evans DB. Universal health coverage. *Eastern Mediterranean Health Journal* 2013; 19: 305–306.

An editorial in the *Lancet* also provides an important perspective on the scale of the challenge:

Editorial. The struggle for universal health coverage. *Lancet* 2012; 380: 859.

Comparison of healthcare systems is a big and important field in global health and the evaluative sciences. Good starting points for following up the material in the chapter are

Weber S, Brouhard K, Bernan P. *Synopsis of health systems research across the World Bank Group from 2000 to 2010.* Washington, DC: World Bank, 2010.

and the reports by the OECD that have looked at individual countries in depth, for example,

Organisation for Economic Cooperation and Development (OECD). *Review of Health Systems: Mexico.* Paris: OECD, 2016.

The World Bank and the OECD produce many reports on different aspects of health systems to enable comparisons. The OECD analyses of performance are particularly valuable, for example,

Organisation for Economic Cooperation and Development (OECD). *Health at a Glance: OECD Indicators, 2015.* Paris: OECD, 2015.

One source makes a judgement on the feature that is best covered by systems of different countries:

Britnell M. *The Perfect Health System: A Comprehensive Assessment of Healthcare Systems across the Globe.* London: Palgrave MacMillan, 2015.

The postwar development of the British welfare state, including the NHS, is very thoroughly and clearly covered in

Timmins N. *The Five Giants: A Biography of the Welfare State.* New ed. London: Harper Collins, 2001.

The Griffiths management review, a key development that we discuss, can be found in

Griffiths R. *NHS management inquiry report (the Griffiths Report).* London: Department of Health and Social Security, 1983.

An excellent and readable account of the 2010–2015 United Kingdom Coalition Government's reorganization (seen by many as a debacle) can be found in

Timmins N. *Never Again? The Story of the Health and Social Care Act 2012.* London: The King's Fund and the Institute for Government, 2012

and raises big questions about the rationale and disruptive effect of reorganizations.

CHAPTER 7: QUALITY AND SAFETY OF HEALTHCARE

There is no single internationally accepted and agreed way of defining, viewing or approaching the question of quality in healthcare. As a result, different approaches to defining, measuring and improving it have developed over time. Some of them are now of historical importance, having laid the foundations for modern thinking; others coexist alongside alternatives. It is fundamental to understanding healthcare quality to know about this. We have referred to the different approaches as 'schools of thought' and described their nature and relevance in the first section of the chapter. A large body of literature has assembled around these, some dealing with practical experience, some modifying the approach and some critiquing or contesting the central idea. For each, we give a key reference that can be a starting point for further study:

Donabedian Triad: Donabedian A. Evaluating the quality of medical care. *Milbank Mem Fund Q* 1966; 44: 166–206.

Deming and Total Quality Management: Deming WE. *Out of the Crisis.* Cambridge, MA: MIT Press, 1982.

Clinical Governance: Scally G, Donaldson LJ. Clinical governance and the drive for quality improvement in the new NHS in England. *BMJ* 1998; 317: 61–65.

RAND and the Concept of Appropriateness: Brook RH. Redefining health systems. Santa Monica, CA: RAND Corporation, 2015.

McMaster and the Evidence-Based Medicine Movement: Sackett DL, Rosenberg WMC, Muir Gray JA, Haynes RB, Richardson WS. Evidence-based medicine: What it is and what it isn't. *BMJ* 1996; 312: 71–72.

Toyota Tradition: Scoville R, Little K. *Comparing Lean and quality improvement. Institute for Healthcare Improvement white paper.* Boston: Institute for Healthcare Improvement, 2014.

Six Sigma: Chassin MR. Is healthcare ready for Six Sigma quality? *Milbank Quarterly* 1998; 76: 565–591.

Clinical Standards and Audit: Burgess R. *New Principles of Best Practice in Clinical Audit.* Oxford: Radcliffe, 2011.

Institute for Healthcare Improvement: Berwick, D. The science of improvement. *JAMA* 2008; 299: 1182–1184.

Standardization and Checklists: Gawande A. *The Checklist Manifesto.* New York: Metropolitan Books, 2009.

Pronovost PJ, Needham D, Berenholtz SM, et al. An intervention to decrease catheter related bloodstream infection in the ICU. *New England Journal of Medicine* 2006; 355: 2725–2732.

We begin the section of the chapter on patient safety by mentioning two official reports, one in the United States,

Kohn K, Corrigan J, Donaldson M. *To Err Is Human.* Washington, DC: National Academy Press, 2000.

and one in the United Kingdom,

Chief Medical Officer. *An Organisation with a Memory: A Report on Learning from Adverse Events in the NHS.* London: The Stationery Office, 2000.

They sparked programmes of action to improve the safety of healthcare. Both are important source documents for anyone wanting to fully understand the underlying concepts in patient safety, how accidents and errors happen and the ways to mitigate and prevent them. A number of textbooks of patient safety subsequently emerged and are a further valuable source through which to appreciate the subject in the round, for example,

Vincent C. *Patient Safety.* 2nd ed. Chichester: John Wiley & Sons, 2010.

The next section of the chapter describes the burden of harm and mentions studies of the 'prevalence' of error in hospital care. To read about these, the following references are relevant:

Brennan TA, Leape LL, Laird NM, et al. Incidence of adverse events and negligence in hospitalized patients – Results of the Harvard Medical Practice Study I. *New England Journal of Medicine* 1991; 324 (6): 370–376.

Wilson RM, Harrison BT, Gibberd RW, Hamilton JD. An analysis of the causes of adverse events from the Quality in Australia Health Care Study. *Medical Journal of Australia* 1999; 170: 411–415.

Vincent C, Neale G, Woloshynowych M. Adverse events in British hospitals: Preliminary retrospective record review. *BMJ* 2001; 322: 517.

Bates DW, Cullen DJ, Laird N, et al. Incidence of adverse drug events and potential adverse drug events. Implications for prevention. ADE Prevention Study Group. *JAMA* 1995; 274: 29–34.

Understanding the importance of 'systems' to safety is essential, not just in healthcare but also in many other safety-critical industries. We devote a section of the chapter to this, the centrepiece of which is a description of Professor James Reason's Swiss cheese metaphor of causation. Reason's books are an invaluable source of further depth of discussion of this area:

Reason J. *Human Error.* Cambridge: Cambridge University Press, 1990.

Reason J. *The Human Contribution: Unsafe Acts, Accidents, and Heroic Recoveries.* Aldershot: Ashgate Publishing, 2008.

Another way to understand the importance of systems is to study investigative reports of catastrophic accidents or failures. We describe several of these in the chapter. The investigation of the death of a teenager due to a medication error is a classic in the field of patient safety and merits reading in its entirety:

Toft B. *External Inquiry into the Adverse Incident that Occurred at Queen's Medical Centre, Nottingham 4th January 2001.* London: Department of Health, 2001.

The Tenerife air disaster was a turning point in attitudes to safety in the airline industry:

Weick KE. The vulnerable system: An analysis of the Tenerife air disaster. *Journal of Management* 1990; 16: 571–593.

The Canadian rail accident is described in sufficient detail in the text. The most recent thinking about systems has focused on the concept of resilience. We explain it in the chapter. A very good introduction to this subject can be found in

Weick KE, Sutcliffe KM. *Managing the Unexpected: Resilient Performance in an Age of Uncertainty.* 2nd ed. San Francisco: Jossey-Bass, 2007.

Another important strand in the consideration of safety is *human factors*. We discuss this in the chapter. The idea is very long-standing (the previous term, which is still used, is *ergonomics*), and most of the conceptual thinking and practical applications have been developed in fields outside healthcare. Many of the authoritative sources of further reading are quite technical, but they are valuable to dip into; see, for example,

Chapanis A. *Human Factors in Systems Engineering.* New York: John Wiley & Sons, 1996.

We discuss the culture of organizations and its importance to safety. There are many facets to this, but a key area is avoiding blame and retribution if learning from error is to take place. A seminal reference here is

Leape LL. Error in medicine. *JAMA* 1994; 272: 1851–1857.

The measurement of cultures is increasingly important in patient safety, and a good example of the approach can be found in

Sorra JS, Nieva VF. *Hospital Survey on Patient Safety Culture.* Rockville, MD: Agency for Healthcare Research and Quality, 2004.

We also cover in the chapter the importance of reporting of patient safety incidents as a source of learning. Many patient safety programmes around the world include a requirement to gather information on errors and harm. The principle of learning from what goes wrong in order to prevent a similar event in the future appears to be a sound one, but it has not proved straightforward, as we discuss in the chapter. An excellent overview of patient safety data, their value and limitations can be found in

Vincent C, Burnett S, Carthey J. *The Measurement and Monitoring of Safety.* London: The Health Foundation, 2013.

whilst an example of the use of data to identify underlying causes of harm is in this article:

Donaldson LJ, Panesar SS, Darzi A. Patient-safety-related hospital deaths in England: Thematic analysis of incidents reported to a national database, 2010–2012. *PLoS Medicine* 2014; 11 (6): e1001667.

We conclude in the chapter that the evidence base to reduce harm is not as strong as is needed. To read further about this, the following comprehensive analysis is very informative:

Shekelle PG, Pronovost PJ, Wachter RM, et al. Advancing the science of patient safety. *Annals of Internal Medicine* 2011; 154 (10): 693–696.

Most modern programmes on patient safety include patients and family members in their work. Patient stories in particular have been vital in galvanizing commitment around the world. We describe the human impact of unsafe care at various points in the chapter. There are many excellent accounts in the literature to facilitate further study, for example,

McIver S, Wyndham R. *After the Error: Speaking Out about Patient Safety to Save Lives.* Toronto: ECW Press, 2013.

Most of the parts of the chapter dealing with harm concern error in weak systems. We also cover the less common source of harm: factors related to the competence and performance of doctors and other health professionals. This can be due to error in the execution of procedures using technical skills. Simulation training in surgery and other fields of medicine has been a growth area in education and will expand further with technological advance. Patients can also come to harm from the conduct and performance of individual practitioners. Further reading in these areas can be found in the following journal articles:

Cook DA, Hatala R, Brydges R, et al. Technology-enhanced simulation for health professions education: A systematic review and meta-analysis. *JAMA* 2011; 306: 978–988.
Donaldson LJ. Doctors with problems in an NHS workforce. *BMJ* 1994; 308: 1277–1282.
Donaldson LJ, Panesar SS, McAvoy PA, Scarrott DM. Identification of poor performance in a national medical workforce over 11 years: An observational study. *BMJ Quality and Safety* 2014; 23: 147–152.

CHAPTER 8: MATERNAL AND CHILD HEALTH

Maternal, newborn and child health is one of the most extensively documented fields of global health. The inclusion of targets in the Millennium Development Goals led to the establishment of monitoring systems and compilation of data to assess progress. Such data are publicly available through reports and websites of the United Nations agencies, the World Bank and nongovernmental organizations with an interest in this field. Many reports and initiatives are joint agency endeavours, for example,

World Health Organization, UNICEF, United Nations Fund for Population Activities, World Bank, United Nations Population Division. *Trends in Maternal Mortality 1990–2015.* Geneva: WHO, 2015.

The same group of agencies also monitor infant and child mortality and make their data openly available, as well as producing regular reports.

Nour NM. An introduction to Maternal Mortality. *Reviews in Obstetrics & Gynecology* 2008; 1 (2): 77–81.

provides a simple overview of the key issues and concepts when considering maternal mortality in a global context.

In the twenty-first century, big philanthropic foundations have taken a much greater role in global health – not just as funders, but also as strategists and leaders. The best example is the Bill and Melinda Gates Foundation. This organization has a maternal, newborn and child health programme of its own. The Foundation produces excellent reports and analyses, and reviews of evidence of effectiveness (accessible through its website). Read alongside reports from the United Nations agencies, this gives an unrivalled overview of the scope of the problems and the main challenges to be overcome, particularly in the poorest parts of the world.

The UK context for maternal and child health is very different to the global one and forms a major part of the chapter. Standard statistics on maternal, newborn and child mortality, as well as population fertility and abortion, are collected, analysed and made publicly available by the Office for National Statistics. We have used this source for such statistics throughout the chapter. The United Kingdom has a long tradition of especially collecting data on maternal and infant mortality in order to identify potentially avoidable causes that can then be used to design interventions and action plans. This has been based on the *confidential enquiry* model whereby clinicians and experts give their opinion on causation as frankly as possible. Data are then aggregated so that individual patients and clinicians cannot be identified; this method emphasizes learning over the long term and avoids litigation intruding and threatening the viability of the surveys. The organization of the databases and their analysis and interpretation have largely been in the hands of professional bodies and academic institutions, although they have been funded and coordinated by the NHS. Changes to administrative arrangements have led to bewildering and complex acronyms. However, the methodologies have remained strong. Examples of these important reports are

MBRRACE-UK. *Perinatal Mortality Surveillance Report: UK Erinatal Deaths for Births from January to Ecember 2014*. Oxford: Oxford University, National Perinatal Mortality Unit, 2015.

Knight M, Tuffnell D, Kenyon S, Shakespeare J, Gray R, Kurinczuk JJ (eds.). *Saving lives, Improving Mothers' care. Surveillance of Maternal Deaths in the UK 2011–13 and Lessons Learned to Inform Maternity care from the UK and Ireland Confidential Enquiries into Maternal Deaths and Morbidity 2009–13*. Oxford: Oxford University, National Perinatal Epidemiology Unit, 2015.

In the chapter, we mention that the level of well-being of children in the United Kingdom compares unfavourably with that of some other European countries. This is part of a regular survey, but the methodology is well described in

Bradshaw J, Richardson D. An index of child well-being in Europe. *Child Indicators Research* 2009: 319–351.

Throughout the second decade of the twenty-first century, there has been mounting concern about the quality of child and adolescent mental health services. This is reviewed in

House of Commons Health Committee. *Children's and Adolescents' Mental Health and CAMHS*. Third report of Session 2014–15. London: The Stationery Office, 2014.

The question of female genital mutilation has become a public health issue during the twenty-first century and has led to action in both the United Kingdom and globally. We discuss this in the chapter and mention strategies to address it. The following are useful sources to explore the topic further:

United Nations Fund for Population Activities–UNICEF. 2014 *Annual Report of the Joint Programme on Female Genital Mutilation/Cutting: Accelerating change*. New York: UNICEF, 2015.

World Health Organization (WHO) (with other agencies and partners). *Global Strategy to Stop Health-Care Providers from Performing Female Genital Mutilation*. Geneva: WHO, 2010.

CHAPTER 9: MENTAL HEALTH

The framework of this chapter emphasizes the modern concept of public mental health and its potential value to improve levels of well-being in societies, as well as reducing the occurrence of mental disorders and improving the quality of care and lives of those who suffer from them. Jonathan Campion, professor of population health at University College London, has been a leading thinker in this field, producing groundbreaking work in defining and conceptualizing public mental health. His work has helped greatly in framing the content of this chapter. References to his work are an important source of further reading, for example,

Campion J, Fitch C. *Guidance for the Commissioning of Public Mental Health Services*. London: Joint Commissioning Panel for Mental Health, 2012.

Campion J. Public mental health: The local tangibles. *Psychiatrist* 2013; 37: 238–242.

Campion J, Bhui K, Bhugra D. European Association guidance on prevention of mental disorder. *European Psychiatry* 2012; 27: 68–80.

and in sources to figures and tables. He was also involved in preparing the policy statement by the Royal College of Psychiatrists:

Royal College of Psychiatrists. *No Health without Public Mental Health: The Case for Action*. London: Royal College of Psychiatrists, 2010.

The case for a strong commitment to global mental health is strongly made in the report of the proceedings of a gathering of the world's mental health leaders that we describe at the beginning of the chapter:

Salzburg Global Seminar. *New Paradigms for Behavioural and Mental Health Care*. Session 536. Salzburg: Salzburg Global Seminar, 2015.

The data we cite on the global burden of mental disorder can be looked at in the context of the Salzburg seminar's conclusions in

Whiteford HA, Degenhardt L, Rehm J, et al. Global burden of disease attributable to mental and substance use disorders: Findings from the Global Burden of Disease Study 2010. *Lancet* 2013; 382: 1575–1586.

and in

World Health Organization (WHO). *Mental Health Atlas 2014*. Geneva: WHO, 2015.

Data for mental disorder (e.g. suicide rates) in the United Kingdom are derived from the Office for National Statistics. Data on the prevalence of particular mental disorders are derived from a periodic national population survey of so-called psychiatric morbidity,

McManus S, Meltzer H, Brugha T, Bebbington P, Jenkins R. *Adult Psychiatric Morbidity in England, 2007*. Leeds: NHS and Social Care Information Centre, 2009.

and related reports from the same cluster of surveys. Data on mental health service usage are derived from *NHS Digital*. We also quote data from the regular survey of suicide and homicide among people with mental illness:

Appleby L (ed.). *National Confidential Inquiry into Suicide and Homicide by People with Mental Illness*. Annual report, 2015. Manchester: University of Manchester, 2015.

Public Health England also leads the Mental Health Dementia and Neurology Intelligence Network, which publishes interactive data online.

An important aspect of public mental health is the subject of mental health inequalities and social determinants of mental health. There is a section of the chapter on this, and some good sources for further reading are

Patel V, Lund C, Heatherill S, et al. Social determinants of mental disorders. In: Blas E, Sivasankara Kurup A (eds.), *Priority Public Health Conditions: From Learning to Action on Social Determinants of Health*. Geneva: World Health Organization, 2009.

Friedli L. *Mental Health, Resilience, and Inequalities*. Copenhagen: WHO Regional Office for Europe, 2009.

Campion J, Bhugra D, Bailey S, Marmot M. Inequality and mental disorders: Opportunity for action. *Lancet* 2013; 382: 183–184.

The important, and often overlooked, bidirectional relationship between mental and physical health is considered in another section of the chapter. Good sources of further reading on this are the Royal College of Psychiatrists report on public mental health referred to earlier,

Royal College of Psychiatrists. *No Health without Public Mental Health: The Case for Action*. London: Royal College of Psychiatrists, 2010.

and

Naylor C, Parsonage M, McDaid D, Knapp M, Fossey M, Galea A. *Long-Term Conditions and Mental Health: The Cost of Co-Morbidities*. London: The King's Fund and Centre for Mental Health, 2012.

Kolappa K, Henderson DC, Kishore SI. No physical health without mental health: Lessons unlearned? *Bulletin of the World Health Organization* 2013; 91: 3–3A.

Rethink Mental Illness. *20 years too soon*. London: Rethink Mental Illness, 2012.

In the introduction to the chapter, we mention the concept of *parity of esteem*, the goal that mental health must be accorded the same priority for high-quality care as physical health. In the English NHS, this was enshrined in law through the *Health and Social Care Act 2012*. The strategy and vision for mental health services to achieve this are set out in

Department of Health (DH). *No Health without Mental Health: Implementation Framework*. London: DH, 2012.

Such aspirational statements of commitment by governments and health system leaders are important, but they do not define how to plan and deliver the right care to meet a population's needs. Indeed, clinicians and public health professionals of long standing have seen many strategies produced at the national level with little change on the ground. In the final third of the chapter, we give a description of the key features of mental health services in the United Kingdom, bearing in mind that precise patterns of care vary around the country. For those who wish to explore further the question of how to provide high-quality care for people with mental disorders, an excellent source is the suite of publications produced by the Joint Commissioning Panel for Mental Health (JCPMH). This is an entity established to raise the standard of mental healthcare in the NHS and to promote well-being by producing guidance for those commissioning mental health services, particularly clinical commissioning groups. It is cochaired by the Royal College of Psychiatrists and the Royal College of General Practitioners. It involves 17 leading organizations within the mental health field. Guidance reports cover both general and specialist aspects of mental health provision. They are clearly written and contain key messages, assessments of the state of current services and a description of what constitutes good care. A good starting point is the report on acute care:

Joint Commissioning Panel for Mental Health (JCPMH). *Guidance for Commissioners of Acute Care – Inpatient and Crisis Home Care.* London: JCPMH, 2013.

The reader can then move on to the guides for other fields, which include child and adolescent services, black and ethnic minorities, dementia services, eating disorders, drug and alcohol services, perinatal mental health services and forensic mental health services. Although written in an easy-to-read rather than an academic style, the guides are well referenced to enable anyone to follow up on the policy context or particular aspects of provision.

It is much more difficult to generalize about the design and orientation of mental health services worldwide, except to say that they vary greatly and are heavily influenced by attitudes to mental illness within the society concerned. In a section towards the end of the chapter, we highlight the need to develop models of care in low- and middle-income countries that start afresh and are not drawn from Western psychiatry traditions. Many leading academics and mental health groups are making strong calls for investment in access to mental health services, particularly in the poorer parts of the world. The article

Patel V, Chisholm D, Parikh R, et al. Addressing the burden of mental, neurological, and substance use disorders: Key messages from *Disease Control Priorities*, 3rd edition. *Lancet* 2016; 387: 1672–1685.

presents the evidence and makes the case on public health, economic and moral grounds. We mention the work of a group supported by the World Health Organization that has developed tools to close the gap between what is current provision in low- and middle-income countries and what is needed:

World Health Organization (WHO). *Mental Health Gap Action Programme (mhGAP): Scaling up Care for Mental, Neurological and Substance Abuse Disorders.* Geneva: WHO, 2008.

Other sources of further reading can be found in the source citations for figures and tables presented in the chapter.

CHAPTER 10: DISABILITY

Two important initiatives have shaped the content of this chapter. Both reflect the changing attitudes towards disability and disabled people.

First, the World Health Organization classification produced at the beginning of the twenty-first century aimed to conceptualize health and disability differently, mainstreaming the experience of disability and recognizing it as a universal human experience. The main classification can be found in

World Health Organization (WHO). *International Classification of Functions, Disability, and Health.* Geneva: WHO, 2001.

A useful short report describes the thinking behind the classification:

World Health Organization (WHO). *Towards a Common Language for Functioning, Disability, and Health.* Geneva: WHO, 2002.

A standardized framework for assessment has been developed to support the classification:

World Health Organization (WHO). *WHO Disability Assessment Schedule (WHODAS 2.0).* Geneva: WHO, 2014.

Second, in 2011, the World Health Organization and the World Bank jointly produced the first global report on disability. It is a very important source book for explanations of the key concepts, a wide range of data, strategies, policies and influences regarding disability. It is an essential starting point for further reading:

World Health Organization (WHO) and World Bank. *World Report on Disability.* Geneva: WHO, 2011.

The chapter also discusses specific areas of disability. In relation to learning disability, a national plan led by NHS England,

NHS England. *Building the Right Support.* London: NHS England, 2015.

is a useful reference to gain an understanding of changing approaches to assessing and meeting the needs of people with a learning disability and their families. Excellent topic-specific analyses and reviews are regularly produced by the Scottish Learning Disability Observatory based in the University of Glasgow and a similar body hosted by Public Health England. Regular publications by the charity Mencap are also invaluable sources of material for further study. The chapter also draws attention to serious concerns about access to NHS care and failures in standards of care in England. This whole area was the subject of an independent enquiry. Its report is a good source for understanding the concerns, how they arose and the policy and legislative context:

Michael J. *Health Care for All; Report of the Independent Enquiry into Access to Healthcare for People with Learning Disabilities.* London: Independent Enquiry, 2008.

Sections of the chapter on sensory impairment are supported by data collated by the Royal National Institute of Blind People (RNIB) and a variety of organizations representing deaf people's interests.

CHAPTER 11: HEALTH IN LATER LIFE

This chapter covers the ageing of populations, the concepts and measures of healthy and unhealthy ageing, the health problems associated with the ageing process and the kinds of care services required to respond to the needs generated.

The chapter uses demographic and health statistics extensively to frame the various themes. These are largely drawn from publicly available data provided by the Office for National Statistics, the World Health Organization, the United Nations and the European Union. Certain statistically based reports were referred to:

United Nations, Department of Economic and Social Affairs, Population Division. *World Population Prospects: The 2012 Revision, Key Findings and Advance Tables*. New York: United Nations, 2013.

Office for National Statistics. *Older Workers in the Labour Market, 2012*. London: Office for National Statistics, 2012.

Kinsella K, He W. *An aging world 2008*. Washington, DC: National Institute on Aging and U.S. Census Bureau, 2009.

There is a big literature on healthy ageing in journals and official reports. Key sources used in the chapter were

Rowe JW, Kahan RL. Successful aging. *Gerontologist* 1997; 37: 433–440.

Baltes PB, Baltes MM. Psychological perspective on successful aging: The model of selective optimization with compensation. In: Baltes PB, Baltes MM (eds.), *Successful Aging: Perspectives from the Behavioral Sciences*. New York: Cambridge University Press, 1990.

World Health Organisation (WHO). *World Report on Ageing and Health*. Geneva: WHO, 2015.

WHO Regional Committee for Europe. *Strategy and Action Plan for Healthy Ageing in Europe, 2012–2020*. EUR/RC62/10 Rev. 1. Geneva: WHO, 2012.

World Health Organisation (WHO). *The Global Strategy and Action Plan on Ageing and Health*. Geneva: WHO, 2016.

The following reference addresses healthy and unhealthy ageing in relation to ethnicity and has an extensive reference list that enables further exploration of the evidence base in this area:

Wohland P, Rees P, Nazroo J, Jagger C. Inequalities in healthy life expectancy between ethnic groups in England and Wales in 2001. *Ethnicity & Health* 2015; 20 (4): 341–353.

Similarly, this reference on dementia is a valuable source for further study:

Matthews FE, Arthur A, Barnes LE, et al, on behalf of the Medical Research Council Cognitive Function and Ageing Collaboration. A two-decade comparison of prevalence of dementia in individuals aged 65 years and older from three geographical areas of England: Results of the Cognitive Function and Ageing Study I and II. *Lancet* 2013; 382: 1405–1412.

A project in the UK government's Foresight Programme,

Foresight Programme. *Future of an Ageing Population*. London: Government Office for Science, 2013–2015.

provides a very rich source of publications of expert reviews and policy discussion papers.

A variety of policy documents and plans to improve services for older people continue to be produced by the NHS headquarters and the Department of Health:

Department of Health (DH). *A National Service Framework for Older People*. London: DH, 2001.

Department of Health (DH). *A New Ambition for Old Age: Next Steps in Implementing the National Service Framework for Older People*. London: DH, 2006.

NHS England. *Safe, Compassionate Care for Frail Older People; Using an Integrated Care Pathway*. London: NHS England, 2014.

Department of Health (DH). *Heatwave Plan for England – Protecting Health and Reducing Harm from Severe Heat and Heatwaves*. London: DH, 2015.

Other key references are cited as sources in figures and tables, and they too can be used to explore the subject matter in more depth.

CHAPTER 12: ENVIRONMENT AND HEALTH

We open this chapter with the book that many consider the point of awakening of the modern environmental movement:

Carson R. *Silent Spring*. Boston: Houghton Mifflin, 1962.

Some readers may be interested in reading about the controversy that surrounded the original publication and Carson's vilification by companies like Monsanto. She was eventually vindicated by the Science Advisory Committee established by President John F Kennedy, and the U.S. government brought in tight regulation of DDT use. An account of these events and Carson's life can be found in

Griswold E. How *Silent Spring* ignited the environmental movement. *New York Times Magazine*, 21 September 2012.

A key theme in considering the relationship between the environment and health is sustainability. We quote the definition of sustainability formulated in an early United Nations report. Although it did not major on health specifically, this report is a valuable source to understand how the concept of sustainability would later be developed and become a universal concern rather than an academic subject. Its scope is wide, with individual chapters dealing with population, energy, the growth of cities, species and ecosystems and industrial production. It can be found at

United Nations. *Report of the World Commission on Environment and Development (the Brundtland Commission)*. New York: United Nations, 1987.

The increasing political attention that followed can be gauged by the attendance of so many of the world leaders at the subsequent conference in 1992. This became known as the Earth Summit. We draw attention in the chapter to the action plan on sustainability that resulted from it, Agenda 21:

United Nations Conference on Environment and Development. *Agenda 21: A Programme of Action for Sustainable Development*. New York: United Nations, 1992.

Other meetings convened by the United Nations have followed most recently:

United Nations (UN). Paris Agreement on Climate Change. New York: UN, 2015.

In addition to this big-picture aspect of sustainability, many healthcare systems have embraced the principle of addressing their impact on the environment, especially their carbon footprint. The NHS in the United Kingdom has done a great deal of work in this area. In the chapter, we quote statistics and list the interventions and action that can be taken by healthcare organizations to ameliorate their impact on the environment. This information was drawn largely from

NHS Sustainable Development Unit. *Carbon Footprint Update for the NHS in England 2012*. Cambridge: NHS Sustainable Development Unit, 2013.
NHS Sustainable Development Unit. *Saving Carbon, Improving Health*. Cambridge: NHS Sustainable Development Unit, 2010.

The sustainable development agenda is now dominated by concerns about, and controversy over, climate change. We take a large section in the chapter to discuss this. In general terms, the report of the Intergovernmental Panel on Climate Change, which we draw from in the chapter, is essential reading to understand how judgements are made and the kinds of action that governments need to take:

Intergovernmental Panel on Climate Change (IPCC). *Climate Change 2014: Synthesis Report*. Geneva: IPCC, 2015.

The report includes a consistent evaluation and assessment of uncertainties and risks; integrated costing and economic analysis; regional aspects; changes, impacts and responses related to water and earth systems, the carbon cycle including ocean acidification, the cryosphere and sea level rise; and treatment of mitigation and adaptation options within the framework of sustainable development. Those working in the field of public health will sometimes be drawn into discussion with those who dispute the conclusion that climate change is resulting from human activities. We have cited Professor David MacKay's book,

Mackay DJC. *Sustainable Energy without the Hot Air*. Cambridge: UIT, 2009.

as a very useful and easily understandable source for further reading on the facts of climate change, the scientific responses to the common points made by sceptics and the ideas behind alternative energy policy.

The potential health effects of climate change are also summarized in the same section of the chapter. The following are good sources of further reading on this subject:

Interagency Working Group on Climate Change and Health. *A Human Health Perspective on Climate Change*. Washington, DC: Environmental Health Perspectives and National Institute of Environmental Health Sciences, 2010.
Wellcome Trust. *Health Consequences of Climate Change*. London: Wellcome Trust, 2008.
Wang H, Horton R. Tackling climate change: The greatest opportunity for global health. *Lancet* 2015; 386: 1798–1799.

In other parts of the chapter, references are tied into figures and tables and serve as sources for further study.

CHAPTER 13: HISTORY OF PUBLIC HEALTH

The content of this chapter is a synthesis of many different sources. For those who wish to read further on the history of public health, it is indeed a fascinating subject. The following suggestions for further reading are aimed at the generalist who wishes to deepen his or her knowledge of areas covered in the chapter. For someone who wishes to specialize in public health history, we recommend a formal course of study that will include instruction in the methods of historical research, including how to use appropriately primary and secondary sources.

We would point to a range of sources.

First, there are a number of comprehensive accounts in books that date back to the mid-twentieth century. Many are now out of print but are easily obtainable, relatively cheaply, from Internet networks of second-hand booksellers. Some are labelled as 'history of medicine', but most of these have the main public health content. They are generally factual and chronologically laid out, and therefore their content is usually still valid, even though they were published some time ago. For example, see

Rosen G. *A History of Public Health*. New York: MD Publications, 1958.
Sigerist HE. *Landmarks in the History of Hygiene*. London: Oxford University Press, 1956.
Sigerist HE. *The History of Medicine*. New York: MD Publications, 1960.

A more recent book that is an excellent source for further study is

Berridge V, Gorsky M, Mold A. *Public Health in History*. Maidenhead: Open University Press, 2011.

Second, there rather more books dealing with the Victorian sanitary reforms. Here, analysis and interpretation of events, policies and actions differ author to author. The following is a valuable source:

Wohl AS. *Endangered Lives: Public Health in Victorian Britain*. London: JM Dent and Sons, 1983.

Some of the biographies listed below also contain much material on public health in the time of the sanitary reforms. The following are very informative on the role of statistics to underpin public health advocacy and action:

Eyler JM. *Victorian Social Medicine: The Ideas and Methods of William Farr*. Baltimore: Johns Hopkins University Press, 1979.
Greenwood M. *Medical Statistics from Graunt to Farr*. Cambridge: Cambridge University Press, 1948.

Third, there are the biographies of key historical figures. Here again, interpretation of the role and personality of the central characters in relation to major events and their life and times is dependent on the research undertaken by the author and his or her view of the subject after doing so. In biography, later writers can come in with revisionist accounts that sometimes differ greatly in the assessment of the character than earlier ones. With major figures, there is quite a 'cottage industry' in writing new biographies of them. Good examples outside the health field are Lord Nelson and Bob Dylan – very different subjects, but each a source of many biographical accounts, reflecting public and professional interest in them, as well as a source of profitability.

No public health figure has attracted this degree of wider celebrity, although Florence Nightingale has proved a subject of continuing interest to modern biographers, helped by the rich source of material. Famous people are either 'scatterers' or 'hoarders' of their personal papers. Miss Nightingale was firmly in the second category. The early biographies of Miss Nightingale were detailed and factual, such as

Cook ET. *The Life of Florence Nightingale*. Vols. 1 and 2. MacMillan and Co., 1913.

but a modern biography has used apparently new evidence to claim that there were government cover-ups that sucked her in:

Small H. *Florence Nightingale: Avenging Angel*. London: Constable, 1998.

Other biographical works relevant to the chapter's content are

Lambert R. *Sir John Simon and English Social Administration 1816–1904*. London: MacGibbon and Kee, 1963.
Fraser WM. *Duncan of Liverpool*. London: Hamish Hamilton, 1947.
Finer SE. *The Life and Times of Sir Edwin Chadwick*. London: Methuen and Co., 1952.
Fisher RB. *Edward Jenner*. London: Deutsch, 1991.

A newer genre is the popular science-type account of historical events. These often have a stronger narrative thread and may introduce a new angle. Good examples of these, relevant to the content of the chapter, are books that deal with the stories of scurvy,

Bown SR. *The Age of Scurvy: How a Surgeon, a Mariner, and a Gentleman Helped Britain Win the Battle of Trafalgar*. West Sussex: Summersdale, 2003.

and of John Snow and the Broad Street pump:

Johnson S. *The Ghost Map*. London: Penguin-Allen Lane, 2006.

Other specific references mentioned in the chapter are

Boccaccio G. *The Decameron: Translated with an Introduction by Rebhorn WA*. New York: WW Norton and Co., 2013.
Smith A. *The Wealth of Nations: With an Introduction by Tom Butler-Bowden*. Chichester: Capstone, 2010.
Defoe D. *A Journal of the Plague Year: Edited with Notes by Louis Landa*. Oxford: Oxford University Press, 2010.

Index